This book is due for return on or before the last date shown below.

ORTHOPAEDIC SURGERY ESSENTIALS

FOOT AND ANKLE

ORTHOPAEDIC SURGERY ESSENTIALS

FOOT AND ANKLE

Series Editors

PAUL TORNETTA, III, MD
Professor and Vice Chairman
Department of Orthopaedic Surgery
Boston University Medical Center
Director of Orthopaedic Trauma
Boston University Medical Center
Boston, Massachusetts

THOMAS A. EINHORN, MD
Professor and Chairman of Orthopaedic Surgery
Boston University School of Medicine
Chief of Orthopaedic Surgery
Boston Medical Center
Boston, Massachusetts

Book Editor

DAVID B. THORDARSON, MD
Professor
Department of Surgery
Division of Orthopaedics
Cedars-Sinai Medical Center
Beverly Hills, California

Wolters Kluwer | Lippincott Williams & Wilkins
Health

Philadelphia · Baltimore · New York · London
Buenos Aires · Hong Kong · Sydney · Tokyo

Acquisitions Editor: Brian Brown
Product Manager: Elise M. Paxson
Production Manager: Bridgett Dougherty
Senior Manufacturing Manager: Benjamin Rivera
Marketing Manager: Lisa Lawrence
Design Coordinator: Doug Smock
Production Service: S4Carlisle

Printed in China

Library of Congress Cataloging-in-Publication Data

Foot and ankle / [edited by] David B. Thordarson.—2nd ed.
     p. ; cm.—(Orthopaedic surgery essentials)
  Includes bibliographical references and index.
  Summary: "Foot and Ankle, Second Edition, the best selling volume in the Orthopaedics Essentials Series, delivers the fundamental information residents need to excel during their foot and ankle surgery rotations. Expert coverage of relevant anatomy, biomechanics, physical examination, and orthotics—followed by vital information on the diagnosis and treatment of specific problems encountered in the foot and ankle clinical are included. The reader-friendly format lets you read the book cover to cover during a rotation or use it as a quick reference before a patient work-up or operation. This comprehensive reference contains clinically focused information, preparing you for the challenges of trauma, infection, and reconstructive surgery"—Provided by publisher.
  ISBN 978-1-4511-1596-3 (hardback)—ISBN 1-4511-1596-2 (hardback)
  I. Thordarson, David B.   II. Series: Orthopaedic surgery essentials.
  [DNLM: 1. Foot—surgery.   2. Ankle—surgery.   3. Orthopedic Procedures—methods.   WE 880]
  617.5'85—dc23
                              2012018968

Care has been taken to confirm the accuracy of the information presented and to describe generally accepted practices. However, the authors, editors, and publisher are not responsible for errors or omissions or for any consequences from application of the information in this book and make no warranty, expressed or implied, with respect to the currency, completeness, or accuracy of the contents of the publication. Application of the information in a particular situation remains the professional responsibility of the practitioner.

The authors, editors, and publisher have exerted every effort to ensure that drug selection and dosage set forth in this text are in accordance with current recommendations and practice at the time of publication. However, in view of ongoing research, changes in government regulations, and the constant flow of information relating to drug therapy and drug reactions, the reader is urged to check the package insert for each drug for any change in indications and dosage and for added warnings and precautions. This is particularly important when the recommended agent is a new or infrequently employed drug.

Some drugs and medical devices presented in the publication have Food and Drug Administration (FDA) clearance for limited use in restricted research settings. It is the responsibility of the health care provider to ascertain the FDA status of each drug or device planned for use in their clinical practice.

To purchase additional copies of this book, call our customer service department at (800) 638-3030 or fax orders to (301) 223-2320. International customers should call (301) 223-2300.

Visit Lippincott Williams & Wilkins on the Internet: at LWW.com. Lippincott Williams & Wilkins customer service representatives are available from 8:30 am to 6 pm, EST.

10 9 8 7 6 5 4 3 2 1

To my wonderful wife, Bo, my children, Caela, Kirsten, Blake, Dustin, Samantha, Katrina, and Dean, and my parents who started it all.

CONTENTS

CONTRIBUTING AUTHORS

Eva Asomugha, MD
Resident Physician
Department of Orthopaedic Surgery
The Cleveland Clinic Foundation
Cleveland, Ohio

Umur Aydogan, MD
Director
ECEM Foot and Ankle Clinic
Karsiyaka-Izmir, Turkey

Aaron A. Bare, MD
Shoulder and Knee Specialist
OAD Orthopaedics
Warrenville, Illinois

Gregory C. Berlet, MD
Attending Physician
Department of Orthopaedics
Orthopaedic Foot and Ankle Center
Westerville, Ohio

Michael J. Botte, MD
Orthopaedic Surgeon
Scripps Clinic
La Jolla, California

Eric Breitbart, MD
Orthopaedic Surgeon
Hospital for Special Surgery
New York, New York

Michael E. Brage, MD
Associate Professor
Department of Orthopaedics and Sports Medicine
University of Washington
Orthopaedic Surgeon
Department of Orthopaedics and Sports Medicine
Harborview Medical Center
Seattle, Washington

Chad B. Carlson, MD
Orthopaedic Surgeon
Bone and Joint Surgeon
Bismarck, North Dakota

Jonathan T. Deland, MD
Orthopaedic Surgeon
Hospital for Special Surgery
New York, New York

Constantine A. Demetracopoulos, MD
Orthopaedic Surgeon
Hospital for Special Surgery
New York, New York

Mark E. Easley, MD
Associate Professor of Orthopaedic Surgery
Co-Director, Foot and Ankle Fellowship
Duke University Medical Center
Durham, North Carolina

Richard D. Ferkel, MD
Orthopaedic Surgeon
Department of Orthopaedic Surgery and Sports Medicine
Southern California Orthopedic Institute
Van Nuys, California

Orrin Franko, MD
Orthopaedic Surgeon
Scripps Clinic
La Jolla, California

Ryan C. Goodwin, MD
Orthopaedic Surgeon
The Cleveland Clinic
Cleveland, Ohio

Steven L. Haddad, MD
Senior Attending Physician
Illinois Bone and Joint Institute, LLC
Glenview, Illinois

Jeffrey D. Jackson, MD
Orthopaedic Surgeon
Salt Lake Orthopaedic Clinic
Salt Lake City, Utah

Anish R. Kadakia, MD
Clinician Educator
Department of Orthopaedic Surgery
University of Chicago Pritzker School of Medicine
Chicago, Illinois
Attending Physician
Department of Orthopaedic Surgery
Illinois Bone and Joint Institute
Glenview, Illinois

Todd A. Kile, MD
Assistant Professor
Department of Orthopaedic Surgery
Mayo Medical School
Rochester, Minnesota
Consultant
Department of Orthopaedic Surgery
Mayo Clinic
Phoenix, Arizona

Christopher Y. Kweon, MD
Resident
Department of Orthopaedics
Banner Good Samaritan Orthopaedic Residency
Phoenix, Arizona

Sheldon S. Lin, MD
Orthopaedic Surgeon
Hospital for Special Surgery
New York, New York

Jeffrey A. Mann, MD
Private Practice
Oakland, California

Ellis K. Nam, MD
Assistant Professor
Department of Orthopaedic Surgery
University of Illinois
Attending Surgeon
Department of Surgery
Illinois Masonic Hospital & St. Joseph Hospital
Chicago Orthopaedics & Sports
Chicago, Illinois

David E. Oji, MD
Chief Resident
Department of Orthopaedic Surgery
Johns Hopkins University School of Medicine
Baltimore, Maryland

Lew C. Schon, MD
Assistant Professor
Department of Orthopaedic Surgery
Johns Hopkins University School of Medicine
Chief, Foot & Ankle Fellowship and Orthobiologic
Laboratory
Division of Foot and Ankle
Department of Orthopaedic Surgery
Union Memorial Hospital
Baltimore, Maryland

James J. Sferra, MD
Orthopaedic Surgeon
Cleveland Clinic
Department of Orthopaedic Surgery
Head, Section of Foot and Ankle Surgery
Orthopaedic and Rheumatologic Institute
Cleveland Clinic
Cleveland, Ohio

G. Alexander Simpson, MD
Orthopaedic Surgery Resident
Department of Orthopaedics
OhioHealth Doctors Hospital
Columbus, Ohio

David B. Thordarson, MD
Professor
Department of Surgery
Division of Orthopaedics
Cedars Sinai Medical Center
Beverly Hills, California

Keith L. Wapner, MD
Clinical Professor
Department of Orthopaedic Surgery
Perelman School of Medicine at the University of
Pennsylvania
Philadelphia, Pennsylvania

PREFACE

Foot and ankle surgery is a burgeoning field in orthopaedics. Twenty-five years ago, most general orthopaedic surgeons had little interest in taking care of problems of the foot and ankle. More recently, however, many orthopaedic surgeons have begun to appreciate the complexity and challenge of taking care of patients with foot and ankle pathology. The American Orthopaedic Foot and Ankle Society has grown from a membership of around 600 in 1994 to almost 1,800 today.

Because the goal of *Orthopaedic Surgery Essentials: Foot and Ankle* is to give orthopaedic residents their first exposure to the field, the contributors were chosen based on their active involvement in resident education. The content is not meant to be encyclopedic. Rather, it is intended to cover almost all aspects of orthopaedic foot and ankle surgery in an introductory fashion to help residents prepare for treatment of most foot and ankle problems as well as for the orthopaedic in-service examination and the American Board of Orthopaedic Surgery written examination. Although surgical techniques are presented, the focus is on the essential information needed to evaluate and diagnose a patient's foot and ankle condition and to begin treatment planning.

Foot and ankle surgery is an exciting, constantly evolving field that comprises all aspects of orthopaedics—trauma, infection, reconstructive surgery with fusion, joint replacement, osteotomies, and tendon transfers. Welcome to the field of foot and ankle surgery. I am sure you will enjoy it.

—David B. Thordarson, MD

ANATOMY AND BIOMECHANICS OF THE FOOT AND ANKLE

CONSTANTINE A. DEMETRACOPOULOS ■
JONATHAN T. DELAND

An understanding of the functional anatomy of the foot and ankle is mandatory if any meaningful attempt at addressing the pathoanatomy is to be undertaken. This chapter provides basic anatomy and biomechanics of the foot and ankle as a basis for treating its disorders.

TERMINOLOGY

Understanding the terminology used to describe the various positions of the foot and ankle is necessary for effective communication. Unfortunately, there are ambiguities in the literature as different terms are used to describe the same positions and motions. In most descriptions of extremity position and motion, the midsagittal plane of the body is used as a reference when describing varus, valgus, abduction, and adduction. In the foot, hallux varus and hallux valgus are consistent with this convention (Fig 1.1). In terms of describing abduction or adduction of the hallux, the reference shifts to the longitudinal axis of the foot defined as a plane through the mid axis of the second metatarsal to the heel. Movement of the hallux away from this axis is termed *abduction*, whereas the opposite motion is termed *adduction*.

Motion and position of the foot and ankle are most easily defined using a familiar triaxial orthogonal coordinate system (Fig 1.2).

■ *Pronation* of the foot refers to the triplanar motion of the foot combining abduction, eversion, and dorsiflexion, resulting in elevation of the lateral border of the foot.
■ *Supination* refers to the triplanar motion combining adduction, inversion, and plantarflexion, resulting in elevation of the medial border of the foot.

The position of the heel (i.e., the calcaneus) is described relative to the talus using the ankle coordinate system. The positional terms *equinus* and *calcaneus* are sometimes used and are synonymous with calcaneal plantarflexion and dorsiflexion, respectively.

ANATOMY OF THE FOOT AND ANKLE

Skin and Subcutaneous Fascia

The skin on the dorsum of the foot is thin, loosely connected to its underlying fascia, and nearly void of subcutaneous fat. This makes the skin relatively mobile, giving some leeway in dorsal surgical exposures and making palpating the underlying structures relatively easy. In contrast, strong vertical fibrous elements of the heel, medial and lateral borders, and ball of the foot tightly bind the skin on the plantar surface of the foot. These vertical fibers form adipose-filled chambers, or *septa*, that are enlarged under the heel and ball of the foot, acting as shock absorbers. Traumatic or surgical destruction of the septa or atrophy of the adipose tissue by steroid injection can permanently impair their shock-absorbing function, leading to pain. The robust blood supply of the plantar skin originates mainly from the medial and lateral plantar arteries and the common plantar digital arteries, allowing the surgeon substantial leeway as to the orientation and number of incisions that can safely be made in this region. The superficial intradermal and subdermal venous system anastomoses with a dorsal system medially and laterally. Lymphatic drainage from the plantar aspect of the foot flows to the dorsal aspect through the webspaces, accounting for why infections in the plantar surface of the foot can cause swelling dorsally.

Bony and Joint Anatomy

The foot has 26 bones, a variable number of sesamoids (usually two) and accessory ossicles, with 34 joints. Classically, the foot is divided into the forefoot, midfoot, and hindfoot.

Forefoot

The forefoot contains 5 metatarsals and 14 phalanges, and extends up to the tarsometatarsal joint (Lisfranc joint). By

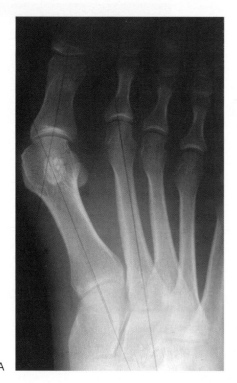

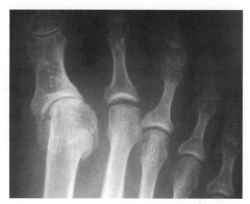

Figure 1.1   Hallux valgus (**A**) and hallux varus (**B**) as referenced from the midsagittal plane of the body.

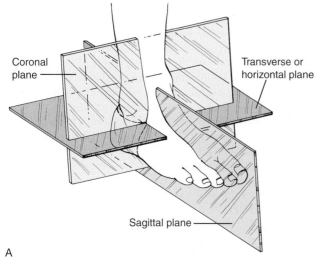

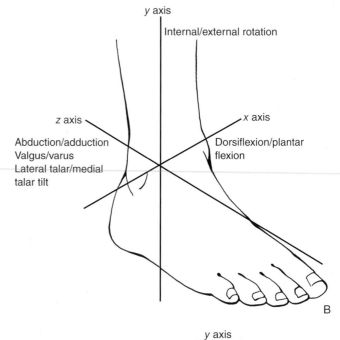

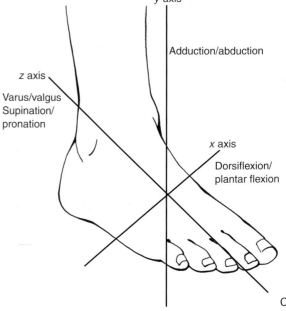

Figure 1.2   (**A**) The three orthogonal planes are represented: coronal or frontal plane (*x–y*), sagittal plane (*y–z*), transverse or horizontal plane (*x–z*). Motion in the sagittal plane is around the *x* axis, motion in the coronal plane is around the *z* axis, and motion in the transverse plane is around the *y* axis. (**B**) The axes of the ankle and respective rotations about these axes are shown. (**C**) The axes of the ankle and respective rotations about these axes are shown.

convention, sequential numbering of the toes and their associated metatarsals (or "rays") starts medial at the hallux, designated number 1, to lateral, designated number 5. Similarly, the intermetatarsal spaces and webspaces are numbered from 1 to 4 from medial to lateral, respectively. The hallux has 2 phalanges, whereas the lesser toes each have three. Approximately 15% of people have only 2 phalanges in their fifth toe. Metatarsals 1, 2, and 3 each have an associated cuneiform at their base. The metatarsals 4 and 5 have an articulation with the cuboid at their base. The metatarsals are unique in that they are the only long bones to support weight perpendicular to their longitudinal axis. The distal metatarsal epiphysis (metatarsal head) has two plantar enlargements called *condyles*. The lateral (fibular) condyle is more prominent than the medial (tibial) condyle. The lengths of the metatarsals vary. Most commonly, the first metatarsal is shorter than the second with a progressive cascade of shortening in the remaining rays. All of the metatarsals incline to some extent with respect to the weight bearing surface. The first metatarsal has the highest inclination (15° to 25°), with the remaining metatarsals demonstrating decreasing angles from medial to lateral: second metatarsal at 15°, third metatarsal at 10°, fourth metatarsal at 8°, and fifth metatarsal at 5°. In normal stance, the metatarsal heads rest evenly on a flat surface. The first ray bears two-fifths of the weight distribution, whereas the four lesser rays share the remaining three-fifths. The fourth, and first and to a lesser extent the first metatarsals are mobile in the sagittal plane, whereas

the second and third are relatively fixed in position by stable articulations at their respective cuneiforms.

The trapezoid-shaped base of the first metatarsal and the distal surface of the medial cuneiform comprise the first tarsometatarsal joint. A facet on the lateral base of the first metatarsal that articulates with the medial base of the second metatarsal is sometimes present. The medial inclination of this joint in the transverse plane varies but is usually between 8° and 10°. Greater angles may correlate with varus alignment of the first metatarsal. The angle between the first and second metatarsals (the first intermetatarsal angle) is typically less than 10° (Fig 1.3). Motion at the first tarsometatarsal joint does not lie directly in the sagittal plane but rather from dorsomedial to plantar lateral. The plantar first metatarsal cuneiform ligament provides the major restraint for dorsiflexion. Plantar intermetatarsal ligaments interconnect the bases of metatarsals two through five. The first ray, however, has no such connection to the second ray. The absence of an intermetatarsal ligament allows the first ray more mobility in the sagittal plane. Hypermobility of the first tarsometatarsal joint has been implicated in hallux valgus and metatarsus primus varus and is sometimes a component of adult acquired flatfoot deformity.

Hallux and First Metatarsophalangeal Joint
The first metatarsophalangeal (MTP) joint of the hallux is a shallow ball-and-socket type joint with a passive arc of motion between 40° to 100° in dorsiflexion and 3° to 43°

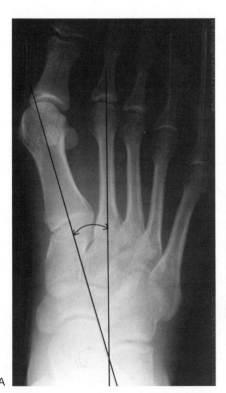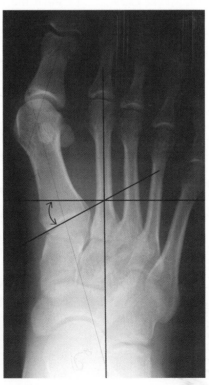

Figure 1.3 (A) Anteroposterior X-ray of the foot with arrow demonstrating first tarsometatarsal joint angle. (B) Weight-bearing X-ray films of the foot demonstrating the first intermetatarsal angle. It is preferable to obtain weight-bearing films for more accurate measure because this angle tends to widen with weight bearing.

in plantarflexion. Motion in abduction and adduction, however, is limited. The head of the first metatarsal is cam-shaped and somewhat larger than the base of the proximal phalanx. Therefore, motion of this joint is more complex than that of a simple hinge, in that the center of rotation is dynamic. Fan-shaped ligaments originating from the medial and lateral epicondyles of the metatarsal head constitute the medial and lateral collateral ligaments responsible for static restraint to valgus and varus stress, respectively. Plantarly, the strong fibrocartilaginous *plantar plate* provides additional stability to the MTP joint. It is formed by the confluence of the plantar fascia and the plantar portion of the MTP joint capsule. The plantar plate attaches firmly to the base of the proximal phalanx, but only loosely at the plantar aspect of the metatarsal neck as part of the joint capsule. It is designed to withstand both tensile force in line with the plantar fascia as the MTP joint goes into dorsiflexion, and compressive force from the metatarsal head during weight bearing. The MTP joint capsule itself is a confluence of ligaments and tendons, including the collateral ligaments, the plantar plate, the metatarsosesamoid and phalangeosesamoid ligaments, the abductor and adductor hallucis (AH) muscles, the extensor digitorum brevis (EDB), and the flexor hallucis brevis (FHB).

Two longitudinally oriented cartilage-covered grooves separated by a rounded ridge called the *crista* run along the plantar surface of the head. The FHB muscle consists of the medial and lateral portion each with a tendon insertion onto the plantar base of the proximal phalanx of the hallux. Contained in each tendon is a sesamoid bone that articulates with its respective overlying groove. The articulating surface of the sesamoid is also covered with hyaline cartilage. Interconnecting the two sesamoids is a thick intersesamoid ligament that maintains the relationship of the

sesamoids and the proper course of the FHB tendons. The presence of these sesamoids gives the tendon a mechanical advantage when pulling at an angle (i.e., when the hallux is in a dorsiflexed position). Morphologically, the size and shape of the sesamoids vary widely. More than 10% of medial (or tibial) sesamoids are bipartite and should not be confused with a fracture. This finding is bilateral in 90% of cases and is seen far more commonly in the medial sesamoid than in the lateral (or fibular) sesamoid. The medial sesamoid can be divided into three or four parts as well, whereas the lateral sesamoid is rarely divided into more than two. The sesamoids are the attachment sites for a number of structures (Fig 1.4).

Lisfranc Joint

Separating the forefoot from the midfoot is the Lisfranc joint complex. The Lisfranc joint is composed of the five metatarsals articulating with the three cuneiforms and the cuboid. It is through this complex joint that the forefoot is attached to the midfoot.

Three columns are described in the foot:

1. Medial column, consisting of the first metatarsal and the medial cuneiform
2. Intermediate or middle column, consisting of the second and third metatarsals and the middle and lateral cuneiforms
3. Lateral column, consisting of the fourth and fifth metatarsals and the cuboid

Several factors contribute to the stability of the Lisfranc complex. The base of the second metatarsal is recessed between the medial and lateral cuneiforms and rigidly attached to the middle cuneiform (Fig 1.5). This configuration forms a "keystone" mortise, which adds stability in

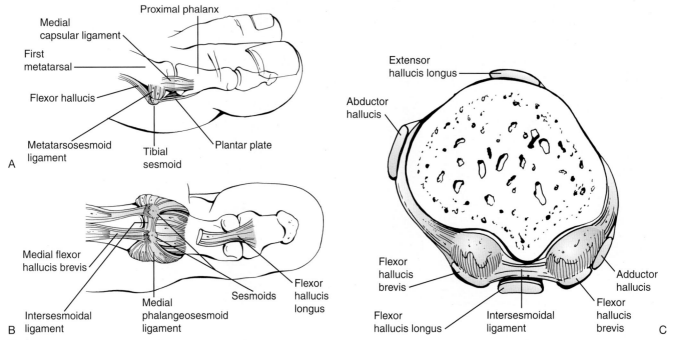

Figure 1.4   (A) Anatomy of the first metatarsophalangeal joint. (B) Plantar perspective. (C) Cross-sectional anatomy through the first metatarsophalangeal head.

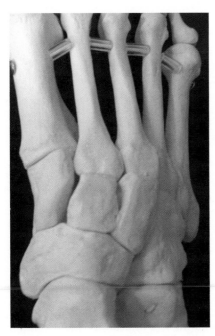

Figure 1.5   Foot model demonstrating the recessed base of the second metatarsal between the medial and lateral cuneiforms.

the transverse plane. The relative immobility of the second ray coupled with the potential stress risers of the flanking medial and lateral cuneiforms are likely factors resulting in the characteristic stress fractures seen at the base of the second metatarsal in dancers. Stability in the coronal plane is enhanced by the arch configuration created by the trapezoidal shape of the cuneiforms and the second and third metatarsal bases (Fig 1.6). Furthermore, stability is further enhanced by the plantar and dorsal tarsometatarsal ligaments (the former being significantly stronger) and the plantar intermetatarsal ligaments. Because of the bony configuration and the strong plantar ligaments, the metatarsal bases are much more likely to displace dorsal than plantar. The second metatarsal, instead of being attached to the base of the first metatarsal, is secured to the medial cuneiform by Lisfranc ligament. This ligament is the strongest

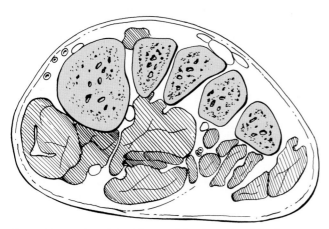

Figure 1.6   Wedge-shaped bases of the second and third metatarsals create a "keystone" effect that stabilizes the arch in the coronal plane.

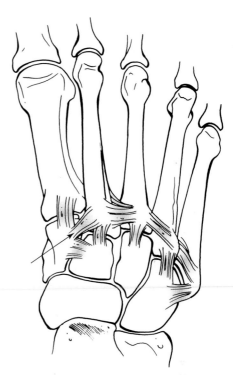

Figure 1.7   Plantar tarsometatarsal ligaments and plantar metatarsal ligaments. Note the absence of a plantar metatarsal ligament between the base of the first and second metatarsals. Lisfranc ligament (*arrow*) runs obliquely from the medial cuneiform to the base of the second metatarsal.

of the Lisfranc joint complex, has a relatively broad attachment on the plantar surface of the medial cuneiform, and runs obliquely to insert onto the plantar aspect of the base of the second metatarsal (Fig 1.7). Disruption of this complex can lead to an avulsion fracture of the base of the second metatarsal. The fragment, still attached to the Lisfranc ligament, can be seen on plain X-ray study (the Fleck sign).

Midfoot

The five bones of the midfoot are relatively immobile with respect to one another. As a unit, they provide a mechanical link between the forefoot and the hindfoot. Furthermore, the midfoot provides protection for the passage of neurovascular structures as well as tendons from the ankle to the foot. The midfoot contains the navicular, the cuboid, and the three cuneiforms and extends from the tarsometatarsal (Lisfranc) joint distally to the transverse tarsal (Chopart) joint proximally.

The navicular has a concave posterior surface where it articulates with the talus and a convex anterior surface, divided into three facets, where it articulates with each of the three cuneiforms. The medial portion possesses a tuberosity that is the main insertion site of the posterior tibial tendon. The plantar surface provides the attachment sites for the *superomedial calcaneonavicular ligament* and the *inferior calcaneonavicular ligament* (spring ligament complex). The superomedial component of the spring ligament also attaches medially directly deep to the posterior tibial tendon. The dorsal surface provides attachments for a number of ligaments including the talonavicular ligament, the dorsal cuneonavicular ligaments, and the dorsal cuboideo-navicular ligaments. The dorsal surface receives the medial slip of the bifurcate ligament (calcaneonavicular part), a strong Y-shaped ligament arising from the superior aspect of the anterior process of the calcaneus.

The navicular is largely responsible for transmitting forces from the hindfoot to the forefoot. For this reason and because there is a relatively poor blood supply to its central third, it is subject to stress fractures and avascular necrosis. Furthermore, the talonavicular joint is most sus-ceptible to non-union after a triple arthrodesis (talonavicu-lar, calcaneocuboid, and subtalar joints).

The cuboid is part of the lateral column of the foot, posi-tioned between the anterior surface of the calcaneus and the bases of the fourth and fifth metatarsals. Posteriorly, it forms a saddle-shaped joint with the calcaneus. Anteriorly, two facets separated by a slight ridge allow a mobile articu-lation with the base of the fourth and fifth metatarsals. The medial surface has an articulating surface for the lateral cuneiform and sometimes for the navicular. The cuboid is stabilized to the calcaneus dorsally by the lateral slip of the bifurcate ligament (from the calcaneus) and the dor-sal calcaneocuboid ligament. Plantar stabilizing structures include the plantar calcaneocuboid ligament (short plantar ligament) and the deep fibers of the long plantar ligament. A groove (or sulcus) is found on the plantar aspect of the cuboid. The superficial fibers of the long plantar ligament, on their way to the second, third, and fourth metatarsal bases, pass over the peroneal groove, converting it to a fibroosseous canal (cuboid tunnel) through which the per-oneus longus (PL) tendon passes.

The cuneiforms articulate with the navicular posteri-orly and their respective metatarsals anteriorly. The medial cuneiform is the largest of the three and is oriented with the thin edge of its wedge shape pointing dorsally. It also serves as the partial insertion site for several tendons including the PL, the posterior tibial tendon, and the ante-rior tibial tendon, as well as Lisfranc ligament.

The middle and lateral cuneiforms are rigidly attached to the bases of the second and third metatarsals, respec-tively. These wedge-shaped bones fit like the stones of a Roman arch to provide the inherent bony stability to the medial longitudinal arch of the foot. Slips from the poste-rior tibial tendon find attachment sites on the plantar sur-faces of both bones.

Transverse Tarsal Joint (Chopart Joint)

The midfoot is separated from the hindfoot by the trans-verse tarsal joint (*Chopart* joint), which includes the talo-navicular and calcaneocuboid joints.

The talonavicular joint is a ball-and-socket type joint that is the key part of a complex motion system called the *acetabulum pedis*. The acetabulum pedis is a deep socket that receives the head of the talus formed by the navicular, the anterior and middle facets of the calcaneus, the super-omedial and inferior calcaneonavicular ligaments (spring ligament complex), and the calcaneonavicular slip of the bifurcate ligament (Fig 1.8). In conjunction with the cal-caneocuboid joint, the acetabulum pedis allows motion in both the longitudinal and transverse planes. These motions contribute to the shock-absorbing ability and the stability

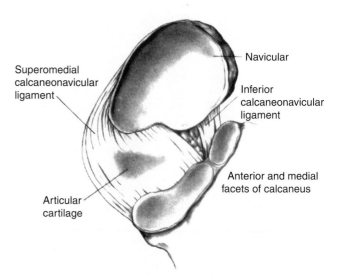

Figure 1.8 The acetabulum pedis from a dorsal view with the head of the talus removed.

of the foot during weight bearing. Additionally, it allows for appropriate alignment between the forefoot and hindfoot when walking on uneven terrain.

The spring ligament complex consists of three anatomic components: the superomedial calcaneonavicular ligament (the largest and strongest portion of the spring ligament complex), the inferior (or plantar) calcaneonavicular liga-ment, and the third ligament. The superomedial component includes the medial talonavicular capsule and is confluent with the tibionavicular portion of the superficial deltoid liga-ment. It is triangular in shape and contains fibrocartilage as a result of its articulation with the talar head. The superficial fibers of the superomedial calcaneonavicular ligament have additional attachments to the posterior tibial tendon. The inferior calcaneonavicular ligament is a narrower, entirely fibrous structure that lies in the plantar-most aspect of the acetabulum pedis. The third ligament is distinct from the superomedial calcaneonavicular ligament. It originates from the notch between the anterior and middle facets of the cal-caneus and attaches to the navicular tuberosity. The spring ligament complex, particularly the superomedial component, is considered the primary static restraint to deformity of the talonavicular joint. Insufficiency of this ligament is a major contributing factor to adult acquired flatfoot deformity.

Any motion of the talonavicular joint or subtalar joint must involve the calcaneocuboid joint. The anterior cal-caneal articular surface is concave vertically and convex transversely. The posterior aspect of the cuboid features a reciprocal undulating surface. Congruency of the two opposing surfaces is at a maximum when the heel is in varus and the forefoot supinated, which is the position of the foot during pushoff.

Hindfoot

The hindfoot contains the calcaneus (os calcis) and the talus. The calcaneus is the largest tarsal bone and forms the heel of the foot. Its complicated shape has six surfaces:

1. The superior aspect articulates with the talus via three articular surfaces (the anterior, middle, and posterior facets).

2. The anterior surface articulates with the cuboid.

3. The posterior surface is the insertion site of the Achilles tendon.

4. The medial surface has a bony shelf called the sustentaculum tali, which supports a part of the talar head through the middle facet and is the attachment site to a number of ligaments.

5. The lateral surface features a bony prominence called the peroneal tubercle, which separates the PL and peroneus brevis (PB) tendon.

6. The inferior surface is the major weight-bearing surface for the hindfoot, which serves as an attachment site for the plantar fascia and a number of intrinsic muscles and ligaments.

The talus is the second largest tarsal bone and is divided into three regions: the head, neck, and body. The neck of the talus connects the body to the head. The neck projects anteriorly, plantarward, and medially from the body, which is important to realize for reconstruction after fracture. The *sulcus tali* is a deep groove on the inferior portion of the neck oriented obliquely in an anterolateral, to posteromedial direction. Where the talus articulates with the superior surface of the calcaneus, the sulcus tali aligns with a corresponding groove (*sulcus calcanei*) to form a bony canal called the *sinus tarsi*. Attached to the sulcus tali and inserting onto the sulcus calcanei is the strong bilaminar interosseous talocalcaneal ligament.

Most of the talar body is covered with articular cartilage. Superiorly it articulates with the tibial plafond, and medially and laterally with the respective malleoli. Inferiorly, it articulates with the posterior facet of the calcaneus.

Almost the entire head of the talus is covered with articular cartilage. It articulates with the tarsal navicular anteriorly and the anterior and middle facets of the calcaneus inferiorly.

The posterior aspect of the talus has two bony prominences: the medial and lateral talar tubercles, between which passes the flexor hallucis longus (FHL) tendon. The lateral tubercle is more prominent and may ossify separately from the rest of the talus, forming an accessory ossicle called the *os trigonum*. It is the second most common accessory bone of the foot and may play a role in posterior ankle impingement syndromes. The lateral talar tubercle can fracture (Shepherd fracture) and mimic an os trigonum.

The lateral talar process is a bony projection located inferiorly on the lateral surface of the talus. Its underlying surface articulates with the posterior articular surface of the calcaneus. This process can fracture (snowboarder's fracture) and is part of the differential diagnosis for lateral ankle pain.

The talus has no tendon or muscle insertions or origins.

Subtalar Joint

The subtalar joint is the articulation of the inferior surface of the talus as it sits "sidesaddle" medially over the superior surface of the calcaneus. This articulation consists of three facets: an anterior facet located on the superomedial

aspect of the anterior process, a middle facet on the sustentaculum tali, and a posterior facet, which is the largest of the three. The anterior and middle facets are often one contiguous joint surface. A groove in the calcaneus which separates the anterior and middle facets from the posterior facet forms the floor of the sinus tarsi. The anterior process may be involved in a congenital anomaly whereby it is joined to the lateral aspect of navicular by a fibrous or bony bridge (calcaneonavicular *tarsal coalition*). Similarly, a coalition may occur in the middle facet (talocalcaneal tarsal coalition). These account for more than 90% of all tarsal coalitions and occur with almost equal frequency.

The deltoid ligament, the calcaneofibular ligament (CFL), the lateral talocalcaneal ligament (LTCL), the cervical ligament (CL), the interosseous ligament (IO), and the inferior extensor retinaculum (IER) stabilize the subtalar joint. The lateral structures have been categorized as superficial, intermediate, and deep (Fig 1.9 and Box 1.1). With progressive inversion of the heel, the lateral ligaments rupture in the following order: CFL, LTCL, and then the IO. The role of the CFL as primary lateral stabilizer of the subtalar joint is a matter of some debate. The orientation of its fibers as well as other anatomic variations (e.g., the LTCL is absent in more than 40%) in this region either contribute to or detract from its role. Subtalar joint range of motion is estimated to be 24°; however, there is wide variability among the population and it is difficult to measure clinically. Furthermore, what constitutes laxity or instability is not clearly defined. One study demonstrated that sectioning the CL or the IO increased subtalar motion a maximum of 2.6°. Because the range of subtalar motion is small to begin with, this increase may be significant,

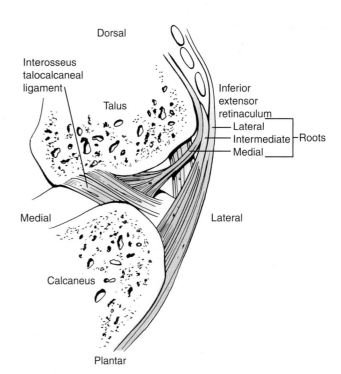

Figure 1.9 Lateral stabilizers of the subtalar joint. (Adapted from Harper MC. The lateral ligamentous support of the subtalar joint. Foot Ankle Int 1991;11:354–358.)

clinically manifesting as symptoms of instability or sinus tarsi syndrome.

Ankle Joint

The body (or dome) of the talus resides in an articulation created by the distal tibia and fibula. This *mortise* is formed by the *tibial plafond* (flat roof) or pilon superiorly and the medial and lateral malleoli. The posterior flare of the distal tibial metaphysis is often referred to as the posterior malleolus. The medial malleolus is the distal-most extension of the tibia and is divided by a longitudinal groove into a small anterior and larger posterior *colliculus*. The inner surface is lined with hyaline cartilage and articulates with the medial aspect of the talus. In a similar fashion, the distal-most aspect of the fibula articulates with the lateral portion of the talus. More proximally, the fibula is set in a tibial recess posterolaterally. The ligaments of the ankle are divided into three groups: syndesmotic ligaments, lateral ligaments, and medial ligaments.

Tibiotalar Syndesmosis

The syndesmosis, located at the level of the tibial plafond, maintains the relationship between the fibula and tibia and comprises four ligaments:

1. anterior inferior tibiofibular ligament (AITFL)
2. posterior inferior tibiofibular ligament (PITFL)
3. transverse tibiofibular ligament (TTFL)
4. interosseous tibiofibular ligament (ITFL)

The AITFL originates from the anterior tibial tubercle and inserts onto the anterior fibula. Occasionally, a slip from this ligament may insert quite distally on the anterior aspect of the fibula (Baxter ligament), causing symptoms as it impinges against the anterolateral aspect of the talus. The PITFL originates on the posterior aspect of the fibula and is the strongest component of the syndesmosis. The TTFL originates deep and inferior to the PITFL on the fibula, extending to the posterior margin of the medial malleolus. In between it forms a posterior labrum that articulates with the posterolateral aspect of the talar body, effectively deepening the tibiotalar joint. The ITFL

spans the area between the distal medial shaft of the fibula and the distal lateral shaft of the tibia just proximal to the talofibular articulation. This strong ligament prevents the proximal migration of the talus between the fibula and the tibia and is the primary restraint to transverse motion at the tibiofibular joint. Proximally it is continuous with the interosseous membrane.

This ligament complex allows for fibular translation, rotation, and proximal migration in ankle dorsiflexion when the widened anterior aspect of the talus rotates into the mortise. This dynamic relationship allows the fibula to share approximately 16% of the axial load.

Lateral Ligament Complex of the Ankle

The lateral ankle ligament complex comprises the anterior talofibular ligament (ATFL), the CFL, and the posterior talofibular ligament (PTFL). The ATFL originates on the anterior aspect of the lateral malleolus and passes anteromedially to insert onto the lateral aspect of the talar neck just distal to the articular facet. The ligament is between 15 and 20 mm long, 6 to 8 mm wide, and 2 mm thick. Its fibers blend with the anterolateral capsule of the ankle joint. The ATFL is the weakest and most commonly injured component of the lateral ligament complex.

The CFL is a rounded ligament measuring 20 to 25 mm long and 6 to 8 mm thick. It originates from the anterior tip of the lateral malleolus distal to the ATFL and extends inferiorly and posteriorly deep to the peroneal tendons to insert on the upper part of the lateral calcaneus. This ligament is extraarticular and spans both the tibiotalar and subtalar joints.

The PTFL is deeply situated, running from the posteromedial aspect of the lateral malleolus to the lateral talar tubercle. The PTFL is 3 cm long, 5 mm wide, and 5 to 8 mm thick. It is the strongest component of the three. The *tibial slip* is an extension off the superior border of the PTFL that attaches to the posterior margin of the distal tibia. The PTFL experiences increasing strain with dorsiflexion of the ankle. The clinical significance of injury to this ligament is unclear. It is uncommonly injured and rarely, if ever, ruptured.

Medial Ligament Complex

The deltoid ligament is the medial collateral ligament of the ankle. It is divided into two portions: the superficial and deep layers. The superficial layer is a broad, fan-shaped, continuous structure arising from the anterior colliculus of the medial malleolus. The superficial deltoid has no discrete bands but is divided into three components based on their insertion sites for descriptive purposes. The anterior part (*talonavicular component*) attaches to the navicular medially and blends with the fibers of the superomedial component of the spring ligament. The central component of the deltoid (*tibiocalcaneal component*) runs vertically inferior to insert onto the sustentaculum tali of the calcaneus. The third component of the superficial deltoid (*posterior tibiotalar component*) extends posterolaterally to attach to the medial tubercle of the talus.

The deep portion of the deltoid is anatomically separate from the superficial portion. This portion is thick and short and is divided into two distinct ligaments: the anterior and posterior deep tibiotalar ligaments. Both are intraarticular but extrasynovial. The anterior component arises from the lateral anterior colliculus and inserts on the medial aspect of the talus just distal to the articular surface. The posterior component, the strongest of the entire deltoid complex, arises from the posterior colliculus and travels inferiorly and posteriorly to attach to the medial talus as well.

The deep and superficial portions of the deltoid ligament act equally to resist valgus tilting of the talus. The deep deltoid provides the greatest restraint against lateral translation. The deltoid acts as a secondary restraint against anterior translation (the lateral ligaments being the primary restraint).

Muscles and Tendons

The foot has an intrinsic and an extrinsic muscle system. The intrinsic muscles lie entirely within the foot. The extrinsic muscles are in the leg but their tendons insert and function in the foot.

Intrinsic Muscle System

The EDB is the only intrinsic muscle on the dorsum of the foot. It originates on the anterior process of the calcaneus and inserts into the dorsal aponeurosis of the lesser toes lateral to the extensor digitorum longus (EDL). The *extensor hallucis brevis* (EHB) is a distinct muscle belly of the EDB and inserts on the base of the hallux. Hypertrophy of the EHB muscle belly can be seen as a mass in the first intermetatarsal space. The EDB acts to extend the MTP joints.

The plantar intrinsic muscles are conveniently divided into four anatomic layers based on depth. The first and most superficial layer includes (from medial to lateral) the abductor hallucis, the flexor digitorum brevis (FDB), and the abductor digiti minimi (ADM) as well as the plantar aponeurosis to which the first layer muscles are deep. All structures in this layer arise from the calcaneus and insert onto the proximal phalanges forming the truss in the windlass mechanism of the foot. The abductor hallucis tendon attaches to the medial base of the hallux where it blends with the medial capsule of the first MTP joint. In hallux valgus deformities, this tendon insertion slides inferiorly with respect to the joint, converting this muscle from an abductor to a flexor and pronator of the hallux. The FDB gives off four tendons, one to each of the lesser toes. These tendons travel through vertical septa to insert onto the bases of their respective middle phalanges. Distally the tendon splits to allow the passage of the flexor digitorum tendon. Contraction of the FDB causes flexion of the proximal interphalangeal (PIP) joint and winds up the windlass mechanism. The ADM inserts onto the lateral aspect of the plantar plate of the fifth toe.

The second layer contains the tendons of the FHL and the flexor digitorum longus (FDL), the quadratus plantae (QP) muscle, and the four lumbricals. The QP originates as two muscle bellies on the medial and lateral inferior surface of the calcaneus and attaches to the lateral border of the FDL tendon just proximal to where the FDL splits into four separate tendons. The QP acts as a "helper" in flexing the lesser toes. The FHL and FDL tendons attach to the base of the distal phalanges and flex the toes at the distal interphalangeal (DIP) joint. The lumbricals arise from the medial border of each of the four separate FDL tendons. They insert onto the medial aspect of the extensor hood after having passed under the transverse metatarsal ligaments. The action of the lumbricals is to flex the MTP joint while extending the PIP and DIP joints.

The third layer contains the short intrinsic muscles of the hallux and fifth toe. The FHB originates from two heads of origin (the plantar surfaces of the cuboid and lateral cuneiform as well as the plantar surfaces of the middle and medial cuneiform) and inserts as two distinct tendons at the base of the proximal phalanx. The *flexor digiti minimi brevis* (FDMB) arises from the plantar base of the fifth metatarsal and inserts onto the proximal phalanx. The AH has two heads: oblique and transverse. The *oblique head* is the larger of the two and originates from the bases of the second, third, and fourth metatarsals. It runs distomedially and eventually blends with the transverse head. The *transverse head* originates from the plantar plates and intermetatarsal ligaments of the third, fourth, and fifth MTP joints. It runs medially to unite with the oblique head. The two heads form a short single tendon that blends with the lateral head of the FHB and lateral (or fibular) sesamoid. The confluence of the abductor hallucis tendon, the lateral head of the FHB, and the intermetatarsal ligament is often referred to as the *conjoined tendon* particularly in the literature pertaining to hallux valgus correction.

The fourth and deepest layer contains seven interosseous muscles (four dorsal and three plantar), the insertions of the posterior and anterior tibial tendons, and the insertion of the PL tendon. The bipennate dorsal interossei abduct the toes with respect to the midaxis of the foot (defined as the second metatarsal) and the unipennate plantar interossei adduct. (This can be remembered using the acronym *dorsal ab*duct, or DAB, and *plantar ad*duct, or PAD.) Therefore, the first dorsal interosseous muscle inserts onto the medial side of the second toe. Dorsal interosseous muscles two, three, and four insert on the lateral side of their respective toes. The three plantar interosseous muscles insert on the medial base of the third, fourth, and fifth toes. When both dorsal and plantar interossei contract, the MTP joint is flexed while the PIP joint is extended through the action of the dorsal expansion.

Extrinsic Muscle System

The extrinsic muscle system originates within one of the four compartments in the leg (anterior, lateral, superficial posterior, and deep posterior). The anterior compartment contains the extensors of the foot, namely the EDL, the *extensor hallucis longus* (EHL), and the *tibialis anterior* (TA) muscles innervated by the deep peroneal nerve. The TA is the only extensor tendon to possess a synovial sheath. The lateral compartment contains the PL and PB muscles innervated by the superficial peroneal nerve. The deep posterior compartment contains the *tibialis posterior* (TP), the *FDL*, and the *FHL* muscles. The superficial posterior compartment contains the *soleus* and the *gastrocnemius* muscles. Both posterior compartments are innervated by the posterior tibial nerve.

Anterior Compartment.   Above the ankle joint, the muscle tendons of the anterior compartment are arranged in the following order from lateral to medial: EDL, EHL, and TA. The anterior tibial artery and deep peroneal nerve are located between the tendons of the EHL and TA above the ankle. As these structures run distally across the ankle joint, this relationship changes. The EHL crosses over the neurovascular bundle to lie medial to it. Before crossing the ankle joint, all structures of the anterior compartment pass deep to the *superior extensor retinaculum*. This tough fibrous structure is anchored to the anterior aspect of the tibial shaft and anterior fibular shaft, and prevents "bowstringing" when the tendons are under tension.

The TA is the primary dorsiflexor of the ankle and also acts as a foot inverter. The EHL inserts onto the dorsal base of the distal phalanx of the hallux. Its action is to dorsiflex the MTP and IP joints of the hallux. It also aids in ankle dorsiflexion. The EDL tendon splits into four distinct tendons as it passes underneath the inferior extensor retinaculum of the foot. These tendons insert onto the dorsal aspects of their respective middle and distal phalangeal bases of the lesser toes via the dorsal expansion. The EDL also aids in ankle dorsiflexion.

Lateral Compartment.   When approached laterally, the PL lies superficial to the PB and its tendon forms more proximally than that of the PB. The tendons of the PL and PB course around the lateral malleolus deep to the *superior peroneal retinaculum*. At this level, the PB is found anterior to the PL and is in direct contact with the posterior surface of the lateral malleolus. This anterior position of the PB makes it more susceptible to attritional tears. Injury to the retinaculum may lead to symptomatic subluxation or dislocation of these tendons.

In the foot, the PL tendon passes inferior to the peroneal tubercle (a protuberance on the lateral aspect of the calcaneus) and then courses through the cuboid tunnel (described earlier). At this point, the tendon turns medially to insert onto the plantar base of the first metatarsal and medial cuneiform. A sesamoid bone called the *os peroneum* is sometimes located within the PL tendon as it turns from the lateral border of the foot. The PL everts the foot and is capable of plantarflexion of the ankle and especially the first metatarsal. The PB courses superior to the peroneal trochlea to insert onto the fifth metatarsal base. It is the primary everter of the foot.

Deep Posterior Compartment.   The tibialis posterior, FDL, as well as the FHL occupy the deep posterior compartment of the leg. The tibialis posterior tendon passes directly posterior to the medial malleolus, then inferomedial to the spring ligament before finding its primary insertion on the navicular bone. This tendon sends extensions to all the tarsal bones except the talus. Furthermore, extensions from the tibialis posterior can be found at the base of the second, third, and fourth metatarsals. The tibialis posterior inverts the foot as well as assists with plantarflexion of the ankle.

The FDL tendon passes superficially over the tibialis posterior tendon proximal to the ankle joint. It then runs posterior to the tibialis posterior tendon as it crosses posteriorly around the medial malleolus. It passes through the tarsal tunnel and then runs obliquely and laterally into the

sole of the foot as it passes deep to the abductor hallucis and FDB. The FDL tendon then crosses superficially over the FHL tendon in the plantar medial aspect of the foot at the knot of Henry. Anatomically, this crossover occurs at the level of the base of the first metatarsal. The FDL then divides into four tendons, one for each of the lesser four toes, which insert onto the base of each distal phalanx.

The FHL tendon passes within its own fibroosseous tunnel as it courses over the posterior surface of the distal tibia as well as the posterior surface of the talus and inferior to sustentaculum tali. The configuration of the three tendons of the deep posterior compartment as they pass posterior to the medial malleolus can be remembered using the mnemonic "Tom, Dick, and Harry" (**TP, FDL, FHL**). All three structures pass deep to the flexor retinaculum, which forms the roof of the tarsal tunnel.

The FHL tendon crosses distally in the sole of the foot past the knot of Henry to insert onto the base of the distal phalanx of the hallux. The FHL tendon usually provides tendon slips, which attach to the medial aspect of the FDL tendons, typically of the second and third toes. The actions of the FHL are to plantarflex the hallux and assist in plantarflexion of the foot at the ankle joint.

Superficial Posterior Compartment.   The superficial posterior compartment contains the *triceps surae*, three muscles that converge into the Achilles tendon to provide the primary plantarflexion power during gait. This muscle complex comprises the medial and lateral heads of the gastrocnemius and the soleus muscles. The gastrocnemius is also capable of knee joint flexion because it originates on the posterior aspects of the femoral condyles, proximal to the knee joint. Arising from the posterior aspects of the fibula, tibia, and interosseous membrane and lying deep to the gastrocnemius is the soleus muscle. Within the triceps surae is the plantaris muscle. This small muscle originates adjacent to the lateral head of the gastrocnemius on the lateral femoral condyle. Its short muscle belly gives rise to a long tendon that courses inferomedially between the soleus and the medial belly of the gastrocnemius to insert medial to the Achilles tendon. It is a vestigial tendon that is useful for tendon grafts. The plantaris tendon is absent in 7% of the population.

The Achilles tendon is the confluence of the tendinous components of the gastrocnemius and soleus muscles, with the gastrocnemius component being the longer of the two contributions. The two tendons fuse into one at about 5 to 6 cm proximal to insertion. The width of the Achilles varies between 1.2 and 2.5 cm. Approximately 12 to 15 cm proximal to its insertion, its fibers start a gradual internal rotation of about 90° whereby the medial fibers rotate posteriorly and the posterior fibers rotate laterally. This ropelike twisting may provide an elastic quality that allows the tendon to better absorb strain. The tendon inserts onto the posterior aspect of the calcaneus distal to the posterosuperior calcaneal tuberosity.

Between the posterosuperior tuberosity and the tendon just proximal to its insertion is the retrocalcaneal bursa. Subcutaneously, between the skin and the distal aspect of the tendon lies a retroachilles bursa. Retrocalcaneal bursitis, subcutaneous Achilles bursitis, and insertional Achilles tendinosis have been associated with a prominence of the posterosuperior tuberosity (so-called Haglund deformity or pump bump).

The Achilles tendon is enveloped not by a true synovial sheath but by a paratenon composed of a single layer of cells. Anteriorly, the paratenon consists of a vascular mesenteric-type tissue responsible for a large portion of the blood supply for the tendon. Other sources of blood supply come from the musculotendinous junction and from the osseous insertion. The blood supply is most tenuous from 2 to 6 cm proximal to its insertion and correlates with the region that is most commonly ruptured.

Nerve Supply of the Foot and Ankle

All of the motor nerves and most of the sensory nerves in the foot are of sciatic nerve origin. The only femoral nerve branch is the *saphenous nerve*, which supplies sensation to the medial aspect of the ankle and sometimes into the foot. The sciatic nerve terminates as two branches, the larger, more medial *tibial nerve* and the *common peroneal nerve*.

The *posterior tibial nerve* carries fibers from L4, L5, S1, S2, and S3. It runs vertically through the popliteal fossa deep to the popliteal artery and vein, past the arc of the soleus into the deep posterior compartment of the leg. While within the popliteal fossa, the posterior tibial nerve provides innervations to both heads of the gastrocnemius, the soleus, and the plantaris, in addition to giving rise to the sural nerve. In the upper portion of the deep compartment, the posterior tibial nerve travels between the tibialis posterior and FDL muscle bellies. In the lower portion of the leg, it travels between the FDL and FHL tendons before entering the tarsal tunnel. The tarsal tunnel is a fibroosseous structure located behind the medial malleolus created by the tibia anteriorly and the posterior process of the talus and calcaneus laterally. It becomes a tunnel as a result of the flexor retinaculum enclosing the structures, which creates a closed space. The posterior tibial nerve terminates as three branches: the *medial calcaneal nerve*, the *medial plantar nerve*, and the *lateral plantar nerve*. In 93% of cases, this branching occurs within the tarsal tunnel.

The medial calcaneal nerve supplies sensation to the plantar heel and medial portion of the proximal sole of the foot. The medial plantar nerve, the largest of the tibial nerve branches, courses deep to the abductor hallucis and then deep to the FDB. It provides the medial hallucal nerve and three common plantar digital nerves. Together they provide sensation to the medial two-thirds of the sole of the midfoot and forefoot as well as medial, lateral, and plantar sensation to the hallux and second and third toes, and medial sensation to the fourth toe analogous to the median nerve in the hand (Fig 1.10). The medial plantar nerve supplies motor innervation to a number of intrinsic muscles of the foot (Table 1.1).

The lateral plantar nerve courses more obliquely and lateral, deep to the abductor hallucis, FDB, and ADM while remaining superficial to the QP and adjacent to the lateral plantar artery. The first branch of the lateral plantar nerve (nerve to ADM or Baxter's nerve) passes between the lateral fascia of the abductor hallucis and the medial fascia of the QP muscle. Here it may become entrapped, causing medial heel pain. The lateral plantar nerve then divides into two branches at the base of the fifth metatarsal: a deep and superficial branch. The deep branch dives deep to the QP muscle and continues as an arch across the proximal aspects of the fourth, third, and second metatarsals. The superficial branch of the lateral plantar nerve passes between FDMB and ADM. Table 1.1 lists the sensory and muscle innervations of the tibial nerve and its branches.

Four *common plantar digital nerves* course longitudinally in the sole of the foot. The nerves are numbered one to four from medial to lateral. Nerves one through

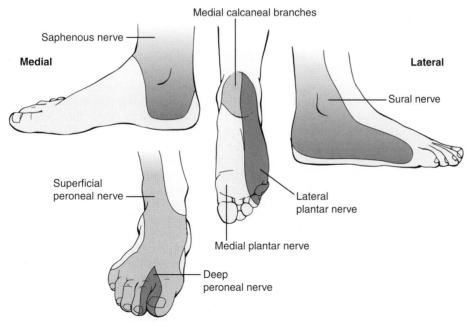

Figure 1.10 Cutaneous nerve distribution in the foot and ankle.

TABLE 1.1 MOTOR AND SENSORY NERVE DISTRIBUTIONS IN THE FOOT

Nerve	Motor Innervation	Sensory Distribution
Posterior tibial (L4, L5, S1, S2, S3)	*Superficial posterior compartment:* gastrocnemius (S1), soleus (S1), plantaris (S1) *Deep posterior compartment:* popliteus (L5, S1), FHL (S1), FDL (S1, S2), tibialis posterior (L4, L5)	See medial and lateral plantar nerve and medial calcaneal nerve
Medial plantar (L4, L5)	FDB, abductor hallucis, FHB, first lumbrical	Medial two-thirds of sole of the midfoot and forefoot; plantar aspect of toes 1, 2, and 3; plantar medial half of fourth toe; tarsal and metatarsal joints (analogous to median nerve in hand)
Lateral plantar (S1, S2)	Quadratus plantae, ADM; *Deep branch:* first, second, third plantar interosseous; second, third, fourth lumbricals; adductor hallucis	*Superficial branch:* lateral third of the sole of the midfoot and forefoot; plantar lateral half of fourth toe; plantar aspect of fifth toe (analogous to ulnar nerve in hand) *Deep branch:* tarsal and metatarsal joints
Medial calcaneal (S1, S2)	None	Plantar heel
Nerve to ADM	ADM	No cutaneous distribution but some deep sensory fibers
Common peroneal (L4, L5, S1, S2)	See deep and superficial peroneal nerves	Articular branches to knee; anterolateral aspect proximal leg (via lateral sural nerve)
Deep peroneal	Tibialis anterior, EDL, EHL, peroneus tertius	*Medial branch:* Dorsal first web space, lateral hallux, medial second toe
	Lateral branch: EDB	*Lateral branch:* tarsal and metatarsal joints
Superficial peroneal	Peroneus longus and brevis	Anterolateral distal two-thirds of leg; dorsum of foot and toes
Sural (S1, S2)	None	Lower lateral calf, lateral heel, lateral border of foot, lateral fifth toe
Saphenous (L3, L4)	None	Medial side of leg and foot up to first MTP joint

FHL, flexor hallucis longus; FDB, flexor digitorum brevis; FDL, flexor digitorum longus; tibialis posterior, tibialis posterior; FHB, flexor hallucis brevis; ADM, abductor digiti minimi; EDL, extensor digitorum longus; EHL, extensor hallucis longus; EDB, extensor digitorum brevis; MTP, metatarsophalangeal.

three are branches of the medial plantar nerve, whereas the fourth nerve is a branch of the superficial branch of the lateral plantar nerve. At approximately the level of the metatarsal head and deep to the transverse intermetatarsal ligament, each common plantar digital nerve terminates as a pair of *proper plantar digital nerves* that pass on the plantar aspect of each side of their respective lesser toes. Swelling and scarring of the nerve can occur at this junction, most commonly in the third webspace causing pain (Morton's neuroma).

Proximally, the common peroneal nerve winds around the lateral aspect of the fibular neck and pierces the PL muscle belly before it divides into two branches: the deep and superficial peroneal nerves. The common peroneal nerve carries fibers from L4, L5, S1, and S2. The *deep peroneal nerve* runs deep in the anterior compartment of the leg just anterior to the interosseous membrane and supplies all the muscles in this compartment. It courses between the EDL and TA in the proximal third of the leg and the EHL

and TA in the middle and distal thirds of the leg, running parallel and lateral to the anterior tibial artery throughout its entire course. Just proximal to the ankle joint, the nerve passes deep to the EHL tendon and is then located between the EHL and EDL on the dorsum of the foot. The deep peroneal nerve passes anterior to the ankle joint deep to the inferior extensor retinaculum and then divides into medial and lateral terminal branches. The medial branch runs lateral to the dorsalis pedis artery in the dorsal space between the first and the second metatarsals. It supplies sensation to the first dorsal webspace and the lateral and medial aspects of the hallux and second toe, respectively. Clinically, this is a convenient way to test deep peroneal nerve function.

The *superficial peroneal nerve* runs within the PL muscle belly proximally and innervates this muscle as well as the PB. It exits the lateral compartment anteriorly an average of 12.5 cm proximal to the tip of the lateral malleolus. The nerve then divides into medial and intermediate branches about 6.5 cm proximal to the tip of the fibula to supply

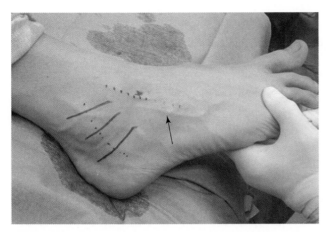

Figure 1.11 Plantarflexion of the fourth toe demonstrating the subcutaneous course of the intermediate branch of the superficial peroneal nerve *(arrow)*.

sensation to the dorsal aspect of the foot. Both branches pass superficial to the superior and inferior extensor retinaculum. The medial branch is the larger of the two and runs parallel to the EHL tendon. It gives off communicating branches to the saphenous nerve to form the dorsomedial cutaneous nerve to the hallux (which is at risk in bunion correction surgery) before dividing into two dorsal digital nerves. The intermediate branch crosses the extensor tendons of the fourth and fifth toe, communicates with the sural nerve, and heads toward the third webspace before dividing into two dorsal digital branches. Plantarflexion of the fourth toe can often demonstrate the subcutaneous course of the intermediate branch (Fig 1.11). Clinically this can be useful in avoiding nerve injury with placement of the anterolateral arthroscopy portal.

The fibers of the saphenous nerve (L3, L4) are purely sensory and originate entirely from the femoral nerve. It becomes superficial at the level of the knee and descends within the subcutaneous fat over the medial aspect of the leg where it is in close association with the saphenous vein. The nerve often bifurcates approximately 15 cm proximal to the tip of the medial malleolus into two branches that run together along the anterior aspect of the medial malleolus.

The *sural nerve* is a superficial sensory nerve formed by the confluence of the lateral and medial sural nerves in the distal third of the leg. The lateral sural nerve arises from the common peroneal nerve and the medial sural nerve arises from the tibial nerve proximal to the fibular head. This "common" sural nerve begins its course essentially in the posterior midline of the leg, then gradually drifts laterally as it descends. Distally its branching pattern is complex, giving off two or three lateral calcaneal branches and often bifurcating over the peroneal tendons distal in the foot. The sural nerve is a common source of nerve graft and biopsy specimen.

Technique for Ankle Block

Regional anesthesia has many advantages in foot and ankle surgery. It can provide pain control for 12 hours or more after surgery, allowing the patient to titrate oral pain control

medications as the block wears off. The unpleasant side effects of general anesthesia are avoided. Regional anesthesia is also well suited for this era of cost-efficient care and the trend toward outpatient surgeries. Furthermore, these techniques can be useful in an emergency department setting when rapid, safe, and effective analgesia is required.

The patient is positioned supine with the leg free to rotate internally and externally. Often the surgery is limited to a certain region in the foot, so only the appropriate nerves need to be blocked. A 25G or 27G needle is used. Mild sedation is helpful because establishing blocks can be quite uncomfortable for the patient. A total of 15 to 20 mL per ft is required for a complete ankle block, whereas 2 to 3 mL is required for a toe block. We use a 1:1 ratio of 2% lidocaine and 0.5% or 0.75% bupivacaine. This allows for fast onset while also providing a long duration of action. The addition of 10 μg per mL of clonidine to lidocaine increases the duration of the block. Some authors advocate the use of a dilute concentration (1:200,000) of epinephrine to the analgesic; we, however, opt to use analgesics without epinephrine. Also, use of epinephrine causes vasospasm, which should be avoided below the ankle, if possible. The maximum safe dose of lidocaine without epinephrine in a healthy adult should not exceed 4.5 mg per kg. This translates into approximately 31 cc of 1% (10 mg per mL) lidocaine in a 70-kg patient. For bupivacaine, the maximum safe dose should not exceed 2.5 mg per kg, which translates to 35 mL of 0.5% (5 mg per mL) bupivacaine in a 70-kg patient. The effects of lidocaine and bupivacaine are additive; therefore, if a 1:1 ratio is used, the maximum safe dose for each agent is halved.

Block of the posterior tibial nerve is done with the knee flexed and the leg externally rotated to expose the posteromedial portion of the ankle. Positioning the leg on a pillow to elevate the ankle allows easier access. A point that is 2 cm proximal to the tip of the medial malleolus is marked and a horizontal line made back to the medial border of the Achilles tendon. The needle is inserted adjacent to the medial border of the Achilles directed anteriorly and advanced until contact is made with the posterior cortex of the tibia; then the needle is withdrawn about 2 mm. At this level, the posterior tibial nerve is directly under the medial border of the Achilles tendon and the artery is just medial (Fig 1.12A, B). Aspiration is performed before injecting 10 cc of local analgesic to ensure the injection is not made into the adjacent artery or vein. The opposite thumb is used to palpate the flexor retinaculum distally. One should feel swelling as the fluid is injected, which indicates instillation into the correct plane.

Block of the deep peroneal nerve is accomplished first by palpating the location of the EHL and EDL tendons. The medial border of the EDL is marked and the dorsalis pedis artery is palpated. Distal to the ankle joint, the medial branch of the deep peroneal nerve runs lateral to the artery. If the block is performed distal to the ankle joint, the needle is directed perpendicular to the skin lateral to the dorsalis pedis artery, advanced to the underlying tarsal bone, and then withdrawn about 2 mm as the nerve is superficially located (Fig 1.12C). Aspiration is performed before injecting 5 mL of local anesthetic. If the block is

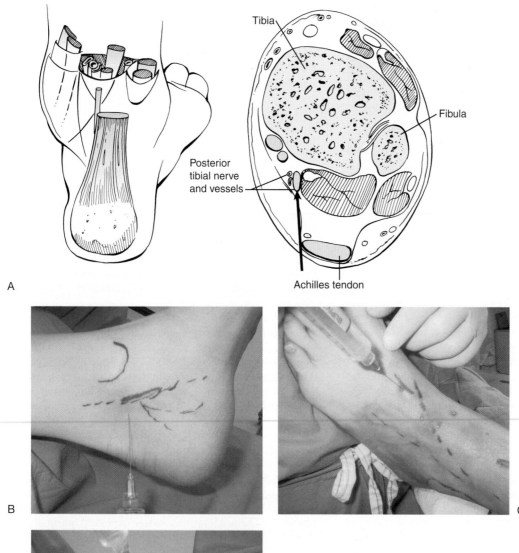

Figure 1.12   Ankle block technique. (**A**) Cross-sectional schematic drawing demonstrates relationship of deep peroneal nerve to surrounding structures. (**B**) Posterior tibial nerve block. (**C**) Deep peroneal nerve block distal to the ankle joint. (**D**) Deep peroneal nerve block proximal to the ankle joint.

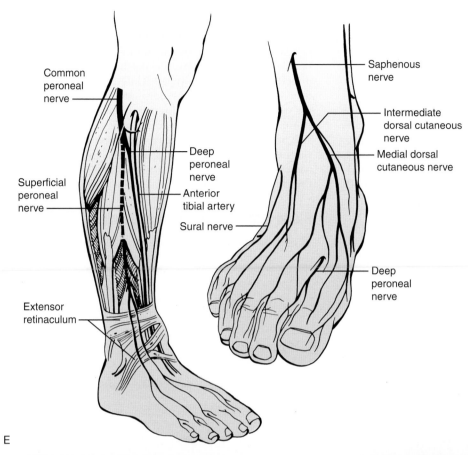

Common
peroneal
nerve

Deep
peroneal
nerve

Superficial
peroneal
nerve

Anterior
tibial artery

Sural nerve

Extensor
retinaculum

Saphenous
nerve

Intermediate
dorsal cutaneous
nerve

Medial dorsal
cutaneous nerve

Deep
peroneal
nerve

E

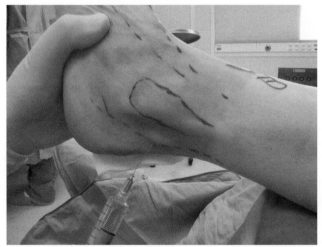

F

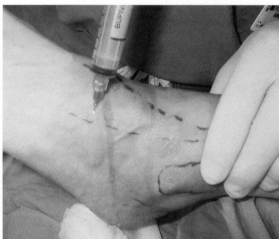

G

Figure 1.12 (*continued*) (**E**) Schematic depiction of sensory nerves to the dorsal aspect of the foot. (**F**) Sural nerve block. (**G**) "Ring" block.

performed proximal to the ankle joint, the needle is again positioned perpendicular to the skin and advanced medial to the artery but lateral to the EHL until bone contact is made, which is much deeper than on the dorsum of the foot with the anterior cortex of the tibia (see Fig. 1.12D). The needle is withdrawn 2 mm and aspirated before injection.

The saphenous, sural, and superficial peroneal nerves run in the subcutaneous tissue of the foot. They are blocked with a subcutaneous ring of local analgesia extending across the anterior aspect of the ankle from the lateral border of the Achilles tendon to the medial malleolus. This ring is located just proximal to the tips of the malleoli but can also be performed in the midfoot if desired. A subcutaneous wheal should be easily visualized if injection is occurring in the correct plane (Fig 1.12E–G). Approximately 5 mL of local analgesia is required.

A digital block of the toe can be accomplished with two needle sticks. Initially, a small subcutaneous wheal is created dorsomedially at the base of the digit. The needle is advanced plantarward until the plantar skin is reached. A "column" of analgesic is created by injecting while withdrawing the needle from plantar to dorsal, returning the needle tip to its starting position. Without removing the needle tip from the skin, the needle is redirected to face directly lateral and advanced while infiltrating. Once the needle tip has reached the dorsolateral corner of the digit, the needle is removed and reinserted at this point directed plantarward. Again, the needle is advanced to the plantar skin and then withdrawn, leaving a column of local analgesia (Fig 1.13). Epinephrine is *never* used when performing a digital block to avoid vasospasm, which may compromise the vascularity of the toe.

Blood Supply of the Foot and Ankle

The blood supply to the foot comprises three vessels: the *anterior tibial artery*, the *posterior tibial artery*, and the *peroneal artery*. The popliteal artery bifurcates into the

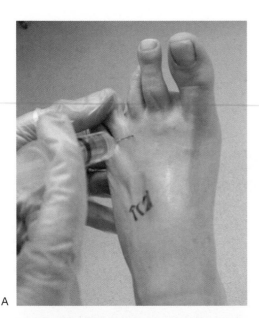

A

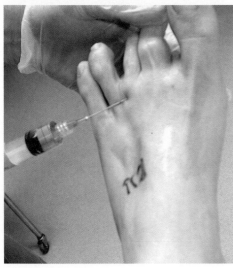

B

Figure 1.13   Toe-block technique. (A) The same site is used to infiltrate analgesia along the lateral base of the toe (B) and the dorsal aspect of the toe by redirecting the needle. (C) The needle is then inserted into a site already infiltrated with analgesia.

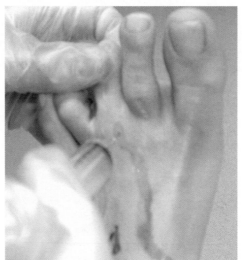

C

anterior and posterior tibial arteries just distal to the popliteus muscle in the popliteal fossa. About 3 cm distal to this bifurcation, the peroneal artery branches off the posterior tibial artery in the deep posterior compartment of the leg.

The anterior tibial artery enters the anterior compartment of the leg by passing over the superior edge of the interosseous membrane. The artery descends with and immediately medial to the deep peroneal nerve. Before crossing the ankle joint, it gives off the *anterior lateral malleolar artery* (which anastomoses with the perforating branch of the peroneal artery) and the *anterior medial malleolar artery* (which anastomoses with the posterior tibial artery). The anterior tibial artery then passes under the superior and inferior extensor retinaculum to become the *dorsalis pedis artery*. In its course across the dorsum of the foot, the dorsalis pedis artery gives off the following branches from proximal to distal: *lateral tarsal artery, medial tarsal artery, arcuate artery*, and the *first dorsal metatarsal artery*.

The arcuate artery runs in the dorsal midfoot across the bases of metatarsals two through five deep to the extensor tendons. It gives off *dorsal metatarsal arteries* that run in the second, third, and fourth intermetatarsal spaces.

The posterior tibial artery, the larger of the two popliteal artery terminal branches and the main blood supply to the foot, descends inferomedially in the deep posterior compartment of the leg medial to the tibial nerve. The artery crosses anterior to the nerve before entering the tarsal tunnel, where it passes posterior to the medial malleolus as part of the neurovascular bundle. It emerges to bifurcate into its terminal branches: the *medial plantar artery* and the *lateral plantar artery*. Each branch runs with its respective medial and lateral plantar nerve. Before this bifurcation, the posterior tibial artery gives off a *posterior medial malleolar artery* (that anastomoses with the corresponding anterior medial malleolar artery), medial malleolar branches, and medial calcaneal branches.

The plantar arterial arch is a continuation of the lateral plantar artery that runs in the sole of the foot extending from the base of the fifth metatarsal to the proximal first intermetatarsal space. Perforating branches from the arch extend dorsally through the proximal intermetatarsal spaces to communicate with the dorsal blood supply, which can be damaged with displaced Lisfranc injuries.

The peroneal artery courses deep to the FHL to run lateral to the fibula in the deep flexor compartment. It gives off branches to the FHL, PT, PB, PL, and soleus muscles. Before terminating in the heel as multiple lateral calcaneal branches, the peroneal artery gives off a perforating branch, a communicating branch, and a posterior lateral malleolar branch. The perforating branch pierces the distal interosseous membrane to run through the anterior compartment of the leg to communicate with the anterior lateral malleolar artery. Ultimately, it anastomoses with the lateral tarsal branch of the dorsalis pedis artery. Approximately 5 cm proximal to the ankle joint over the posterior aspect of the distal tibial metaphysis, the communicating branch anastomoses with a corresponding communicating branch from the posterior tibial artery. The posterior lateral malleolar

branch communicates with the anterior lateral malleolar branch of the anterior tibial artery. The peroneal artery is responsible for the blood supply to the skin overlying the lateral aspect of the calcaneus. This fact is of considerable clinical relevance when a posterolateral approach is used for operative fixation of calcaneal fractures.

Although a detailed review of the arterial supply of each bone in the foot and its five angiosomes is beyond the scope of this chapter, certain anatomic regions are discussed further because of their particular relevance in clinical practice.

Spontaneous avascular necrosis of the first metatarsal head is rare; however, this complication has been reported after hallux valgus surgery. This is particularly true after a distal metatarsal chevron osteotomy. Three arteries supply the first metatarsal head. The *first dorsal metatarsal artery* and the *first plantar metatarsal artery* run dorsolaterally and plantar-laterally to the first metatarsal, respectively. The latter arises from the deep perforating branch of the dorsalis pedis artery. The *superficial branch of the medial plantar artery* runs plantar-medially. These three vessels form a network of anastomoses around the head of the first metatarsal that is most robust dorsally and laterally, where the first dorsal metatarsal artery provides several branches. The plantar cruciate anastomosis is an extensive complex proximal to the sesamoids and metatarsal head, providing blood supply plantar-medially and plantar-laterally to the head. The first metatarsal head also receives an intraosseous blood supply.

Fractures at the metaphyseal–diaphyseal junction at the base of the fifth metatarsal (so-called Jones fracture) are notorious for their nonunion rate. The extraosseous blood supply is provided by the fourth dorsal metatarsal artery and the plantar arch. The confluence of these vessels medially at the junction of the proximal and middle thirds of the metatarsal creates a vascular watershed zone. A nutrient artery, part of the intraosseous blood supply, penetrates the medial cortex in this same region. An osteotomy or extensive surgical dissection in this region can lead to nonunion.

An understanding of the blood supply to the talus is important because of the high rate of avascular necrosis associated with displaced talar neck fractures. The blood supply to the talus comes from five vessels: the artery of the tarsal canal (a branch of the posterior tibial artery), the artery of the tarsal sinus, dorsal neck branches from the dorsalis pedis artery, the posterior tubercle vessels, and the deltoid branches from the posterior tibial artery. The majority of the surface area of the talus is covered by hyaline cartilage. Blood supply to the talus is provided by entry sites in the talar neck, the medial surface of the body, the sinus tarsi, and the posterior tubercle. The talar body receives a majority of its blood supply from an anastomotic sling along the inferior neck between the artery of the tarsal canal and the artery of the tarsal sinus. Fractures of the neck disrupt this crucial anastomosis. However, there is a dense anastomotic network of vessels around the posterior tubercle of the talus comprising contributions from the posterior tibial and peroneal arteries. These vessels supply the talar body in an anterograde fashion. Branches of the dorsalis pedis, which are a minor source of blood supply to the head, enter the neck dorsally. The deltoid branch travels between the tibiotalar and talocalcaneal portions of the deltoid ligament to supply the medial portion of the talar body.

BIOMECHANICS OF THE FOOT AND ANKLE

In general, the reason a patient seeks a physician for foot and ankle problems can be divided into four categories: pain without instability, pain with instability, instability without pain, and pain from distorted biomechanics. Pain can be caused by the pathologic process itself (e.g., tendinosis, arthritis, infection, tumor, fracture), the result of biomechanical instability (e.g., Lisfranc joint incompetence, posterior tibial tendon insufficiency, transfer lesion from a hypermobile first ray), or distorted biomechanics (e.g., tight Achilles tendon contributing to plantar ulcers, metatarsalgia resulting from a long metatarsal). Patients with instability may present with no pain symptoms, as is seen in Charcot-Marie-Tooth disease. Identifying the etiology of the patient's symptoms with attention to the aforementioned categories is a critical first step in treatment. Once a biomechanical cause is identified, an appropriate treatment can be rendered that requires a basic understanding of foot and ankle biomechanics.

Kinematics

For the student of foot and ankle kinematics, a comprehensive description of the dynamic range of motion of each of the joints in the foot and ankle during gait would be so overwhelming that key concepts could easily be lost. For this reason, simplified approaches to this topic are usually used. The complexity is diminished by making certain assumptions, such as limiting joint range of motions to a single plane or axis or assuming that otherwise less mobile joints (or collection of joints) have no motion at all and are treated as rigid segments or links.

The axis of rotation of the tibiotalar joint consists of a functional series of instant centers of rotation. However, for most clinical purposes, this axis can be considered as passing through the distal tips of both malleoli. This places the axis in 20° to 30° of external rotation in the transverse plane and approximately 8° of varus in the coronal plane (Fig 1.14). Therefore, the axis of rotation is not perpendicular to the tibial axis. This relationship has important consequences with regard to tibial rotation and subtalar motion. As the ankle dorsiflexes, the tibia internally rotates. Conversely, when the foot plantarflexes, the tibia externally rotates (Fig 1.15).

The rotation of the tibia is coupled with the motion of the subtalar joint. It is this coupled motion that allows the tibia to internally and externally rotate during the phases of gait (Fig 1.16). The concept of coupled motion is an important recurrent theme in joint kinematics. Joints have a primary motion (such as dorsiflexion and plantarflexion in the case of the ankle joint) and secondary motions associated with the primary motion (such as internal or external rotation). Disruption of a secondary motion can interfere with a primary motion.

Using the model, one can imagine that rotation of the vertical component around a more horizontally oriented hinge (or subtalar joint axis) would translate to greater

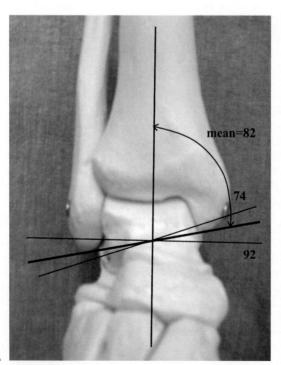
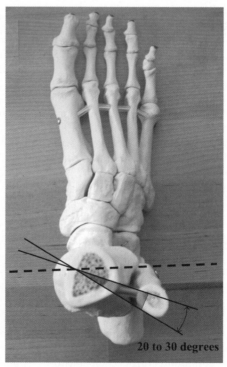

Figure 1.14   (A) Ankle joint axis of rotation viewed from the coronal plane. (B) Ankle joint axis of rotation viewed from the transverse plane.

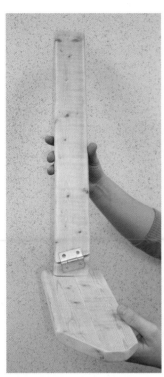

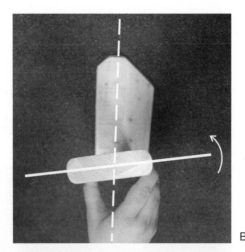

B

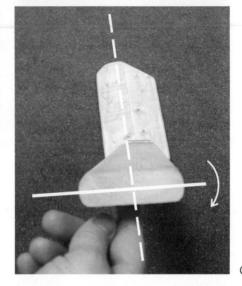

C

A

Figure 1.15 (**A**) Model depicting the effect of obliquely placed ankle axis. Dorsiflexion results in internal rotation of the tibia (**B**), whereas plantarflexion results in tibial external rotation (**C**).

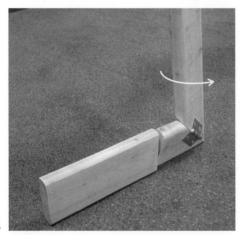

A

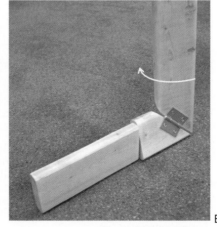

B

Figure 1.16 Motion of the subtalar joint has been likened to a mitered hinge. The vertical component of the model represents the tibia, the short proximal horizontal component represents the hindfoot, and the distal horizontal component, the forefoot. A peg separating the proximal and distal horizontal components is analogous to the transverse tarsal joint. (**A**) Internal rotation of the tibia is associated with valgus hindfoot motion. (**B**) External rotation of the tibia is associated with varus hindfoot motion.

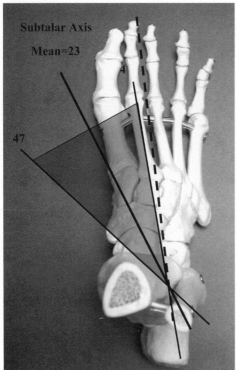

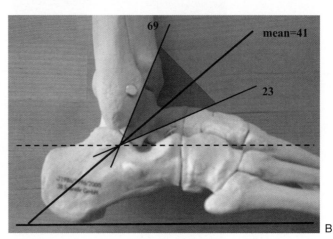

Figure 1.17   (A) Subtalar transverse axis of motion ranges between 4° and 47°. (B) The sagittal axis of motion of the subtalar joint ranges between 21° and 69°. Wide variations exist between individuals. (Adapted from Isman RE, Inman VT. Anthropometric studies of the human foot and ankle. Bull Prosthet Res 1969;10:97.)

A   B

rotation of the horizontal component. The reverse is true with a more vertically placed hinge. Patients with asymptomatic flatfeet have a more horizontally positioned subtalar joint and clinically greater subtalar motion than those with "average" feet. Conversely, the more vertically aligned subtalar axis in a cavus foot tends to be stiffer. Unlike the kinematics of the ankle joint, which are somewhat predictable given the relatively straightforward geometry of the talus and mortise articulation, the kinematics of the subtalar joint are difficult to estimate given the complex geometry of its multiple joints (Fig 1.17).

The talonavicular joint and calcaneocuboid joint (i.e., the transverse tarsal joint) allow the hindfoot to pivot while the forefoot component remains stationary. This relationship is facilitated by a region known as the acetabulum pedis, the anatomy of which has been described earlier. The primary motion is that of abduction and adduction, followed by a substantial amount of dorsiflexion and plantarflexion. Pronation and supination also occur. Anatomically, when the heel is in an everted position, the joint surfaces of the talonavicular joint and calcaneocuboid joint are parallel. Functionally, this allows flexibility in the transverse tarsal joint. When the heel is inverted, the once parallel relationship of these joint surfaces changes to an unparallel relationship, which stiffens the transverse tarsal joint preparing the foot for push-off (Fig 1.18).

Adding to the stability of the foot is the plantar aponeurosis. The function of this structure has been likened to a Spanish windlass mechanism (Fig 1.19). As the heel rises, the MTP joints dorsiflex, pulling the plantar aponeurosis over the metatarsal heads. The plantar aponeurosis tightens, raising the height of the longitudinal arch by depress-

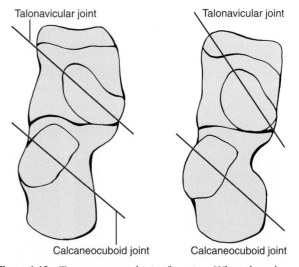

Figure 1.18   Transverse tarsal joint function. When the calcaneus is everted, the talonavicular joint and calcaneocuboid joints are parallel, permitting mobility across the joint complex. Inversion of the calcaneus causes the axes to become unparallel, stiffening the transverse tarsal joint.

ing the metatarsals. This action is most pronounced in the first metatarsal and decreases with progression toward the fifth metatarsal. A secondary action is to draw the calcaneus into further inversion.

The posterior tibial tendon plays a critical role in influencing hindfoot inversion during gait through its action across the transverse tarsal joint. By adducting the trans-

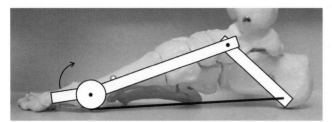

Figure 1.19   Spanish windlass mechanism. The truss is shown superimposed on a foot skeleton model. As the toes dorsiflex, the windlass winds up and tightens the plantar fascia, helping to stabilize the foot.

verse tarsal joint, the navicular rotates medially over the head of the talus, inverting the subtalar joint. The ability to perform a complete heel rise depends on the ability of the posterior tibial tendon to stabilize the transverse tarsal joint into an adducted position. This coupled motion between the transverse tarsal joint and the subtalar joint has implications when arthrodesis is considered. Arthrodesis of the talonavicular joint decreases subtalar motion to 9% of its original motion. In turn, arthrodesis of the subtalar joint decreases motion of the transverse tarsal joint. The triceps surae, through the action of the Achilles tendon, is the strongest hindfoot inverter. However, for the Achilles to act as an inverting force, the hindfoot must be positioned in varus (Fig 1.20). External rotation of the tibia at heel rise, the obliquity of the metatarsal cascade (the metatarsal break), the pull of the plantar aponeurosis windlass mechanism, and the pull of the posterior tibial tendon act to place the hindfoot into varus so that the powerful triceps surae can "lock" the heel into this position. A rigid platform for forward propulsion is the result.

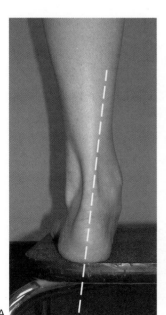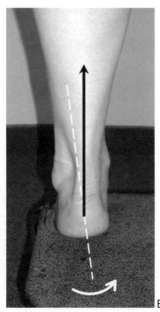

A   B

Figure 1.20   (A) Heel positioned in valgus during stance. (B) In toe-rise, the heel swings across the line of action of the Achilles (*black arrow*) into varus, allowing the triceps surae to become a strong inverter of the hindfoot.

Gait

A complete gait cycle is defined as the motions between one foot-strike to the successive foot-strike on the same side. The *stance phase* of gait begins when the foot strikes the ground to when the toes of the same side push off. This represents 62% of the cycle. *Swing phase* is from when the toes leave the ground to when the foot strikes the floor again and represents the remaining 38% of the gait cycle. Each phase of gait is divided into three periods: initial double-limb support, single limb stance, and second double-limb support for stance phase and initial swing, midswing, and terminal swing for swing phase. The cycle is broken down further into segments that are defined by functional episodes within the cycle (Fig 1.21).

Thorough gait analysis requires the use of a gait laboratory where kinematic data, dynamic electromyography (EMG) data, and foot pressure data can be acquired. Kinematics measures the motion of a joint or segment using variables of velocity, acceleration, and displacement. Standardized skin markers are tracked by cameras that yield data allowing three-dimensional analysis of motion. Knowledge of muscle activity can be important in determining the cause of a problem and critical in deciding which muscles or tendons should be recruited for transfer. The EMG data in normal gait (Fig 1.21) can be summarized as follows: at heel strike, the anterior muscles of the leg are active in controlling the descent of the foot to a foot flat position. This eccentric contraction of the anterior muscle group, primarily the TA, also serves an energy-absorbing role. Activity of the extensor muscles is then largely replaced by activity of the flexor muscle groups starting with the posterior tibialis. The posterior tibial tendon stabilizes the foot and helps initiate heel rise. The peroneal tendons become active, providing varus stability as the ankle goes into dorsiflexion during single-limb stance. The triceps surae is activated, which causes the heel to rise while other plantarflexors are recruited. At initial swing phase, the plantarflexors cease firing and the extensors act to bring the foot into dorsiflexion to allow foot clearance and prepare the foot for the next heel strike. As the foot progresses from foot strike to toe-off, the progression of the center of load under the foot proceeds rapidly from the heel distally toward the first metatarsal head region and eventually across the hallux (Fig 1.22).

Ligamentous Stability of the Ankle

The ligaments about the ankle have a difficult task. They must provide stability for the tibiotalar and subtalar joints without interfering with the complex motion of these joints. Inman likened the talus to a cross section of a cone in which the medial side is oriented toward the apex and the lateral side toward the base (Fig 1.23). The fan-shaped deltoid ligament complex is suitable for stability of the medial side where the apex of the deltoid meets the apex of the cone. On the lateral side, the area of rotation is larger and therefore the ligaments need to be more spread out, making the task of stabilizing the ankle more difficult. An understanding of the relationship of the lateral ligaments to one another and to the tibiotalar and subtalar joints is necessary to understand their function as stabilizers.

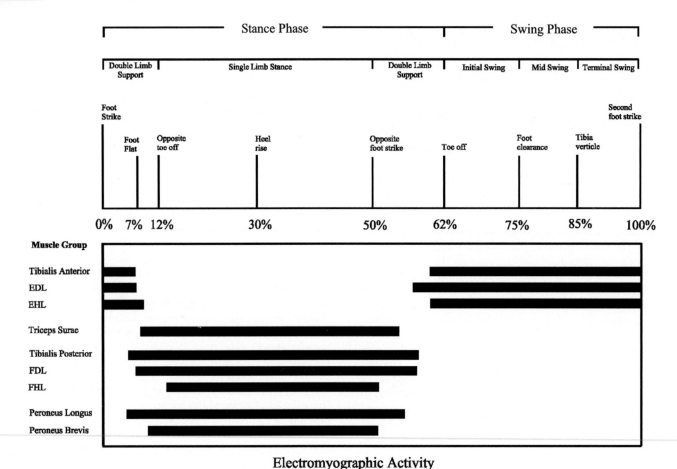

Electromyographic Activity

Figure 1.21   Schematic of a normal gait cycle correlated with electromyographic activity. (Adapted from Sutherland DH, Kaufman KR, Moitoza JR. Kinematics of normal human walking. In: Rose J, Gamble JG, eds. Human walking, 2nd ed. Baltimore: Williams & Wilkins, 1994:23–44.)

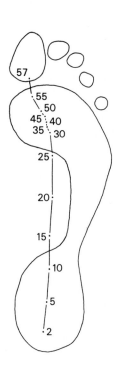

Figure 1.22   Progression of the center of load. The points across the sole represent the summation of forces under the foot through stance phase at a given time expressed as a percentage of the gait cycle. Notice the rapid progression of load across the heel and sole indicated by the wide spacing of points. Also notice the disproportionate time the load spends in the metatarsal head region. (Reproduced with permission from Hutton WC, Stott JRR, Stokes JAF. The mechanics of the foot. In: Klenerman L, ed. The foot and its allied disorders. Oxford, UK: Blackwell Scientific, 1982:42.)

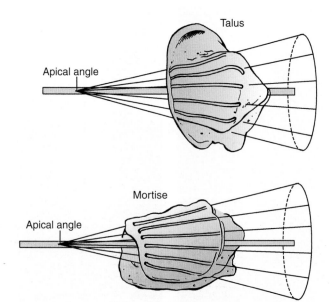

Figure 1.23   The talus as the cross section of a cone with the apex on the medial side supported by the deltoid ligament complex. (Adapted from Inman VT. The joints of the ankle. Baltimore: Williams & Wilkins, 1976.)

Lateral ankle stability depends on the ATFL and CFL. In neutral position, both ligaments contribute to stability. As the ankle is plantarflexed, however, the orientation of the ATFL fibers becomes more vertical, allowing it to provide most of the lateral stability. Conversely, the fibers of the CFL become more horizontal, rendering the ligament ineffective as a stabilizer. The roles are reversed in dorsiflexion. In the sagittal plane, the angle produced by these two ligaments is an average of 105°. However, variation is considerable with angles ranging between 70° and 140°. There may be biomechanical implications at the extreme ranges of this variation. If one imagines these two ligaments passing through an arc of motion, at some point, in certain ligament configurations, neither may be oriented to act as a true collateral ligament. This anatomic variability may account for why some people are susceptible to chronic ankle sprains. Furthermore, persons with "ligamentous laxity" may in fact not be lax at all, but rather they may possess a certain ligament orientation that does not provide optimal stability in the position tested.

SUGGESTED READING

Elftman H. The transverse tarsal joint and its control. Clin Orthop 1960;16:41.

Hamilton WG. Clinical symposia: surgical anatomy of the foot and ankle, vol 37, no 3. New Jersey: Ciba-Geigy, 1985.

Hicks JH. The mechanics of the foot. II. The plantar aponeurosis and the arch. J Anat 1954;88:25.

Inman VT. The joints of the ankle. Baltimore: Williams & Wilkins, 1976.

Mann R, Coughlin M, eds. Surgery of the foot and ankle, 7th ed. St. Louis: Mosby, 1999.

Sarrafian SK. Anatomy of the foot and ankle: descriptive, topographic, functional, 2nd ed. Philadelphia: JB Lippincott, 1993.

2 PHYSICAL EXAMINATION AND ORTHOTICS

RYAN C. GOODWIN
JAMES J. SFERRA
EVA ASOMUGHA

PHYSICAL EXAMINATION

A thorough history and physical examination constitute the cornerstone of any medical encounter that ultimately leads to a correct diagnosis and appropriate treatment. This chapter focuses on physical examination elements specific to the foot and ankle and underscores the fact that a systematic approach provides consistent, reproducible information in an effort to minimize missed diagnoses and simultaneously optimize efficiency. General principles of orthotic management and specific examples related to the foot and ankle are discussed.

PATIENT HISTORY

The importance of a carefully obtained history can never be overstated. Even though a comprehensive history is helpful, certain key historical aspects specific to the foot and ankle are essential. Patient age, gender, occupation, and recreational activities provide a foundation for the patient encounter. Occupational requirements and shoe-wear preferences are also helpful.

The patient's chief complaint should always be elicited. Pain is typically the primary complaint for which people seek care; however, other complaints such as deformity, swelling, instability, and stiffness may be the patient's main concern. Precipitating and relieving factors that affect the patient's symptoms should be sought, as should the timing of symptoms (e.g., worse in the morning or progression over weeks to months). The presence or absence of sensory disturbances including numbness, burning, or tingling and any associated radiation of symptoms should be elicited and may indicate neurologic pathology. Prior therapies and their efficacies should also be noted.

Associated relevant medical history is important because various systemic illnesses may render the foot and ankle more susceptible to certain problems. Specifically, patients should be questioned about a history of diabetes mellitus, vascular disease, inflammatory arthritis, and neurologic conditions. Current medications and medical allergies should be noted. A prior surgical history—specifically prior foot and ankle procedures—is also helpful. Patients should also be questioned regarding a history of trauma. Prior adverse reactions to anesthetics should be noted in patients who are candidates for surgery.

History of tobacco use, specifically cigarette smoking, and alcohol use should be routinely obtained because they can significantly affect the outcomes of both surgical and nonsurgical therapies. Pending litigation and worker's compensation claims may influence the diagnostic approach, the treatment plan, and ultimately the patient outcome.

History taking in the athlete deserves special mention as a thorough, focused history on injury mechanism, chronicity of symptoms, and compensatory mechanisms may provide important clues to the diagnosis. With acute injuries, details should be elicited, including the position of the foot or ankle relative to the body during injury; whether there was any particular sensation experienced including a pop, locking, or crunching; whether weight-bearing was possible immediately after the injury; and whether any reduction maneuvers had to be performed immediately after the injury. For chronic symptoms, athletes may be questioned on previous treatments; whether symptoms were initiated by a distant trauma, experienced only with athletic activity, or were exacerbated by external factors such as shoe wear or athletic pads. Precipitating athletic activity such as cutting, jumping, or running may also provide important clues.

INITIAL PRIMARY EXAMINATION

A systematic and reproducible primary examination should be performed on every patient to gather accurate and complete objective information consistently. This overview may provide insight that may not be specifically related to the patient's chief complaint. Following a reproducible primary survey, a more focused physical examination can be undertaken based on the patient's complaints and other findings. By performing the same primary examination with each patient, critical omissions are avoided.

Inspection and Observation

Shoe Wear

Inspection of the patient's shoe wear can be valuable in various foot and ankle disorders and should not be omitted. Improper shoe wear and shoe size have been implicated as causative factors in various foot pathologies. Studies have demonstrated significant discrepancies between actual measured foot size and the patient's perceived shoe size in certain populations. Furthermore, many patients will have an actual mismatch in shoe size between the right foot and left foot, which is often unaccounted for in footwear sizing.

Specific patterns of shoe wear may be observed:

- An oblique as opposed to a transverse crease in the shoe's forefoot may suggest hallux rigidus.
- Scuffing of the toe box may indicate a drop foot.
- A significant flatfoot deformity may result in broken medial shoe counter.
- Excessive in-toeing or high-arched feet may create excessive lateral sole wear.

Standing Inspection

The remainder of the initial examination should proceed in a systematic manner, beginning with standing inspection of the foot and ankle from both anterior and posterior.

- The patient's legs should be exposed from the knee to the toes.
- Overall alignment of the hindfoot and forefoot should be assessed as should any focal deformity.
- The status of the longitudinal arch should be noted. Quantitative clinical indices of arch height have been described such as the Staheli, Chippaux-Smirak, truncated arch, and arch length indices; however, these are primarily for research purposes. Navicular height and normalized navicular height (normalized to foot length) have been shown to be the most accurate clinical measures of arch height.
- The importance of the standing, weight-bearing examination cannot be overemphasized.
  - ☐ The foot structure may appear normal while sitting, but can be strikingly different when subjected to weight-bearing forces, as may be the case with hypermobile flatfoot deformity, flexible toe deformities, and hypermobile metatarsophalangeal (MTP) joints.
- The "too many toes" sign is indicative of hindfoot valgus (Fig. 2.1).
- Examination of gait is an essential part of the initial primary examination.
- Observations should include assessment of any side-to-side asymmetry, ability to achieve a plantigrade foot, foot placement, and general flow of the heel strike, foot flat, toe-off progression as well as any avoidance patterns.

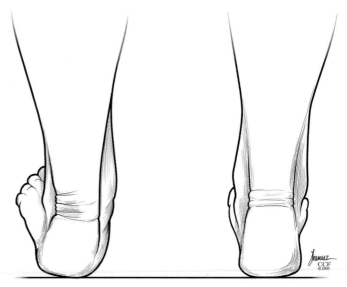

Figure 2.1   Malalignment of the "acquired flat foot" with tibialis posterior tendon rupture (*left foot*) and a "too many toes" sign. (Reprinted with permission of the Cleveland Clinic.)

- Single- and double-limb heel rises should be observed from behind the patient with the knees extended.
- Side-to-side comparison is helpful in identifying pathology.
- The inability to perform a single-limb heel rise or lack of symmetrical inversion of the hindfoot strongly suggests tibialis posterior tendon pathology (Fig. 2.2).

Seated Evaluation

- The vascular evaluation includes palpation of the dorsalis pedis and posterior tibial pulses.
  - ☐ The dorsalis pedis pulse is typically located between the extensor hallucis longus (EHL) and the extensor digitorum longus tendons, just proximal and lateral to the dorsal prominence of the first metatarsal base and medial cuneiform.

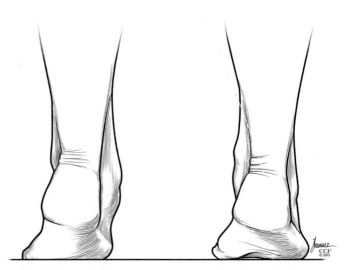

Figure 2.2   Double heel rise test. Calcaneal inversion is normal on the right and absent on the left. (Reprinted with permission of the Cleveland Clinic.)

☐ The posterior tibial pulse is palpable behind the medial malleolus, approximately one-third of the distance to the medial border of the Achilles tendon.

☐ If pulses are weak or absent, a more comprehensive vascular evaluation is warranted, especially if surgery is being considered or if the patient has an open wound.

☐ This evaluation may include pulse volume recordings with toe pressures or transcutaneous oxygen levels.

■ Skin and nail abnormalities are noted.

☐ The presence of callosities may be indicative of regions of increased loading and are strong clues to abnormal foot mechanics.

☐ Skin changes indicative of vascular disease, edema, and erythema are also noted.

■ A gross sensory evaluation helps prevent omission.

☐ Light-touch sensation is evaluated grossly at the dorsal first and fourth web spaces (deep and superficial branches of the peroneal nerve) as well as the plantar surface of the foot (tibial nerve).

☐ The medial and lateral aspects of the foot should also be briefly tested (saphenous and sural nerves).

☐ More specific neurologic testing can be carried out later during the examination.

■ A brief range of motion examination with the patient in the sitting position may also provide insight into the presence of possible foot and ankle pathology.

☐ Passive and active motions can be briefly and easily tested and should be part of the routine initial primary examination.

☐ Normal passive ankle motion is approximately 20° of dorsiflexion to 50° of plantarflexion.

☐ Subtalar motion can also be tested with the patient seated.

☐ The examiner grasps the patient's hindfoot with one hand while the other hand passively ranges the subtalar joint.

☐ Normal range is approximately 15° in both subtalar inversion and eversion and is usually referenced as a fraction of the uninvolved side.

☐ Ankle motion should be tested with the patient's knee flexed to eliminate the effect of the gastrocnemius with the hindfoot held in neutral alignment to prevent dorsiflexion through the transverse tarsal joints (Fig. 2.3).

☐ Forefoot abduction and adduction are tested with the hindfoot stabilized and passive force applied to the forefoot.

☐ Normal range of forefoot motion is 20° of adduction and 10° of abduction.

☐ Limitation of passive motion or pain with passive motion may indicate degenerative disease of a particular joint, prior fusion, or other pathology associated with that joint.

☐ Active motion is grossly assessed by having the patient trace a circular pattern in the air with his or her toes. Alternatively, having patients walk on their toes and on the medial and lateral borders of their feet is also an indicator of whether a relatively normal range of motion is present.

☐ Resistance strength testing should be performed in all major planes of active motion of the foot and ankle. This may provide insight into tendon, muscle, or nerve pathology.

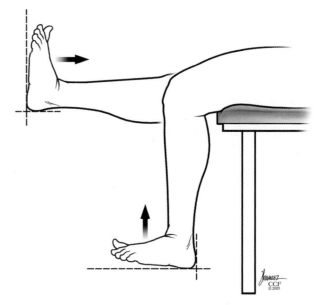

Figure 2.3 Ankle dorsiflexion—knee extended and knee flexed. The hindfoot must be held in neutral alignment.

This brief initial primary examination provides an excellent foundation for the remainder of a problem-focused physical examination. A basic assessment of the patient's overall alignment, appearance, neurovascular status, range of motion, and strength can be obtained in a relatively short period without omission of any critical elements. Problem-focused physical examination can then proceed in a concise and orderly fashion.

FOCUSED EXAMINATION

Skin and Nails

■ The integrity of the soft-tissue envelope about the foot and ankle is important to note in any foot and ankle examination, especially if surgery is contemplated.

☐ Prior surgical scars should be noted, as should the overall quality of the skin.

☐ Trophic changes and hair loss may indicate peripheral vascular disease.

☐ Dependent rubor is indicative of poor perfusion to the foot.

☐ Venous insufficiency may manifest with pigmentation in the supramalleolar region.

☐ Swelling, erythema, and increased skin temperature may be due to a number of causes including cellulitis, inflammatory arthritis, or neuropathic joints.

☐ Ulcerations should be noted and characterized based on their location and appearance.

■ Callosities may form in regions subjected to higher than normal axial or shear load.

☐ Although the function of callosities is to prevent blistering and protect deeper structures, they may become pathologic in that they paradoxically lead to increased pressure, especially in the neuropathic patient, frequently leading to ulceration.

☐ Viral agents can cause plantar warts, which produce callosities that may be difficult to distinguish from mechanically induced callus. Trimming the overlying callus usually reveals punctate black capillaries at the base of a wart. Pinching a wart usually causes significant pain, whereas it is relatively pain free with calluses.

- ☐ Skin prints diverge around warts, whereas they course through a callosity.
- ▪ Malignant melanoma is the most common primary malignant tumor of the foot.
  - ☐ Pedal lesions may be subtle and may present as a small area of subungal or epidermal discoloration. In the absence of recent trauma, a high index of suspicion is necessary to prevent delayed treatment or misdiagnosis.
- ▪ Toenail disorders are often the cause of patient concern.
  - ☐ The closed environment of shoe wear can predispose the toenails to problems not seen in the hand. Eponychia, paronychia, and onychomycosis are common infectious processes seen in the toenail and are easily diagnosed by inspection alone.
  - ☐ *Eponychia* is an infection of the proximal nail fold, whereas *paronychia* refers to an infection of either the lateral or medial nail fold. These are commonly referred to as *ingrown toenails*.
  - ☐ *Onychomycosis* refers to a fungal infection of the nail and results in thickening, yellow-brown discoloration, discoloration, splitting, pitting, or ridging of the nail plate.
  - ☐ Pitting of the nail is also seen with psoriasis.

Bones and Soft Tissues

Bones

Because pain is frequently the patient's chief complaint, localization and reproduction of the patient's pain is invaluable in achieving a correct diagnosis. Much of the bony and soft-tissue anatomy of the foot and ankle is subcutaneous and relatively easy to palpate. With a thorough knowledge of the anatomy, localization of the painful structure is usually relatively straightforward.

- ▪ The examination should be focused on the region of the patient's complaint.
- ▪ Asking the patient to point with one finger to the area of maximal pain is a simple way to begin a focused examination.
- ▪ Pain can typically be reproduced by palpation of one or more bony or soft-tissue structures.

Bony landmarks that are easily palpable on the *medial aspect* of the foot include the first MTP joint, first metatarsal, medial cuneiform, navicular tuberosity, talar head, sustentaculum tali, medial malleolus, and medial calcaneus.

- ▪ The first MTP joint is frequently associated with a bunion deformity or degenerative changes.
- ▪ The navicular tuberosity is the primary attachment for the tibialis posterior tendon, and pain with palpation may indicate insertional pathology.
- ▪ Avascular necrosis of the navicular or stress fracture may lead to tenderness.
- ▪ The talar head can be more prominent in a pes planus deformity.
- ▪ The medial malleolus is easily palpable and is the medial buttress for the tibiotalar joint.

- ▪ The sustentaculum tali is located approximately one fingerbreadth below the medial malleolus. It may not be palpable, but it is important in that it serves as the attachment for the spring ligament and provides support for the talus.

Bony landmarks that are easily palpable on the *lateral aspect* of the foot include the fifth MTP joint, the fifth metatarsal, base of the fifth metatarsal, the cuboid, lateral calcaneus, including the anterior process and peroneal tubercle, lateral malleolus, and the talar dome and neck.

- ▪ The base of the fifth metatarsal provides the insertion for the peroneus brevis tendon, and tenderness could indicate insertional pathology or a fracture.
- ▪ The peroneal tubercle is palpable on the lateral aspect of the calcaneus below the lateral malleolus and serves as the point where the peroneal tendons (longus and brevis) separate as they turn around the lateral calcaneus.
- ▪ The lateral malleolus provides a lateral buttress to the ankle joint.
  - ☐ It extends further distally than the medial malleolus and slightly posteriorly, allowing the ankle mortise to occupy a position of approximately 15° of external rotation relative to the long axis of the tibia.
  - ☐ It is susceptible to fracture.
- ▪ The talar dome is palpable just anterior to the lateral malleolus with the foot held in plantarflexion and slight inversion.
  - ☐ Tenderness here may suggest an ostechondral lesion, fracture, or synovitis.
- ▪ The sinus tarsi region is the soft spot that is easily palpable on the lateral aspect of the hindfoot and is the site most specific for subtalar joint pathology.
- ▪ Deep palpation may reveal tenderness at the anterior process of the calcaneus, a potential site of fracture or arthrosis.
- ▪ The lateral process of the talus can be palpable and may be a site of injury (snowboarder's fracture).
- ▪ The lateral neck of the talus may also be palpable in some patients. Areas of edema, tenderness, or pain should be noted and deep palpation should be applied on the lateral aspect of the talar neck. If pain is elicited, further imaging with CT or MRI should be obtained to rule out an occult fracture if there is a history of trauma. Up to 39% of ankle and midfoot fractures may be missed on initial examination and radiographic evaluation. Palpation of the *posterior aspect* of the foot is performed with the patient seated.
- ▪ Grasping the calcaneus and applying gentle compression may elicit pain indicative of a calcaneal stress fracture.
- ▪ The retrocalcaneal bursa can be palpated with the thumb and fingers in the depressions adjacent to the Achilles tendon.
- ▪ The medial tubercle of the calcaneus is palpable on the medial plantar surface and serves as the attachment for the abductor hallucis and flexor digitorum brevis, and is a common source of heel pain in adults.
- ▪ Tenderness to palpation centrally along the plantar surface of the calcaneus may indicate a periostitis.
- ▪ The posterior aspect of the calcaneus may be a site of tenderness in children as a manifestation of an

apophysitis (Sever disease) or insertional Achilles tendinitis in adults.

- The bony landmarks to examine on the *plantar surface* of the foot include the sesamoid bones and the metatarsal heads.
- Deep palpation at the plantar surface of the first MTP joint reveals two palpable sesamoid bones.
  - □ These sesamoid bones lie within the substance of the flexor hallucis brevis tendons and help distribute weight borne by the first ray, as well as provide mechanical advantage for the flexor hallucis brevis tendons.
  - □ Tenderness may reveal a sesamoiditis, stress fracture, or avascular necrosis.
  - □ Their location may be altered with hallux valgus.
- The lesser metatarsal heads are easily palpable on the plantar surface of the forefoot and may be tender if poorly padded or with MTP synovitis.
- Callosities may be present in areas of overuse.
- Tenderness at the metatarsal heads can be due to avascular necrosis (Freiberg disease).

Soft Tissues

Palpation of the soft tissues should likewise proceed in a systematic and focused fashion based on the patient's complaints.

- At the *forefoot medially*, the first MTP joint is a common source of pathology, especially if hallux valgus deformity is present.
  - □ Bursal formation at the first MTP joint may be present and may be tender to palpation at the medial aspect of the joint.
  - □ Gouty tophi may be present and painful.
  - □ Callus formation and tenderness may be present in a longstanding pes planus deformity.
- On the *medial side of the hindfoot and ankle*, the deltoid ligament is typically palpable beneath the medial malleolus (Fig. 2.4).
  - □ The soft-tissue depression between the medial malleolus and the Achilles tendon includes the tibialis posterior tendon, flexor digitorum longus tendon,

neurovascular bundle (posterior tibial artery and tibial nerve), and flexor hallucis longus tendon.
  - □ The tibialis posterior tendon is most readily palpable from behind the medial malleolus to its insertion on the navicular tuberosity.
  - □ The flexor hallucis longus is typically not palpable because of its deep location.
  - □ A Tinel sign is present if paresthesias along the distal course of the tibial nerve are elicited by tapping on the nerve, possibly indicating the presence of tarsal tunnel syndrome.
- On the *dorsum of the foot*, the tibialis anterior (TA) tendon is easily palpable along the medial aspect of the ankle, extending to its insertion at the medial base of the first metatarsal.
  - □ The EHL tendon is lateral to the TA tendon and can be traced distally along the first ray.
  - □ Tenderness may indicate tendon pathology.

A lump beneath the extensor retinaculum along the ankle may represent a ruptured anterior tibialis tendon.

- Along the *lateral aspect of the ankle*, the three primary lateral ankle ligaments—the anterior talofibular ligament, posterior talofibular ligament, and calcaneofibular ligament—are palpated (Fig. 2.5).
  - □ Tenderness may indicate injury to the lateral ligaments.
- The peroneal tendons are palpable along the lateral aspect of the ankle.
- *Distally*, the head of the fifth metatarsal may be a site of bursal formation resulting from a bunionette.
- The *Achilles tendon* is the largest tendon in the human body and is palpable in the subcutaneous hindfoot down to its insertion into the calcaneus.
  - □ A defect may be palpable in cases of rupture.
  - □ Nodularity may be present and tender in cases of chronic inflammation or tendinosis.
  - □ The retrocalcaneal and calcaneal bursae may be tender on the anterior and posterior surfaces of the Achilles tendon, respectively.

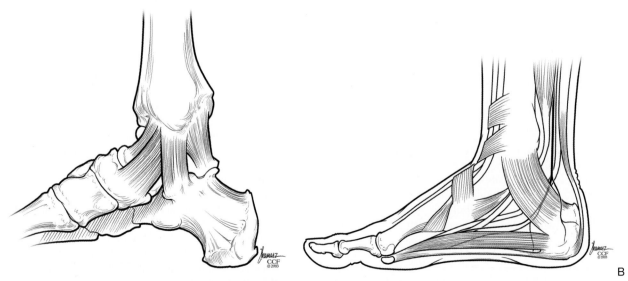

A   B

Figure 2.4   Medial view of the ankle. (**A**) Deep layer—deltoid ligament. (**B**) Superficial layer—retinacular/tendon structures. (Reprinted with permission of the Cleveland Clinic.)

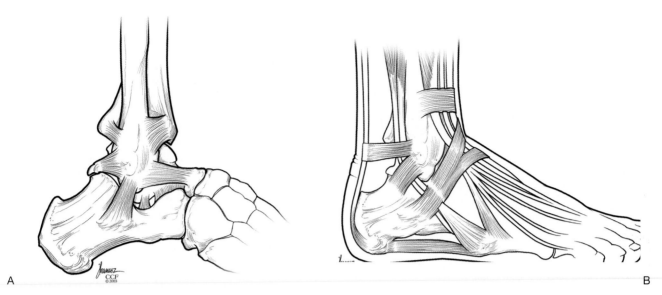

Figure 2.5 Lateral view of the ankle. (**A**) Deep layer—lateral ligaments. (**B**) Superficial layer—retinacular/tendon structures. (Reprinted with permission of the Cleveland Clinic.)

■ The *plantar fascia* is also palpable from its insertion at the medial tubercle of the calcaneus and along its course on the plantar medial surface of the foot. Tenderness may indicate inflammation, and nodularity may be present with plantar fibromatosis.

Nerves

Certain complaints, symptoms, and concurrent medical conditions mandate a more thorough neurologic examination than is done in the initial primary assessment.

■ Peripheral neuropathy due to a systemic process such as diabetes mellitus may be present.
■ Decreased or absent sensation is present symmetrically in a stocking distribution.
■ Absence of the Achilles reflex and decreased vibratory sensation may indicate peripheral neuropathy.
■ The ability to detect a 5.07 (10-g) Semmes–Weinstein monofilament is typically indicative of the presence of protective sensation.

More specific peripheral nerve pathology such as nerve entrapment or a surgical or traumatic lesion should be sought in cases of neurologic complaints.

■ The common peroneal nerve may become entrapped at the fibular neck, producing symptoms of numbness on the dorsum of the foot and weakness in foot and toe dorsiflexors.
■ The superficial branch of the peroneal nerve can become entrapped just anterior to the fibula as it penetrates the superficial fascia approximately 8 to 10 cm above the ankle joint (Fig. 2.6).
  ☐ Percussion along the course of the nerve may elicit paresthesias or pain.
■ The posterior tibial nerve and its branches may become entrapped in the tarsal canal posterior to the medial malleolus (Fig. 2.7).
  ☐ Patients typically complain of burning, aching, or numbness on the plantar surface of the foot.

☐ Tenderness and a positive Tinel sign with propagation of paresthesias with percussion aid in the diagnosis of tarsal tunnel syndrome.

Isolated peripheral nerve injuries are often the result of trauma, sometimes the consequence of a prior surgical procedure.

■ The sural nerve is at risk with lateral hindfoot approaches resulting in numbness of the lateral border of the foot.

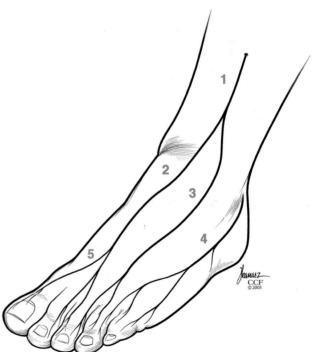

Figure 2.6 Nerves—dorsolateral view. (*1*) superficial peroneal nerve (the numeral is located where the nerve may be entrapped as it passes through the investing fascia); (*2*) dorsal medial cutaneous nerve; (*3*) dorsal intermediate cutaneous nerve; (*4*) sural nerve; and (*5*) dorsal hallucal nerve. (Reprinted with permission of the Cleveland Clinic.)

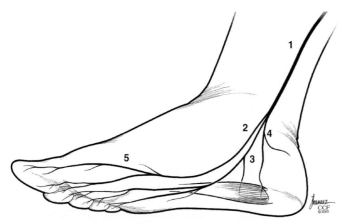

Figure 2.7 Nerves—plantar medial view. *(1)* Tibial nerve; *(2)* medial plantar nerve; *(3)* lateral plantar nerve; *(4)* medial calcaneal nerve; *(5)* medial plantar hallucal nerve. (Reprinted with permission of the Cleveland Clinic.)

- The dorsal cutaneous nerves can be injured as a result of anterior approaches to the ankle or dorsal approaches to the midfoot.
  - ☐ Longitudinal incisions minimize the risk of iatrogenic injury.
- The dorsal cutaneous nerve can be injured with dorsal approaches in bunion procedures.
- The medial calcaneal nerve can be damaged with a medial incision during a procedure for plantar fascia release.
- Incisional cutaneous hypersensitivity, point tenderness along the course of a nerve, distal anesthesia, and percussion-induced paresthesias are all signs of a damaged peripheral nerve.
- Charcot arthropathy may occur in patients with peripheral neuropathy, leading to bone and joint destruction.
  - ☐ It may occur spontaneously or, more commonly, following a minor trauma.
  - ☐ On physical examination, the affected region appears edematous, erythematous, and warm; sometimes mildly tender, which can be confused with cellulitis.
  - ☐ When Charcot changes are present in the midfoot region, a rocker bottom deformity may develop, with collapse of the midfoot ultimately leading to ulceration over abnormal bony prominences.

Musculotendinous Complexes

The gastrocnemius–soleus (GCS) complex and Achilles tendon provide powerful plantarflexion to the foot.

- Because the muscle group is powerful, a weakened complex may still easily overcome the examiner's strength in manual testing.
- Subtle side-to-side differences are best appreciated by observing fatigability on repeated single-limb heel rises.
- Shortening of the GCS complex has been implicated in several disorders—through its pathologic effect of increasing plantar pressures during normal gait—including metatarsalgia, plantar fasciitis, forefoot ulceration, and Charcot midfoot breakdown. Manual testing of the tibialis posterior is best done with resistance to inversion in the plantar-flexed and pronated foot.

- If the patient is able to perform a single-limb heel rise, the heel should invert slightly with an intact tendon.
- Failure of hindfoot inversion with a single- or double-limb heel rise suggests tibialis posterior incompetence; this is the most sensitive test on physical examination to confirm the diagnosis.
- Isometric subtalar inversion and forefoot adduction strength are reduced by 20% and 30%, respectively, in patients with type II posterior tibial tendon dysfunction (PTTD) compared with controls.
- In the absence of trauma, the posterior tibial edema (PTE) sign refers to pitting edema along the course of the tendon and is highly sensitive and specific for PTTD. The TA is the prime foot and ankle dorsiflexor.
- A slapping gait may indicate TA dysfunction.
- Resisted ankle dorsiflexion is perhaps the best manual test of TA function.
- Its tendoncan be palpated over the dorsal medial ankle during resistance testing. The peroneal tendons (longus and brevis) act as evertors of the foot.
- Strength is tested by resisting active eversion.
- Subluxation or dislocation of the peroneal tendons from their groove behind the fibula should be inspected during resisted eversion with the ankle in dorsiflexion.

Articulations

The first MTP joint provides dorsiflexion and plantarflexion predominantly, with adduction and abduction possible as well.

- Ankle position during testing may be important in that a tight flexor hallucis longus tendon may limit dorsiflexion, especially if the ankle is held neutral or is slightly dorsiflexed.
- Conversely, a tight EHL tendon may limit plantarflexion of the first MTP joint if the ankle is plantarflexed.
- If motion is limited, it should be tested with the ankle in both positions.
- Pain and limitation of passive motion suggest underlying pathology, such as hallux rigidus or synovitis.
- Abduction and adduction of the hallux can be measured relative to the long axis of the first ray, but is usually only relevant as a measure of flexibility of a varus or valgus deformity.

The subtalar joint, talonavicular joint, and calcaneocuboid joint constitute the hindfoot joints.

- Limitation at any of these three joints can result in significant reduction of motion of the entire complex.
  - ☐ Examples include selective arthrodesis of one of the three joints or tarsal coalition in the adolescent patient.
- The ankle should be passively dorsiflexed to neutral to lock the talus in the ankle mortise, thus preventing tibiotalar rotation, which could increase the effective motion observed.
- The heel is grasped with one hand and with the other the foot is passively inverted and everted (Fig. 2.8).
- Because the ankle is in neutral, theoretically a tight Achilles tendon limits motion somewhat in this position. If this is the case, a prone examination may also be effective with the examiner's fingers placed on the posterior facet joint line to palpate specific subtalar motion.

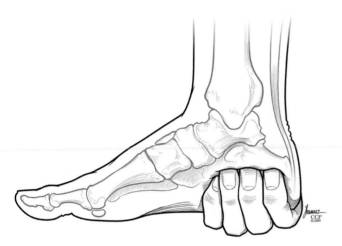

Figure 2.8 Calcaneal inversion and eversion. (Reprinted with permission of the Cleveland Clinic.)

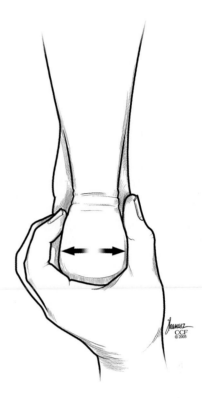

- The talonavicular joint is also easily palpable while placing the complex through a gentle range of motion and can give a better idea of absolute transverse tarsal joint motion.
- Hindfoot motion is usually recorded as a fraction of the uninvolved side.

The ankle joint is essentially a hinge joint with motion restricted to the sagittal plane. Loss of ankle motion can have a profound effect on the overall gait cycle and gait mechanics.

- Normal passive ankle motion is typically 20° of dorsiflexion to about 50° of plantarflexion.
  - □ This measurement is obtained between the mechanical axis of the tibia and a line parallel to the plantar aspect of the foot.
- The two most common causes of restricted ankle motion, especially dorsiflexion, are degenerative changes of the ankle joint and a tight Achilles tendon.
- Comparing ankle dorsiflexion first with the knee flexed and then with the knee extended with hindfoot in neutral elicits the contribution of the gastrocnemius tightness to limited dorsiflexion, which is also known as the Silfverskiold test (see Fig. 2.3).
- If passive dorsiflexion increases significantly with knee flexion, a gastrocnemius contracture is the cause of decreased motion, which is especially important in patients with a pes planus deformity.
- Because excessive subtalar eversion may provide the appearance of additional ankle dorsiflexion, it is important to hold the hindfoot locked in neutral to slight supination to eliminate this deformity.
- The anterior drawer test can be performed to determine the presence of ligamentous laxity of the ankle.
  - □ One hand immobilizes the distal tibia while the other grasps the heel to control the hindfoot with the ankle in plantarflexion.

- □ The heel is then gently translated forward and any subluxation is noted (Fig. 2.9).
- □ Side-to-side comparison with the uninjured ankle is vital in detecting abnormalities.
- The anterolateral drawer test has been described on cadaveric specimens and is thought to better evaluate the anterolateral rotatory nature of talar displacement.
  - □ The ankle is placed in plantarflexion while the talus is palpated and an internal rotational force is applied. Any opening or discrepancy between sides is suggestive of lateral ankle instability or ligament rupture.

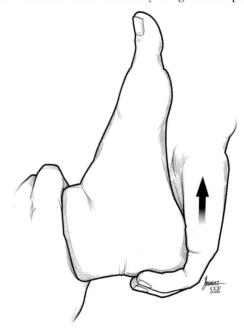

Figure 2.9 Anterior drawer test. (Reprinted with permission of the Cleveland Clinic.)

Injury to the anterior tibiofibular ligament or "high ankle sprain" is less common than a lateral ankle sprain.

☐ Reproduction of this mechanism by stabilizing the leg and externally rotating the foot reproduces pain in these cases.

☐ A "squeeze test," in which the tibia and the fibula are compressed together in the midleg, may also yield ankle pain.

☐ The "heel-thump test" has also been described for the diagnosis of tibiofibular ligament or syndesmotic injuries. The patient is seated with the knee in 90° of flexion and the ankle in a natural equinus position. The leg is stabilized with one hand while the other hand delivers a thump to the center of the heel. A positive test reproduces pain along the anterior, posterior, or distal leg corresponding to injury to the anterior tibiofibular, posterior tibiofibular, or interosseous ligaments, respectively.

Forefoot

Hallux Valgus

▨ A valgus deformity of the first MTP joint is invariably noted.

▨ The deformity may or may not be passively correctable (Fig. 2.10).

▨ The valgus deformity is usually associated with pronation of the hallux (Fig. 2.11).

▨ Some patients may exhibit a valgus deformity distal to the first MTP joint or hallux valgus interphalangeus. It is important to make this distinction because the surgical treatment of hallux valgus interphalangeus differs from other bunion procedures.

▨ In addition to routine hallux valgus radiographs, other methods of clinical diagnosis and evaluation have been suggested. These include goniometric assessment, measurement of forefoot girth, and standardized photography.

☐ The Manchester scale is a noninvasive method of clinically grading the severity of the deformity by comparing the patient's bunion with four standardized images. This may be most useful for research purposes.

▨ Hallux valgus may coexist with degenerative changes at the first MTP joint, restricting motion and producing pain. Hallux rigidus and first MTP osteoarthritis, however,

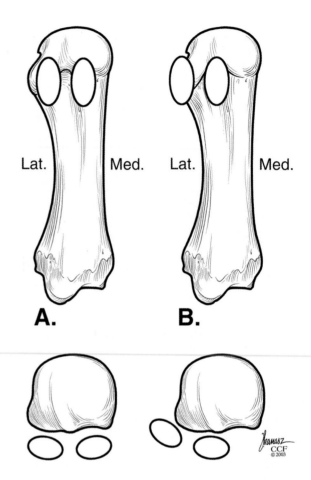

A.   **B.**

Figure 2.11   (**A**) Neutral alignment of the sesamoids. (**B**) Subluxed sesamoids with hallux pronation. (Reprinted with permission of the Cleveland Clinic.)

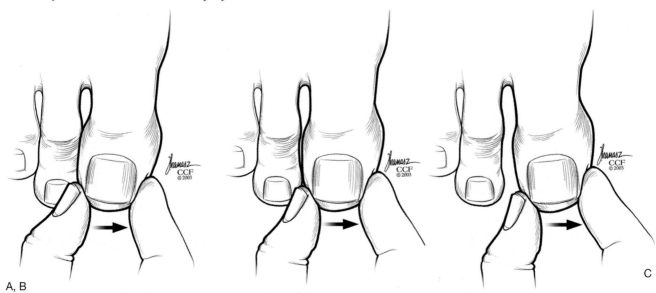

A, B   C

Figure 2.10   Passive correction of hallux valgus. (**A**) Not correctable. (**B**) Correctable to neutral. (**C**) Overcorrectable. (Reprinted with permission of the Cleveland Clinic.)

are distinguished by the near complete absence of dorsi-flexion in the former.

☐ The first MTP grind maneuver may also elicit pain in a patient with hallux rigidus, which is performed by axially loading the first MTP joint through a range of motion in all planes, including rotation, which is frequently painful in affected patients.

☐ Dorsal osteophytes may be palpable.
☐ Hypermobility of the first ray may be a component of hallux valgus pathology.
  ☐ It can be assessed by grasping the lesser metatarsals in one hand and translating the first metatarsal dorsally and plantarly with the ankle in neutral position (Fig. 2.12).

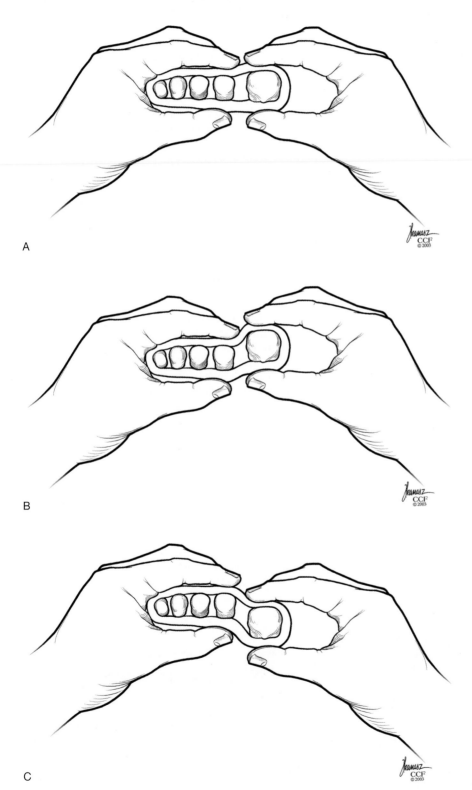

A

B

C

Figure 2.12 Assessing first tarsometatarsal hypermobility. (**A**) No hypermobility. (**B, C**) Hypermobile first ray. (Reprinted with permission of the Cleveland Clinic.)

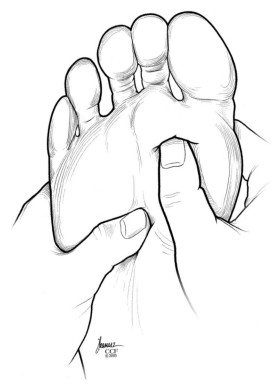

Figure 2.13 Location of sesamoid tenderness. Fibular tenderness pictured. (Reprinted with permission of the Cleveland Clinic.)

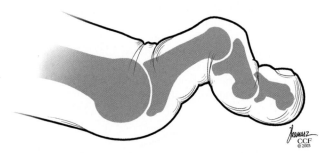

Figure 2.15 Hammer toe. (Reprinted with permission of the Cleveland Clinic.)

- Flexible claw toe deformities are typically a result of shoe wear. Eventually they become rigid.
- A more rigid claw toe deformity can result from entities such as Charcot–Marie–Tooth disease, instability due to rheumatoid disease, or following a deep compartment syndrome producing a contracted flexor digitorum longus tendon.
- A deformity that is passively correctable with the ankle plantarflexed but rigid with the ankle dorsiflexed may be due to a tight flexor tendon.
- Calluses may form on the tips of the toes with rigid deformities.

Hammer toe deformity is defined as flexion of the PIP joint with extension deformity of the DIP joint (Fig. 2.15).

- The MTP joint is typically held in neutral or extension.
- Painful callus formation is common on the dorsum of the PIP joint.
- This deformity is similar to a boutonniere deformity in the finger, and it may be flexible or rigid.
- The metatarsal heads become prominent and may become painful with callus formation.

Mallet toe is defined as a flexion deformity of the DIP joint with the PIP in neutral or slight extension (Fig. 2.16).

- The MTP joint is usually neutrally aligned.
- Pain and callosities typically develop over the tip of the toe and the DIP joint, and the deformity may be rigid or flexible.
- Extrinsic contracture of the flexor digitorum longus tendon may play a role in the flexibility of the deformity, warranting examination with the ankle in both dorsiflexion and plantarflexion.

    □ Hypermobility may necessitate a first tarsometatarsal joint fusion.
   □ Plantar pain in the region of the first MTP joint is also common in hallux valgus deformity in that sesamoid subluxation occurs as part of the deformity.
   □ Overload of the sesamoids can cause pain and the sesamoids should be palpated (Fig. 2.13).

Lesser Toes

Claw toe is defined as a flexion deformity of both the distal interphalangeal (DIP) and the proximal interphalangeal (PIP) joints of a given toe (Fig. 2.14).

- The deformity may be flexible or rigid.
- The MTP joint may be uninvolved or in extension.
- Dorsal calluses may form and can be painful.

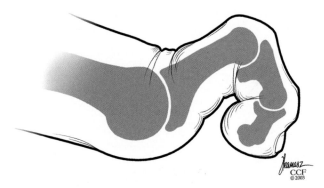

Figure 2.14 Claw toe. (Reprinted with permission of the Cleveland Clinic.)

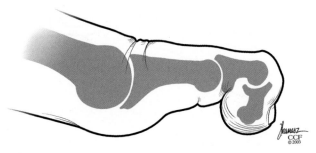

Figure 2.16 Mallet toe. (Reprinted with permission of the Cleveland Clinic.)

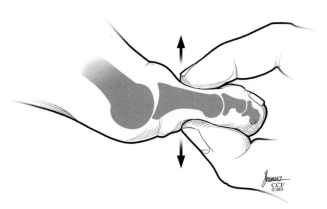

Figure 2.17   Toe translation test. Stage 1: subluxable. (Reprinted with permission of the Cleveland Clinic.)

Crossover deformity of the lesser toes may occur with MTP joint instability.

■ The second toe is most commonly involved.
■ Attenuation of the capsular structures develops as a result of the mechanical imbalance of the MTP joint.
■ Sometimes, systemic pathology (e.g., rheumatoid disease) may be causative.
■ Examination will often reveal dorsomedial deviation of the second toe. A drawer test should be performed to elicit any instability. A positive drawer sign is thought to be the first objective sign of MTP joint instability.
■ Second toe crossover of the hallux usually occurs with severe cases of hallux valgus. Gaps between the toes, especially in the second web space, may be an early indicator of impending crossover deformity.
■ As the deformity progresses, subluxation and eventual dislocation of the MTP joint can occur.
■ Symmetrical laxity with toe translation (Fig. 2.17) may be indicative of generalized laxity. Chronic irritation of the skin at adjacent portions of two neighboring toes may produce a hyperkeratosis referred to as a *corn*.
■ Soft corns are commonly found in the web spaces and can become macerated because the environment between the toes when shoes are worn is relatively moist.
■ Corns are usually caused by the irregular pressures caused by bony prominences abutting each other on adjacent toes (Fig. 2.18).

Metatarsalgia

Pain localized to the plantar aspect of the MTP joints is termed *metatarsalgia*. It has many causes. The etiology can be either intra-articular (capsulitis, capsular injury, degenerative changes, and avascular necrosis) or extra-articular (interdigital neuroma, flexor tenosynovitis, and metatarsal stress fracture).

■ Patients with MTP capsulitis have tenderness to palpation over the affected metatarsal heads.
  □ The capsule degenerates and ultimately ruptures, resulting in painful instability with a positive toe translation/drawer test.
  □ Crossover deformity may result in instability.
■ Arthritis or synovitis leads to local tenderness, which is typically dorsal in nature because the articular cartilage loss begins dorsally.

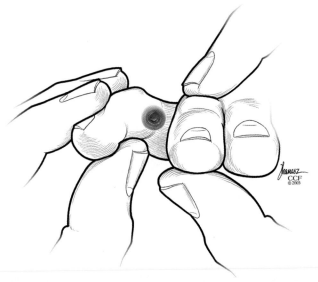

Figure 2.18   Soft interdigital corn between toes. (Reprinted with permission of the Cleveland Clinic.)

  □ Freiberg disease or avascular necrosis of the metatarsal head can produce both dorsal and plantar pain with palpation.
■ Flexor tenosynovitis can mimic capsulitis because patients have plantar tenderness over the affected ray.
  □ Capsulitis can sometimes be distinguished by the presence of tenderness over the flexor tendons as well as pain with resisted plantarflexion.
■ Interdigital neuromas may present as web space (most commonly third) pain and numbness with tenderness on examination (Fig. 2.19).

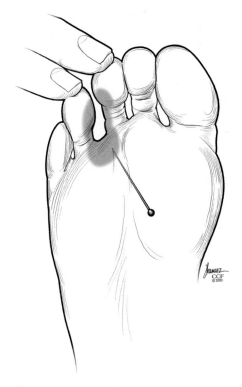

Figure 2.19   Sensory distribution of interdigital nerve. (Reprinted with permission of the Cleveland Clinic.)

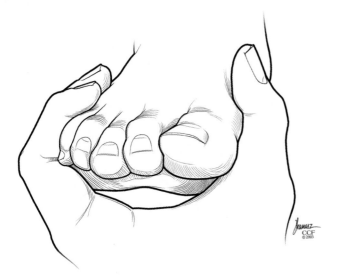

Figure 2.20   Forefoot squeeze for Mulder click. (Reprinted with permission of the Cleveland Clinic.)

☐ A palpable clunk when squeezing the forefoot (Mulder click) may be suggestive but not diagnostic (Fig. 2.20).

☐ Relief of symptoms with a diagnostic injection of local anesthesia is the most reliable confirmatory test.

☐ If the patient has a history of prior surgical neurectomy, recurrent or persistent symptoms are not infrequent. Symptoms typically recur within the first 12 months after surgery and may represent an incomplete neurectomy or recurrence because the nerve stump is near the plantar weight-bearing surface of the foot.

■ Metatarsal stress fracture causes localized tenderness over the fracture site as well as local warmth and edema.

Heel Pain

■ The etiology of heel pain has been categorized as arthritic, traumatic, mechanical, neurologic, and other.

■ The most common cause of plantar heel pain is biomechanical stress on the plantar fascia causing plantar fasciitis.

■ Pain to palpation over the medial tubercle of the calcaneus at the origin of the plantar fascia is virtually pathognomonic of plantar fasciitis.

☐ Swelling of the heel pad may also be present.

☐ Other clinical indicators include a tight Achilles tendon, increased BMI, and pain exacerbated with inappropriate shoe wear.

☐ The quality and height of the plantar fat pad should also be assessed, as it may be a major contributor to heel pain.

☐ The pain may be reproducible with performance of the Windlass test (described as extension of either the first MTP joint or all MTP joints), which places the plantar fascia on stretch.

■ Posterior heel pain typically indicates Achilles tendon pathology. An abnormal contour of the Achilles

tendon may indicate chronic inflammatory changes or tendinosis.

■ With the patient seated, the Achilles tendon is palpated along its course, noting any tenderness, thickening, or nodularity.

☐ Either global or localized tenderness and swelling may be present at the insertion in cases of tendinitis.

☐ Palpable defects are indicative of a chronic or acute rupture depending on the patient's history. A Thompson test may be performed with the patient in the prone position and the calf squeezed, which should elicit ankle plantarflexion with an intact tendon. Sagging of the ankle into more dorsiflexion compared with the uninjured side in the prone position is also indicative of an Achilles rupture.

■ A Haglund deformity (a bony prominence of the posterior superior calcaneal tuberosity) with or without retrocalcaneal bursitis should also be considered, particularly in women between 20 and 30 years of age. Typically, symptoms are aggravated with shoe wear. On examination, tenderness is lateral to the Achilles tendon with a palpable posterolateral prominence.

■ In the adolescent population, calcaneal apophysitis (Sever disease) is more commonly seen with tenderness to palpation over the calcaneal apophysis posteriorly (Fig. 2.21B).

■ An insidious onset of heel pain with a sudden increase in activity may suggest a stress fracture.

☐ The heel squeeze test reproduces the patient's pain and is virtually diagnostic of a calcaneal stress fracture.

■ Plantar fibromas that are located in the plantar fascia may be present throughout the plantar foot, but are usually present in the midarch region.

☐ Patients with plantar fibromas may also have a Dupuytren contracture, thus warranting inspection of the hands.

■ Neurogenic heel pain may also be a cause of the patient's symptoms. Pain to palpation over the center of the plantar calcaneus may indicate central heel pain syndrome (see Fig. 2.21A), which may have a neurologic cause.

☐ The nerves that may cause symptoms through entrapment or a neuroma include the posterior tibial (tarsal tunnel syndrome), medial calcaneal (heel neuroma), medial plantar, lateral plantar (entrapment of the branch to the abductor digit minimi), and the sural including the lateral calcaneal branch.

☐ Abnormal sensory testing and a positive Tinel sign (tapping along the distribution of the nerve reproducing the patient's symptoms) may be present.

☐ The dorsiflexion–eversion test with or without MTP joint extension of all the toes has been shown to increase strain in the tarsal tunnel and plantar nerves. A test is considered positive if passive ankle dorsiflexion, followed by eversion and extension of all MTP joints reproduces plantar heel pain. However, some research indicates that this test may not be specific for nerve-related pathology.

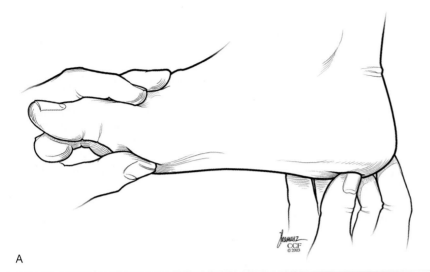

A

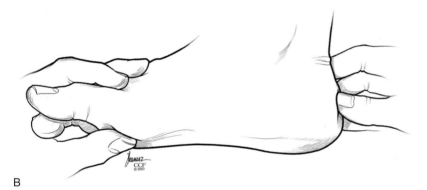

B

Figure 2.21 Heel palpation. (**A**) Inferior. (**B**) Posterior. (Reprinted with permission of the Cleveland Clinic.)

Tendon Disorders

- Tendinopathy usually presents with a gradual onset of pain in the region of the affected tendon.
  - □ Overuse of the affected tendon aggravates pain.
  - □ Start-up pain may be present.
  - □ Local swelling, warmth, tenderness, weakness, and pain with passive stretch of the tendon may be present.
  - □ A static deformity may develop.
- The Achilles tendon is palpated for tenderness or thickening (Fig. 2.22).
  - □ Putting the Achilles tendon on gentle stretch may also produce some discomfort.
  - □ If there is a question that the Achilles tendon has been ruptured completely, the Thompson test should be performed with the patient lying prone on the examination table with the toes hanging over the edge of the table.
    - □ The affected calf muscle belly is gently squeezed, which leads to passive tensioning of the tendon and produces ankle plantarflexion with an intact Achilles tendon.
    - □ If no plantarflexion occurs, the Achilles tendon is incompetent (Fig. 2.23).

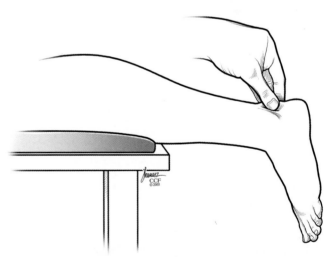

Figure 2.22 Achilles tendon palpation. (Reprinted with permission of the Cleveland Clinic.)

- Whereas acute ruptures of the tibialis posterior tendon are rare, gradual degeneration is a common entity that ultimately leads to an acquired flatfoot deformity.
  - □ As the standing patient is viewed from behind, the affected hindfoot is typically in valgus, and the "too

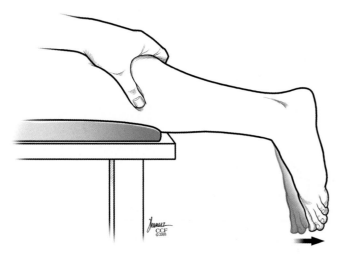

Figure 2.23 Thompson squeeze test. (Reprinted with permission of the Cleveland Clinic.)

many toes sign" is present with forefoot abduction, which is usually asymmetric (see Fig. 2.1).

☐ Failure of hindfoot inversion with a single- or double-limb heel rise suggests tibialis posterior incompetence; it is the most sensitive test on physical examination to confirm the diagnosis.

☐ The course of the tibialis posterior tendon to its main insertion on the navicular tuberosity is palpated for tenderness.

☐ Tibialis posterior function can be evaluated with resisted adduction and inversion of the affected foot with it held in plantarflexion, which may make the tendon visible or elicit pain.

☐ Comparison with the unaffected side can be helpful in determining the severity of the pathology.

▪ TA tendon rupture or tendinitis is rare, but it can easily be missed.

☐ Patients may describe pain and swelling along the anterior ankle with or without a specific injury.

☐ The TA tendon is essentially subcutaneous and is palpable from the superomedial ankle to its insertion at the base of the first metatarsal.

☐ The TA tendon should be easily seen with active dorsiflexion, and its absence suggests rupture. A history of systemic or local steroid use may be present in cases of rupture.

☐ Tendinosis tends to occur in overweight elderly women and typically presents with burning medial midfoot pain and swelling over the distal portion of the insertion.

▪ Peroneal tendinitis leads to lateral ankle or hindfoot pain that is activity related.

☐ Palpation along the course of the tendons produces tenderness in the retromalleolar area or less commonly at the insertion of the peroneus brevis on the fifth metatarsal base.

☐ Swelling along the lateral wall of the calcaneus and pain with passive stretch of the tendons may be present.

☐ Subluxation of the peroneal tendons may be the source of the patient's complaints.

☐ Resisted active eversion and abduction with the ankle in dorsiflexion may reproduce painful subluxation of the peroneals around the lateral malleolus (Fig. 2.24).

☐ Similarly, a peroneal compression test may be performed with forceful eversion and dorsiflexion of the ankle, and is considered positive if any pain, crepitus, or popping occurs at the distal fibula.

▪ Tendinitis of the flexor hallucis longus is most often seen in dancers.

☐ The flexor hallucis longus tendon can become inflamed following repetitive motion in the groove between the medial and lateral tubercles of the posterior process of the talus.

☐ Pain with resisted active hallux flexion is indicative.

☐ Advanced cases can produce a stenosing tenosynovitis with catching or triggering of the great toe.

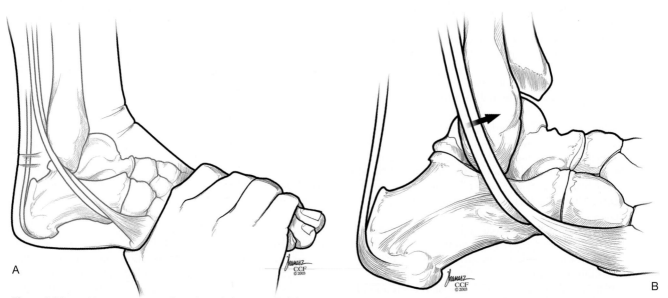

A   B

Figure 2.24 Subluxating peroneal tendons. (**A**) Reduced. (**B**) Subluxated. (Reprinted with permission of the Cleveland Clinic.)

☐ Rarely a functional hallux rigidus may develop because the scarred proximal flexor hallucis longus can render the first MTP joint relatively motionless despite relatively normal articulation.

PHYSICAL EXAMINATION IN THE ATHLETE

The examination of the athlete must incorporate additional aspects that may not be necessary or possible when examining the general population. Particularly in chronic conditions in those symptoms that are elicited only with activity, the athlete may need to be observed while performing the activity. This may include jumping, dancing, cycling, cutting, or sprinting. If this is not possible, reviewing a recording of the athlete to view any pathologic compensatory mechanisms or any eliciting positions may be useful. Observing for muscle fatigue with repetitive testing rather than one-time strength testing may also be beneficial.

An important consideration in the athlete is that any positive physical findings may have a distant traumatic origin. For example, a hallux valgus deformity or dorsiflexed hallux may be secondary to a previous plantar plate disruption, or injury to the medial collateral ligament, medial head of the flexor hallus brevis, or medial sesamoids. Similarly, a fifth metatarsal stress fracture may be secondary to a chronic traumatic injury to medial soft-tissue structures.

ORTHOTICS

DESCRIPTION

An orthotic device is most simply defined as an external device that applies biomechanical forces to the body. Devices such as casts, splints, and off-the-shelf braces as well as custom-made devices can all be classified as orthoses. When prescribing an orthosis, certain goals of treatment should be kept in mind. The benefits of orthotics include control of motion (prevention or limiting), correction of deformity, compensation for weakness, and partial axial unloading.

Even though many eponyms have been used for specific orthoses, standard nomenclature has been established to accurately describe an orthotic device in terms of the body segment to be incorporated and the biomechanical controls that are desired. For example, an *AFO* is an *ankle–foot orthosis*, which begins at the toes, crosses the ankle, and terminates at the calf.

Apart from the body segment to be incorporated, each orthosis can further be described by the degree of biomechanical control it provides at any particular joint. The five degrees of control are defined in Table 2.1. The orthosis can be more specifically described by adding one of the modifiers

TABLE 2.1 FIVE DEGREES OF ORTHOTIC CONTROL

Degree	Description
Free	Unrestricted motion permitted in a given plane
Assist	An external force is applied to increase the range, force, or velocity of any desired motion
Resist	An external force is applied to minimize undesired motion (the reverse of assist)
Stop	Prevents motion in one direction
Hold	Immobilizes the body segment in each plane

listed in Table 2.2. This nomenclature describes the exact functional outcome expected with an orthotic device. An orthotist can fabricate an appropriate device using a variety of available materials to meet the biomechanical needs of a particular patient as long as they have an accurate, descriptive prescription from the treating physician.

Foot orthoses (FOs) are suitable for the management of many commonly encountered problems of the foot and ankle, and are readily accepted by most patients because they fit inside most shoe wear. The design of most foot orthotics is based on the following principles:

- Providing total surface contact
- Providing foot support in a biomechanically corrected position
- Limiting excessive motion
- Compensating for restricted motion or fixed deformity
- Attenuating impact

Total surface contact is inherent in all custom-molded orthoses. The concept of distributing weight to the largest possible surface area decreases the pressure at any specific area. With impaired sensation, total contact inserts in particular help decrease localized pressure when combined with materials such as Plastazote, which attenuates impact. An orthotic can limit hypermobility such as hyperpronation by supporting the longitudinal arch. Fixed deformities cannot be corrected with orthotics, but can be accommodated with appropriately constructed ones, essentially providing support between a rigid deformity and the floor, yielding a plantigrade surface for ambulation.

TABLE 2.2 MODIFIERS TO DESCRIBE ORTHOTICS

Modifier	Description
Lock	A removable type of hold
Degree	Selects stop endpoints for motion in a given plane
Variable	An adjustable stop
Axial unloading	Transfer of axial loads from skeleton to soft tissues

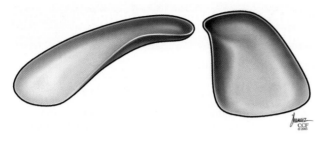

Figure 2.25 Longitudinal arch supports. (Reprinted with permission of the Cleveland Clinic.)

Foot orthotics can be divided into three basic categories: accommodative, or soft, devices; semirigid devices; and corrective, or rigid, devices.

- *Accommodative* FOs cradle or cushion deformed, dysvascular, or neuropathic feet and as such can be used in a protective fashion.
  - Most over-the-counter inserts designed for minor aches and pains such as metatarsalgia are accommodative in nature and are constructed of soft, resilient materials (Fig. 2.25).
- *Semirigid* orthotics are useful because they can be constructed from layers of different materials, providing varying degrees of control, thus making them versatile for use in a wide variety of problems.
  - Semirigid designs are easily modified by adding metatarsal pads or posting.
- *Corrective* designs made of rigid materials are more difficult to successfully apply and require strict attention to detail as well as an initial weaning period to improve patient compliance (Fig. 2.26).
  - Skin problems may develop when using rigid materials, but they are excellent for controlling flexible deformities.
  - Caution should be used when applying a rigid device to a patient with sensory impairment or history of skin ulceration.

Posting is a modification of an orthotic whereby a small wedge can be added under either the medial or the lateral edge. Typically, these are limited to approximately one-eighth of an inch, or else the orthotic becomes too large

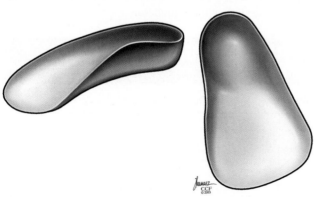

Figure 2.26 University of California Biomechanical Laboratory foot supports. (Reprinted with permission of the Cleveland Clinic.)

to fit inside a shoe. When more correction is necessary, a wedge can be added to the sole of the shoe. Larger correction can thus be placed on the bottom of the shoe, with up to ¼ in being well tolerated by most patients.

In recent years, a considerable amount of research has been performed comparing custom or semicustom orthotics with prefabricated orthotics. Elucidating differences in the efficacy of these orthotics could amount to savings of hundreds of dollars to the patient. A recent review on the use of custom FOs in comparison with a variety of other treatment options including sham orthotics, prefabricated, surgery, or night splints in a variety of painful foot conditions was performed. The authors concluded that in rheumatic metatarsalgia, plantar fasciitis, and hallux valgus, custom orthotics may improve foot pain; however, in metatarsalgia and plantar fasciitis, they may not give any added benefit compared with noncustom orthotics.

A cadaveric study investigating the effects of custom and semicustom foot orthotics on bone strain across the second metatarsal during dynamic gait simulation demonstrated that custom orthotics allowed greater reductions in bone strain relative to the semicustom orthotics.

In support of the use of custom orthotics, a prospective study evaluated the efficacy of custom shoes on pain and foot pressure reduction in patients with degenerative foot disorders. The data demonstrated significant reductions in both plantar and perceived foot pain across five different activities with semicustom shoes.

Although the data remain somewhat inconclusive regarding the superiority of custom orthotics over prefabricated inserts, they have been shown to provide improvement both biomechanically and symptomatically. Custom-molded orthotics have the advantage of allowing the treating practitioner with the opportunity to tailor an orthosis to the patient's specific anatomy and pathology. Some guidelines for the orthotic management of common foot and ankle pathologies are provided below.

Achilles Tendonitis

The primary role of the orthotic in the treatment of Achilles tendonitis is to minimize stresses on the tendon. This is accomplished in two ways. First, pressure on the tendon is relieved by stabilizing the foot in a relatively plantigrade position. This is straightforwardly accomplished with heel posting. It is recommended that at least a 3-mm heel lift is utilized. Up to 0.5 in can be accommodated in a closed heel shoe before the foot is lifted out of the heel counter. Second, in a foot with otherwise normal mechanics, the orthotic should also act to minimize subtalar rotational stresses on the tendon by correcting any reducible varus or valgus positioning of the calcaneus. This is readily achieved with a deep heel cup (16-mm deep) with extrinsic varus or valgus posting as dictated by the patient's deformity. The orthotic should be semirigid and terminate just proximal to the metatarsal heads to place the forefoot below the axis of the hindfoot during ambulation, aiding further in forefoot plantarflexion.

Pes Planus

Pes planus deformity correction requires a very thoughtful approach given the many resultant manifestations of the deformity. In most moderate-to-severe cases, correction must be obtained throughout the forefoot, midfoot, and hindfoot, which generally calls for a semirigid orthotic. In the forefoot, the pathologic valgus positioning may be corrected with an extrinsic wedge located inferior to the metatarsal heads to create a more varus position. Along the arch, medial posting is typically required to support the fallen arch and unload the stressed, medial structures. Finally, given the intrinsic valgus heel position that occurs with worsening deformity, a varus rearfoot post may be added with a deepened heel cup (approximately 20 mm) for correction.

Hallux Rigidus

Although moderate-to-severe hallux rigidus typically improves most dramatically with operative intervention, orthotics may be used as a temporizing measure prior to planned surgical treatment or in patients who are not operative candidates or for those deferring surgery. The primary role of the orthotic is to minimize motion through the arthritic first MTP joint by splinting the joint along its plantar surface. This is best accomplished with a rigid extension, or shank, which extends distal to the pathologic joint. This is most often achieved through a rigid Morton extension. This acts to absorb the dorsiflexion moment across the joint during the gait cycle. This extension may be incorporated into a full insert that spans the foot from the heel. These rigid extensions require the patient to select shoe wear that is accommodative of the insert, which may prove challenging to some patients. As such, semiflexible inserts may be better tolerated.

Plantar Fasciitis/Heel Pain

In pathologic heel conditions, the role of the orthotic is 2-fold: to provide cushioning along the heel to offload inflamed soft tissues or painful bony spurs and to improve any hindfoot malalignment producing undue tension on hindfoot structures. In the case of plantar fasciitis, this is successfully accomplished with a gel-like heel cushion with at least 3 mm of cushioning. Heel spur pathology may be better managed with a horseshoe-shaped pad, which acts to elevate any painful bony spurs. In advanced cases, both types of cushions may be attached to a thin extension that spans the entire foot and is placed within a deep heel cup, which has the added benefit of neutralizing any pathologic subtalar motion contributing to the inflammation.

Metatarsalgia

Metatarsalgia is a common condition that presents as a manifestation of a variety of foot pathologies such as cavovarus feet, hallux rigidus, hammer toes, or any other condition that causes a transfer of foot pressure to the lesser metatarsal heads. Treating metatarsalgia with orthotics often provides patients with drastic improve-

ments in their foot pain. Attempts should be made to have patients localize the site of maximum pain, if possible. Patients can be instructed to mark the site of their discomfort prior to their visit so as to guide proper placement of the orthotic. The insert is then made with a metatarsal pad, which cushions the affected metatarsal heads or spans the entire ball of the foot. A 3-mm cushion is often sufficient and well tolerated. The ideal insert is total contact, which allows load transfer to neighboring osseous structures and unloads the painful metatarsal heads. If using isolated pads, patients must be cautioned to place the pad just proximal to the area of tenderness as it may otherwise increase the pain as a result of plantarflexing the pathologic area.

Pes Cavus/Cavovarus

In pes cavus or cavovarus deformities, imbalances in the forces across the foot result in a high arch and often an accompanying varus deformity of the forefoot. The goals of the orthotic are therefore multiple and include reducing midfoot and forefoot supination, increasing total plantar surface contact and thereby unloading lateral structures, and stabilizing the hindfoot. A semirigid, total contact orthosis would therefore be most beneficial. The orthosis should span most of the width of the foot and fully contact the arch to distribute plantar pressures. For the cavus deformity, lateral posting and cushioning will be useful to lift and unload the lateral structures. Forefoot varus may be managed with a valgus forefoot extension to resist forefoot supinatory forces. A deep heel cup with a heel lift of at least 3 mm will address the hindfoot instability. An excavation over a plantarflexed first metatarsal head may also relieve pressure and help correct flexible heel varus.

Ankle–Foot Orthoses

For more extensive deformities where bridging of the ankle is necessary, AFOs may be used. Most of these devices are constructed of lightweight plastic materials (polypropylene) that fit into most shoe wear. They are similar to a posterior splint with contact on the posterior aspect of the leg and plantar aspect of the foot (Fig. 2.27). Perhaps the most important aspect of AFO design is patient compliance. Appropriate means should be undertaken to ensure that the patient or family is compliant with use of an appropriate orthotic.

AFOs, like other orthoses, should provide one of the following benefits: control of motion, correction of deformity, compensation for weakness, and partial axial unloading. An AFO may also indirectly influence remote body locations. For example, a floor reaction AFO (a rigid plastic AFO with the ankle locked in slight dorsiflexion and a padded anterior segment to stabilize the tibia) controls ankle motion with rigidity, but it also accentuates knee extension during midstance, compensating for a weak GCS complex with relatively good quadriceps function such as the one that occurs in myelodysplasia, incomplete spinal cord injury, and poliomyelitis. In cases of foot drop, a hinged AFO with spring-loaded dorsiflexion-assist mechanism can compensate for a weak TA. Occasionally, partial axial

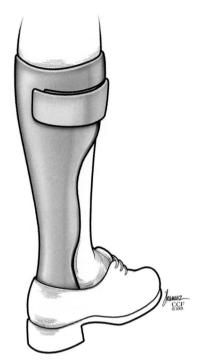

Figure 2.27   Solid molded plastic ankle–foot orthosis. (Reprinted with permission of the Cleveland Clinic.)

unloading is desirable, rather than complete axial loading. Thus, a portion of the axial load from the foot is shifted to the proximal tibial condyles, in order to partially unload the foot. Rigid AFO's may also be useful in arthritic conditions of the ankle or subtalar joint, where restriction of motion of the involved joint may alleviate symptoms.

Adult acquired flat foot deformity (AAFD), more commonly known as PTTD, requires special mention given the many recent advances in the devices used for nonsurgical management. The exact pathology in AAFD can be found in later chapters. Briefly, the primary initiating event is an attenuation of the posterior tibial tendon (PTT). The PTT maintains a rigid midfoot and forefoot, which acts to counteract the ground reaction force dorsiflexion moment and redistribute it to the ankle. Progressive failure of the medial soft tissues eventually leads to bony malalignment and degeneration of articular surfaces particularly in the ankle and hindfoot. Torque-absorbing AFOs may be utilized and act by transferring some of the dorsiflexion force generated in the late stance to the material of the AFO. Rigid or semirigid devices may be used. Other considerations include whether the AFO is articulating or nonarticulating.

Nonarticulated devices restrict motion along the ankle joint and theoretically allow more load sharing. However, some ankle motion is necessary for proper biomechanics during gait; therefore, some practitioners prefer articulated devices that allow some ankle dorsiflexion while still allowing load sharing. Examples of torque absorbing AFOs are the Arizona lace-up AFO and UCBL (University of California Biomechanics Laboratory) AFO. Proximal weight-bearing AFOs deserve mention, although rarely used given their bulky design and patient dislike. These include calf lacers or the patella tendon bearing AFOs that are designed to transmit the patient's body weight directly to the floor, circumventing the ankle and foot completely.

PRESCRIBING

It is important that an appropriate prescription be written for orthotics of any kind. An accurate diagnosis should be a component of any prescription. If one has an excellent orthotist, specific instructions should be reserved for situations in which specific requirements need to be achieved. A prescription that reads "articulating plastic AFO with neutral plantarflexion stop" precludes the orthotist from considering other alternatives that may accomplish the same goal. A request for direct discussion facilitates communication with the orthotist to ensure that the proper treatment goals are achieved.

Finally, when prescribing an orthotic device, appropriate follow-up is necessary to ensure proper fit and function of the device. Patients must be educated on the importance of a break-in period where they gradually increase the wear of their devices. Typically, patients may start with wearing their orthotic for a few hours once or twice a week. Wear should progressively increase until patients are using the device during the majority of their active hours. Patients should hone in to any problematic areas such as regions causing increased pressure on bony prominences or rubbing of soft tissues that are painful and may preclude regular use.

SUGGESTED READING

Alexander IJ. The foot examination and diagnosis, 2nd ed. New York: Churchill Livingstone, 1997.
Goldberg B, Hsu JD. Atlas of orthoses and assistive devices, 3rd ed. Philadelphia: Mosby-Year Book, 1997.
Hoppenfeld S. Physical examination of the spine and extremities. East Norwalk: Appleton-Century–Crofts/Prentice Hall, 1976.
Michael JW. Overview of orthoses. In: Spivak JM, ed. Orthopaedics—a study guide. New York: McGraw-Hill, 1999.

NEUROMUSCULAR DISORDERS

MICHAEL J. BOTTE
ORRIN FRANKO

Neuromuscular disorders that cause foot deformities are often divided into two main types: *spastic* and *paralytic*. Spasticity develops from injury to the *upper* motor neurons of the central nervous system (involving the brain or spinal cord). These injuries include traumatic brain injury (TBI), stroke, spinal cord injury (SCI), and cerebral palsy (CP). Conversely, paralysis or paresis (weakness) commonly develops from injury to lower motor neurons (involving the peripheral nerves). A classic example is Charcot–Marie–Tooth (CMT) disease (peroneal muscular atrophy), which involves peripheral nerve demyelination and degeneration. Peripheral nerve lacerations and polio also involve the lower motor neurons and result in paralysis, not spasticity.

Whether an affliction results in spasticity or paralysis, the net result is muscle imbalance in the limb. With significant muscle imbalance, the stronger, more active, or mechanically advantaged muscles overpower the weaker or paralytic muscles and pull the limb into a deformity (Fig. 3.1). This leads to the several common foot and ankle deformities seen in neuromuscular disorders, including equinus, varus, equinovarus, cavus, and various toe deformities. Because of the differences of etiology, associated deformities, and methods of treatment, this chapter is divided into two sections: disorders of spasticity and disorders of paralysis.

Although the emphasis of the text is placed on the foot, the interdependence of the hip and knee for function and operative planning must also be appreciated and is discussed in association with these problems. Evaluation of the whole patient must be kept in mind and the multidisciplinary team approach is stressed.

DISORDERS OF SPASTICITY

PATHOGENESIS

Etiology

TBI is commonly caused by a direct blow to the skull, penetrating injury, or an anoxic episode. A direct blow results in immediate local neural disruption, which can be compounded by subsequent ischemia from subdural or epidural hematoma. Common events associated with TBI are motor vehicle and motorcycle accidents, assaults, and gunshot wounds. Anoxic injuries are caused by near drowning, chemical asphyxia, drug overdose, and myocardial infarction. Brain damage is global in these patients and the prognosis is often poor. Near-drowning accidents are the most common cause of acquired spasticity in children. In addition, brain injury can occur from severe inflammation, infection, neoplasm, metabolic causes, or other vascular afflictions or malformations that result in neuron death.

Stroke or cerebrovascular accident (CVA) is the result of interruption of the oxygenation of the brain by thrombosis, emboli, or hemorrhage. Cerebral thrombosis accounts for nearly three-fourths of patients with stroke. Arteriosclerosis and smoking history are known predisposing factors for thrombosis. The risk of ischemic stroke in current smokers is about double that of nonsmokers after adjustment for other risk factors. Spontaneous intracerebral or subarachnoid hemorrhage, for which hypertension is a predisposing factor, accounts for approximately one-sixth of patients sustaining CVAs. Emboli account for one-tenth of cases of CVA and are usually associated with extracranial pathology such as atherosclerosis or arrhythmias. Atrial fibrillation increases the risk of stroke by about 5-fold.

In the case of SCI, the most common cause is trauma, usually from direct injury, compression, or hematoma following fractures or dislocations of the spine. Common causes by percentage of SCI are motor vehicle accidents (40% to 48%), falls (8% to 21%), acts of violence (15% to 37%), sports injuries (14% to 15%), and miscellaneous causes (3%). Of the sports injuries, diving and surfing comprise about 70% of injuries, followed by football, snow skiing, gymnastics, wrestling, and horseback riding. Other causes include compression from neoplasm and myelopathy from infection, inflammation, or vascular disorders.

Spastic CP includes a spectrum of brain injury caused before or during birth or in the immediate postnatal period. These injuries are associated with hypoxia, trauma, metabolic or infectious causes, and congenital malformations. Injuries of hypoxia that occur before birth include those from interruption of blood flow through the umbilical cord (associated with prolapse or torsion), placental

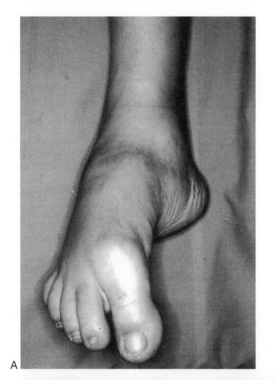

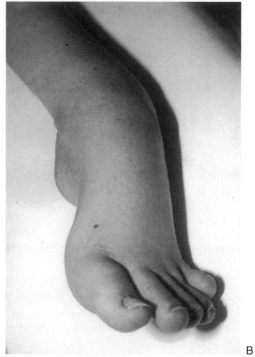

A

B

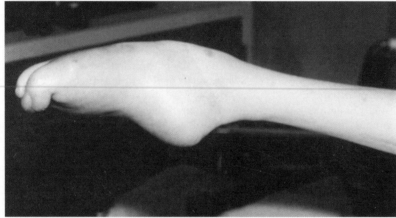

C

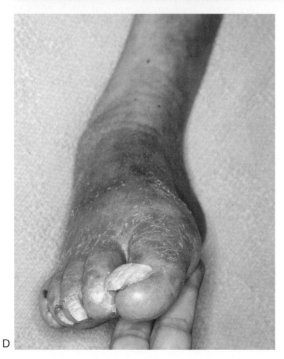

D

Figure 3.1 Photographs of foot deformities seen in patients with acquired spasticity. The most typical deformities are equinovarus with toe flexion deformities. (**A**) Young man with equinovarus and toe flexion following traumatic brain injury from gunshot wound. (**B**) Young woman with equinovarus following a closed head injury from assault. (**C**) Severe spasticity and rigidity following anoxic brain injury from near drowning. Note the degree of equinus and toe flexion deformity. Deformities were bilateral. (**D**) Elderly man with equinovarus following cerebrovascular accident.

abnormalities (e.g., placenta previa or placental infarction), coagulopathies, and maternal cardiopulmonary disease. At birth, a difficult delivery can result in brain injury from trauma or from a hypoxic episode. Birth hypoxia has been estimated by the Center for Disease Control (CDC) to account for less than 10% of CP cases. A difficult delivery is more common with abnormal fetal position or presentation, or prolonged labor. Neonatal apnea (failure to breathe after birth) can be related to prematurity, hypoxia during pregnancy or delivery, or fetal cardiopulmonary insufficiency (from atelectasis, bronchial obstruction, pulmonary edema, or anatomic malformation). Fetal injury may also occur from toxic injury, toxic accumulation of naturally occurring substances (e.g., Rh incompatibility), abnormal metabolic conditions (e.g., maternal uremia and diabetes), or infectious causes. Infection of the placental membranes (chorioamnionitis) may account for 12% of spastic CP among children born full term and 28% born prematurely.

Epidemiology

Epidemiologic aspects of these neuromuscular diseases demonstrate the magnitude of these problems and their importance to so many patients, their families, and society in general.

The Centers for Disease Control and Prevention estimated in 2011 that 1.7 million people in the United States sustain TBI annually. Of these, 52,000 do not live, leaving a large number of survivors with spasticity. TBI is the leading cause of acquired spastic limb deformity in young adults. It is also the cause of death in 55% of multiple trauma patients dying within the first 2 days of hospitalization. Males between 15 and 25 years of age are the most common victims of TBI, with children aged 0 to 4 and adults older than 65 years comprising other common age groups. Despite the severe deficits sustained, many patients with TBI survive long enough and achieve adequate function to justify aggressive rehabilitation and operative reconstruction. Because most traumatic injuries to the brain occur in young adults, those who survive commonly have a normal life span despite the injury. Foot and ankle deformities and gait disturbances are frequent problems in this population.

The CDC estimated in 2011 that 795,000 people in the United States have a stroke annually. About half of these survive each year. Approximately 610,000 of these are first or new strokes, and about 185,000 people who survive a stroke go on to have another. Nearly three-quarters of all strokes occur in people older than 65 years, although stroke can occur at any age. Stroke is the third leading cause of death in the United States (behind heart disease and cancer) and is the leading cause of adult hemiplegia. More than 2 million people currently have permanent neurologic deficits following stroke, and the average patient who survives a stroke beyond the first few months has a life expectancy greater than 5 years. It has been estimated that 10% of stroke patients have spastic deformities that could benefit from surgery, providing a patient population of 20,000 to 25,000 new surgical candidates per year. In addition, there are already approximately 2.5 million surviving stroke patients in the United States, adding to this large number of patients who could benefit from operative management.

The Foundation for Spinal Cord Injury Prevention, Care, and Cure notes that SCI occurs in 12,000 people per year in the United States, with 200,000 people currently living with SCI in the United States. Reported average ages at injury are 16 to 30 years, with a median age of 28.7 years. Males comprise 80% of cases. Motor vehicle accidents, falls, acts of violence, sports injuries, and miscellaneous causes account for the majority of SCI. Occurrence of SCI increases with increased daylight hours and with increased temperature, usually associated with summer seasonal activities and outdoor sports. Fifty-three percent of all injuries occur on weekend days (Friday through Sunday). Gunshot spinal cord injuries appear to have a higher incidence in undeveloped and developing countries. In sports injuries, about 5% of SCIs have resulted in incomplete paraplegia, 4% in complete paraplegia, 47% in incomplete quadriplegia, and 45% in complete quadriplegia.

The most common motor disability acquired during childhood is CP. Population-based studies from around the world report prevalence estimates of CP ranging from 1.5 to more than 4 per 1,000 live births. Regional estimates show that CP occurs in 1.7 to 2 per 1,000 one-year-olds in the United States, 0.93 to 1.28 per 1,000 in China, and 2.08 per 1,000 in Europe. Usually, one in seven children with CP does not survive the first year of life. Males are involved 1.2 times more frequently than girls. Spastic CP is the most common type of CP, found among approximately 80% of CP children. Spastic diplegia occurs in 7% to 36% of cases. In 2006, 56% of children with CP were able to walk independently, whereas 33% had limited or no walking ability. About 20% of CP children have severe intellectual deficits that contribute to their inability to walk. Prematurity and associated low birth weight are associated with higher incidences of CP; in infants weighing less than 1,500 g at birth, the rate of CP was more than 70 times as high as that in infants weighing 2,500 g or more.

Pathophysiology

Spasticity develops from interruption of upper motor neuron inhibitory pathways from the brain to the spinal cord (Fig. 3.2). With the loss of the inhibitory pathways, the muscle reacts more to the influence of the spinal reflex, resulting in spasticity, which can cause muscle imbalance and lead to extremity deformities. In the foot and ankle, the most common deformity is equinus and varus.

Dynamic Nature of Spasticity

In disorders of acquired spasticity (TBI, CVA, and incomplete SCI), there is an initial dynamic (i.e., changing) nature, which is important to appreciate for proper planning and timing of surgical procedures. In these disorders, immediately following the initial central nervous system insult, there is usually a brief period (from hours to weeks) of flaccid paralysis or paresis, hypotonia, and depression of stretch reflexes of the neurologically impaired limb. The neural injury, which disrupts the inhibitory pathways of the brain to the muscles, allows the muscles to become influenced by or come under the control of the spinal reflex arc. When influenced by the reflex arc, the muscles become hypersensitive to passive stretch, resulting in reflexive contraction.

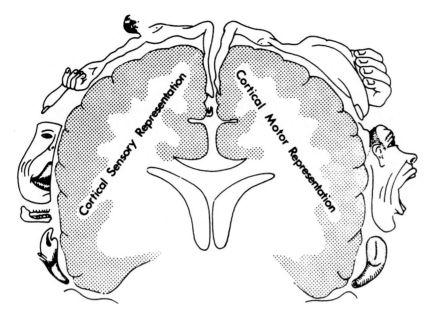

Figure 3.2 Illustration of brain showing the parts of the brain that control motor and sensory functions. The foot and ankle are controlled by the portion in the midsagittal cortex. The anterior cerebral artery supplies this area, and, if afflicted by thrombosis or hemorrhage, a selective deficit in the foot and ankle can occur. More often, direct penetrating injury, subdural hematoma, or cerebrovascular accidents involve both the lateral and midsagittal cortices, resulting in both upper and lower extremity deficits. Anoxic episodes and near drowning produce global brain injury and result in bilateral upper and lower extremity deformities, often producing rigidity.

Therefore, following the initial period of hypotonia, there is a period of increasing muscle tone. The stretch reflexes return and there is a progression to hyperactive reflexes, which culminate in spasticity. Muscle tone and hyperreflexia reach a peak within a few days or weeks. Besides increased tone, muscles may exhibit hyperreflexia, clonus, or rigidity. Clonus is an abnormal repetitive rhythmic muscle contraction following initial stretch. Volitional control is often impaired, and there may be overall residual weakness and loss of dexterity. Spastic paralysis is seen in severely afflicted muscles.

Because upper motor neurons have some capacity to recover, there is a long period of spontaneous neurologic improvement during which spasticity improves and muscles return to a more normal, less hypertonic state. Strength, coordination, and volitional control as well as sensory and cognitive function all improve to varying degrees during this recovery phase. The duration of recovery varies among the different types of acquired spasticity (Table 3.1).

Operative procedures for reconstruction should usually be delayed until a patient is no longer neurologically recovering (or making improvement in a rehabilitation program). Thus the data listed in Table 3.1 can act as a rough guide for timing the surgical procedures if deformity exists and recovery has reached a plateau (discussed further under surgical treatment).

TABLE 3.1 NEUROLOGIC RECOVERY TIMES IN DISORDERS OF SPASTICITY

Disorder	Recovery Time
CVA	6 mo
Incomplete spinal cord injury	12 mo
TBI	18+ mo
Cerebral palsy	Static

Limb Deformity from Spasticity

With spasticity, the stronger or more hyperactive muscles or those with mechanical advantage overpower the weaker or paralytic muscles and pull the limb into a deformity. This leads to the common foot and ankle deformities seen in neuromuscular disorders, most often equinus or equinovarus along with toe flexion deformities (Figs. 3.1 and 3.3). The equinus component of the deformity is usually from spasticity of the gastrocnemius and soleus, with additional contributions from the tibialis posterior, flexor hallucis longus (FHL), and flexor digitorum longus (FDL). The majority of the varus component of deformity is from the tibialis anterior (in TBI or CVA) or from the tibialis posterior (in CP) and is possibly worsened in both by any associated weakness of the peroneus longus and brevis. The differences in the tibialis anterior contribution to the varus in TBI and CVA compared with the tibialis posterior contribution in CP are important because these muscle differences have implications in operative correction when addressing the specific muscles at fault. Cavus deformity is less often seen in TBI, CVA, and CP, and is usually associated with weakness of the intrinsic muscles of the foot (seen more commonly in paralytic disorders; see later discussion).

Anatomic Correlations between Area of Brain Injured and Severity of Limb Involvement

Different clinical presentations result from different areas of brain involvement. The midcortex of the brain in the sagittal plane controls sensory and motor functions predominantly in the lower extremity and foot (see Fig. 3.2). The anterior cerebral artery supplies this area. A stroke involving the anterior cerebral artery usually results in hemiplegia with deficits in the lower extremity. Severe foot deformities can occur from injuries to this part of the brain (Figs. 3.1 and 3.3). More commonly, however, a CVA involves the middle cerebral artery, which supplies the cerebral cortex, which controls the face, upper extremity, and trunk. These patients have hemiplegia with more speech and upper extremity deficits than lower extremity involvement, but lower extremity

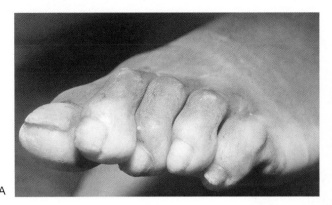

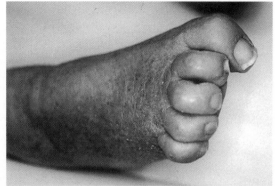

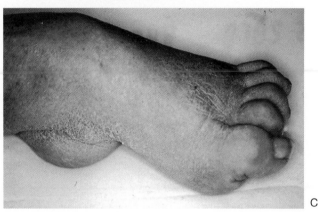

Figure 3.3 Photographs of spastic toe flexion deformities seen following cerebrovascular accidents (**A**) and traumatic brain injury (**B, C**).

involvement may also be significant. Often, TBI also involves this area of the cerebral cortex, and a patient can have similar deficits as those with a CVA (Fig. 3.4). Anoxic injuries, which are usually more global cerebral insults, produce a wide spectrum of bilateral upper and lower extremity deficits. The entire brain and brainstem may be involved, producing the most severe clinical picture of spastic quadriplegia and mental retardation. In CP, because of the many possible etiologies and mechanisms for brain injury, several clinical presentations and various dyskinesias can develop, including athetosis and ataxia. *Athetosis* is marked by continuous slow, involuntary writhing movements, especially in the hands. *Ataxia* is exemplified by loss of muscular coordination, irregularity of muscular action, intention type tremor, and marked unsteadiness in standing or ambulation. Ataxia is commonly seen with cerebellar involvement.

Classification

Spastic disorders can be grouped using several classification schemes and descriptive terms. These are based on acquired versus static spasticity and the limb or limbs involved. In addition, spasticity has been classified according to the degree of spasticity, the muscle groups involved, the type of movement disorder, and the types of deformities present.

Classification Based on Acquired versus Static Spasticity
The acquired spasticity group includes TBI, stroke, and SCI, where spasticity is *acquired* in a previously normal limb. The static spasticity group includes CP, in which the neurologic insult occurs at birth or in the perinatal period. Acquired spasticity differs from static spasticity in that the acquired

spasticity may change (decrease) over time as a result of neurologic recovery following the initial brain or spinal injury. The spasticity of CP is static and does not usually change over time. (Deformities in CP, however, may change over time, especially during periods of rapid growth or as a result of chronic effects of spasticity on the immature skeleton.)

Classification Based on Extremity Involved
Spasticity can be described as spastic *monoplegia* or *monoparesis* involving one extremity, *paraplegia* or *paraparesis* involving both lower extremities, *quadriplegia* or *quadriparesis*, and *tetraplegia* or *tetraparesis* involving all four extremities. The suffixes *plegia* and *paresis* denote paralysis and weakness, respectively. The term *diplegia* is often used to describe more involvement in the lower extremities than in the upper extremities. *Hemiplegia* and *hemiparesis* denote involvement of one upper and lower extremity on the same side. In CP, diplegia accounts for about 50%, hemiplegia for about 30%, and quadriplegia for about 20% of those with spasticity.

Classification Based on Degree of Deformity
Goldner originally classified CP according to degrees of deformity to include mild, moderate, and severe types. A *mild* deformity implies slight spasticity in the gastrocsoleus muscle group, voluntary action of the tibialis anterior, and minimal or no muscle imbalance owing to muscle weakness caused by cortical cell damage. Minimal spasticity of the adductors and mild tightness of the hamstrings may coexist with equinus. A *moderate* deformity indicates a greater degree of muscle tension, significant soft tissue, or fixed contracture in the calf muscles; unequal activity or overactivity of the invertors or evertors of the foot; and no voluntary

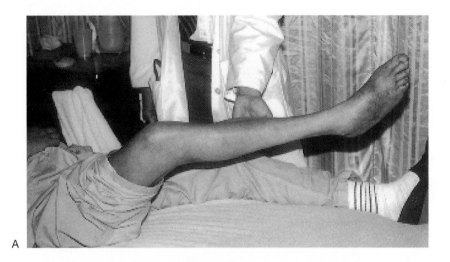

A

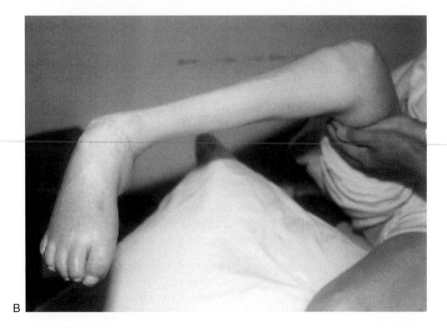

B

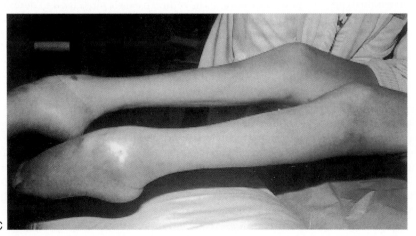

C

Figure 3.4   Photographs of spastic hip and knee flexion deformities seen in cerebrovascular accidents (**A**), traumatic brain injury (**B**), and anoxic brain injury (**C**). Involvement is unilateral with hemiplegia in the patients with cerebrovascular accidents and traumatic brain injury; involvement is bilateral in the patient with global brain injury from anoxia. Equinovarus deformities can also be seen.

control of the dorsiflexors of the foot. A *severe* deformity indicates fixed contracture of the calf muscles, atrophy of the muscle mass, equinus uncorrectable by manipulation, muscle imbalance with overpull of the invertors or evertors, and no voluntary or involuntary action of the dorsiflexors. The hip flexor muscles and adductor muscles are often contracted, along with the hamstring muscles, producing hip flexion, adduction deformity, and knee flexion contracture.

Classification of Cerebral Palsy Based on Movement Disorders

More recently, CP has been classified on the basis of the type of movement disorder. This classification places the patients into two main groups: those with spasticity (about 80%) and those with extrapyramidal or dystonic movements (about 20%). The extrapyramidal group includes those with injury to the basal ganglia of the brain, who exhibit athetosis, chorea, ballismus, ataxia, or hypotonia (Table 3.2). *Athetosis* consists of involuntary persistent writhing movements, usually of the hands and trunk. *Chorea* is characterized by a ceaseless involuntary variety of rapid, highly complex, jerky movements. *Ballismus* involves dyskinetic flinging or violent movements usually caused by contractions of proximal limb muscles. *Ataxia* is noted by loss of coordination and notably impaired balance with associated gait disturbances. *Hypotonia* is an abnormal loss or decrease in muscle tone. This classification is clinically relevant in that classic spasticity responds more to conventional methods of muscle relaxants (e.g., benzodiazepines) and to muscle lengthening or recession, whereas the extrapyramidal movement patterns may react less predictably to either medical or operative management.

Classification Based on Deformity

Spastic foot deformities are usually classified as equinus, varus, equinovarus, valgus, and planovalgus. Equinovarus is the most common form. Associated toe deformities are variable, but can be grouped into intrinsic minus (claw toe deformity, characterized by extension at the metatarsophalangeal [MTP] joint, and flexion of the proximal and distal interphalangeal [DIP] joints), hammer toe deformity (characterized mainly by extension at the MTP joint and flexion

at the proximal interphalangeal [PIP] joint), and mallet toe deformity (characterized chiefly by flexion at the DIP joint).

DIAGNOSIS

History and Physical Examination

It is important to establish the etiology and type of neurologic involvement as well as the time elapsed (days, months, or years) from the original affliction. Note whether the affliction is one of acquired or static spasticity. The patient's cognitive involvement (with memory problems, agitation, or retardation) may require the assistance of family members and healthcare workers as well as a review of the patient's medical record. If the spasticity is acquired (e.g., from TBI or stroke), one should determine whether the patient is still neurologically recovering or has reached a plateau in improvement (see Table 3.1).

When gathering the history, determine the rehabilitation treatment and the results received to date, including type and amount of physical therapy, use of splinting and orthoses, current or past medications or injections (*Botulinum* or phenol) used to decrease spasticity, and any previous operative management.

For specific foot and ankle involvement, functional capabilities can, in part, be established from the history, such as whether the patient has retained volitional control of the foot and whether the patient is able to ambulate, perform transfers, dress, place the foot plantigrade on the wheelchair footrest or floor, or bear weight. Determine whether the contracture is painful.

Establish whether an orthosis can be worn, whether shoe wear is prevented, whether the foot can be placed on a plantigrade wheelchair footrest, and whether there are problems with calluses or skin breakdown.

Clinical Features

The most frequent foot and ankle deformities in spasticity disorders are equinus of the ankle and varus of the hindfoot, thus resulting in the commonly seen equinovarus deformity. Various toe deformities often coexist and usually include toe flexion attitudes. The hallux is often flexed at the MTP and interphalangeal joints. The hallux may, however, develop an extension deformity at the MTP joint with flexion of the interphalangeal joint, producing a type of claw toe or "cock-up deformity." Less common deformities are foot planovalgus or cavus, or various toe extension deformities. The hip and knee are often afflicted as well in spasticity disorders. The most common hip deformities are flexion and adduction. Flexion of the knee is the most common knee deformity.

Several clinical problems develop from these deformities. Functional problems include impairment of ambulation or stance for wheelchair transfers, problems with positioning the foot on the wheelchair footrest (Fig. 3.5), inability to wear shoes or protective shoe wear, and difficulty dressing. The deformities can lead to development of painful callosities, skin maceration, and pressure sores; difficulty in patient hygiene; and extremity pain. Equinovarus often results in painful callosities of the lateral plantar foot from concentrated pressure beneath the fifth metatarsal

TABLE 3.2 EXTRAPYRAMIDAL MOVEMENT DISORDERS SEEN IN CEREBRAL PALSY

Disorder	Description
Athetosis	Involuntary persistent writhing movements, usually of the hands and trunk
Chorea	Ceaseless involuntary variety of rapid, highly complex, jerky movements
Ballismus	Dyskinetic flinging or violent movements usually caused by contractions of proximal limb muscles
Ataxia	Loss of coordination and notably impaired balance with associated gait disturbances
Hypotonia	Abnormal loss or decrease in muscle tone

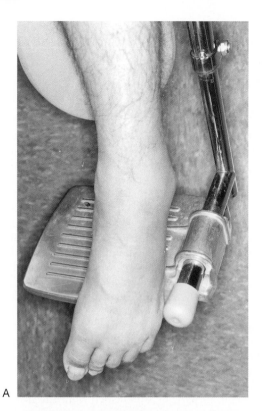

A

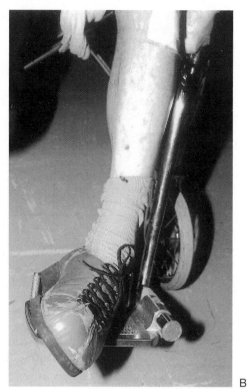

B

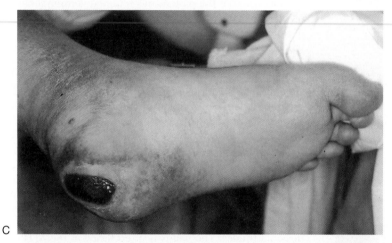

C

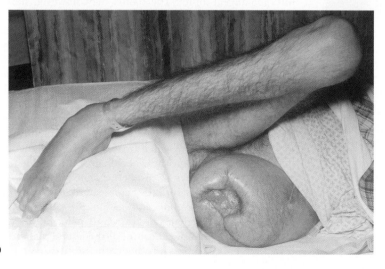

D

Figure 3.5   Problems associated with spastic equinovarus deformities. (**A**) Spastic equinovarus deformity causing problems with positioning and foot placement on a wheelchair footrest. (**B**) Patient with acquired spasticity from cerebrovascular accident in which deformity prevents plantigrade foot placement on the wheelchair platform. Skin breakdown developed when correction with an ankle–foot orthosis was attempted (note the bandage on proximal lateral calf). (**C**) Skin breakdown in hemiplegic patient with diabetes. Chronic hindfoot pressure from knee flexion deformity contributed to skin breakdown. (**D**) Spastic quadriplegic patient in whom osteomyelitis and necrotizing infection developed from contracture-related skin breakdown; the patient subsequently required amputation. Problems with skin breakdown should be preventable with proper patient positioning, padding, frequent turning, and correction of contractures. Problems associated with contractures cannot be overemphasized, and operative management is indicated as an adjunct to prevent these problems.

head or metatarsal styloid process of the fifth ray. Callosities also develop on the tips of the toes from toe flexion deformities where the toes press against the floor. Callosities may develop on the dorsum of the PIP joints where extension at the MTP joint or acute flexion of the PIP joint may result in increased pressure against the shoe. Severe varus can produce maceration and skin breakdown within the skin folds of the medial foot. Long-standing deformities, if not mobilized, lead to fixed soft-tissue contractures. Joint subluxation and dislocation can occur with chronic imbalance. Severe foot deformities that prevent use of shoe wear for comfort or protection may also be so severe as to preclude the fitting of orthotic devices. Pressure sores of the hindfoot, lateral foot, and between the toes have led to development of osteomyelitis and amputation.

Besides the functional problems, foot deformities are of concern to the patient and family for physical appearance and social acceptance. Cognitive deficits, aggressive behavior, and other personality changes, often seen following TBI or CVA, further contribute to the difficulty in clinical assessment and treatment.

Clinical evaluation of motor impairment includes assessment of muscle tone, presence of patterned reflexes or volitional control, and development of clonus, rigidity, or fixed contractures. Assessment is made of motor strength, muscle phasic activity, and degree of flexibility, with active and passive range of motion. If spasticity is mild, quantitative evaluation of muscle strength can be assessed.

Dynamic electromyography (EMG) provides information on phasic muscle activity (Fig. 3.6). Electrical activity

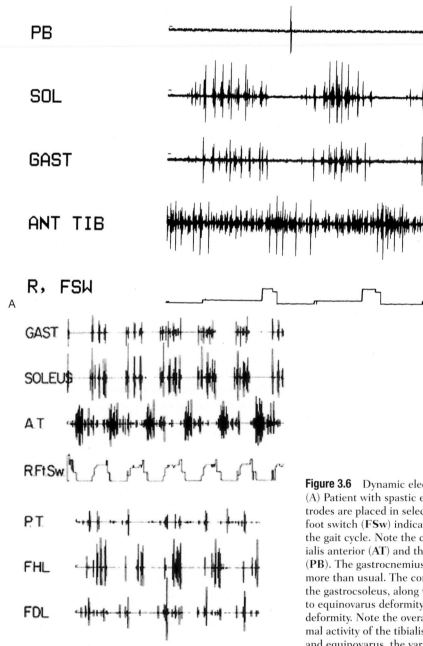

Figure 3.6 Dynamic electromyograms of patients with acquired spasticity. (A) Patient with spastic equinovarus from traumatic brain injury. Electrodes are placed in selected muscles. The patient then ambulates. The foot switch (**FSw**) indicates the heel strike and weight-bearing portion of the gait cycle. Note the constant muscle contraction (spasticity) of the tibialis anterior (**AT**) and the silent (paralytic) activity of the peroneus brevis (**PB**). The gastrocnemius (**Gast**) and soleus (**Sol**) muscles are also firing more than usual. The combination of spasticity of the tibialis anterior and the gastrocsoleus, along with the weakness of the peroneus brevis, leads to equinovarus deformity. (B) A similar patient with spastic equinovarus deformity. Note the overactivity of the tibialis anterior (**AT**) and the minimal activity of the tibialis posterior (**PT**). In adults with acquired spasticity and equinovarus, the varus component is usually produced by the tibialis anterior. Conversely, in children with cerebral palsy, the varus component is usually produced largely by the tibialis posterior.

(Continued on next page)

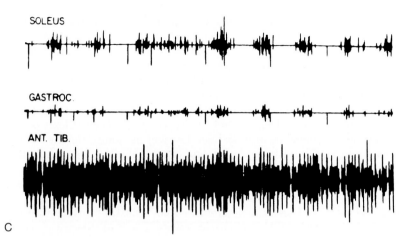

SOLEUS

GASTROC.

ANT. TIB.

C

Figure 3.6 (*Continued*) (C) Patient with traumatic brain injury and spastic equinovarus. Note the constant activity of the tibialis anterior. (Courtesy of Jacquelin Perry, MD, and the Pathokinesiology Laboratory, Rancho Los Amigos Medical Center, Downey, California.)

is recorded as the patient ambulates. The test shows the presence of normal (phasic), overactive (spastic), or silent (paralytic) activity. Dynamic EMG is particularly useful to evaluate activity of muscles difficult to assess by physical examination alone. It is useful in determining which muscles are contributing to a deformity, especially when multiple muscles may be responsible.

A fixed limb deformity may be caused by severe spasticity or by fixed soft-tissue contracture, which may be difficult to differentiate. Deformity caused by spasticity may exhibit clonus with sudden stretch or show some correction over a few minutes with prolonged stretch. Deformity caused by soft-tissue contracture does not show noticeable correction with passive stretch. Additional determination may be achieved with a lidocaine nerve block to the involved muscles with deformity caused by muscle spasticity improving after a block. Nerve blocks can be given to the femoral nerve for hip flexion, obturator nerve for hip adduction, and tibial nerve at the level of the knee for equinovarus and toe flexion.

Evaluation of the potential to ambulate, stand, or sit is an important aspect of the clinical assessment. Following a stroke, 20% to 30% of patients regain normal ambulation, and 75% return to some level of ambulation. Requirements for ambulation in an adult with acquired spastic hemiplegia include the following:

- Voluntary hip flexion
  - ☐ Active hip flexion to 30° is usually required for limb advancement.
  - ☐ Occasionally, adductors can substitute for weak flexors to assist limb advancement, which is an important consideration before the release of the adductor muscles for hip adduction deformity.
- Adequate sitting and standing balance
  - ☐ Patients often lean over the unaffected side to support the body with a cane held in the unaffected hand. Because of upper extremity involvement in hemiplegia, use of a walker is often not feasible.
  - ☐ The double limb support standing test popularized by Perry assesses balance by noting alignment of the trunk and the amount of spontaneous support given by the hemiplegic limb as the patient stands with the aid of a cane. Even with severe hemiparesis, a patient should be able to stand by shifting the body weight over to the unaffected side. Falling toward the

hemiparetic side suggests a problem known as *body neglect* rather than limb disability as the cause of inability to ambulate.
  - ☐ Balance may also be impaired when there is loss of proprioception at the hip or knee.
- Limb stability
  - ☐ Stability at the hip, knee, and ankle must be adequate to support body weight during stance phase.
  - ☐ Single limb stance on the hemiparetic limb is carefully tested, while protecting the patient in case of limb collapse.
  - ☐ Forward lean of the trunk implies weakness of the hip extensors. Flexion of the knee with ankle dorsiflexion may be indicative of soleus weakness. Knee flexion during stance also demonstrates good preservation of quadriceps strength, when the quadriceps are able to support the body weight on the flexed knee. Hyperextension of the knee usually indicates weakness of the quadriceps or occurs with an ankle equinus contracture.
  - ☐ Even though a patient may not be able to ambulate, standing is an important function for wheelchair transfers or dressing. Prerequisites for stable upright posture in stance are plantigrade feet and ankles, ability to extend the knee and hip, and adequate balance of the trunk, head, and neck.

Sensibility of the foot can be severely impaired following stroke or brain injury. Evaluation is performed with touch, pinprick, monofilament testing, and proprioception evaluation. Sensibility evaluation is often difficult in the patient with cognitive deficits who is unable to fully cooperate. Sensibility deficits add to the risk of skin breakdown.

Persistent extremity pain is a common sensory aberration following brain injury or stroke. Although poorly understood, this pain is often referred to as "pain of central origin"—characterized by diffuse, poorly localized, and at times severe leg or foot pain on the affected side. Ipsilateral upper extremity pain may also be present. Pain of central origin may represent a form of a complex regional pain syndrome (previously referred to as *reflex sympathetic dystrophy*) or a variant of other regional pain syndromes. Other causes of foot pain include muscle pain from chronic tension or chronic joint position from spasticity or contracture, joint subluxation from muscle imbalance, heterotopic ossification (HO; seen in the hip or knee; rare in the foot and ankle), occult acute or stress fractures, and peripheral neuropathy from nerve stretch in a deformed limb. Pain in an extremity should be evaluated with appropriate examination, standard radiographs, and imaging and electrodiagnostic studies as appropriate. Testing for sympathetic nerve dysfunction includes lumbar sympathetic nerve blocks and triple-phase technetium bone scan. Suspected HO can be further assessed by technetium bone scan or by measuring serum alkaline phosphatase levels.

Body neglect is a clinical condition seen in TBI or CVA patients where a portion of the side of the patient's body is not recognized. Evaluation is made by examining the hemiplegic patient during standing or attempted ambulation. Ambulation is difficult when the patient does not accommodate the weight of the unrecognized side. Patients often fail to look across their midline toward the affected side, and they have a tendency to lean or fall toward that side. Self-drawings sketched by these patients usually show omissions of extremities on the neglected side. Body neglect usually has a poor prognosis for ambulation.

Assessment of cognitive impairment of a patient with neuromuscular foot deformities is helpful in selecting those who are candidates for aggressive rehabilitation and in determining realistic goals, prognosis, and expectations. Cognitive abilities (in TBI and CVA) are evaluated by appropriateness of response to questions, ability to follow commands, psychological testing, and direct testing of learning ability in a rehabilitation setting. Decreased learning ability and loss of short-term memory may become apparent only with testing. Cognitive deficits may be severe in patients with frontal lobe injury who otherwise have few motor or sensory deficits. These patients show clinical features similar to senility, with lack of attention span and little motivation for recovery.

Aphasia is the loss of the ability to communicate. It may be expressive or receptive, and commonly occurs with lesions of the left cerebral cortex. Receptive aphasia has a poor prognosis for some aspects of rehabilitation (such as ambulation retraining) because the patient cannot understand instructions. Expressive aphasia, however, may be compatible with rehabilitation, if the patient is able to comprehend instructions.

Apraxia is the impairment of execution of a learned purposeful movement in the absence of motor impairment. It is characterized by a loss of ability to perform a routine task, such as tying shoelaces, ambulating, or using stairs. Apraxia occurs more often with right hemispheric involvement. The prognosis for ambulation with severe apraxia is usually poor.

Behavioral and psychological aberrations occur following CVA and TBI, including hostility, resentment, depression, withdrawal, or emotional instability. The behavior is often a reflection of premorbid personality traits, such as aggressive behavior. Psychiatric consultation assists evaluation. An understanding of premorbid states helps in coping with the difficult patient and establishing a functional prognosis from a psychological standpoint.

Radiologic Features

- Standard AP, lateral, and oblique radiographs of the foot and ankle are usually obtained to assess and document the degree of deformity.

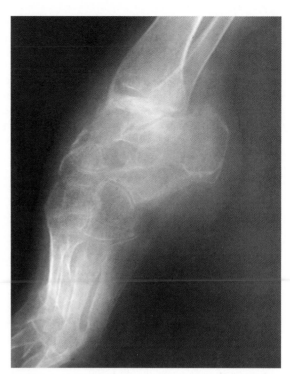

Figure 3.7 Standard lateral ankle radiograph of patient with severe fixed acquired equinovarus deformity. Note the degree of equinus. Osteopenia is present because of the patient's inability to bear weight on this involved extremity. Weight-bearing views are often not possible.

- Weight-bearing views are often difficult and may require assistance from the radiologic technician to support or position the patient (Fig. 3.7).
- Standard radiographs are also used to assess other skeletal causes of the deformity. These are particularly indicated if the patient has a rigid fixed deformity, has had prior operative procedures on the foot and ankle, or has sustained concomitant lower extremity skeletal trauma.
- Standard radiographs of the hip and knee can establish the presence of neurogenic HO in fixed contractures. Neurogenic HO is rare in the foot and ankle, but relatively common in the hip and occasionally in the knee with TBI and SCI.
- Computed axial tomography (CAT scan) is occasionally done for further evaluation if there is concomitant skeletal injury, if there is concern regarding integrity of joint surfaces, or if the patient has had previous operative procedures.
- CT scans of the hip and knee are also helpful in establishing the three-dimensional extent of HO. Please confirm whether it should be CT or CAT scan in this instance
- Three-phase technetium bone scans are helpful in establishing the presence of coexisting complex regional pain syndromes.
- Technetium bone scans, along with serum alkaline phosphatase levels help establish the maturity or activity level of neurogenic HO.
- MRI of the foot and ankle is seldom obtained in the patient with spasticity because it can be difficult

for the patient to remain still or to tolerate the test. An MRI is occasionally done if the integrity of specific soft tissues (such as tendons or ligaments) is in question.

- Arteriograms of the limb can be obtained if integrity of the posterior tibial or dorsalis pedis artery is in question, especially when the patient has sustained previous trauma or has had prior operative procedures. Many adult patients with CP will have had several previous foot and ankle procedures in childhood.

TREATMENT

Nonsurgical Treatment

- General rehabilitation strategies (Algorithm 3.1)
  - ☐ Initial treatment is usually nonoperative, especially when the patient is in the recovery phase of the neurologic insult (see Table 3.1).
  - ☐ Nonoperative treatment consists of a comprehensive rehabilitation program that usually includes physical

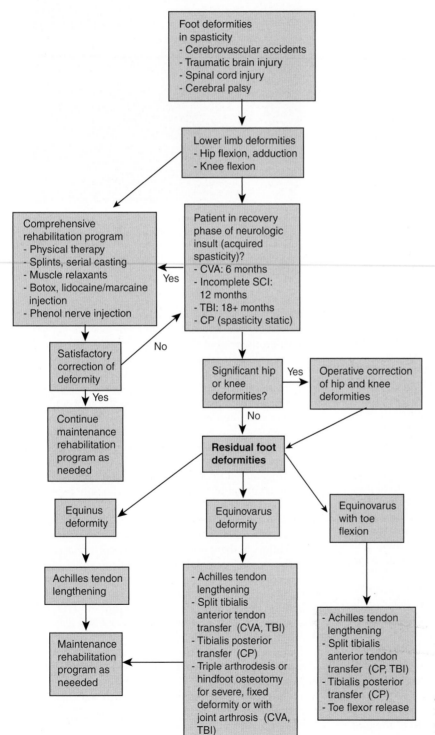

Algorithm 3.1   Algorithm for acquired spastic foot deformities. CVA, cerebrovascular accident; SCI, spinal cord injury; TBI, traumatic brain injury; CP, cerebral palsy.

therapy, splinting or serial casting of deformities, muscle relaxants, and nerve blocks.

- ☐ When nonsurgical efforts are not successful in preventing problematic contractures and the patient is beyond the period of neurologic recovery, operative management is considered.

■ Physical therapy
- ☐ Physical therapy provides passive stretching, strengthening of weak antagonistic muscles, static splinting (including static progressive splinting), corrective or serial casting, biofeedback, functional retraining (for balance, stance, transfers, and ambulation), and desensitization of the painful limb.
- ☐ Adjunct therapy includes functional electrical muscle stimulation and can be used to strengthen weak antagonist muscles, assist mobilization of the joints, and inhibit the spastic agonist.

■ Muscle relaxants
- ☐ Baclofen, dantrolene sodium, and diazepam are common muscle relaxants that are effective initial methods for decreasing mildly spastic muscle tone.
- ☐ Baclofen is usually given orally, but can be administered intrathecally when spasticity is severe.
- ☐ Diazepam has potent muscle relaxant properties; however, side effects of lethargy and somnolence and the potential addictiveness make its use less optimal in many patients, especially when long-term therapy is needed.
- ☐ These medications also have potential hepatotoxicity and warrant periodic liver function tests.

■ Mobilization, splinting, and orthoses
- ☐ Mobilization and splinting provide the most important initial steps in a comprehensive rehabilitation program to treat spastic deformities.
- ☐ Contractures do not develop in a joint that is passed through a full range of motion daily. Range of joint motion exercises that elongate shortened muscles should be performed several times daily.
- ☐ In equinovarus deformities, stretching is performed by passive mobilization into maximal dorsiflexion and hindfoot valgus. Extending the knee during ankle mobilization further stretches the gastrocnemius. During Achilles tendon stretching for equinus, the hindfoot should be "locked" by placing the foot in inversion to prevent midfoot collapse and resulting in a rocker bottom foot. The stretching should be gentle, prolonged, and maintained. A "stretch and hold" method is an effective method, commonly used by physical and occupational therapists.
- ☐ Muscle strengthening with active motion against resistance is incorporated when there is adequate volitional control.
- ☐ The ankle is maintained in proper position by static splinting with well-padded bivalved casts, molded splints, or static ankle–foot orthoses (AFOs; Fig. 3.8). The double-upright metal and leather AFO is often needed for the more severe spasticity; the lightweight synthetic AFO is feasible when spasticity is mild. The well-padded "boot" type orthoses are also effective and readily available in several sizes to fit the patient.

- ☐ Toe flexion deformities can be minimized with daily stretching and maintained by the incorporation of a well-padded toe plate into the AFO.
- ☐ Static splints and "inhibitive casts" also decrease spastic muscle tone by decreasing motion, which lessens stimulation to the stretch reflex and, in turn, decreases spasticity.
- ☐ Dynamic splints or traction devices must be used with caution in the spastic limb because the continuous stretch may provide stimulation that increases spasticity or perpetuates clonus.
- ☐ Several commercial dynamic splints are available for ankle and knee deformities, allowing a set amount of traction to be placed across a joint.
- ☐ Dynamic splints are usually more effective when a fixed contracture exists but spasticity is minimal. Even though they are well designed and well padded, these devices must be closely monitored for pressure areas or potential skin breakdown, especially when contractures are severe.

■ Serial casting
- ☐ If a fixed joint contracture has developed, serial casting can be an effective means of slowly stretching soft tissues to correct a deformity.
- ☐ In fixed equinovarus deformities, the limb is passively stretched, then held in the position of maximum correction while a well-padded short-leg cast is applied.
- ☐ Optimally, each week the cast is removed, the skin is inspected for pressure areas, the patient undergoes additional passive joint mobilization, and a new cast is applied with additional correction. This uses the "stretch–hold" manual technique, followed by static progressive correction with the cast.
- ☐ Over a 6- to 8-week period, many contractures can be significantly improved as the shortened muscles, ligaments, or tendons are gradually stretched.
- ☐ Lidocaine nerve block to the tibial or sciatic nerve before stretching and cast application should provide spastic muscle relaxation and may help gain correction. Serial nerve blocks may be helpful for decreasing overall spasticity or unwanted patterned contractions.

■ Phenol nerve blocks
- ☐ Dilute phenol (3% to 5% solution) nerve block produces a temporary but long-acting block to decrease spasticity for several months. These motor nerve blocks provide muscle relaxation during the period of neurologic recovery. The temporary abolition of spasticity facilitates limb mobilization for contracture prevention.
- ☐ These blocks usually have more application in the treatment of the brain-injured patient because of the longer associated neurologic recovery period.
- ☐ The duration of a phenol nerve block is variable and is dependent on the accuracy of the initial injection and on the distance and time required for regenerating axons to reach the respective motor end plates. Successful blocks last 6 weeks to 3 months.
- ☐ Several phenol motor blocks to the spastic lower extremity have been described.

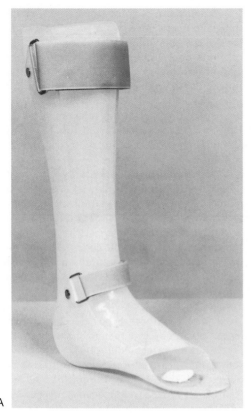
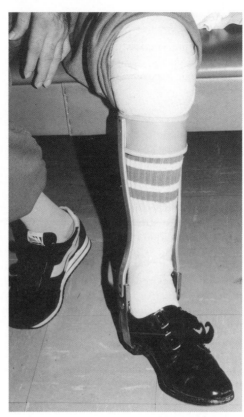

A B

Figure 3.8 Common ankle–foot orthoses (AFOs) used in patients with neuromuscular disorders. (**A**) Lightweight synthetic AFO, often used for spastic equinus deformities. The orthosis can correct or sustain correction in mild, flexible equinovarus. The AFO also has application in paralytic afflictions such as polio or Charcot–Marie–Tooth disorders, in which the orthosis helps to support the foot if the gastrocsoleus muscle is weak and a foot drop has developed. A hinge can be placed at the ankle to allow motion, and with a paralytic foot drop, a spring-loaded device can be added to help bring the foot back to a neutral position. (**B**) A more rigid double-upright AFO made of leather with metal uprights. This type of AFO is used for more severe deformities of acquired spasticity when a lightweight orthosis is not adequate. Ankle motion can be blocked to provide stability or to correct or control deformity. Alternatively, various amounts of ankle motion can be allowed to accommodate the specific amount of spasticity or weakness.

☐ Femoral nerve motor branch to the rectus femoris helps decrease hip flexion.

☐ Obturator nerve block helps with hip adduction spasticity.

☐ Sciatic nerve motor branch block to the hamstring muscles decreases knee flexor spasticity.

☐ Tibial nerve motor branch to the gastrocnemius and soleus decrease equinovarus deformity.

☐ Blocking the motor branches to the FHL and FDL decreases toe flexion spasticity.

☐ The phenol nerve blocks are given in either a closed or an open fashion, depending on the anatomic accessibility and motor–sensory composition of the nerve.

☐ If a nerve has primarily motor fibers (e.g., femoral or obturator nerves), the entire nerve can be injected in the closed fashion, aided with the needle guided by a nerve stimulator or ultrasound.

☐ Nerves with large amounts of mixed sensory and motor fibers (e.g., main sciatic or tibial nerve trunks) should, in general, not be injected in the closed fashion because of the associated loss of protective sensibility and possible resulting painful paresthesias occurring from the sensory components.

☐ An open block with these mixed nerves is usually preferable, where the motor branches are surgically exposed and injected separately as they enter each muscle, thus avoiding sensory components (Fig. 3.9).

☐ Open blocks usually provide a more complete and longer-lasting block than do closed blocks because of the greater accuracy of direct nerve branch injection.

☐ Open blocks can also be used when closed blocks are not adequate or are short lived.

■ Botulinum toxin

☐ Intramuscular botulinum toxin type A injection (onabotulinumtoxin A, Botox [BTX], Allergan, Inc., Irvine, California) effectively decreases muscle tone.

☐ The toxin is a neurotoxin produced by *Clostridium botulinum* that interferes with the release of acetylcholine at the nerve synapse, thereby producing a functionally denervated (relaxed) muscle. This method reduces spasticity and provides muscle relaxation for months, similar to phenol.

☐ Botox is injected directly into the muscle belly, and, even though it is injected in the vicinity of the myoneural junction, it does not require as precise motor nerve injection as is required for phenol.

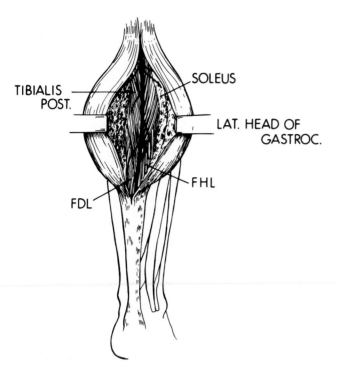

Figure 3.9 Exposure of the motor branches of the tibial nerve for phenol nerve block. *FDL,* flexor digitorum longus; *FHL,* flexor hallucis longus; *Tibialis post.,* tibialis posterior; gastroc., gastrocsoleus. Alternatively, Botox injections directly into the muscle bellies of the involved muscles can be given, without need for individual motor nerve injection. (Reproduced with permission from Botte MJ, Keenan MA. Brain injury and stroke. In: Gelberman RH, ed. Operative nerve repair and reconstruction. Philadelphia: JB Lippincott, 1991:1444.)

☐ Botox effects on muscle are usually seen in 12 to 72 hours postinjection and usually last for 3 to 6 months.

☐ Reported improvement occurs in about 80% of patients. If deformity persists or recurs, injections may be repeated after 2 or more weeks. Up to six injections may be given at one site until adequate muscle relaxation is achieved.

☐ Botox is more expensive than phenol and, in general, the blocks may not last as long as well-directed phenol blocks. However, the ease of application and the avoidance of an open (surgical) procedure have helped promote the popularity of botulinum injections.

☐ Although Botox injection is a relatively new technique compared with phenol, its safety and efficacy appear to be well established to treat muscle spasticity. It is replacing the use of phenol in many rehabilitation medical centers.

Surgical Treatment

Surgical management of a spastic limb deformity in the patient with acquired spasticity is indicated when problematic deformities have not responded to a comprehensive multidisciplinary rehabilitation program. Disfigurement alone is usually not an indication for surgical intervention, unless function, hygiene, or positioning is impaired

as well. If a patient is still in the recovery period when spontaneous improvement can still be expected, Botox intramuscular injection or phenol nerve blocks are usually considered before operative management. If a patient is beyond the recovery period and no spontaneous limb recovery is expected, operative correction is considered. Reconstructive surgery should not, in general, be performed on patients who are still in the recovery phase and who continue to show improvement in a comprehensive therapy program. This often means waiting for 6 months after a stroke event or for 18 months after TBI.

Goals of surgery include improvement of function, relief of pain from chronic deformity due to spasticity or contracture, prevention or treatment of painful foot callosities, facilitation of hygiene, ease of positioning and dressing, and prevention of pressure sores. Corrective surgery can allow the use of shoes or AFOs that will otherwise not be feasible. Reconstructive surgery should also be considered in the nonambulatory patient when hygiene, positioning, and pressure sores are a problem.

Each of the lower extremity joints is discussed separately; the entire lower limb must be taken into consideration for operative planning. Severe hip and knee deformities are often addressed at a separate procedure before correction of foot deformity, so that the foot can be positioned more optimally on the operating room table for later reconstructive surgery.

Operative Management of Hip Deformity

The major problems associated with the hip are adductor and flexor spasticity and their associated myostatic contractures. There is no practical orthosis available to treat these deformities. Initial nonoperative management includes mobilization and intermittent positioning in a prone position in a physical therapy program. Botox muscle injections, serial obturator lidocaine and marcaine nerve blocks, or closed phenol nerve blocks alleviate adductor spasticity and facilitate stretching exercises. Adductor spasticity in a hemiplegic patient seldom causes problems with hygiene when the deformity is unilateral, and adequate motion of the contralateral hip allows skin care. Scissoring, however, is the action of hip adduction that causes the limb to cross over the midline, impeding ambulation and standing for transfers. With prolonged scissoring, skin maceration and breakdown can develop in the groin skin folds.

Definitive operative procedures for adduction deformity are selective adductor release and obturator neurectomy. The adductor longus and gracilis are usually addressed and can also include a portion of the adductor brevis. Care must be taken to avoid complete adductor release or neurectomy in a patient whose adductors are the sole means of limb advancement. Such a patient walks with the lower extremity externally rotated. Diagnostic lidocaine nerve block to the obturator nerve simulates adductor release or neurectomy and allows preoperative evaluation of ambulation before operative management. Dynamic EMGs are also helpful in these instances. In adults with TBI and CVA with adductor spasticity, adductor release alone is usually sufficient. In pediatric patients with CP, obturator neurectomy is usually described as an adjuvant to the adductor release when severe spasticity is present. Adductor release of the hip is often combined with ipsilateral hip flexor release and knee flexor release (discussed later).

Flexion deformity of the hip is initially treated with passive mobilization and prone positioning. Splinting of the hip for flexion deformity is difficult. Botox intramuscular injections or phenol motor nerve block to the hip flexor muscles include the rectus femorus, sartorius, iliopsoas, and tensor fascia lata. If persistent deformity persists or recurs, and the flexion deformity causes groin maceration, positioning problems, or a flexed attitude during ambulation, operative release is indicated. Hip flexion deformity is often accompanied with knee flexion deformity and can lead to pressure sores on the posterior heel or sacrum, or overlying the greater trochanter. Operative release is also performed as a precursor to foot deformity correction, to allow positioning and access to the foot for later surgical reconstruction. The hip flexor muscles addressed operatively include the rectus femoris, sartorius, tensor fasciae latae, and iliopsoas. These rectus femorus, sartorius, and tensor fascia lata can be released or lengthened using a muscle origin recession through a single anterior incision. The iliopsoas can be released or lengthened in the tendinous portion close to the insertion into the lesser trochanter. In a nonambulatory patient, hip flexor release assists patient dressing and patient positioning to prevent pressure sores. Ipsilateral hip and knee flexion deformity can be corrected simultaneously, often being combined with hip adductor release.

Stiffness of the hip in the patient with TBI may also be due to neurogenic HO. Ankylosis of the hip may occur from the HO. Evaluation by standard radiographs is usually diagnostic. Evaluation for bone maturity before resection can be further studied with serum alkaline phosphatase levels or technetium bone scans. A CAT scan of a hip is used as a further preoperative study, and will show the osseous mass in three dimensions to aid operative planning.

Operative Management of Knee Deformity

The most common deformity of the knee is flexion caused by spasticity of the hamstring muscles. Usually both the medial and the lateral hamstrings are involved. Alternatively, some patients have the opposite (knee extension) deformity, presenting as a straight leg deformity or a limb with inability to flex the knee. This deformity is caused by spasticity of the quadriceps.

Knee flexion deformity causes several problems. In the nonambulatory patient, pressure sores on the heel, sacrum, or over the greater trochanter can develop. In the ambulatory patient, increased quadriceps demand is required to stabilize the knee in the flexed position during stance. Energy consumption is greatly increased. Increased hip extensor demand is also required to stabilize the hip. Initial management includes stretching exercises, splinting, or corrective serial casting. Intramuscular Botox injections or phenol motor nerve blocks to the hamstring muscles are an important adjuvant. If problematic deformity persists or recurs, operative management is considered. In the nonambulatory patient, treatment usually consists of distal release of the hamstring muscles (Fig. 3.10). The posterior knee capsule is usually not released to preserve joint stability. Any residual capsular contracture can be treated later

by stretching or serial casting following muscle release. In the ambulatory patient (or potentially ambulatory patient), musculotendinous junction or Z-lengthening of each hamstring muscle is performed in an effort to preserve some active knee flexion. If hip flexion attitude is also present, it is desirable to preserve the hip extensor function of the hamstrings. This can be accomplished with distal transfer of the hamstring muscles from the proximal tibia to the distal femur, as described by Eggars.

Stiff-legged gait is a dynamic problem of spastic quadriceps activity. The quadriceps contracts during terminal stance phase and early swing phase to extend the knee, causing a stiff-legged gait and preventing normal knee flexion. This is an opposite deformity of the knee flexion contracture and occurs much less commonly. In the stiff-legged gait, the patient must hike the pelvis and circumduct the limb so that the foot clears the floor. Botox injections can be given to the quadriceps muscles, and phenol nerve injections to the motor branches can be considered. In general, nonoperative treatment for this deformity can be difficult. EMG studies have shown that the abnormal activity may be restricted to the rectus femoris and vastus intermedius, or, in some cases, all four of the quadriceps muscles may be involved. If only the rectus femoris and vastus intermedius are responsible for the deformity, selective release of these muscles should relieve the stiff-legged gait and allow knee flexion (Fig. 3.11).

If all four heads of the quadriceps are overactive, as seen by dynamic EMG studies, release of the rectus femoris and vastus intermedius is often not sufficient. However, release of all four heads is not optimal because some extensor function must be preserved to stabilize the knee. There is currently no universally effective procedure to correct this difficult problem. One solution with severe spasticity involves release of the involved muscles to relieve the stiff-legged component and then bracing of the knee with a knee–ankle–foot orthosis if there is residual quadriceps weakness. An alternative is to release the rectus femoris and vastus intermedius (and a small portion of the vastus lateralis and vastus medialis, if needed) and to accept some residual stiff-legged gait abnormality.

Operative Management of Ankle and Foot Deformities

Deformities of the foot and ankle in disorders of spasticity usually comprise ankle equinus, equinovarus, or hindfoot varus. Rarely, hindfoot planovalgus may occur. Equinovarus is the most common. Equinus is caused by spasticity of the gastrocnemius and soleus with contributions from the FHL, FDL, and tibialis posterior. In the adult with acquired spasticity from brain injury or stroke, the varus component is usually predominantly due to overactivity of the tibialis anterior, with contributions from the FDL and FHL. The involvement of the tibialis posterior is variable in adults with acquired spasticity; however, in the pediatric CP patient with spastic equinovarus, the varus component is often mostly due to overactivity of the tibialis posterior. Because of these differences, operative procedures in pediatric patients are often directed toward transfer or lengthening of the tibialis posterior, whereas in the adult with brain injury or stroke, procedures more commonly use transfer of the tibialis anterior.

HAMSTRING RELEASE

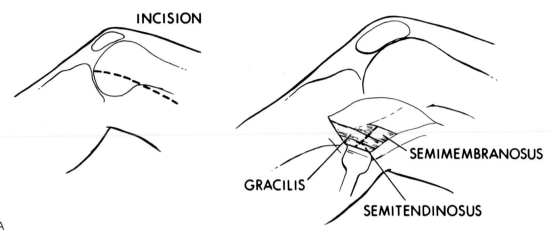

INCISION

SEMIMEMBRANOSUS

GRACILIS

SEMITENDINOSUS

A

HAMSTRING RELEASE

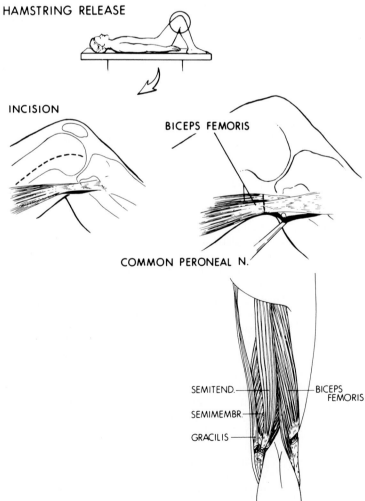

INCISION

BICEPS FEMORIS

COMMON PERONEAL N.

SEMITEND.

SEMIMEMBR.

GRACILIS

BICEPS FEMORIS

FRACTIONAL LENGTHENING

B

Figure 3.10 Release or lengthening of medial (**A**) and lateral (**B**) distal hamstring muscles. On the medial side, the semitendinosus, semimembranosus, and gracilis are released or lengthened. On the lateral side, the two heads of the biceps femoris are released or lengthened. (Reproduced with permission from Botte MJ, Keenan MA. Brain injury and stroke. In: Gelberman RH, ed. Operative nerve repair and reconstruction. Philadelphia: JB Lippincott, 1991:1442–1443.)

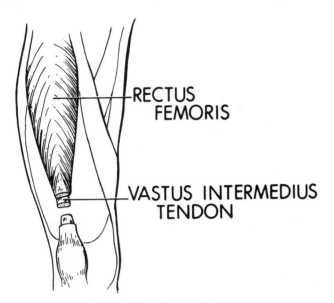

Figure 3.11   Distal release of the rectus femoris and vastus intermedius tendon.

Toe flexion deformities are also common in brain injury and stroke, and depending on the specific muscle imbalance, different deformities occur. Flexion at the MTP, PIP, and DIP joints results in a curly toe deformity. Extension of the MTP with flexion at the PIP and extension of the DIP results in a hammer toe. Extension of the MTP and flexion at both PIP and DIP joints results in a claw toe deformity. When there is paralysis of the intrinsic muscles of the foot (with spasticity of the extrinsic muscles), the claw toe deformity is more common. A foot that has been left untreated in the equinus position develops contracture of the extrinsic toe flexors, and toe flexion deformity can be accentuated by the tenodesis effect when the ankle equinus is corrected. As the foot is passively brought out of equinus, tension increases on the toe flexors.

Initial management of foot deformities is, as discussed for nonoperative options, comprising a rehabilitation program with physical therapy for soft-tissue stretching, muscle relaxants to decrease spasticity, and maintenance using a locked AFO, bivalved casts, or intermittent casting combined with passive mobilization. Static splints are generally preferred over dynamic spring-loaded devices, which may aggravate spasticity or perpetuate clonus. If bracing alone cannot control deformity and the patient is in the recovery phase of spasticity, Botox intramuscular injections or phenol motor nerve blocks to the gastrocsoleus, tibialis posterior, FHL, and FDL may be helpful. If spasticity is no longer present but a residual fixed soft-tissue contracture exists, dynamic splints and serial casting are instituted.

If nonsurgical efforts are not successful in preventing problematic contractures and the patient is beyond the period of neurologic recovery, operative management can be used to correct the deformity. Indications for operative management of the equinovarus foot include deformity that causes functional problems, difficulty in shoe or brace wear, difficulty in foot positioning, and skin problems such as callosities or pressure ulcers. More specific indications for foot and ankle reconstruction include a deformity that is

so severe that an AFO cannot be fitted or a residual deformity that interferes with ambulation despite the use of an AFO. In addition, some patients who ambulate well with an AFO with adequate proprioception and calf strength may become brace free following reconstruction. Operative reconstruction should also be considered in the nonambulatory patient when correction may allow the foot to be placed on the wheelchair platform or allow protective shoe wear. The varus component may also contribute to callosities or skin breakdown on the lateral aspect of the foot over the styloid process or over the lateral head of the fifth metatarsal.

Operative reconstruction of the equinovarus foot in TBI and CVA is usually accomplished with tendo Achilles lengthening (TAL) combined with the split tibialis anterior tendon transfer (SPLATT). Transfer of FHL and FDL to the calcaneus as described by Keenan is also performed to address and augment plantarflexion strength, which is often weak following Achilles tendon lengthening. Reconstruction in the equinovarus foot in the pediatric patient with CP is usually with TAL combined with transfer or lengthening of the tibialis posterior.

Occasionally, posterior capsule release of the ankle is required for adequate correction of severe, long-standing equinus. TAL can be accomplished by Z-lengthening, fractional lengthening, and percutaneous triple hemisection tenotomy. In a patient who has not had a prior tendon lengthening, the percutaneous triple hemisection tenotomy is reliable and effective. This procedure involves minimal incisions, provides adequate safety, and is sufficient when both the gastrocnemius and soleus are involved. If only the gastrocnemius is spastic, then selective fractional lengthening of this muscle can be performed. In the patient who has had a previous lengthening and has a recurrent deformity, open lengthening is preferable because the previous lengthening produces adhesions that can interfere with percutaneous lengthening.

■ TAL with percutaneous triple hemisection tenotomy (Fig. 3.12)
   □ Three tenotomy cuts are made with a no. 11 scalpel and placed through small stab incisions at approximately 3-cm intervals.
   □ The distal and proximal incisions are located medially to help decrease the varus component that is usually present with the equinus.
   □ Approximately one-half of the tendon is incised at each level in this closed fashion.
   □ The foot is passively dorsiflexed to about 5° of dorsiflexion, causing the tendon to lengthen.
   □ The SPLATT, toe flexor release (TFR), and transfer of the FHL and FDL to the calcaneus are often performed at the same setting.
   □ Lengthening the Achilles tendon, although necessary to correct the equinus, further weakens the gastrocnemius–soleus (GCS) muscle group. Transfer of the FHL and FDL to the calcaneus augments the strength of the surgically lengthened GCS muscle complex. This transfer also helps correct concomitant toe flexion deformities by release of the extrinsic toe flexors. The released tendons are attached to the calcaneus through a drill hole and can be secured with an interference screw.

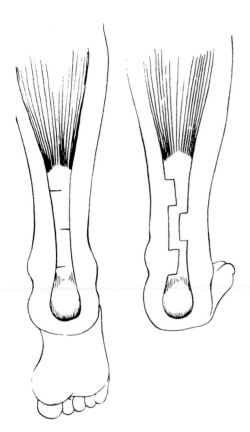

Figure 3.12 Achilles tendon lengthening using the percutaneous triple hemisection technique.

- The incision is dressed and a short leg, well-padded cast applied.
- Care should be taken to prevent overcorrection, which may lead to calcaneus gait.
- Postoperative management includes immobilization in the short leg cast for 6 weeks.
- If the procedure is performed in combination with the SPLATT procedure, protection is continued in a locked AFO and night splint used for 4 to 5 months following the initial period of cast immobilization.
- TAL: open Z-lengthening
  - An 8-cm longitudinal incision is placed along the lateral or medial aspect of the Achilles tendon.
  - The sural nerve located posteriorly and laterally should be protected from injury.
  - A Z-step incision is placed in the tendon with adequate length to accomplish correction.
  - Because of the twisting orientation of the tendon, the anterior two-thirds of the tendon distally near the insertion is divided while 3 inches proximally, dividing the medial two-thirds of the tendon.
  - Alternatively, the posterior half of the tendon can be released proximally and the anterior half of the tendon distally to place the exposed raw surface of the tendon proximally, where it is covered by thick subcutaneous tissue.
  - The knee is extended and the foot is gently passively dorsiflexed to a corrected position as the tendon slides to an appropriate length.
  - In a tendon that has undergone previous lengthening,

the entire incision of the Z-step cut is made with a scalpel because previous adhesions may prevent adequate sliding of the tendon to length.

- The tendon is repaired at the corrected length with 2-0 or 3-0 nonabsorbable suture. Overlengthening must be avoided to prevent calcaneal deformity from occurring.
- Transfer of the FHL and FDL to the calcaneus to augment the surgically lengthened (and weakened) GCS complex can be performed at the same setting, as noted above.
- Occasionally, posterior capsule release of the ankle is needed for adequate correction of severe long-standing equinus deformities.
  - Following Z-tenotomy of the Achilles tendon, dissection is continued toward the posterior ankle.
  - The FHL crosses the posterior aspect of the ankle in a lateral-to-medial direction.
  - The tendon is retracted and a transverse capsulotomy of the posterior ankle is performed. In TBI and CVA, posterior capsulotomy is seldom needed and adequate correction is usually accomplished with TAL alone.
  - Postoperative care is the same as above for percutaneous TAL.

If the gastrocnemius alone is causing the equinus, this muscle can be selectively lengthened using either fractional lengthening at the myotendinous junction or proximal recession at its origin. Determination of the sole involvement of the gastrocnemius muscle is made by noting resolution of the equinus when the gastrocnemius is relaxed by flexing the knee. In general, recession or lengthening of the gastrocnemius at the proximal level or at the myotendinous junction is seldom used because the other methods that address lengthening at the tendon level are simpler and more effective, and require less operative exposure. In addition, EMGs during gait in patients with CP and equinus deformity usually show increased activity of both the gastrocnemius and soleus. Therefore, lengthening at the tendon level addresses both muscles.

- Gastrocnemius fractional lengthening
  - A longitudinal incision is placed on the middle third of the posterior calf.
  - The deep fascia is opened to expose the gastrocnemius muscle.
  - The aponeurotic tendon of the muscle is divided transversely just proximal to the point where it joins with the soleus fibers.
  - The muscle is separated from the underlying soleus by blunt dissection.
  - The foot is passively dorsiflexed to the neutral position, and the retracted aponeurotic tendon is sutured to the underlying soleus.
  - Postoperatively, the ankle is immobilized for 4 weeks, followed by physical therapy for mobilization and strengthening.

Ankle and hindfoot varus in TBI and CVA are usually caused mainly by spasticity of the tibialis anterior. If in question, preoperative EMG studies help determine which specific muscles are responsible for the varus deformity.

The FHL, FDL, soleus, and tibialis posterior muscles can all contribute to the deformity.

The SPLATT procedure is used to correct the varus component. The procedure consists of transfer of the lateral half or two-thirds of the tibialis anterior to the cuboid or lateral cuneiform, thus converting the deforming force to a corrective force. Overcorrection is prevented by the remaining nontransferred portion of the tendon. The SPLATT is usually combined with a TAL to correct an equinovarus deformity and with FHL and FDL transfer to the calcaneus to augment plantar flexion strength (see above). TFR is also used to correct toe flexion deformity.

Although the tibialis anterior is usually the major deforming force producing the varus in TBI and CVA, the tibialis posterior may become secondarily contracted, preventing adequate correction. Z-lengthening or fractional lengthening of the tibialis posterior is then considered and performed at the time of the SPLATT. In addition, residual tightness may be due to capsular contracture of the medial joints (talonavicular and naviculocuneiform joints) necessitating a capsulotomy.

- SPLATT (Figs. 3.13 and 3.14)
  - ☐ The procedure is performed through three incisions: one over the base of the first metatarsal to detach the portion of the tibialis anterior; the second about 8 cm proximal to the ankle, used to pass and redirect the transferred tendon, and the third over the cuboid and lateral cuneiform to reattach the tendon.
  - ☐ The tibialis anterior insertion is identified in the first incision.

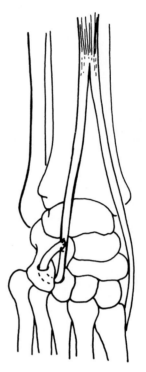

Figure 3.13 Split tibialis anterior tendon transfer (SPLATT) to correct varus deformity caused by spasticity of the tibialis anterior muscle. The lateral half of the tibialis anterior tendon is transferred to the lateral aspect of the foot to provide a correction force. The tendon is attached to the cuboid or cuboid and third cuneiform. (Reproduced with permission from Botte MJ, Keenan MA. Brain injury and stroke. In: Gelberman RH, ed. Operative nerve repair and reconstruction. Philadelphia: JB Lippincott, 1991:1445.)

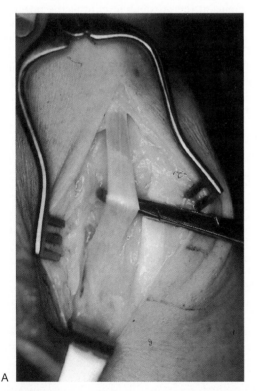 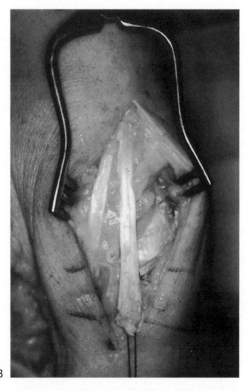

Figure 3.14 Intraoperative photographs of the split tibialis anterior tendon transfer. (**A**) Incision over insertion of tibialis anterior of the left foot in preparation for splitting the tendon. The tendon is held in the probe. (**B**) The tendon is split longitudinally, and the lateral half of the tendon is detached from its insertion. A suture has been placed in the tendon to facilitate sliding the tendon under the skin.

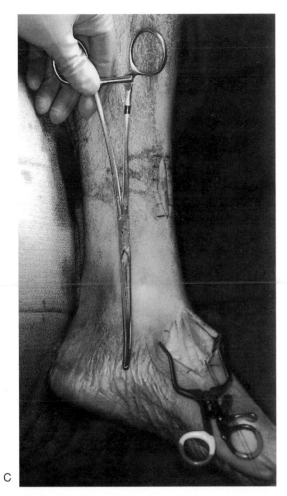

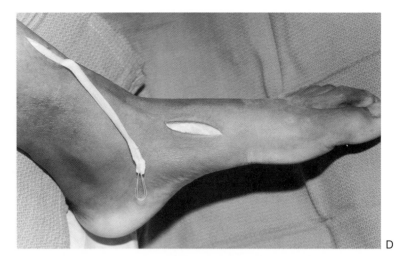

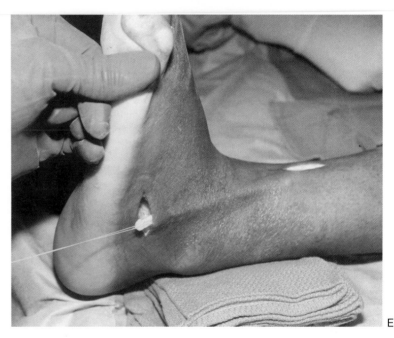

C

D

E

Figure 3.14 (C) A long clamp is used to facilitate pulling the split tendon from the first incision to the second incision. (D) The split tendon has been transferred to a second incision over the distal anterior calf and is now ready to transfer the third incision. (E) The tendon is transferred to a third incision over the cuboid. (F) Close-up photograph of third incision, with the tendon passed through a drill hole in the cuboid. (G) The tendon is sutured back onto itself.

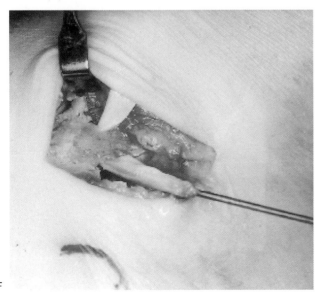

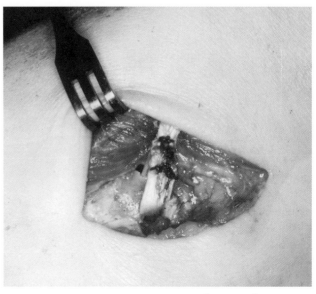

F

G

(continued on next page)

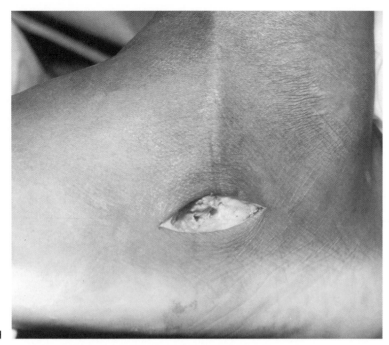

H

Figure 3.14 (*continued*)   (H) Photograph showing transferred tendon secured into the cuboid. Note the slight tension of the transferred tendon that can be seen passing under the skin. An interference screw can be used to augment fixation of the tendon into the drill hole.

□ The lateral half to two-thirds of the tendon is detached from its insertion, a suture is placed in the end of the split, detached tendon, and the tendon is split longitudinally along its fibers.

□ The clamp is passed subcutaneously, superficial to the extensor retinaculum, from the second (tibial) incision to the first incision.

□ The clamp grasps the detached tendon, pulling it into the second incision, further splitting the tendon.

□ The tendon is then passed subcutaneously to the third incision, using the long clamp passed from the third incision to the second incision.

□ The tendon is then attached to the lateral aspect of the foot through a 4-mm drill hole in the cuboid or lateral cuneiform. It is sutured to itself using 2-0 nonabsorbable suture with the foot held in a corrected position. Alternatively, an interference screw can be used to achieve or augment fixation of the tendon to the bone.

■ Toe flexor release (Fig. 3.15)

□ A 2-cm longitudinal incision is placed at the proximal flexion crease of each toe.

□ The neurovascular bundles are protected. The flexor tendon sheath is opened.

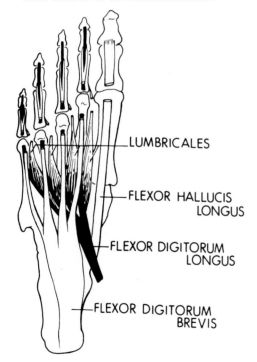

LUMBRICALES

FLEXOR HALLUCIS LONGUS

FLEXOR DIGITORUM LONGUS

FLEXOR DIGITORUM BREVIS

A

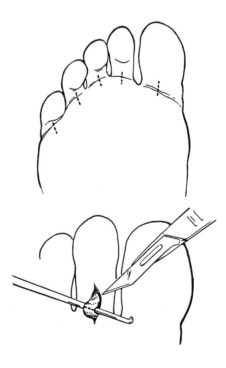

B

Figure 3.15   Toe flexor release. (**A**) Release of the extrinsic and intrinsic toe flexor tendons. (**B**) Incisions are placed on the plantar base of each involved toe. The tendon is delivered into the incision and incised.

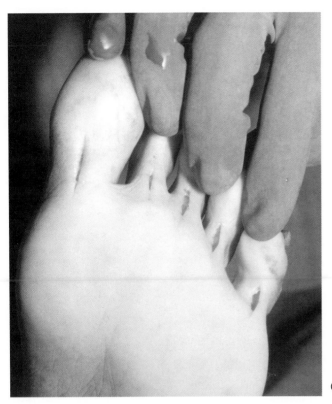

C

Figure 3.15 (*continued*) (C) Photograph showing incisions and correction obtained following toe flexor release. (**A** and **B** reproduced with permission from Keenan MA, Gorai AP, Smith CW, et al. Intrinsic toe flexion deformity following correction of spastic equinovarus deformity in adults. Foot Ankle 1987;7:333–337.)

- ☐ A small right-angle retractor facilitates retrieval of the tendon and pulls it superficially for the tenotomy.
- ☐ The flexor digitorum brevis is identified first and usually consists of two tendon slips.
- ☐ If the incision was placed distally in the region of the middle phalanx, the flexor digitorum brevis tendons may be located at the medial and lateral margins of the larger, more centrally located FDL.
- ☐ Before tenotomy, each tendon is inspected under loupe magnification for adherent neurovascular structures (which can occur with long-standing deformity).
- ☐ A 1-cm portion of each tendon is excised. If needed for adequate correction, the intrinsic tendons are released as well.
- ☐ Postoperatively following the TAL, SPLATT, and TFR, the foot and ankle are immobilized in a cast for 6 weeks, followed by continued protection in an AFO for an additional 4.5 months.
- ☐ By approximately 6 months after surgery, patients progress in therapy to a brace-free status if they are physically able.

The tibialis posterior can also be lengthened using fractional lengthening at the myotendinous junction. This method is recommended by Hoffer in the management of equinovarus in CP. It is also feasible in TBI and CVA, and does preserve function, especially when a relatively small amount of lengthening is needed. In general, a long

Z-lengthening allows a greater amount of correction and may be more optimal if minimal volitional control exists in a severe deformity.

TAL, SPLATT, and TFR are well-established procedures to correct equinovarus and toe flexion (Fig. 3.16). However, approximately 60% to 70% of patients still require use of an AFO because of residual gastrocsoleus weakness, most apparent during late stance phase when the body mass is anterior to the ankle joint. Weakness of the gastrocsoleus is, in part, the result of paresis that accompanies these spastic disorders, along with the additional weakness caused by the lengthening of the Achilles. The additional transfer of the long toe flexors—FHL and FDL—to the calcaneus augments strength of the gastrocsoleus group and helps stabilize the ankle. This transfer is performed at the time of TAL and SPLATT. As studied by Keenan, 70% of patients were brace free at follow-up when the extrinsic toe flexors were transferred to the calcaneus, compared with 30% of patients when the toe flexors were not transferred. Besides adding plantarflexion strength, transfer of the FHL and FDL can also help correct toe flexion deformities.

Others advocate anterior transfer of the long toe flexors to the dorsum of the foot to provide additional correction to an Achilles tendon lengthening. The transferred toe flexors thus assist dorsiflexion or function as a tenodesis to augment correction. The transfer of the long toe flexors is optimally indicated for equinus of the foot with persistent activity of the toe flexors, which produces curling of the toes during the swing phase of gait or a fixed flexion deformity.

In a child with CP, reconstruction of equinovarus often addresses the tibialis posterior instead of the tibialis anterior. EMGs help determine the muscles most responsible for the deformity and help in planning operative correction accordingly. If the tibialis anterior is most active in stance and swing phase of gait, the SPLATT procedure combined with the TAL as described for TBI and CVA is used. However, if EMGs during gait show the tibialis posterior to be continuously overactive or overactive in stance and during swing phase of gait, the tibialis posterior is lengthened using fractional lengthening. In the less common situation in which the tibialis posterior is active exclusively in swing, the muscle is either transferred anteriorly through the interosseous membrane to the dorsum of the foot or is split, and a portion is transferred to the lateral foot through the peroneus brevis tendon.

Transfer of the tibialis posterior both eliminates the deforming varus force of the tibialis posterior and transforms it into a dorsiflexor to help balance the equinus deformity. Before transfer of the tibialis posterior, adequate passive correction is desirable through physical therapy or serial casting because the transfer alone cannot overcome a rigid deformity.

- ▪ Anterior transfer of the tibialis posterior through the interosseous membrane
  - ☐ Three incisions are made.
  - ☐ The first is placed over the medial aspect of the foot along the course of the tibialis posterior tendon, which is isolated and detached distally.

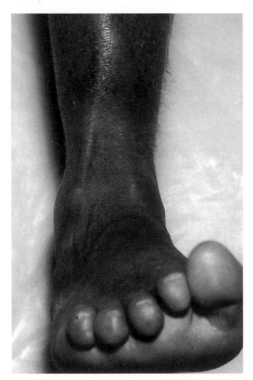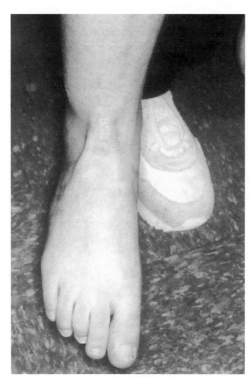

Figure 3.16   Postoperative photographs of patients following Achilles tendon lengthening, split tibialis anterior tendon transfer, and toe flexor release. Note the prominent split tibialis anterior, assisting with correction of varus.

- ☐ The second is placed longitudinally along the posterior border of the tibia, and the tendon is gently pulled and delivered from the first incision to the second incision.
- ☐ The third is placed on the anterior distal leg, and the tibialis anterior is elevated from the anterolateral surface of the tibia together with the anterior tibial artery, deep peroneal nerve, and extensor hallucis longus muscle.
- ☐ A rectangular window is cut in the interosseous membrane large enough to permit easy passage of the tibialis posterior tendon and muscle.
- ☐ Using a tendon passer or clamp placed on the suture on the tendon, the tibialis posterior is passed through the window to reach the anterior compartment. The tendon is then passed deep to the inferior extensor retinaculum.
- ☐ The foot is then held in a neutral position, and the tendon is attached to the base of the second metatarsal through a drill hole and secured with an interference screw or suture anchors into a roughed trough of bone.
- ☐ Alternatively, if insufficient length does not allow attachment to the second metatarsal, the tendon can be transferred to the middle cuneiform through a drill hole or attached with a suture anchor.
- ☐ Postoperatively, the foot is immobilized non–weight bearing for 6 to 8 weeks, followed by a physical therapy program for mobilization and functional retraining.

- ■ Split tibialis posterior tendon transfer to the lateral foot (Fig. 3.17)
  - ☐ The first incision is placed on the medial aspect of the foot, the distal 5 cm of the tibialis posterior tendon is split longitudinally, and the plantar half of the tendon is detached.
  - ☐ A long clamp pulls the split tendon into the second incision along the posterior tibia.
  - ☐ A third incision posterior to the lateral malleolus is made, and the split tendon is then transferred into this incision.
  - ☐ A fourth incision is placed over the peroneus brevis tendon. With the foot held in slight valgus, the split tendon is woven and sutured into the distal peroneus brevis tendon under tension.
  - ☐ Postoperatively, the foot is immobilized in neutral or slight valgus for 6 weeks in a short leg cast. Partial weight bearing is permitted in the cast.
  - ☐ Physical therapy is then initiated for mobilization and gradual strengthening.

If there is a severe, long-standing fixed hindfoot varus deformity, soft-tissue procedures using the described tendon transfers and lengthening may not be adequate for correction, even when combined with capsular release of the posterior ankle or medial joints. This often occurs when the TBI is sustained in a child or adolescent with an immature, developing skeleton. Fixed varus at the subtalar joint or a varus deformity within the calcaneus develops in some of these patients. If most of the deformity originates at the subtalar joint, corrective subtalar arthrodesis with a lateral

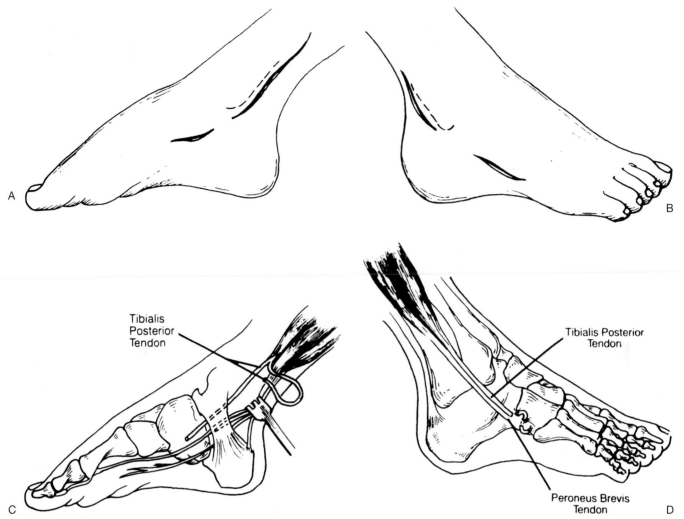

Figure 3.17   Split tibialis posterior tendon transfer as described by Green. (**A**) Two medial incisions are placed over the tibialis posterior. One incision is placed over the insertion, and the other incision is placed over the muscle belly in the medial calf. (**B**) Two lateral incisions are placed over the peroneal tendons for transfer and attachment of split tibialis posterior tendon. (**C**) The tibialis posterior tendon is split longitudinally from its insertion proximally to the musculotendinous junction and passed posterior to the tibia and fibula but anterior to all tendons and neurovascular bundle. (**D**) The split tendon is brought out through the proximal lateral incision, then passed to the lateral distal incision, and sutured to the peroneus brevis tendon. (Reproduced with permission from Hsu JD, Feiwell EN, Hoffer MM. Congenital neurologic disorders of the foot. In: Mann RA, Coughlin MJ, eds. Surgery of the foot and ankle. St. Louis: Mosby, 1993:589.)

closing wedge helps correct a fixed or bone deformity. CT scans or axial views of the calcaneus help evaluate the alignment of the subtalar joint as well as the shape and deformity of the calcaneus.

If the calcaneus is deformed with a varus component and the subtalar joint appears relatively normal and without degenerative changes, a calcaneal sliding osteotomy can be performed.

Results and Outcomes

Correction of the equinovarus foot in acquired spasticity has shown the potential for operative reconstruction. Good to excellent results are usually achieved in more than 80% of patients. It has also been specifically shown that a severe deformity that could not be fitted with an AFO could be improved enough to allow further correction and maintenance in an AFO. In ambulatory patients who preoperatively used an AFO, several patients are able to

become brace free following operative treatment. Some of the nonambulating patients also showed adequate improvement to become ambulatory with the additional help of an AFO. Poor results were associated with inadequate correction, recurrence of deformity, or residual weakness. The results in reconstruction of equinovarus reconstruction in CP have also been similarly satisfactory.

DISORDERS OF PARALYSIS

Polio residuals, CMT disease (hereditary motor–sensory neuropathy [HMSN], peroneal muscular atrophy), and other injuries or afflictions of peripheral nerves produce weakness or paralysis. Weakness (not spasticity) is produced by affliction of the lower motor neurons. Management is therefore directed toward splinting or bracing to support the weak limb and, when indicated, operative procedures to augment or overcome lost function. Even though the following sections discuss and emphasize polio and CMT disease (which are two of the more common types of paralytic disorders), many of the examination findings, deformities, and treatment strategies apply to other types of paralytic deformities as well.

PATHOGENESIS

Etiology

Infection from poliovirus can result in a wide range of clinical symptoms (Table 3.3). Many patients who contract a poliovirus infection are asymptomatic and have no neurologic sequella. However, paralytic poliomyelitis, which targets the anterior horn cells of the spinal cord, can result in permanent motor paresis or paralysis. The range of involvement varies from specific weakness of individual muscle groups to complete limb paralysis.

HMSN is a group of hereditary disorders that includes CMT. CMT disease (HMSN type I) is an inherited autosomal dominant condition involving peripheral nerves. Motor nerves are among the more severely afflicted, resulting in progressive muscular weakness and atrophy. Sensibility defects such as loss of proprioception also occur. HSMN type II is a form of CMT that has not shown a clear inheritance pattern.

Clinical onset of type I usually occurs in the first and second decades of life, and results in severe impairment of nerve conduction times and hypertrophic endoneurial changes seen on nerve biopsy. In type II CMT, age of onset is generally later, usually the third to fifth decade, and involvement more often affects the lower extremity with much less sensory loss than in type I.

Epidemiology

The incidence of poliomyelitis has decreased dramatically in the Western world since the introduction of polio vaccination in the United States in 1954. A large number of adults older than 55 years, however, are still faced with postpolio problems. The lower extremities are involved more often than the upper limbs. In addition, the large number of immigrants to the United States continues to add to the incidence of patients who have sustained poliomyelitis. Outbreaks of poliomyelitis do occur in the developed world, usually in groups of people who have not been vaccinated. Polio often occurs after someone travels to a region where the disease is common. As a result of a massive, global vaccination campaign over the past 20 years, polio exists only in a few countries in Africa and Asia.

One of the most common inherited neurologic disorders is CMT disease, also known as HMSN. The incidence of CMT disease is about 1 in 2,500 people in the United States, as noted by the National Institute of Neurological Disorders and Stroke. Men are afflicted more often than women with CMT. The incidence of cavus foot deformities ranges and progresses from 20% in the first decade of life to 67% among patients past the first decade of life. CMT usually does not shorten the patient's normal life expectancy.

Pathophysiology

Poliomyelitis

The severity of the paralysis is determined by the extent of the neuronal infection and number of neurons affected. The paralysis may therefore involve one or more limbs. Because the anterior horn cells are usually the most significant portion of the spinal cord involved, motor paralysis occurs usually in the absence of sensory deficits. Spasticity does not usually develop. *Postpoliomyelitis*, or *postpolio syndrome*, is a term used to describe a recurrence or increase of weakness and muscle wasting in individuals noted 30 to 40 years after the initial infection. Postpolio syndrome is seen in 20% to 80% of original victims. It does not indicate a recurrence of infection, but rather it reflects physiologic and aging changes and subsequent deterioration of paralytic muscles already burdened by the loss of neuromuscular function. The result is additional weakness and sometimes pain.

Charcot–Marie–Tooth Disease

This disease is characterized by a progressive symmetrical peripheral neuropathy that involves demyelination and loss of axons. Degenerative changes in the spinal cord can also be seen in the later stages. Hypertrophic endoneurial nerve changes are seen on nerve biopsy. The peripheral neuropathy results in progressive loss of motor function, characterized by weakness, muscle atrophy, and limb deformities secondary to muscle imbalance. The peroneal muscles, especially the peroneus brevis, are often initially

TABLE 3.3 CLASSIFICATION OF POLIOVIRUS INFECTIONS

Type of Illness	Occurrence (%)	Involved Tissue	Symptoms
Asymptomatic illness	90	Oropharynx, gut	None
Abortive poliomyelitis (minor illness)	5	Oropharynx, gut	Fever, headache, malaise, sore throat, vomiting
Nonparalytic poliomyelitis (aseptic meningitis)	1–2	Oropharynx, gut, meninges, CNS	Back pain, muscle spasms (+ symptoms of minor illness)
Paralytic poliomyelitis (major illness)	0.1–2	Oropharynx, gut, meninges, CNS	Paralysis (+ above symptoms)

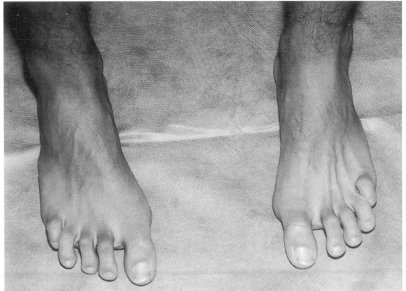

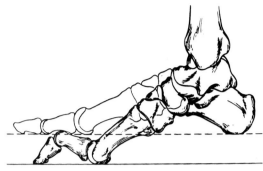

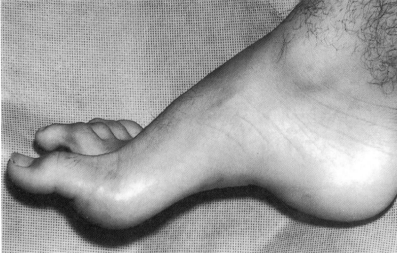

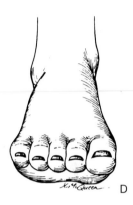

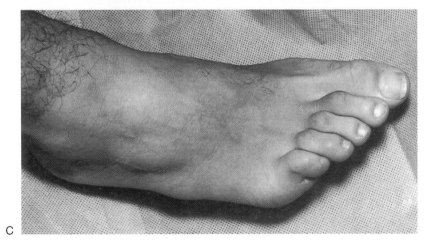

Figure 3.18 (A to C) Photographs of young adult male's feet with Charcot–Marie–Tooth disease showing the cavus foot and claw toe deformities. Note the high arch associated with the cavus foot. There is also plantarflexion of the first ray. Claw toes are characterized by extension at the metatarsophalangeal joints and flexion at the proximal and distal interphalangeal joints. (D) Illustration of cavus foot with plantarflexion of the first ray and claw toes. (D modified from Richardson GE. Neurogenic disorders. In: Canale ST, ed. Campbell's operative orthopaedics. St. Louis: Mosby, 1998:1828.)

involved, thus the former name *peroneal muscular atrophy*. As the disease progresses, symmetrical muscle weakness and atrophy can become apparent in the toe extensors and, subsequently, the tibialis anterior. Weakness of the tibialis anterior leads to a drop foot gait. Intrinsic foot weakness or various combinations of muscle imbalance lead to a cavus foot and claw toes. Often, the peroneus longus is relatively spared compared with the peroneus brevis and tibialis anterior, resulting in a plantar flexed, pronated first metatarsal. Weakness of the peroneus

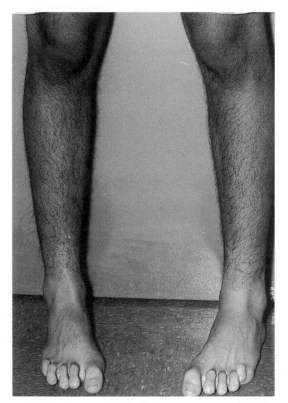

Figure 3.19   Photograph of patient with Charcot–Marie–Tooth disease showing bilateral and symmetrical calf muscle atrophy. Cavus feet and claw toe deformities are also apparent. Muscles proximal to the knee were not afflicted.

brevis and sparing of the tibialis posterior accentuates forefoot equinus and inversion of the foot at the midtarsal joints, leading to varus of the hindfoot (Figs. 3.18 to 3.20). The upper limbs may become involved, being characterized by involvement of the distal muscles, including the hand intrinsic and thenar muscles. In both the lower and upper extremities, the process is usually limited to the more distal muscles. Muscles proximal to the knee or elbow are usually not affected.

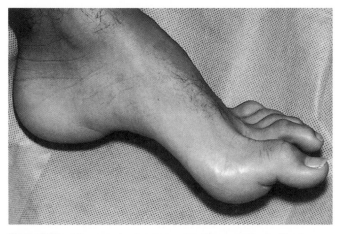

Figure 3.20   Photograph of patient with Charcot–Marie–Tooth disease with equinus contracture secondary to weakness of the tibialis anterior. Muscle imbalance has led to cavus foot, plantarflexion of the first ray, and claw toe deformities.

A variable loss of sensory nerve fibers can result in loss of proprioception and vibratory sensibility. Vibratory loss is usually limited to below the knee. In some patients, the degeneration of sensory nerves can also result in reduced ability to feel heat, cold, and pain. Conversely, some patients may have associated extremity pain, which varies from mild to severe.

Classification

This disease is part of a group of disorders termed HMSN (Table 3.4). There are now up to five forms (CMT types 1 to 4, and CMTX) Classic CMT disease is HMSN type I. A similar but nonhereditary disorder, also considered CMT disease, is HMSN type II. An additional variant of CMT is termed the *neuronal type*, which is characterized by autosomal dominant inheritance and onset in middle age or later and can show foot and ankle muscle weakness and atrophy that is more severe than in the other types of CMT. The intrinsic muscles of the hand are usually not as involved in the neuronal type.

DIAGNOSIS

History and Physical Examination

The main complaints, followed by a chronology of associated problems and treatments, are elicited. Because of the inheritance patterns of CMT disease and related disorders, a family history of neurologic disorders is significant. Many patients with long-standing neurologic disorders are well adapted to the disability, and what may appear as an obvious or severe deformity may not be problematic to the patient and may not require intervention. Specific problems related to pain and functional limitations are among the most important. A knowledge of prior treatment including physical therapy, orthotic and brace management, and prior operative management is important. Patients with a new or progressive sensory or motor loss require evaluation by a neurologist.

Physical examination of the patient with paralytic disorders usually starts with the patient sitting. Appearance of deformity, alignment, and presence of limb length deformity, limb atrophy, and skin callosities or breakdown is observed. Motor examination includes evaluation of strength and coordination. Sensory examination includes gross sensibility with light touch, sharp and dull or hot and cold discrimination, proprioception, and vibratory evaluation. Proprioception and vibratory sensibility are often lost early in CMT disease. Further neurologic examination includes testing for deep tendon reflexes and presence of cerebellar involvement such as tremors, ataxic movements, or loss of coordination. Specific examination of the foot includes active and passive ranges of motion of the ankle, hindfoot, midfoot, and forefoot joints. Deformity is assessed for severity and flexibility. Degree of pes cavus, presence of a hindfoot varus component (Fig. 3.21), plantarflexion of the first ray, and the common coexistence of claw toes of the hallux and lesser toes are noted. Compensatory forefoot valgus may develop in a patient with hindfoot varus.

Examination is then performed with the patient standing to note any change in deformity with weight bearing. Examination from behind enables the examiner to visualize

TABLE 3.4 ETIOLOGY OF PES CAVUS

Classification	Manifestation
Neuromuscular	
Muscle disease	Muscular dystrophy
Afflictions of peripheral nerves and lumbosacral spinal nerve roots	Charcot–Marie–Tooth disease Spinal dysraphism Polyneuritis Traumatic peroneal palsy Intraspinal tumor
Disease of the anterior horn cell of the spinal cord	Poliomyelitis Spinal dysraphism Diastematomyelia Syringomyelia Sprinal cord tumors Spinal musculature atrophy
Long tract and central disease	Friedreich ataxia Roussy–Levy syndrome
Congenital	Idiopathic cavus foot Residual of clubfoot Arthrogryposis
Traumatic	Residuals of compartment syndrome (Volkmann ischemic contracture) Crush injury to lower extremity Severe burns Fracture malunion

Adapted from Ibrahim K. Pes cavus. In: Evarts CM, ed. Surgery of the musculoskeletal system. New York: Churchill Livingstone, 1990:4015–4034; and Wapner KL. Pes cavus. In: Myerson MS, ed. Foot and ankle disorders. Philadelphia: WB Saunders, 2000:919–941.

hindfoot deformities such as varus. Limb length discrepancies (common in polio) are noted with the patient both sitting and standing. With the patient sitting, relative calf shortening may be visually apparent. The knees may appear at different levels. With the patient standing, the relative levels of the knees and the iliac crests can be assessed. The patient is then evaluated with and without shoes during gait.

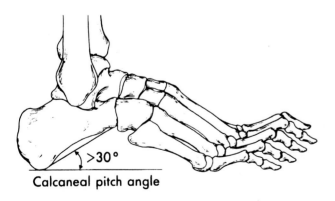

Figure 3.21 Illustration of cavus foot with increased calcaneal pitch angle. An angle of greater than 30° is often associated with a hindfoot varus. (Reproduced with permission from Richardson GE. Neurogenic disorders. In: Canale ST, ed. Campbell's operative orthopaedics. St. Louis: Mosby, 1998:1830.)

Evaluation involves noting stability of the limb during weight bearing, the stride length, and the heel position at heel strike and stance phase. Accentuation of toe deformities is noted. Recurvatum of the knee during stance implies weakness of the quadriceps. Ankle inversion or a tendency of the ankle to collapse may be due to peroneal weakness or lateral ligament dysfunction, or to varus deformity of the hindfoot or a combination of them. Weakness of the tibialis anterior can be noted with an inability to heel walk or a tendency of the foot to slap the floor at heel strike. More severe loss of the tibialis anterior results in a complete drop foot. Extension of the toes during the swing phase of gait may be due to the toe extensors attempting to substitute for weakness of the tibialis anterior. During stance, gastrocsoleus weakness can often be seen when the ankle buckles with forward movement of the tibia on the talus. If severe weakness of the gastrocsoleus exists, a crouch gait may occur. If the patient uses a brace or other orthotic or assistive device, evaluation also includes noting the effect or benefits of the brace.

Electrodiagnostic evaluation includes EMG and nerve conduction velocity (NCV) studies. An abnormal NCV study with prolonged latencies and a minimal decrease in velocity suggests axonal degeneration. Significant slowing of conduction indicates demyelination. If there is anterior horn cell loss (as in polio), EMG studies can show prolonged polyphasics, positive sharp waves, and muscle fibrillations. Neurologic consultation is needed if a definitive diagnosis has not been made.

Clinical Features

Poliomyelitis.   The most common clinical foot problems include loss of dorsiflexion (drop foot), loss of plantarflexion, and cavus foot with claw toes. With unilateral involvement, limb atrophy with limb length discrepancy may exist. Other lower extremity problems can include paralytic subluxation of the hip and angulation deformities of the knee (including valgus, varus, and recurvatum).

The loss of dorsiflexion is usually from weakness of the tibialis anterior and toe extensors. The loss of plantarflexion strength is usually from weakness of the gastrocsoleus. Cavus foot and coexisting claw toes are complex deformities, probably due to relative muscle imbalance between the intrinsic and extrinsic foot muscles. There is often a component of varus hindfoot with the cavus foot. The loss of dorsiflexion and plantarflexion causes obvious functional problems with ambulation. Over time, secondary degenerative problems of the ankle sometimes develop as a result of abnormal joint loading.

In polio and CMT disease as well as other types of cavus deformity, clinical symptoms vary with the specific cause and degree of deformity. Symptoms include generalized fatigue of the foot and discomfort caused by abnormal joint loading (i.e., the loss of subtalar and transverse tarsal motion). Body weight may be concentrated on the hindfoot under the calcaneus and in the forefoot under the metatarsal heads, in part, owing to the high arch, which does not participate in bearing and sharing body weight. Metatarsalgia and callosities can develop in these areas of concentrated weight bearing (see below).

CMT Disease.   The progressive weakness of CMT disease often leads to characteristic limb deformities and associated problems. The progression of weakness commonly involves sequentially the peroneus brevis, toe extensors, tibialis anterior, and foot intrinsic muscles. Initial clinical findings may include loss of foot eversion. With involvement of the tibialis anterior and toe extensors, a drop foot gait with loss of toe extension develops. Intrinsic weakness and subsequent muscle imbalance between the extrinsic foot and ankle muscles can lead to cavus foot and claw toes. Residual strength of the peroneus longus relative to the peroneus brevis and tibialis anterior will result in a plantarflexed, pronated first metatarsal and eventually result in fixed pronation of the forefoot. The cavus foot leads to secondary problems of pressure concentration, associated skin callosities, and possible skin breakdown on the hindfoot and under the metatarsal heads.

With long-standing dropfoot or muscle imbalance with overpull of the gastrocsoleus, an equinus contracture (see Fig. 3.20) and cavus or cavovarus may develop in some patients with CMT. Footdrop and selective progressive muscle weakness cause fixed deformities and contractures in the feet. The overall clinical picture may be one of leg atrophy, footdrop, pes cavus, plantarflexion of the first ray, hindfoot varus, and claw toes. Long-standing deformities, especially in the growing child, result in fixed bone deformities. The hips and knees are usually not involved in CMT, so patients retain the ability to ambulate.

Variable sensibility deficits can occur. Proprioception and vibratory loss is often noted; more severe involvement can lead to loss of protective sensation and contribute to the risks of skin breakdown.

Radiologic Features

- Radiographic evaluation of the patient with paralytic disorders includes standard radiographs of the foot and ankle—weight bearing if possible.
- Radiographs document the presence and degree of deformities as well as any associated degenerative changes.
- Findings such as cavus, varus, and claw toes are well demonstrated.
  - In the cavus deformity, the lateral weight-bearing radiograph demonstrates an upward inclination of the calcaneus, the arch is elevated, the navicular may be positioned at the height of the arch, and there is a downward inclination of the metatarsals (Fig. 3.21).
  - Claw toe deformities, also visualized on the lateral radiograph, are characterized by extension at the MTP joints and by flexion of the PIP and DIP joints.
  - Severe cavus deformity is often accompanied with hindfoot varus, and an upward pitch of the calcaneus of greater than 30° usually indicates marked heel varus (Fig. 3.21). An axial view of the calcaneus helps demonstrate hindfoot varus.
- In patients with paralysis, radiographs also reveal secondary degenerative joint changes that can occur from long-standing abnormal joint loading or joint instability.
- If ankle instability is in question (in the patient with varus deformity and a history of multiple ankle sprains), weight-bearing ankle radiographs of the mortise can assist with the diagnosis.
- Stress radiographs of the mortise with the foot held in inversion and lateral radiographs with an anterior drawer maneuver (pulling the calcaneus and talus forward on the tibia) help to establish the diagnosis.
  - Stress radiographs are usually performed bilaterally for comparison.
- Radiographs are also important in the evaluation of the patient who has undergone previous operative procedures. Many adult patients with paralytic deformities have undergone procedures in childhood, and, often, few or no records or radiographs are available.
- CT is used to further investigate joint congruency or degree of degeneration.
- MRI is useful when soft-tissue or cartilage integrity is in question.
  - Hindfoot varus with ankle instability often leads to recurrent sprains and associated osteochondral defects. These defects and the integrity of the lateral ankle ligaments are further visualized with MRI.

TREATMENT

Nonsurgical Treatment

In disorders of paralysis, the main problems are usually weakness, associated limb instability, subsequent deformity, and degenerative joint arthrosis in long-standing disorders. Treatment strategies usually start with nonoperative options. If these are not successful, operative reconstruction can be considered. Many patients with slowly progressive disorders such as CMT become accustomed to the loss of function despite obvious deformities. Many patients remain

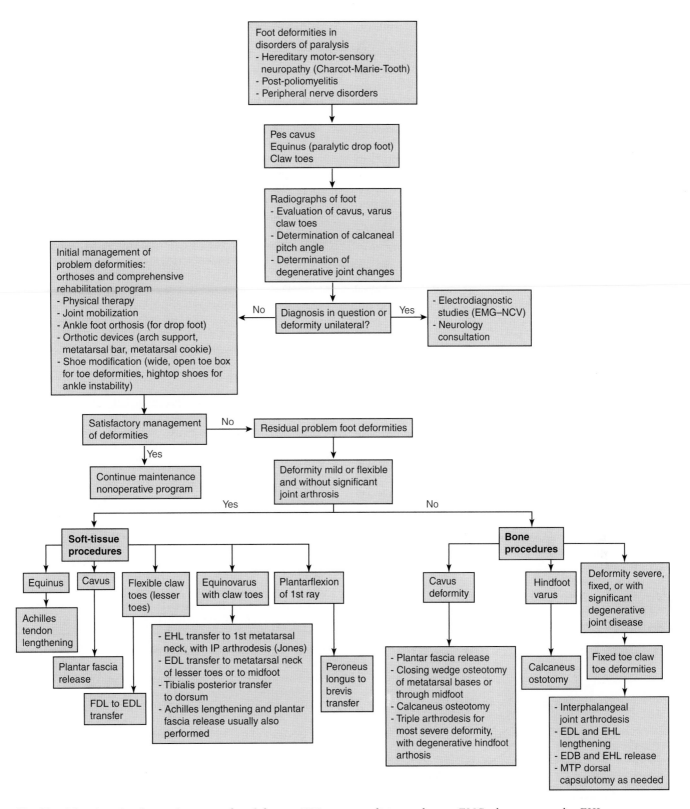

Algorithm 3.2 Algorithm for paralytic cavus foot deformity. EDL, extensor digitorum longus; EMG, electromyography; EHL, extensor hallux longus; FDL, flexor digitorum longus; IP, interphalangeal; MTP, metatarsophalangeal; NCV, nerve conduction velocity.

functional and pain free, and no specific intervention is needed.

Initial nonoperative treatment in paralytic disorders includes a comprehensive rehabilitation program for joint mobilization and bracing to prevent or treat contracture or deformity, strengthening, and functional retraining (Algorithm 3.2). The orthopaedic surgeon works closely with other members of the rehabilitation team including physical and occupational therapists, orthotists, pedorthotists, rehabilitation nurses, neurologists, and physical medicine specialists.

In CMT and polio with mild cavus, cavovarus, and claw toe deformity, nonoperative options include custom orthotic devices and extra-depth shoes that help decrease the areas of concentrated weight on the plantar aspect of the foot and allow ample room for the deformities. These devices increase comfort and function, but do not treat or improve the deformity. Mild flexible varus can be accommodated with a lateral wedge to help stabilize the foot. Early operative treatment of the cavus foot in CMT using soft-tissue procedures when the hindfoot is flexible has several advantages to prolonged nonoperative treatment, possibly delaying the need for more extensive procedures later.

If there is weakness of ankle dorsiflexion or plantarflexion, an AFO can support the ankle and manage footdrop. Dynamic bracing can be added to facilitate function, such as using a spring-loaded component to dynamically add ankle dorsiflexion during the swing phase of gait. If there is lateral ankle instability secondary to a chronic varus hindfoot, initial treatment can include light canvas or synthetic sports braces, high-top athletic shoes, or lateral heel wedges.

Surgical Treatment

Early operative management of the cavus foot in CMT, when the foot is flexible, can delay the need for more extensive reconstructive procedures.

Surgery for the cavus foot can be divided into several categories, with specific operative planning being based on individual deformity. Options include soft-tissue procedures (plantar fascia release, with or without tendon transfers or lengthening), osteotomy to correct or improve the high arch, and hindfoot fusion, usually consisting of triple arthrodesis and performed for more severe unstable or rigid deformity with degenerative joint changes (Fig. 3.22). Soft-tissue procedures are often combined with bone procedures and are individualized. Common soft-tissue procedures are summarized in Table 3.5.

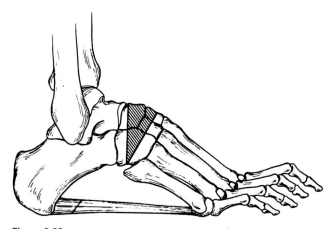

Figure 3.22 Operative management options for the paralytic cavus foot. Initial treatment often consists of plantar fascial release. Note the line of incision in posterior portion of plantar fascia. Closing dorsal wedge osteotomy through the midfoot (or base of the metatarsals) is also depicted. (Reproduced with permission from Richardson GE. Neurogenic disorders. In: Canale ST, ed. Campbell's operative orthopaedics. St. Louis: Mosby, 1998:1840.)

Soft-tissue procedures should be performed when the deformity is flexible. They include plantar fascial release, tendon lengthening, and transfers. The plantar fascia becomes tight secondary to the cavus deformity. It then becomes a contributing factor to plantarflexion of the forefoot and to the varus component.

■ Plantar fascial release
  □ An incision is placed on the medial border of the hindfoot, starting at the distal aspect of the calcaneal fat pad. Care is taken to avoid injury to the medial and lateral plantar nerves.
  □ Dissection is carried out down to the plantar fascia. The superficial subcutaneous fat is dissected free.
  □ The fascia is isolated and incised, taking care to gently separate the fascia from the underlying tendons and neurovascular structures.
  □ A 5-mm strip of fascia can be removed.
  □ Postoperative management includes cast immobilization for about 4 weeks to help maintain or improve correction.
  □ The plantar fascial release is often combined with other procedures that require additional time of immobilization.

Several tendon lengthening and transfer procedures have been described in the reconstruction of the cavus foot deformity (see Table 3.5). In long-standing footdrop imbalance, shortening of the gastrocsoleus can develop and requires TAL. Achilles lengthening can be performed in a variety of ways described earlier. In general, the open Z-lengthening procedure has good application in paralytic deformities because it allows a precise amount of lengthening to be obtained and can be combined with other soft-tissue or bone procedures.

Transfer of the extensor hallux longus (EHL) to the neck of the first metatarsal is indicated when there is a claw toe deformity of the hallux, along with flexible plantarflexion of the first metatarsal. The transfer, often referred to as the *Jones procedure*, is usually combined with interphalangeal fusion of the hallux. The EHL transfer eliminates its contribution to the hallux hyperextension at the MTP joint, and its power is transferred to augment foot dorsiflexion in a dropfoot. The transfer may also help alleviate the plantarflexion deformity of the first metatarsal and thus decrease the cavus of the first ray. The procedure is usually combined with plantar fascia release and transfer of the extensor digitorum longus (EDL) tendons (discussed later).

■ Transfer of the EHL to the first metatarsal, interphalangeal fusion (Jones procedure; Fig. 3.23)
  □ A longitudinal incision is placed on the dorsomedial aspect of the hallux, starting at the distal phalanx and continuing proximally and laterally to the level of the metatarsal neck.
  □ The EHL tendon is released from the distal phalanx and mobilized from the extensor mechanism.
  □ Attention is then directed to fusion of the interphalangeal joint. The capsule is opened and collateral ligaments are released.
  □ The cartilage surfaces of the base of the distal phalanx and head of the proximal phalanx are removed and the surfaces fashioned with a rongeur or power saw so

TABLE 3.5 SOFT-TISSUE PROCEDURES FOR PARALYTIC CAVUS, CAVOVARUS, AND CLAW TOE DEFORMITIES

Procedure	Indications/Comments
Plantar fascia release	A usual first step in cavus reconstruction. The plantar fascia becomes secondarily contracted from long-standing cavus, and release is usually combined with other soft-tissue or bone procedures
Achilles tendon lengthening	Weakness of the TA leads to dropfoot, resulting in Achilles contracture and secondary equinus
EHL transfer to first metatarsal neck	"Jones procedure" helps eliminate EHL contribution to hallux claw toe. EHL power augments foot dorsiflexion, usually combined with hallux IP fusion Transfer to the dorsum of the metatarsal may also help lessen the metatarsal plantarflexion and thus decrease the cavus of this ray
EDL transfer to metatarsal neck of lesser toes	Use of Jones procedure to eliminate EDL contribution of lesser toe clawing Transfer to metatarsal may help lessen plantarflexion of the metatarsal and thus decrease cavus, also helping to augment foot dorsiflexion
EDL transfer to midfoot	Transfer to the lateral cuneiform helps eliminate EDL contribution to claw toe Transfers of EDL adds dorsiflexion force for dropfoot
Peroneus longus to peroneus brevis transfer	Eliminates first ray plantarflexion force and augments (typically weak) foot eversion
Tibialis posterior transfer to dorsum of foot	Helps relieve varus component produced by the TP tendon; augments weak foot dorsiflexion
FDL to EDL transfer of lesser toes	"Girdlestone procedure" is designed for flexible lesser toe deformities Flexor force at distal phalanx is transferred to dorsum of toe to extend distal phalanx

TA, tibialis anterior; EHL, extensor hallucis longus; IP, interphalangeal joint;
EDL, extensor digitorum longus; TP, tibialis posterior; FDL, flexor digitorum longus.
Modified from Wapner KL. Pes cavus. In: Myerson MS, ed. Foot and ankle disorders.
Philadelphia: WB Saunders, 2000:928.

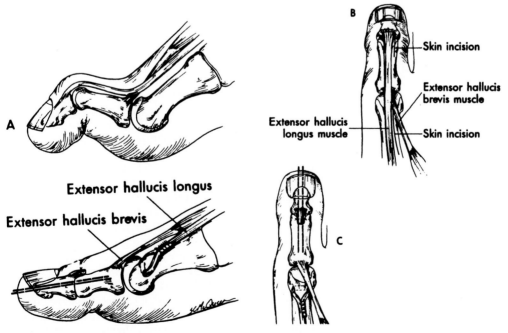

Figure 3.23 Jones type procedure for correction of clawing of the great toe. (**A**, *top*) Lateral view of the claw toe deformity (**A**, *bottom*). Lateral view following transfer of the extensor hallucis longus to the neck of the first metatarsal and combined with arthrodesis of the interphalangeal joint. (**B**) Dorsal view showing skin incisions. (**C**) Dorsal and (**D**) lateral views following transfer of the extensor hallucis and interphalangeal arthrodesis. The procedure corrects the claw toe deformity and (at least theoretically) helps correct plantarflexion of the first ray. (Reproduced with permission from Richardson GE. Neurogenic disorders. In: Canale ST, ed. Campbell's operative orthopaedics. St. Louis: Mosby, 1998:1835.)

that the joint will be fused in about 0° to 5° of flexion. Internal fixation is accomplished with crossed smooth pins, tension band wires, or compression screws.

☐ The free end of the EHL is then passed, from lateral to medial, through a hole in the metatarsal neck.

☐ The foot is then held in about 15° of dorsiflexion, and the tendon is then sutured back onto itself using 2-0 or 3-0 nonabsorbable sutures. An interference screw can also be used to secure the tendon to the metatarsal. The foot is maintained in dorsiflexion throughout the remainder of the procedure.

☐ After wound closure, the foot is placed in a well-padded cast in slight dorsiflexion.

☐ Postoperatively, the tendon transfer is protected in a cast for 4 to 6 weeks. Because of potential swelling, the cast must be well padded and neurovascular function must be monitored closely.

Transfer of the EDL tendons to the midfoot is indicated when there are flexible claw toe deformities and flexible, mild cavus (Fig. 3.24). The EDL tendons are transferred to the third cuneiform or to the third and fifth metatarsals. The procedure helps eliminate the extensor

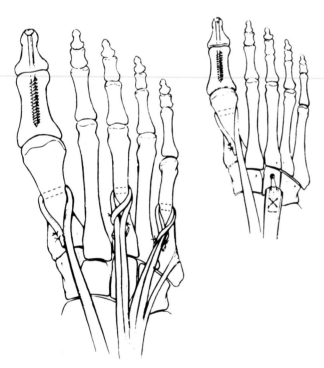

Figure 3.24 Transfer of the extensor digitorum longus (EDL) tendons to the midfoot (combined with Jones procedure). The hallux is addressed by transfer of the extensor hallucis longus combined with arthrodesis of the interphalangeal joint. The EDL tendons are then detached, leaving the extensor digitorum brevis tendons intact. The EDL tendons from the second and third toes are transferred through the drill hole in the third metatarsal, and the tendons from the fourth and fifth toes are transferred through the drill hole in the fifth metatarsal. Alternatively, all four tendons can be transferred into a drill hole placed into the third cuneiform (as described by Hibbs). (Reproduced with permission from Wapner KL. Pes cavus. In: Myerson MS, ed. Foot and ankle disorders. Philadelphia: WB Saunders, 2000:931.)

force at the MTP joint of each toe contributing to the claw toe deformity, and it transfers the force to help augment foot dorsiflexion for drop foot. This procedure is often combined with transfer of the EHL to the first metatarsal (Jones procedure, described earlier).

Transfer of the peroneus longus to the peroneus brevis is indicated when there is weakness of the peroneus brevis and relative overpull of a preserved peroneus longus. The procedure helps eliminate the plantarflexion force of the peroneus longus and helps restore some of the lost foot eversion from peroneus brevis weakness. This procedure is often combined with calcaneal osteotomy and can be performed through the same incision. With the foot held in slight eversion, the slack is removed from the peroneus longus, and the tendons are sutured to each other. The peroneus longus can be released distal to the tenodesis to remove all deforming force of the peroneus longus on the first ray.

Transfer of the tibialis posterior is an additional procedure to help augment dorsiflexion when the tibialis anterior is weak. The tibialis posterior can be transferred through the interosseous membrane to the dorsum of the foot, or it can be split and half of it transferred to the lateral foot into the peroneus brevis (Fig. 3.17). These transfers also help relieve some of the varus component in the cavovarus foot. The operative procedure and postoperative care are as described earlier under spastic disorders. For flexible claw toes, several soft-tissue procedures remain popular. These include flexor tendon releases to decrease the flexion on the distal phalanx, extensor lengthening to decrease the extension at the MTP joint, and the FDL to EDL (Girdlestone) procedure, which transfers the deforming flexion force of the FDL on the distal phalanx into a corrective force at the PIP joint. Although these procedures remain popular, fusion of the PIP joint, especially in the skeletally mature patient, results in a predictable and longlasting correction.

Soft-tissue procedures have their greatest application when the foot and toe deformities are flexible, and they have shown application in younger patients in whom more extensive procedures are avoided until later in life. However, when deformities are no longer flexible, especially in an older patient, bone procedures can be more predictable and can yield a greater amount of correction. There are several basic bone procedures performed (Table 3.6). For the fixed cavus deformity, the abnormally high arch of the cavus foot is improved with closing wedge osteotomy in the midfoot tarsal bones or metatarsals. Plantar fasciotomy is usually included with the midfoot or metatarsal osteotomy. A crescentic osteotomy of the calcaneus can be used to help decrease the calcaneal pitch angle. For fixed varus of the hindfoot, correction using a lateral closing wedge or lateral sliding osteotomy of the calcaneus is performed. For the severe, rigid cavovarus foot, or foot with secondary painful degenerative changes involving the hindfoot joints, triple arthrodesis is performed. Claw toes that are not flexible can be managed with PIP fusion, usually combined with EHL lengthening, extensor digitorum brevis (EDB) tenotomy, and dorsal MTP capsulotomy.

Proximal metatarsal osteotomy has been described for the management of the cavus deformity in CMT disease. The procedure has application in the cavus type foot in other

TABLE 3.6 BONE PROCEDURES FOR PARALYTIC CAVUS, CAVOVARUS, AND CLAW TOE DEFORMITIES

Procedure	Indications/Comments
Metatarsal osteotomies	Closing wedge osteotomy placed at the base of the metatarsal. Can be used only for the first metatarsal or, as needed, for all of the metatarsals. Usually combined with plantar fasciotomy
Midfoot osteotomies	An alternative to the metatarsal osteotomy. Can be individualized and placed where most of the high-arch deformity exists. Usually combined with plantar fasciotomy
Calcaneal osteotomy	Lateral wedge closing osteotomy used for hindfoot varus. Variations include a crescentic osteotomy and an osteotomy combined with subtalar fusion, depending on the nature and location of the deformity. CT scan of the calcaneus helps in selection for calcaneal corrective procedure
Triple arthrodesis	Used in the most severe, rigid deformities. Also used when there is secondary painful degenerative arthrosis of the hindfoot joints from chronic deformity. Variations such as subtalar fusion alone can be used with specific deformities or areas of symptoms
Interphalangeal joint fusions	For fixed claw toe deformities, PIP fusion is usually combined with EDL lengthening, EDB tenotomy, and MTP dorsal capsulotomy

CT, computerized tomography; PIP, proximal interphalangeal joint; EDL,
extensor digitorum longus; EDB, extensor digitorum brevis; MTP, metatarsophalangeal.
Modified from Wapner KL. Pes cavus. In: Myerson MS, ed. Foot and ankle disorders.
Philadelphia: WB Saunders, 2000:928.

disorders too, including idiopathic, posttraumatic, or other neurologic or paralytic conditions. It has particular use when the apex of the cavus deformity is at or near the tarsometatarsal joints or base of the metatarsals. Radiographs can be traced on paper and trial osteotomies placed to simulate correction and estimate the amount of wedge necessary for correction.

A similar alternative to the osteotomies placed at the base of the metatarsals includes osteotomies placed in the midfoot through the tarsometatarsal joints or through the cuboid, cuneiforms, and navicular bone. These procedures should not be performed before skeletal maturity and normal muscle balance should be present.

Calcaneal osteotomy has several variations and is used for persistent or fixed hindfoot varus. It can also correct a component of increased calcaneal pitch angle (dorsiflexion position). These osteotomies are often combined with other bone procedures. A common variation uses a lateral closing wedge to correct the varus (Fig. 3.25). Alternatively, a sliding osteotomy to translate the calcaneus laterally can be performed. A crescentic osteotomy is an additional alternative and, with dorsal translation of the posterior fragment, helps correct severe dorsiflexion inclination of the calcaneus (Fig. 3.26). The crescentic osteotomy can be combined with a translation component to correct the varus also. If there is painful degenerative arthrosis of the subtalar joint, the closing wedge can be incorporated into a subtalar fusion.

The triple arthrodesis is indicated for severe, rigid cavovarus deformities. It is also useful when there are secondary painful degenerative arthritic changes of the hindfoot. The triple arthrodesis includes fusion of the subtalar, calcaneocuboid, and talonavicular joints (Fig. 3.27). In removing cartilage and subchondral bone for the arthrodesis, a closing wedge can be incorporated into the subtalar and calcaneocuboid joints to correct hindfoot varus and inversion, respectively. Incorporating a dorsal closing wedge in the calcaneocuboid and talonavicular joints also helps correct the cavus components (Figs. 3.28 and 3.29). The triple

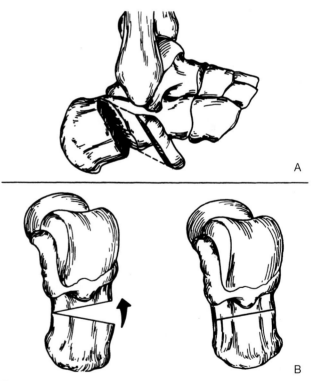

Figure 3.25 Lateral closing wedge calcaneal osteotomy to correct hindfoot varus. This is often referred to as the *Dwyer osteotomy*. (**A**) Lateral view showing removal of bone wedge. (**B**) Dorsal view showing correction of deformity. Technique is as described by Dwyer FC in Journal of Bone and Joint Surgery (Br) 1959;41:80. (Reproduced with permission from Richardson GE. Neurogenic disorders. In: Canale ST, ed. Campbell's operative orthopaedics. St. Louis: Mosby, 1998:1842.)

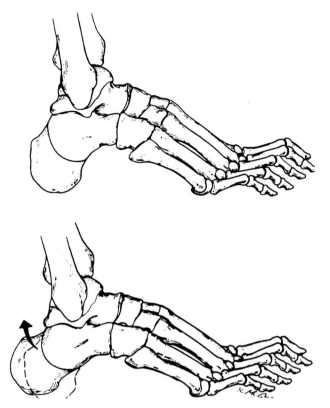

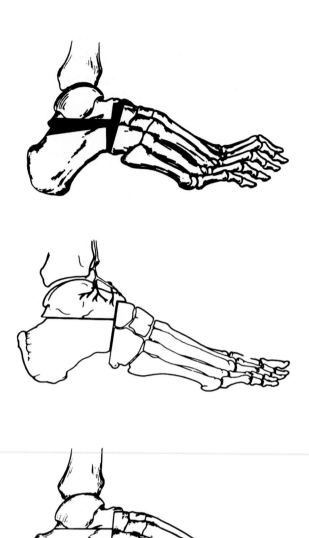

Figure 3.26 Crescentic calcaneal osteotomy to help correct cavus deformity. A crescentic osteotomy is placed through a lateral approach to the calcaneus. The posterior portion is moved dorsally to decrease calcaneal pitch angle and correct deformity. Technique is as described by Bateman JE, ed. Foot science. Philadelphia: WB Saunders, 1976. (Reproduced with permission from Richardson GE. Neurogenic disorders. In: Canale ST, ed. Campbell's operative orthopaedics. St. Louis: Mosby, 1998:1842.)

Figure 3.27 Triple arthrodesis for correction of hind-foot deformity. It has application in the correction of the long-standing or severe cavus deformity, especially if secondary joint degenerative changes are present. Technique is as depicted by Siffert RS, et al. Clinical Orthopaedics 1966;45:101. (Reproduced with permission from Richardson GE. Neurogenic disorders. In: Canale ST, ed. Campbell's operative orthopaedics. St. Louis: Mosby, 1998:1848.)

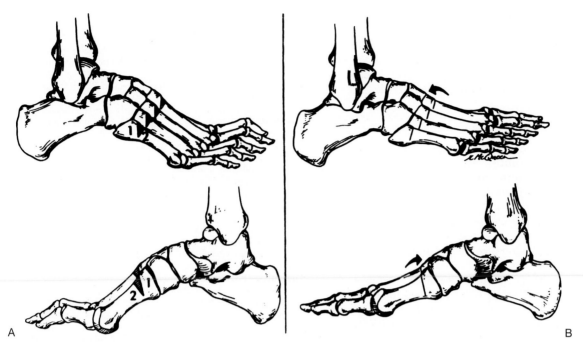

Figure 3.28 Dorsal closing wedge osteotomies of the metatarsals to correct cavus deformity. (**A**) Lateral and medial views showing level configuration of osteotomies. (**B**) The dorsal wedge is closed, decreasing the amount of cavus. Technique is as described by Gould N. Foot and Ankle 1984;4:267. (Reproduced with permission from Richardson GE. Neurogenic disorders. In: Canale ST, ed. Campbell's operative orthopaedics. St. Louis: Mosby, 1998:1836.)

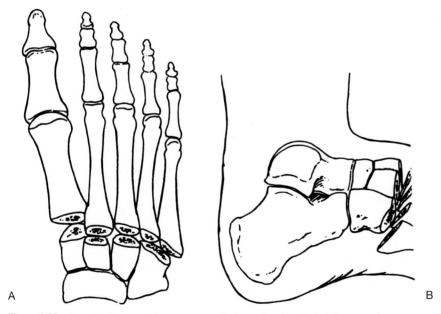

Figure 3.29 Dorsal closing wedge metatarsophalangeal arthrodesis. The procedure is similar to that of the closing wedge osteotomy (see Fig. 3.28), except that the closing wedge is incorporated into the metatarsophalangeal arthrodesis. (**A**) Dorsal view. (**B**) Lateral view. (Reproduced with permission from Wapner KL. Pes cavus. In: Myerson MS, ed. Foot and ankle disorders. Philadelphia: WB Saunders, 2000:933.)

arthrodesis can be combined with other procedures, such as claw toe reconstruction and plantar fascia release.

Fixed, problematic claw toe deformities are managed with PIP arthrodesis, EDL lengthening, EDB tenotomy, and dorsal MTP capsulotomy. This procedure is more effective than soft-tissue procedures when the deformity is not flexible.

Results and Outcomes

Outcomes and long-term results of surgical procedures used for paralytic deformities are difficult to assess because of the multiple causes and degrees of deformity, as well as the variety of procedures used for correction. Combinations of procedures are often used and the need for individualization in the preoperative planning makes statistical analysis difficult. One study noted good results in 90% of patients undergoing combined soft-tissue and bony procedures (excluding arthrodesis). Among the most common problems with soft-tissue procedures was recurrence of the deformity. Despite the later need for triple arthrodesis in many patients, it is generally believed that soft-tissue procedures performed in the young patient with a flexible deformity improves function and delays the need for more aggressive procedures performed later. Several authors studying results of triple arthrodesis have noted 75% to 90% satisfactory to good results in patients with neuromuscular disorders; however, up to 60% of feet in some series were found to be overcorrected or undercorrected. One study noted that only one-half of patients had plantigrade feet at follow-up; however, 75% of patients were symptomatically improved. Most studies involve adolescent patients, and little information is available regarding long-term studies of a primarily adult population. Results of the adolescent population may be skewed, because the population requiring earlier intervention may have a more severe disease process. The lack of results and the lack of uniformity of outcomes attest to the difficult nature of treating these problems and the challenges associated with analyzing the efficacy of those treatments.

SUGGESTED READING

Botte MJ, Bruffey JD, Copp SN, et al. Surgical reconstruction of acquired spastic foot and ankle deformity. Foot Ankle Clin 2000;5:381–416.

Gould N. Surgery in advanced Charcot–Marie–Tooth disease. Foot Ankle 1984;4:276–283.

Graham HK, Aoki KR, Autti-Ram S, et al. Recommendations for the use of botulinum toxin type A in the management of cerebral palsy. Gait Posture 2000;11:67–79.

Hoffer MM, Reiswig JA, Garret AM, et al. The split anterior tibial tendon transfer in the treatment of spastic varus hindfoot of childhood. Orthop Clin North Am 1974;5:31–38.

Hosalkar H, Goebel J, Reddy S, et al. Fixation techniques for split anterior tibialis transfer in spastic equinovarus feet. Clin Orthop Relat Res 2008;466(10):2500–2506.

Keenan MA, Creighton J, Garland DE, et al. Surgical correction of spastic equinovarus deformity in the adult head trauma patient. Foot Ankle 1984;5:35–41.

Keenan MA, Gorai AP, Smith CW, et al. Intrinsic toe flexion deformity following correction of spastic equinovarus deformity in adults. Foot Ankle 1987;7:333–337.

Keenan MA, Lee GA, Tuckman AS, et al. Improving calf muscle strength in patients with spastic equinovarus deformity by transfer of the long toe flexors to the os calcis. J Head Trauma Rehabil 1999;14:163–175.

Namdari S, Park MJ, Baldwin K, et al. Effect of age, sex, and timing on correction of spastic equinovarus following cerebrovascular accident. Foot Ankle Int 2009;30(10):923–927.

Perry J, Waters RL, Perrin T. Electromyographic analysis of equinovarus following stroke. Clin Orthop Relat Res 1978;131:47–53.

Reddy S, Kusuma S, Hosalkar H, et al. Surgery can reduce the nonoperative care associated with an equinovarus foot deformity. Clin Orthop Relat Res 2008;466(7):1683–1687.

Royal College of Physicians of London. Guidelines for the use of botulinum toxin (BTX) in the management of spasticity in adults. Clinical Effectiveness and Evaluation Unit, 2002:1–17.

Wapner KL. Pes cavus. In: Myerson MS, ed. Foot and ankle disorders. Philadelphia: WB Saunders, 2000:919–941.

Waters RL, Perry J, Garland D. Surgical correction of gait abnormalities following stroke. Clin Orthop Relat Res 1978;131:54.

Zigler JE, Capen DA. Epidemiology of spinal cord injury: a perspective on the problem. In: Levine AM, Eismont FJ, Garfin SR, et al, eds. Spine trauma. Philadelphia: WB Saunders, 1998:2–8.

NERVE ENTRAPMENT SYNDROMES

4

ANISH R. KADAKIA
AARON A. BARE
STEVEN L. HADDAD

Pain from nerve entrapment is often misdiagnosed and incorrectly understood. Nerve entrapment disorders of the foot and ankle require an understanding of both anatomy and clinical symptoms to lead the clinician to a correct diagnosis. The differential diagnosis should always include proximal neural lesions from the spine or conditions such as systemic disease. Isolated nerve problems may be static or functional. Functional symptoms are often seen during athletics, when increased activity causes temporary impingement. In this situation, the common workup of radiographs or other imaging studies usually does not assist in making a diagnosis. These diagnoses require dynamic activity with testing. An appreciation of nerve conduction tests as well as their applications often helps to confirm the diagnosis. For entrapment syndromes, the physical examination generally provides sufficient information to institute treatment. Treatment for these disorders is often conservative and entails relieving pressure in the affected region. Surgical management is reserved for refractory cases and requires careful preoperative planning and intraoperative execution to avoid postoperative scarring and complications. Such complications may lead to increased pain and significant patient dissatisfaction.

INTERDIGITAL NEUROMA (MORTON NEUROMA)

The interdigital neuroma was first described in 1845 as a condition involving "the plantar nerve between the third and fourth metatarsal bones." In 1876, Morton related it to the fourth metatarsophalangeal (MTP) joint and hypothesized that this represented a neuroma or possibly hypertrophy of the lateral plantar nerve. The term *Morton neuroma* is used now commonly to describe an interdigital neuralgia of the forefoot.

PATHOGENESIS

Etiology

An interdigital neuroma is thought to evolve as an entrapment neuropathy of the common digital nerve. Chronic pressure on the digital nerve as it courses beneath the transverse intermetatarsal ligament results in perineural and endoneural fibrosis with frequent degeneration of the myelinated fibers as verified histologically. Seldom are the histologic changes seen proximal to the intermetatarsal ligament, which lends further support to a compressive etiology.

The anatomy of the digital nerves was previously considered to predispose a patient to a Morton neuroma in the third web space. Branches from the lateral and medial plantar nerves enter the web spaces as common digital nerves. Traditionally, it was thought that both the medial and the lateral plantar nerves send branches to the third web space creating a nerve tethered over the flexor digitorum brevis that predisposed it to increased microtrauma (Fig. 4.1). However, it has been shown that a medial communicating branch to the third web space is present in only 27% of the population. This study proposed that the middle web space etiology of interdigital neuroma may instead be related to the anatomic finding of increased narrowness of the second and third interspaces.

Metatarsal mobility may also contribute to the pathology. The medial three rays are firmly attached to the cuneiform bones and are more rigidly fixed than the lateral two metatarsal attachments to the cuboid. The third web space is imbalanced by an immobile third ray and a mobile fourth ray, which may lead to abnormal motion within the web space. However, this theory does not explain the prevalence of interdigital neuromata in the second web space.

Narrowed toe box shoes and high heels may also contribute to neuroma formation. Dorsiflexion of the MTP joints causes plantarflexion of the metatarsal heads. Theoretically, as the metatarsal heads translate plantarward, the digital nerve may become tethered beneath the transverse intermetatarsal ligament, resulting in entrapment. High-fashion shoes cause this deformity—making the tethered nerve subject to repetitive trauma through increased compression

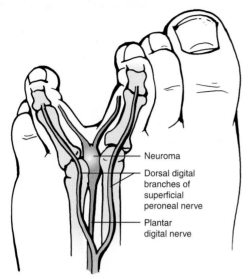

Figure 4.1 The source of a digital neuroma often occurs at the branch site of the plantar digital nerve.

Neuroma

Dorsal digital branches of superficial peroneal nerve

Plantar digital nerve

by the metatarsal heads and stretching over the intermetatarsal ligament. Occasionally, traumatic mechanisms such as falls, penetrating injuries, or crush injuries may lead to neuroma development. Extrinsic factors may also influence neuroma formation. Ganglions or synovial cysts arising from the MTP joint may cause direct pressure on the digital nerve. Degeneration of the MTP joint capsule from inflammatory conditions such as rheumatoid arthritis often causes subluxation of the MTP joint and stretches the nerve. Such distortion of the MTP joint may also compress the bursae surrounding the ligament, resulting in increased pressure on the surrounding tissues, which may cause symptoms in approximately 10% to 15% of patients with interdigital neuromata.

Epidemiology

Women have an 8 to 10 times increased prevalence of interdigital neuromas, which is believed to be secondary to constrictive, high-heeled footwear.

Pathophysiology

Histologic analysis has revealed that the nerve is affected distal to the intermetatarsal ligament. Fusiform swelling of the nerve has generated the term *neuroma*. Chronic entrapment leads to sclerosis and edema of the endoneurium, thickening of the perineurium, deposition of eosinophilic material, and demyelination of nerve fibers distal to the ligament. The culmination of this pathologic process is an increased diameter of the affected nerve through intrasubstance hypertrophy and swelling (Fig. 4.2).

DIAGNOSIS

History and Physical Examination

Classically, a patient with a symptomatic interdigital neuroma complains of pain located on the plantar aspect of the foot at or distal to the metatarsal heads. The pain is described

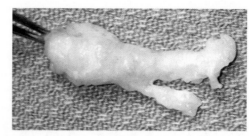

Figure 4.2 A specimen of an interdigital neuroma illustrates its bulbous shape and size, located at the digital nerve branch point.

as burning, often with radiation to the toes. Seldom do the symptoms radiate proximally. More than 50% of patients with a documented Morton neuroma report at least one of the following symptoms: plantar pain that increases by walking (91%), relief of pain by rest of the involved foot (89%), relief of pain by removing the shoe (70%), pain radiating into the toes (62%), and burning pain (54%). Occasionally, a patient may report a feeling of an object "moving around" in the offending area or the feeling of walking on a marble that is thought to be a result of the nerve becoming temporarily entrapped beneath the metatarsal head and then released. The symptoms are generally aggravated by activity or footwear that compresses the forefoot or elevates the heel. Patients often report improvement with wearing of athletic shoes.

The historically reported rate of double neuromas has been 1.5% to 3.0%. This has been recently disputed with a more contemporary reported rate of 8.9%. Although the rate of concurrent neuromas may be higher than previously reported, it is imperative that alternate causes for the forefoot pain be excluded before making this diagnosis.

- Physical examination elicits tenderness in the plantar web space, with radiation to the toe.
- The patient should be examined standing for a hammer toe, claw toe, or crossover toe.
- The presence of an equinus deformity should be determined.
- The web space should be examined for fullness.
  - The examiner can grasp both metatarsal heads adjacent to the suspected neuroma and, with one thumb, apply dorsal pressure to the plantar web space, which displaces the nerve between the metatarsal heads.
  - Increasing pressure is applied on both metatarsal heads in a mediolateral direction, forcing each metatarsal head toward the nerve.
  - With this increased pressure on the nerve, the nerve is forced plantarward, creating a clicking sound as it leaves the interspace.
  - This maneuver, called *Mulder sign* (Fig. 4.3), causes a crunching or clicking perception in the second or third web interspace.
  - If this sensation also creates pain or reproduction of the patient's symptoms, it is diagnostic of an interdigital neuroma.
- Palpation of the plantar aspect of the foot may reveal a ganglion or synovial cyst.
- The overall sensory and vascular examination is typically normal. However, any signs of dysvascularity, including lack of palpable pulses or hair loss should be further evaluated before surgical intervention.

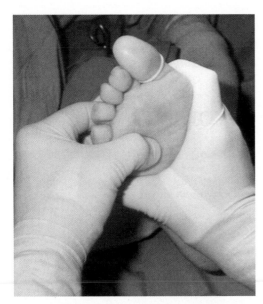

Figure 4.3 Mulder sign can be elicited by palpating the space between the metatarsal head with pressure applied both dorsally and plantar.

- The metatarsal heads should be palpated and checked for fat pad atrophy.
  - ☐ Differentiating between metatarsalgia and interdigital neuromata is critical, and the location of pathology is merely a few millimeters apart.
  - ☐ If pain exists in the web space as well as over the metatarsal heads, care should be taken in diagnosing a Morton neuroma (Box 4.1).
  - ☐ Repeat evaluation or further imaging is warranted.

BOX 4.1 DIFFERENTIAL DIAGNOSIS OF AN INTERDIGITAL NEUROMA

MTP Joint Disorders
- Degeneration of plantar pad or capsule
- Synovitis of MTP joint caused by nonspecific synovitis or rheumatoid arthritis
- Subluxation or dislocation of MTP joint
- Freiberg infraction
- Arthrosis of MTP joint

Pain of Neurogenic Origin Unrelated to Interdigital Neuroma
- Degenerative disk disease
- Tarsal tunnel syndrome
- Lesion of medial or lateral plantar nerve
- Peripheral neuropathy

Lesions of Plantar Aspect of the Foot
- Synovial cysts
- Soft tissue not involving MTP joint (e.g., ganglion, lipoma, synovial cyst)
- Soft tissue tumor (e.g., lipoma)
- Tumor of metatarsal bone

From Mann RA. Disease of the nerves. In: Coughlin MJ, ed. Surgery of the adult foot and ankle. St. Louis: Mosby–Year Book, 1993:507.

Radiologic Features

Most patients with a symptomatic interdigital neuroma can be diagnosed with physical examination and history, without the need for additional studies.

- Three weight-bearing views of the foot can be performed to help rule out any pathologic process of the MTP joint.
- Soft-tissue imaging is not routinely required to obtain the diagnosis of a neuroma. For clinical cases with a questionable diagnosis, some experts have advocated the use of ultrasonography or high-resolution magnetic resonance imaging (MRI).
  - ☐ Ultrasonography has demonstrated a high sensitivity with a variable specificity in the diagnosis of a neuroma. One study noted that ultrasound accurately predicted the size and location of the neuroma in 98% of 55 neuromas without a false-positive reading. However, other studies have demonstrated a 95% sensitivity, with only a 65% specificity rate.
  - ☐ The use of MRI remains controversial. Before the development of high-resolution scanners, the predictive value of MRI was low. Currently, an MRI scan may detect aberrant pathology such as a cyst or ganglion. However, its use for detection and diagnosis of an interdigital neuroma remains open to debate.
  - ☐ In general, the diagnosis is usually made without the use of ultrasound or MRI and should be considered with rare clinical presentations.

Diagnostic Workup

For a patient with a classic presentation, diagnosis of an interdigital neuroma can be made based solely on the history and physical examination. For patients with an inconclusive physical examination, further evaluation is warranted.

- Ultrasonography can be considered.
- Alternatively, a diagnostic injection can be performed.
  - ☐ With the needle penetrating the transverse intermetatarsal ligament, 2 mL of lidocaine is injected into the web space through a dorsal approach. The tip of the needle should abut on the plantar skin and backed off 1 to 2 mm to reliably place the medication adjacent to the nerve, and not through the nerve. The physician should not place his or her opposite hand on the plantar surface of the foot, as the patient may produce a sudden dorsiflexion movement of the ankle during injection, injuring the physician's hand through direct penetration of the injection needle.
  - ☐ A successful injection should result in numbness in the appropriate web space and cessation of pain temporarily. This result, however, should be interpreted with caution because other pathologic processes in the region, such as MTP arthritis or bursal inflammation, can also be partially relieved with local injection owing to spillover of the medication. Injections that result in numbness without relief of pain are not consistent with a neuroma.
  - ☐ Some clinicians advocate the addition of cortisone to the injection; others avoid cortisone in younger patients with a suspected neuroma. The hypothesized effect of cortisone is reduction in the inflammation of the neuroma along with atrophy of the web space tissue to decrease compression. Detractors of cortisone injections believe that the potential for fat pad atrophy,

degeneration or rupture of the plantar plate or collateral ligaments, outweighs the potential benefits of the injection. Such injections can lead to a claw toe or crossover toe deformity developing as a result of weakened tissues. These complications are more closely associated with repeated cortisone injections into the web space.

☐ The success rates with cortisone injections have varied. Retrospective reviews have reported results that range from transient pain relief to 80% resolution of pain at 2 years of follow-up. A recent prospective study utilizing ultrasound guided injections demonstrated complete relief in 28% of patients and significant relief with minor residual pain in 44% of patients at 9 months of follow-up. The authors reported no complications with this injection technique. The use of a single cortisone injection is appropriate in the workup and management of a neuroma and has the potential to provide long-term pain relief with a low reported rate of complications. However, multiple injections can lead to fat pad atrophy and potential soft-tissue disruption and should only be used with caution.

TREATMENT

Nonsurgical Treatment

■ Footwear modification is the hallmark of treatment of an interdigital neuroma.
  ☐ Recommending wider toe box shoes, metatarsal pads to alter the position of the metatarsal heads, and an arch support may help the patient.
  ☐ Patients should avoid shoes that constrict the forefoot or have elevated heels.
  ☐ If a metatarsal pad is used, it is placed proximal to the involved interspace. This device helps to splay the metatarsal heads and decompress the thickened nerve.
■ Cortisone injection is an option for patient's refractory to footwear adjustments (Fig. 4.4).
  ☐ The success of multiple injections has not been clearly elucidated and should be considered with caution because of the potential complications.
■ The use of multiple ethanol injections has also been advocated as a surgical alternative. The basic science behind intralesional alcohol injection is the ability of 20% dehydrated alcohol to inhibit neuron cell function in vitro. Espinosa et al. have recently demonstrated a 22% success rate with an average of 4.1 injections required. This is in contrast to previously reported results that have suggested a 71% to 82% rate of complete pain relief after 1 year of follow-up. No major complications have been reported; however, the injection can result in extreme pain leading to cessation of the injection before completion. Given the variable reported relief and the discomfort associated with multiple injections, this technique is not currently performed by the authors.

Surgical Treatment

When conservative management fails, surgical excision of the neuroma should be considered. The authors do not advocate isolated release of the intermetatarsal ligament secondary to the known histopathologic changes that occur

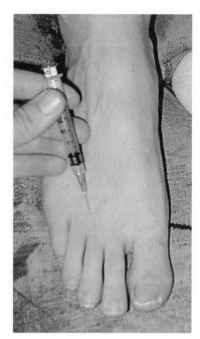

Figure 4.4   Local injection of an interdigital neuroma is performed from the dorsum of the foot, directly over the neuroma, directing the needle between the metatarsal heads.

with a Morton neuroma. Release of the ligament does not correct the pathologic process and thus may not result in cessation of pain. In the setting of adjacent neuromas, the excision of one neuroma and transection of the intermetatarsal ligament of the web space that has a macroscopically normal appearing nerve can be performed to prevent anesthesia of the middle digit. However, if both nerves appear thickened and abnormal, resection should be performed.

Successful results of both the dorsal and the plantar approaches have been reported. A retrospective review performed by Akermark et al. reviewed the results at 2 years from neuroma resection by either a dorsal or a plantar approach in 125 patients. The intermetatarsal ligament was transected with the dorsal approach and left intact with the plantar approach. Confirmation of neuroma resection was performed with histology in all patients. No significant difference with respect to overall satisfaction was identified between the groups. However, the patients who underwent a plantar approach had significantly less complication rates, sensory loss, and sick leave weeks. They did note a 5% missed neuroma resection rate with a dorsal approach and a 5% hypertrophic painful scar formation in the plantar group. The surgeon should utilize the approach that they are most comfortable with, given the similar rates of patient satisfaction for the treatment of a primary neuroma.

A plantar approach is advocated for revision surgery secondary to superior visualization and to allow for more proximal resection. As previously mentioned, advanced imaging studies can be obtained before surgical intervention in patients with failed conservative management and atypical presentation.

■ Both the dorsal and the plantar approaches allow visualization of the intermetatarsal ligament and the involved nerve (Fig. 4.5).
■ The nerve should be completely visualized and transected proximal to the metatarsal heads to help prevent the development of a painful residual stump neuroma.

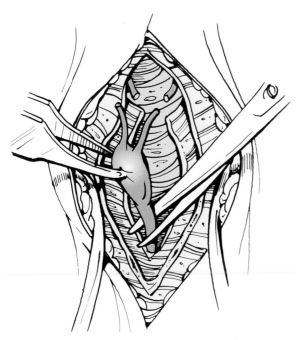

Figure 4.5 Excision of the neuroma begins distally. The proximal segment is gently pulled distal to expose a region of normal nerve. Resection includes several centimeters of healthy nerve to prevent a recurrence.

- The nerve can be released distally first to prevent retraction before amputation.
- Dorsiflexion of the ankle following nerve transection pulls the nerve proximally into the midfoot.
- Meticulous hemostasis before closure is critical for two reasons:
  □ It lessens the risk of postoperative scarring, which may cause entrapment of the nerve.
  □ It lowers the risk of a postoperative hematoma in the "dead space" that may lead to subsequent infection.
- Some clinicians advocate sparing the intermetatarsal ligament if possible to preserve continuity of the metatarsals following nerve transection. This modification of the traditional procedure carries with it the risk of inadequate visualization of the nerve and subsequent insufficient resection with a dorsal approach (Fig. 4.6).
- Postoperatively, a compression dressing is applied over the forefoot, and the patient is allowed to walk in a postoperative shoe.
- Sutures are traditionally removed around 2 weeks following surgery. This, of course, is based on the type of incision closure.
- Transition to an athletic shoe is routinely achieved by 2 weeks. The patient is instructed to perform active and

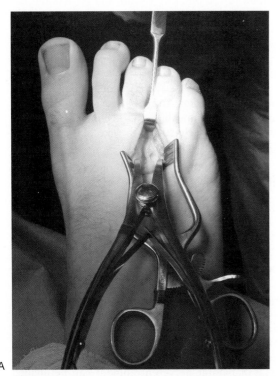

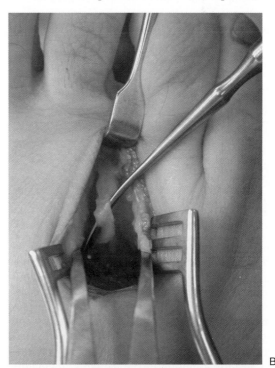

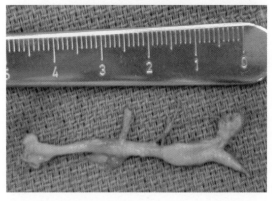

Figure 4.6 (**A**) An incision is made vertically on the dorsum of the foot in the involved web space. (**B**) The neuroma is located deep into the transverse metatarsal ligament, near the metatarsal heads. (**C**) The specimen illustrates the recommended amount of nerve resection proximal to the neuroma that lies just proximal to nerve branch site.

passive ranges of motion exercises of the digits to prevent postoperative contracture.

- Occasionally, physical therapy with ultrasound is required to mobilize proliferative scar tissue, which may cause a secondary nerve entrapment.

Results and Outcomes

Surgical excision of the involved nerve has a success rate ranging from 75% to 90%. Mann and Reynolds reported 71% "essentially asymptomatic" patients and a 14% failure rate more than 1 year following the procedure. The results did not vary with nerve removal from either the second or the third web space. Patients can be expected to have numbness in the interspace as well as plantar numbness adjacent to the interspace.

The most frustrating complication of neuroma surgery is a painful stump neuroma. Recurrence of pain can be attributed to two causes:

1. The nerve was excised as a result of an incorrect diagnosis. Usually, these patients present with recurrent symptoms soon after the surgery was performed.
2. A stump neuroma may develop, leading to similar symptoms. Up to 12 months is required for the development of a symptomatic, painful stump neuroma after the original surgery. Thus, the recurrence of symptoms after more than a year of relief suggests a recurrent neuroma.

Treatment for a recurrent neuroma is similar to index neuroma surgery, although the plantar approach is preferred because it allows improved visualization proximal to the metatarsal heads. Patients should be informed that a secondary exploration for recurrent neuroma through either approach results in poor outcome of 20% to 40% of the time.

TARSAL TUNNEL SYNDROME

Tarsal tunnel syndrome is caused by entrapment of the tibial nerve or one of its terminal branches (the medial or lateral plantar nerve) in the lower leg or ankle region. The flexor retinaculum lies superficial to the path of the tibial nerve, creating the roof of the tarsal tunnel; this structure originates from the posterior medial malleolus and inserts into the calcaneus. The clinical presentation varies depending on the location of entrapment within the tarsal tunnel. Specific attention to the patient's complaints and as an understanding of the involved anatomy helps the physician localize the area of impingement.

PATHOGENESIS

Etiology

The different causes for tarsal tunnel syndrome include the following:

- Trauma: It is the most common identifiable cause of tarsal tunnel syndrome. Fractures of the hindfoot can

reduce the space within the tarsal tunnel. In addition, traumatic synovitis of the flexor tendons decreases the available space within the tarsal tunnel.

- Space-occupying lesions: They can create increased pressure within the tarsal tunnel, such as ganglion cysts, lipomas, neurilemomas, varicosities, accessory muscles, and proliferative synovitis.
- Bony architecture: A talocalcaneal coalition, an enlarged or displaced os trigonum.
- Flexor retinaculum: Covers the tarsal tunnel and may impinge on the tibial nerve.
- Hindfoot deformity: Heel valgus with an abducted forefoot has been demonstrated to increase the tension on the tibial nerve. Heel varus with a pronated forefoot results in a shortened abductor hallucis, and this is hypothesized to increase the diameter of the muscle, therefore decreasing the available space of the distal tarsal tunnel.

Pathophysiology

- The tarsal tunnel comprises a fibrosseous tunnel beginning in the posteromedial leg and traveling behind the medial malleolus.
- The tunnel is bordered by the distal tibia anteriorly and by the posterior border of the talus and calcaneus posteriorly.
- Covering the tunnel is the flexor retinaculum, which begins up to 10 cm proximal to the medial malleolus.
- The contents of the tunnel include the tibial nerve, the posterior tibial artery and vein, the posterior tibial tendon, the flexor hallucis longus tendon, and the flexor digitorum longus tendon.
- Bifurcation of the tibial nerve into the medial and lateral plantar nerves proximal to the tarsal tunnel may predispose patients to tarsal tunnel syndrome. The incidence varies from 4% to 7% of patients and creates a larger cross-sectional area that can lead to compression within the tarsal tunnel.
- The tibial nerve has an extensive blood supply through the course of the tarsal tunnel. Thus, nerve ischemia does not appear to contribute to the clinical picture.
- Symptoms often arise distal to the site of compression, although this is not mandatory.

Classification

Attempts have been made to categorize tarsal tunnel syndrome by location. Tarsal tunnel syndrome can be separated into proximal and distal subsets based on the location of the pathology.

- *Proximal* compression results from compression proximal to the branching of the tibial nerve into the plantar nerves. Therefore, the entire tibial nerve distribution is affected below the ankle.
- The *distal* syndrome results from impingement distal to a terminal nerve branch, commonly at either the medial or lateral plantar nerves.
  - □ Distal or plantar nerve entrapment can be divided into two separate entities—medial and lateral plantar nerve entrapments.
  - □ *Medial* plantar nerve impingement occurs at the fibromuscular tunnel formed by the abductor hallucis

and the navicular tuberosity. Afflicted patients may suffer from pes planovalgus or they may be distance runners, leading to a predisposition for this condition. Often referred to as "jogger's foot," this syndrome causes a burning pain along the medial arch that radiates into the first, second, third, and part of the fourth toes.

☐ *Lateral* plantar nerve entrapment, more common than medial plantar nerve entrapment, occurs as the nerve crosses beneath the foot. One such manifestation is entrapment of the first branch of the lateral plantar nerve, which can lead to significant heel pain. Distal to this nerve branch, the lateral plantar nerve courses obliquely in a separate tunnel across the plantar surface of the foot. The acute bend in this tunnel, along with its relatively decreased vascular supply compared with that of the medial plantar nerve, is believed to lead to its greater incidence.

DIAGNOSIS

History and Physical Examination

The clinical presentation of this disorder can vary significantly. In general, patients describe a diffuse radiating, burning, tingling sensation, or numbness on the plantar aspect of the foot. Eliminating tendon or joint pathology is important in the differential diagnosis. Proximal radiation of the pain occurs in one-third of patients and is termed the *Valleix phenomenon*. Usually, tarsal tunnel symptoms are too diffused to originate from a specific tendon around the ankle. Some patients may generalize their symptoms to the posteromedial ankle or describe global paresthesias of the foot. Symptoms are generally exacerbated by activity or exercise and improve with rest. Some patients may complain of sympvtoms at night from their sleeping posture or from direct pressure on the tunnel.

It is important to ascertain from the history the presence of concomitant injuries or illnesses. Rheumatologic diseases can lead to extensive tenosynovitis within the tarsal tunnel. Lumbar spine disorders, such as herniated nucleus pulposus, can cause lower extremity radiculopathy, mimicking symptoms. Systemic diseases causing nerve damage include, but are not limited to, alcoholism, diabetes, and vitamin deficiencies. Furthermore, the "double crush" phenomenon, which includes a proximal lesion or systemic condition in conjunction with the distal lesion, should be included in the differential diagnosis.

- Percussion of the tibial nerve or its branches within the tunnel should recreate the paresthesias.
- Direct compression of the tibial nerve within the tunnel may recreate plantar symptoms. Often, the compression must be held for 30 seconds or more to duplicate the patient's symptoms.
- The sensory and vascular examinations are usually unremarkable.
- Long-standing symptomatic nerve compression may lead to intrinsic muscle weakness and atrophy, most often manifested as a cavus foot and/or as claw toes.

- Evaluating the patient's stance and gait may reveal pes planovalgus or forefoot abduction, either of which may create increased tension on the tibial nerve within the tunnel.
- Palpation along the entire tunnel may reveal space-occupying lesions, such as ganglia.
- A lumbar spine examination to evaluate for spinal pathology or the double crush phenomenon is mandatory.

Radiologic Features

- Radiographs of the ankle and foot can be obtained to identify primary bone pathology such as an exostosis or a tarsal coalition.
- Computed tomography is useful to further evaluate suspected primary bone pathology.
- MRI may reveal a space-occupying lesion or varicosities creating tunnel impingement. One study found that nearly 90% of patients with clinically diagnosable tarsal tunnel syndrome had identifiable MRI abnormalities.

Electrodiagnostic Studies

Electrodiagnostic studies can have up to 90% accuracy in diagnosing tarsal tunnel syndrome. The complete electrodiagnostic evaluation includes both motor and sensory nerve conduction studies and electromyography. Slowed conduction through and distal to the tunnel as well as fibrillation potentials in the intrinsic musculature are positive findings. Abnormal sensory conduction velocity is a more sensitive (90%) finding compared with abnormal terminal motor latency (54%). Lack of abnormal motor latency therefore is insufficient to rule out tarsal tunnel syndrome. Even though the tests can be accurate, the electrodiagnostic results do not correlate well with the surgical findings or postsurgical clinical results. Therefore, electrodiagnostic testing confirms the suspected clinical diagnosis or rules out a coexisting proximal lesion rather than making the specific diagnosis.

TREATMENT

Nonsurgical Treatment

In general, space-occupying lesions causing tarsal tunnel syndrome respond best to surgical management (Fig. 4.7). For patients without identifiable lesions, conservative management should be attempted before surgical intervention.

- Nonsteroidal anti-inflammatory medications can be used to decrease inflammation and local irritation around the nerve.
- Corticosteroid injection can be helpful with a localized Tinel sign. This injection must be placed carefully to avoid steroid infiltration around the tendons within the tunnel, which may result in tendon rupture. Postinjection immobilization with the use of a removable cast boot for 4 to 6 weeks may decrease the risk of tendon rupture if there is any concern.
- To reduce the tension on the tibial nerve, especially in planovalgus feet, an orthosis that limits pronation can be used. Such an orthosis is especially useful in jogger's

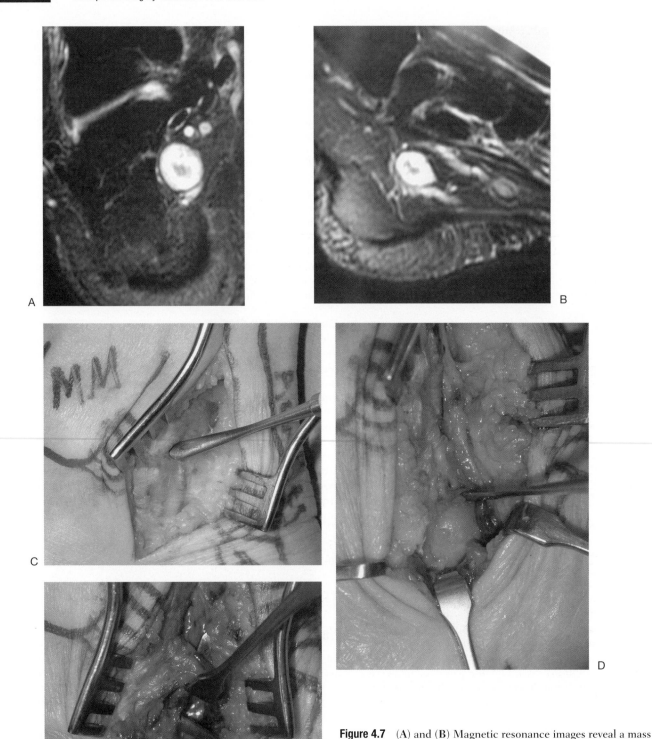

Figure 4.7 (**A**) and (**B**) Magnetic resonance images reveal a mass within the tarsal tunnel. (**C**) The roof of the tunnel is the flexor retinaculum. (**D**) Deep to the flexor retinaculum, a schwannoma is identified. (**E**) The schwannoma is removed and the tunnel is decompressed.

foot. The orthosis should be designed with a medial heel wedge and forefoot support and must accommodate through the arch (without direct support of the arch) to avoid increased pressure on the abductor. Utilizing a medial arch support to correct the deformity can result in increased pain and discomfort.

- A brief period of immobilization can be considered.

- The use of compression stockings to decrease venous congestion can be helpful.
- A 1-in heel lift can be successful in patients whose pain is reproduced with dorsiflexion of the ankle. The lift decreases the tension placed upon the nerve. If a custom orthotic is required for pes planus, the lift can be incorporated into the design.

Surgical Treatment

If entrapment is from the flexor retinaculum and conservative management has failed, surgical release of the tibial nerve should be considered.

- When surgical release is performed, an extensive release is recommended from the origin of the flexor sheath past the nerve bifurcation—beneath the abductor hallucis.
- Proximally, the release may extend into the superficial posterior compartment of the leg.
- Distally, if symptoms suggest that impingement is occurring at the medial plantar nerve, the release should extend to the master knot of Henry.
- If the lateral plantar nerve is specifically involved, the release should extend deep to the plantar fascia (Fig. 4.8).
- Any space-occupying lesion must be removed in addition to release of the flexor retinaculum.

Entrapment of the first branch of the lateral plantar nerve to the abductor digiti quinti usually presents as isolated plantar heel pain. (This condition can coexist with plantar fasciitis and is discussed elsewhere.) Treatment is similar to general tarsal tunnel syndrome and conservative treatment should be maximized.

- Surgical management can be limited to a small incision over the site of entrapment at the abductor hallucis.
- A 2-in incision is made parallel to the posterior border of the tibia along the midfoot.
- The superficial fascia of the abductor hallucis is incised, and the muscle is retracted superiorly. This maneuver will expose the deep fascia of the abductor hallucis, which can then be released, thereby decompressing the nerve.
- It is important to achieve meticulous hemostasis with bipolar electrocautery to limit scarring about the nerve postoperatively. Such scar tissue can compromise the results, leading to difficult revision surgery. Thus, at the completion of the procedure, if a tourniquet is used, it should be deflated to ensure that no active bleeding is present before incision closure.
- Postoperatively, a compression dressing with ankle immobilization in a splint or cast is recommended. Alternatively, use of a cooling compression device limits swelling about the incision and assists with hemostasis.
- Elevation of the extremity for 7 to 10 days and non–weight bearing help to decrease inflammation and incision tension.
- Most patients report symptomatic improvement within 6 weeks of surgery, although it may take as long as 6 months for maximal improvement.

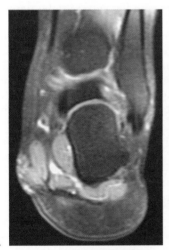
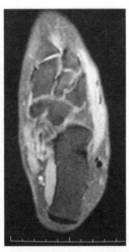
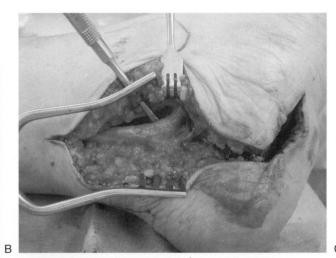
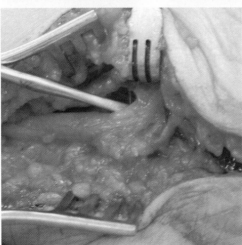
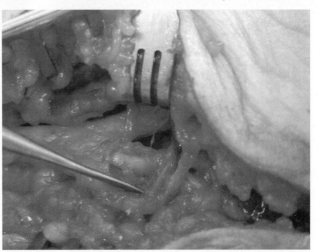

Figure 4.8 (A) and (B) Magnetic resonance images show significant swelling along with plantar fasciitis within the distal tarsal tunnel. Decompression of the tibial (C), medial (D), and lateral (E) plantar nerve relieved the patient's symptoms.

Results and Outcome

It has been documented that the most favorable outcomes following tarsal tunnel release are for removal of space-occupying lesions creating impingement. However, a recent review of 13 patients demonstrated only a 54% satisfaction rate with excision of a space-occupying lesion and concomitant tarsal tunnel release. Success of tarsal tunnel release varies in the literature, with satisfactory results in 45% to 90% of cases, regardless of the etiology. A meta-analysis of more than 120 patients revealed that 69% of patients had complete resolution of their symptoms and 22% had substantial improvement. Others have reported 44% good or excellent results, whereas 38% were clearly dissatisfied. A review of 75 procedures with a mean follow-up of 48 months demonstrated that maximum improvement can take up to 27 months after surgical release. The delay from surgical intervention to maximum improvement must be explained to the patient to minimize postoperative dissatisfaction with the surgery. The authors also demonstrated that patients who had symptoms for less than 1 year showed the greatest improvement in symptoms emphasizing that surgical treatment should not be delayed in the setting of an appropriate clinical diagnosis and failed nonoperative management. The available literature demonstrates that despite clinical and electromyographic evidence of tarsal tunnel syndrome, clinical success from surgical release is moderate at best.

Failure of improvement following surgical release of the tarsal tunnel is usually due to one of three causes:

1. The symptoms may have originated from a different source (i.e., the diagnosis was incorrect).
2. The release may not have included the full area of entrapment. Not extending the release far enough distally is a frequent cause of failed surgery.
3. Development of scar tissue around the nerve following release has been reported.

Patients who initially do well but experience recurrence of symptoms at a later date may have symptomatic scar tissue around the nerve. Results of revision surgery are much less favorable, with those patients who had inadequate initial release of the tunnel as their cause of failure having the best prognosis. Revision surgery is compromised by scar tissue, which can result in inadvertent sectioning of all or part of the nerve. Some surgeons advocate vein wrapping around the nerve in revision cases to create a barrier to recurrent scar adherence.

DEEP PERONEAL NERVE ENTRAPMENT (ANTERIOR TARSAL TUNNEL SYNDROME)

Less common than tarsal tunnel syndrome, anterior tarsal tunnel syndrome involves entrapment of the deep peroneal nerve (DPN). Compression often occurs at the level of the extensor retinaculum or at the level of the extensor hallucis brevis (EHB) muscle. Symptoms generally include paresthesias involving the dorsum of the foot that are worsened with plantarflexion. Motor symptoms may be involved resulting in weak hallux dorsiflexion, depending on the site of entrapment. Treatment remains similar to that for other entrapment syndromes with conservative treatment preceding nerve decompression.

PATHOGENESIS

Etiology

Entrapment of DPN may occur at various locations in the foot and ankle.

- Trauma is the most common contributing factor. Direct trauma to the nerve may occur when a heavy object is dropped on the dorsum of the bare foot.
- A contusion or sprain of the ankle might initiate an inflammatory cascade.
- A cavus foot deformity increases the relative prominence of the talar head placing increased pressure on the DPN.
- A higher incidence of distal branching of the DPN was found in patients who required surgical release of the anterior tarsal tunnel. In patients where the nerve branched distally, the course of the nerve was directly over the prominent central portion of the talar head, as opposed to proximal branching, in which case the nerves are on the less prominent medial and lateral aspects of the talar head.
- The two most common anatomic locations are at the proximal and distal edges of the extensor retinaculum.
  - □ The extensor retinaculum is Y-shaped and has two distinct bands—a superomedial and an inferomedial band.
  - □ The most common site of impingement is the inferior edge of the inferomedial band, followed by the superomedial band.
- Entrapment beneath the EHB muscle is another source of impingement.
- Other causes of the disorder include space-occupying lesions such as ganglion cysts, osteophytes, and chronic edema.
  - □ Footwear increases pressure over any of these space-occupying lesions.

Pathophysiology

The anterior tarsal tunnel is a fibrosseous canal comprising the inferior extensor retinaculum as the roof and the talus and the navicular as the base. Both the DPN and the artery pass through the tunnel deep to the extensor hallucis longus and the extensor digitorum brevis (EDB) tendons. Most commonly, at approximately 1.5 cm proximal to the talonavicular joint, the nerve branches into a medial motor branch as well as a lateral sensory branch. Compression proximal to the branch point, usually at the superior portion of the retinaculum, often leads to both motor (weakness of the EHB and EDB) and sensory deficits. Compression distal to this branch, at the inferior retinaculum, causes only sensory deficits. However, an anatomic study noted that the branch point was distal to the talar head in 2/25 dissected normal ankles. In this case, distal compression may result in combined motor and sensory deficits. Isolated sensory deficits are also seen from injury or hypertrophy to the extensor hallucis brevis, again localized distal to the branch point.

DIAGNOSIS

History and Physical Examination

The most common clinical complaint is a deep ache on the dorsal midfoot, often with tingling or numbness in the first and second toes. The numbness is not necessarily isolated to the first web space. Symptoms are usually aggravated with activity and improve with rest. Restrictive shoe wear or tightly laced shoes exacerbate symptoms. Plantarflexion of the involved foot at night places increased tension on the nerve and can exacerbate symptoms, often awakening the patient. Patients may also give a history of trauma or recurrent ankle sprains.

Specific symptoms depend on the level of entrapment. For proximal compression, paresthesias may be combined with atrophy of the EDB muscle (atrophy of the short toe extensors) and pain referred to the tarsal sinus region. Distal sites of compression past the bifurcation cause only sensory symptoms. Entrapment of the nerve in conjunction with the EHB is distal and produces purely sensory symptoms.

- Physical examination of both feet is important, especially comparing altered sensation on the first and second toes or within the first web space.
- Weakness of the EDB suggests a proximal lesion.
- Ganglion cysts or other masses may be palpated along the course of the nerve, except when the mass is beneath the retinaculum.
- It is important to rule out more proximal pathology by palpation or percussion around the fibular neck for a common peroneal nerve lesion or by seeking signs of tension to assess for lumbar radiculopathy.

Radiologic Features

- Plain radiographs are important when evaluating this condition to locate osteophytes as the potential source of entrapment. In the setting of a dorsal osteophyte, it is critical to differentiate an exostosis from arthrosis of the joints with secondary osteophyte formation. In the setting of degenerative disease, the entire pain or in part may radiate from the diseased joints, and decompression of the nerve will not result in a successful outcome. In that setting, decompression with an appropriate arthrodesis is required.
- MRI is useful to evaluate for a ganglion cyst or other space-occupying lesions, which are often located directly beneath the retinaculum.

Electrodiagnostic Testing

Electrodiagnostic testing can help identify the location of the lesion. Conduction velocities determine proximal lesions around the fibular neck or lumbar spine. This sensitive testing may also determine involvement of the extensor digitorum brevis, suggesting impingement proximal to the inferior extensor retinaculum. Sensory conduction studies are useful for distal lesions and must be compared with the contralateral extremity to confirm the accuracy of the study.

Diagnostic Workup

- After a history and physical examination, removal of tight-laced shoes can be the first step in confirming the diagnosis.

- Radiographs should be obtained, with a focus on the weight-bearing lateral radiograph of the foot looking for dorsal osteophytes.
- Electrodiagnostic studies can give an estimate of the location of impingement and the quantity of sensory disturbance.
- An MRI scan can be obtained if a lesion such as a ganglion cyst is suspected.
- Local anesthetic in the region of the pathology should improve or alleviate symptoms.
- The addition of a corticosteroid to the injection is advocated by some.
- If no transient relief of symptoms is noted after injection, the diagnosis should be questioned and further workup considered.

TREATMENT

Surgical Indications

Surgical decompression may be considered following failure of conservative measures. If the diagnosis has been made correctly, surgical decompression of the anterior tarsal tunnel may be successful.

- The surgical incision is made over the dorsum of the foot adjacent to the base of the first and second metatarsals, extending cephalad to the ankle.
- Various branches of the superficial peroneal nerve (SPN) cross the surgical field superficial to the retinaculum, and the surgeon should avoid damaging these nerve branches.
- The extensor retinaculum is released at the area of entrapment, beginning from distal to proximal. In the setting of symptomatic motor findings, the release should be carried out proximally to the superior portion of the retinaculum proximal to the bifurcation. In patients with a distal bifurcation, proximal release may not be required if the compression is identified distally.
- All osteophytes or soft-tissue lesions are removed.
- If possible, a portion of the retinaculum should be preserved to prevent bowstringing of the extensor tendons. A review of nine patients undergoing release with complete decompression found that no patient had bowstringing of the tendons after a minimum of 1.5 years of follow-up. Preservation of the retinaculum should not come at the expense of an inadequate release of the nerve.
- Partial or complete resection of the EDB is performed if it is found to be involved in the pathology.
- Primary closure of the skin is followed by a minimally compressive dressing.
- Using noncompressive footwear, activity as tolerated is permitted after the postoperative swelling has diminished.

Results and Outcome

In addition, few articles have addressed the outcome following surgical decompression of the anterior tarsal tunnel. One series reported good to excellent results in more than 60 operative decompressions that failed conservative management. Excellent results were found in more than 80% of patients who underwent release of the extensor retinaculum and neurolysis of the nerve with excision of a section of the extensor brevis muscle. In general, if the correct diagnosis is coupled with the proper surgical release, a good to excellent result is likely.

SUPERFICIAL PERONEAL NERVE ENTRAPMENT

PATHOGENESIS

Etiology

Entrapment of the SPN is an uncommon entity. The location of SPN entrapment is believed to be where the nerve exits the deep crural fascia. A fascial defect with muscle herniation can exacerbate the impingement. In some cases, a short fibrous tunnel between the anterior intermuscular septum and the fascia of the lateral compartment can be present, which is theorized to cause a local compartment syndrome.

Another cause of nerve irritation is chronic ankle sprains, which predispose the nerve to chronic tension and stretching. Damage to peripheral nerves has been documented to occur with as little as 10% strain. Under conditions of a simulated ankle sprain, the SPN was found to sustain a mean of 16% strain, well within the range to result in injury to the nerve. An iatrogenic cause occurs after an anterior compartment release for exercise-induced compartment syndrome. In this case, the patient may experience a shift in the fascia, resulting in stretch and impingement of the nerve. Other less common causes of SPN entrapment include fibular fractures, chronic edema, trauma, and space-occupying lesions such as an accessory bone along the course of the nerve (Fig. 4.9).

Epidemiology

The average age range for this condition is 30 to 40 years, although a wider range has been reported. The syndrome is equally common in men as well as in women. Within the athletic population, entrapment is most often seen in runners or those who participate in running sports such as soccer and tennis.

Pathophysiology

- The SPN is a branch of the common peroneal nerve.
  - □ It courses through the anterolateral compartment and innervates the peroneus brevis and longus.
  - □ It travels through the anterolateral intermuscular septum and the fascia of the lateral compartment, piercing the deep fascia approximately 10 to 12 cm above the tip of the lateral malleolus.
- The nerve then travels in the subcutaneous layer and branches into the intermediate and medial dorsal cutaneous nerves approximately 6 to 7 cm proximal to the malleolus.

- The intermediate dorsal cutaneous nerve supplies sensation to the dorsal lateral ankle and the fourth and fifth toes.
- The medial dorsal cutaneous nerve provides sensation to the dorsomedial ankle, the medial aspect of the great toe, and the second and third toes.
- The entrapment often occurs where the nerve becomes subcutaneous, after it traverses the fascia.
- Symptoms are produced distal to the site of the entrapment, rarely radiating proximally.

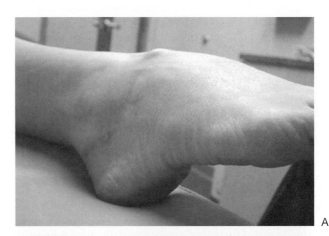

A

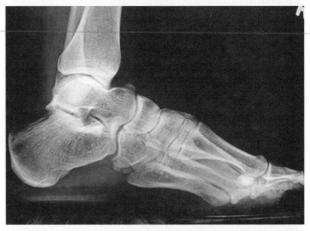

B

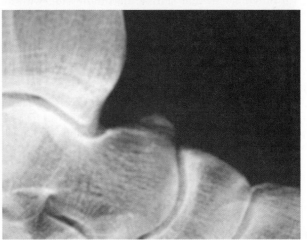

C

Figure 4.9   (**A**) This patient complained of paresthesias over the dorsum of the foot. (**B**) and (**C**) Examination and radiographs reveal an exostosis that caused superficial peroneal nerve irritation.

DIAGNOSIS

History and Physical Examination

Superficial peroneal nerve entrapment usually causes pain radiating across the ankle and the dorsum of the foot. Patients also commonly describe numbness or tingling from the lateral side of the ankle extending into the sinus tarsi or dorsum of the foot. The clinical scenario may accompany exertional compartment syndrome. This additional diagnosis is suggested when an athlete complains that pain worsens with activity and improves with rest. The presence of a bulge over the anterolateral aspect of the leg that occurs only with activity and creates associated symptoms suggests focal herniation of the peroneal musculature through a fascial defect that creates nerve compression. This phenomenon is a focal compression of the SPN and should be differentiated from exertional compartment syndrome.

Nerve tenderness or a Tinel sign is often present where the nerve exits the lateral compartment fascia. This exit point is located approximately 10 to 12 cm proximal to the tip of the distal fibula. Occasionally, muscle herniation through the fascial defect has been reported. Approximately 60% of affected patients have a palpable fascial defect. The sensory examination can be abnormal when compared with the contralateral foot. A sensory deficit on the dorsum of the foot in the distribution of the medial and intermediate terminal branches is common. Overall, muscle strength and reflex testing should be normal. Two provocative tests have been described:

1. With the foot plantarflexed and inverted, the patient may have reproduction of symptoms or their worsening. This maneuver places the SPN on tension, increasing its irritability. In addition, the nerve should be percussed at the site of suspected entrapment. Failure to elicit a Tinel sign does not rule out the diagnosis of nerve entrapment. In a series of eight patients with superficial pereoneal nerve tension neuropathy, all had increased pain with plantarflexion and inversion, as expected. However, none of the patients in the cohort had a positive Tinel sign.
2. Dorsiflexion and eversion of the foot tightens the compartmental fascia and places the nerve under compression. A positive test is recorded when percussion results in pain or paresthesias.

Ankle instability should be assessed as a possible contributing factor. An ankle (talus) that translates forward upon the distal tibia (i.e., a positive anterior drawer test) may place intermittent tension on the SPN, creating symptoms. In addition, an unstable ankle places the patient at increased risk for recurrent ankle injuries that results in a repetitive traction injury to the SPN. Proximal causes of impingement must be evaluated, including the common peroneal nerve as it courses around the fibular head, and the lumbar spine. Pathology to either region may lead to similar symptoms, and thus must be eliminated from the differential diagnostic list.

Radiologic Features

- Although frequently normal, initial evaluation begins with weight-bearing radiographs of the ankle.
- Stress radiographs can be performed by the examiner to evaluate for potential ankle instability.
- An MRI study is warranted if a space-occupying lesion is suspected.

Electrodiagnostic Studies

The role of electrodiagnostic studies is unclear. Conduction studies in one extremity may show a delay in the somato-sensory-evoked potentials compared with those in the other extremity. However, a normal study does not rule out entrapment and in the setting of SPN neuropathy, routine electrodiagnostic evaluation is not recommended in the setting of a strong clinical diagnosis.

Diagnostic Workup

After a thorough history, physical examination, and diagnostic studies, a local injection can be considered. Injection of a local anesthetic with or without corticosteroid at the site of tenderness may provide temporary relief and assist in the diagnosis. In patients with a history of ankle sprains, confounding pain from the ankle joint can be difficult to differentiate from pain secondary to SPN neuropathy. Staggered injections of local anesthetic adjacent to the SPN, and secondarily within the ankle joint, can help to determine the source of symptoms. Patients who have increased relief with an intra-articular injection warrant further evaluation and treatment of the ankle joint itself in addition to considering decompression of the SPN.

TREATMENT

Nonsurgical Treatment

Conservative management should be attempted before undertaking a surgical release of the compartment. Physical therapy for strengthening the lateral muscles of the leg and use of a supportive ankle brace to avoid inversion of the ankle as well as a lateral heel and sole wedge to lessen inversion can be attempted. Treatment of ankle instability and of associated exercise-induced compartment syndrome is appropriate.

Surgical Treatment

For patients without lesions compressing the nerve or ankle instability, conservative care is often of limited value. Surgical decompression is warranted when conservative care has failed.

- Release of the SPN as it exits the fascia at the fibrous tunnel can be performed under regional or general anesthesia.
- The nerve should be identified in the subcutaneous tissue several centimeters proximal to the ankle and traced proximally to its exit point in the fascia (Fig. 4.10).
- Neurolysis with partial compartment fasciotomy is recommended. The nerve should be free of tension with intra operative plantarflexion of the ankle.
- If lateral ankle instability is contributing to the symptoms, lateral ligament reconstruction should be performed simultaneously.

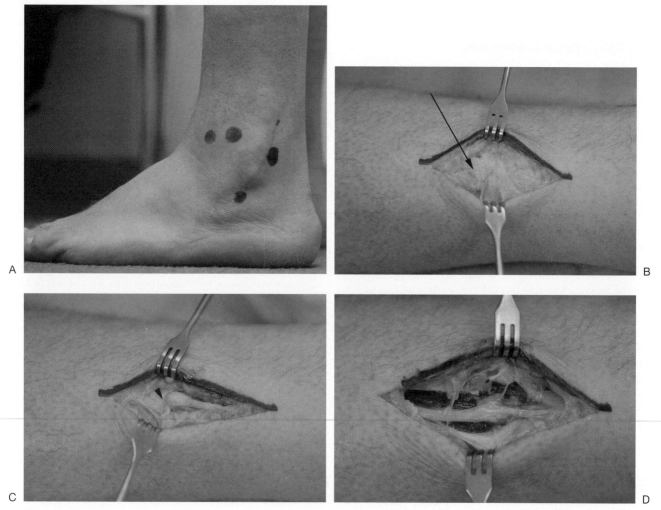

Figure 4.10 (**A**) Clinical photograph demonstrating the location of pain (darkened circles) in a patient with compression of the superficial peroneal nerve. (**B**) "Bulging" of the nerve as it exits the tight fascia *(arrow)*. (**C**) The nerve is focally compressed at the distal aspect of the fascia *(arrowhead)*. (**D**) Release of the fascia removes the compression on the nerve, relieving the patient's symptoms.

- If exercise-induced compartment syndrome is present, a complete lateral compartment fasciotomy is recommended.
- When the procedure is limited to isolated nerve decompression, primary closure is followed by a soft dressing. The use of a removable cast boot simplifies weight bearing and puts less tension on the surgical incision.
- Crutches may be used initially, but after a few days, patients can bear weight as tolerated.
- After the sutures or staples are removed, activity as tolerated can be resumed.

Results and Outcomes

The rarity of this condition is reflected by the limited number of published reports. The largest series evaluated 19 patients with a mean follow-up of 3 years: 9 patients were satisfied, 6 patients were improved but only partially satisfied, and 4 patients had no improvement. The reviewers concluded that operative decompression produces significant improvement in approximately 75% of the affected population, with athletes doing more poorly than the general population. In a smaller series of eight patients, five were noted to have concomitant complex regional pain syndrome (CRPS) in association with SPN tension neuropathy. All patients were treated with sympathetic nerve blocks prior to surgery and given short-term relief of their pain. Despite the presence of CRPS, the authors performed the surgical release and were able to achieve improvement in both the symptoms related to the SPN and the CRPS in four patients with both conditions. Although the sample size is small, surgical release of the nerve may be of benefit in patients who have both diagnoses and have failed nonoperative management.

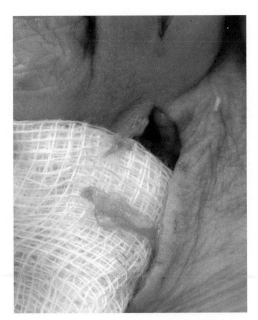

Figure 4.14 A previous percutaneous extensor digitorum longus tenotomy led to a neuroma of a distal branch of the superficial peroneal nerve, which failed conservative treatment and required excision.

within the scar or at its periphery and can be palpated or percussed. Sensation distal to the neuroma should be decreased.

An injection of local anesthetic can help determine whether a neuroma is secondary to nerve transection or from a neuroma in situ. Local injection of a transected nerve produces the same sensory deficit distally when compared with the sensory deficit before the injection. Injection of a neuroma in situ (with a partially intact nerve) increases the numbness following the injection.

TREATMENT

Nonsurgical Treatment

Conservative management includes padding over the involved nerve. Steroid cream to the dorsum of the foot, and the liberal use of oral anti-inflammatory medications, sometimes reduces inflammation surrounding the damaged nerve and alleviates pain. In addition, neuropathic medications such as pregabalin and gabapentin may assist in blunting the severity of nerve pain.

Surgical Treatment

Surgical release or excision of the painful neuroma should be carefully planned. The goal is to remove the painful neuroma without creating a new one. For neuromas in continuity, resection is recommended over neuroma dissection and primary nerve repair. Results have shown that patients with small areas of anesthesia over the dorsum of the foot generally do well, and there is sufficient sensory overlap to limit numbness distal to the area of resection.

- The incision should generally follow the prior incision (if one was made) to avoid skin necrosis.
- If no prior incision has been made, footwear pressure points should be avoided.
- The nerve must be dissected proximal to the site of the lesion. The nerve must be in pristine condition upon visual inspection at the site of the proposed transection.
- After transection of the nerve, the proximal portion must be mobilized and buried beneath an adequate bed of soft tissue or muscle, or inserted into a drill hole made in adjacent bone (Fig. 4.15). Thordarson and Estess have described a simple but effective technique to ensure that affected nerve remains buried within the muscle belly and does not "slip" out. The perineural

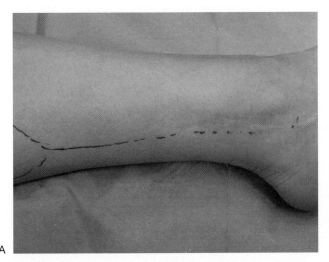
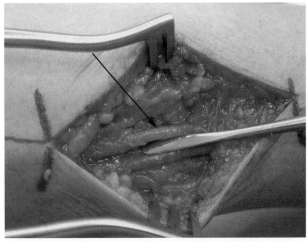

Figure 4.15 (**A**) This patient presented with symptoms consistent with a traumatic sural neuroma following peroneal tendon surgery. The incision is based along the course of the prior incision and extended proximally to identify normal appearing nerve. (**B**) The sural nerve (*arrow*) is identified adjacent to the short saphenous vein. The nerve should be transected proximal to the neuroma in an area of normal nerve as was done in this case.

(continued on next page)

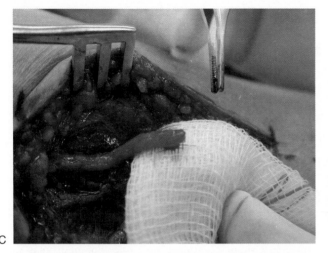

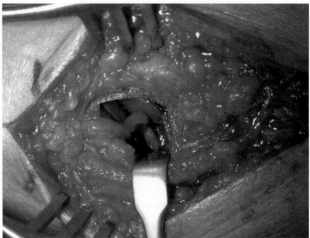

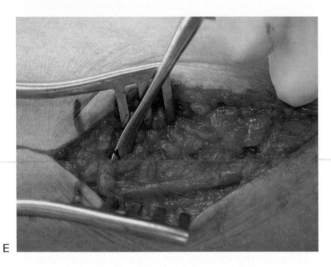

Figure 4.15 (continued) (**C**) Transection of the nerve is performed distally. (**D**) A small incision is made within the fascia and the distal end of the nerve is inserted. (**E**) The fascial incision is closed distally to stabilize distal stump within the muscle. An epineural stitch can also be used to prevent nerve migration.

tissue is ligated with an absorbable suture just proximal to site of transection. A small fascial incision is then made 2 cm proximal to the site of transection. The needle from the suture used for ligation is then taken into the fascial defect from superficial to deep, passing through a significant portion of muscle. The needle should exit through an intact portion of the fascia. The two limbs of the suture are then tied together, with mild tension placed on the nerve to ensure that it remains within the muscle. This technique is optimal for the sural nerve.

■ Results of SPN neuroma resection and burial into the peroneal musculature have demonstrated moderate success. In a review of 15 patients, 36% (4 of 15 patients) had no relief, with an additional 36% having partial relief of their symptoms. Given the unsatisfactory results, the same authors changed their practice to placement of the transected stump into the fibula. In this group of patients, only 7% (1 of 14) had no relief with 79% of patients stating nearly complete or complete resolution of pain. The technique requires a 3.5-mm unicortical drill hole proximal to the site of transection to prevent tension on the nerve. A 5-0 suture is then utilized to grasp the epineurium 1 cm proximal to the site of transection and sutured to the

periosteum after burial into the bone to prevent pull-out of the buried nerve.
■ Following trauma to the SPN branches on the dorsum of the foot, consideration should be made to burying the nerve under the extensor brevis musculature and suturing it to the periosteum without tension.

COMPLEX REGIONAL PAIN SYNDROME

Historically referred to as *reflex sympathetic dystrophy* (RSD), CRPS has replaced RSD as the term to describe sympathetically mediated pain following noxious stimuli. The condition has been described as "the complex clinical entity in which pain exists in the presence of trophic changes and vasomotor instability secondary to inappropriate hyperactivity of the sympathetic nervous system." To date, the etiology and pathophysiology have not been completely agreed upon, but recent articles have focused on certain definitive clinical symptoms and treatment patterns. The key to a successful outcome is early recognition and treatment.

PATHOGENESIS

Etiology and Pathophysiology

Sympathetic nerve dysfunction is believed to be part of a pain dysfunction syndrome. Pain dysfunction syndrome is based on an inciting event. First, a local trigger, such as an ankle sprain or a metatarsal fracture, serves as an organic stimulus. The secondary component, the sympathetic nerve dysfunction, is initiated. The mechanism of this process has yet to be determined. The sympathetically elicited pain is maintained and often gradually worsens following its initiation. It is important to remember that the symptoms following the inciting event are more severe than expected following the stimulus.

Epidemiology

Complex regional pain syndrome is more common in women than in men and occurs more frequently in patients in their fourth and fifth decades. However, the clinical presentation and age distribution varies widely and occasionally occurs in the pediatric population. A fracture is the most common inciting event.

Classification

This syndrome can be categorized into types I and II:

▣ Type I describes an area of sympathetic dysfunction that does not follow the distribution of the peripheral nerve.
  □ After the inciting stimulus, ongoing pain and hyperesthesia develop.
  □ This is followed by classic sympathetic dysfunction, including edema, surface, and blood flow changes.
  □ This is referred to as classic regional pain syndrome.
▣ Type II (causalgia) has a similar clinical picture, but differs from type I in that there is a known nerve injury. This is less common than type I.

DIAGNOSIS

History and Physical Examination

An inciting event involving a noxious stimulus triggers the cascade of hyperactive sympathetic nerve response. Such stimuli include trauma or surgery to the leg, ankle, or foot. By history, pain develops out of proportion to the normal postoperative course (or normal postinjury course). The stimulus may be trivial, something that would normally be expected to resolve quickly. If an unusual amount of pain develops after an injury or surgery, complex regional pain should be considered. The pain is typically continuous in nature, with the patient having significant difficulty finding relief despite elevation and rest.

Although the examination of a patient with CRPS has a variable presentation, the signs of sympathetic hyperactivity should be sought. The use of the Budapest criteria to diagnose CRPS has shown a 99% sensitivity and 68% specificity by combining both the patient's subjective complaints with objective findings (Box 4.2).

BOX 4.2 BUDAPEST CLINICAL DIAGNOSTIC CRITERIA FOR CRPS

1. Continuing pain that is disproportionate to inciting event
2. Must report at least one symptom in three of the following four categories:
   a. Sensory: reports of hyperesthesia and/or allodynia
   b. Vasomotor: reports of temperature asymmetry and/or skin color changes and/or skin color asymmetry
   c. Sudomotor/edema: reports of edema and/or sweating changes and/or sweating asymmetry
   d. Motor/trophic: reports of decreased range of motion and/or motor dysfunction (weakness, tremor, dystonia) and/or trophic changes (hair, nail, skin)
3. Must display at least one sign at the time of evaluation in two or more of the following categories:
   a. Sensory: evidence of hyperalgesia (to pinprick) and/or allodynia (to light touch and/or deep somatic pressure and/or joint movement)
   b. Vasomotor: evidence of temperature asymmetry and/or skin color changes and/or asymmetry
   c. Sudomotor/edema: evidence of edema and/or sweating changes and/or sweating asymmetry
   d. Motor: evidence of decreased range of motion and/or motor dysfunction (weakness, tremor, dystonia) and/or trophic changes (hair, nail, skin)
4. There is no other diagnosis that explains better the signs and symptoms

From Harden RN, Bruehl S, Perez RS, et al. Validation of proposed diagnostic criteria (the "Budapest Criteria") for complex regional pain syndrome. Pain 2010;150:268–274.

▣ Sympathetic overactivity causes a swollen, immobile, and painful limb. The distribution of symptoms is non-anatomic (Fig. 4.13).
▣ Usually an increase in sweating and color changes of the involved extremity occur (Fig. 4.16).
▣ Use of an infrared thermometer may detect differences in the skin temperature between the affected and unaffected limbs.
▣ Allodynia, defined as pain to a normally non-noxious stimulus (e.g., light touch), may be present.
▣ Hyperpathia, or overreaction to a painful stimulus, may be present.
▣ Later in the course of the disease, trophic changes such as smooth, shiny skin, brittle nails, muscle or subcutaneous atrophy, or joint contractures may develop.

Clinical Features

One of the first and earliest signs is cold intolerance. Diffuse pain throughout the lower extremity and skin sensitivity in a nonanatomic region exist. Patients complain of allodynia and hyperpathia that cause significant morbidity in their daily activities. Often, bedsheets are enough to cause severe pain. Frequently, patients do not progress as expected with physical therapy, noting that passive range of motion exercises exacerbate their symptoms.

Radiologic Features
▣ Radiographs often show diffuse osteoporosis involving the affected foot, but this is not specific and has limited application toward the diagnosis.

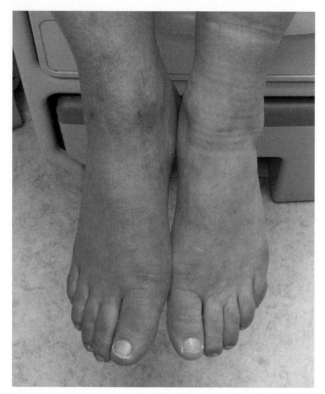

Figure 4.16 A patient with persistent pain after multiple ankle surgeries consistent with complex regional pain syndrome type I on the affected right leg. Note the persistent edema and discoloration compared with the unaffected left lower extremity that does not follow an anatomic distribution.

- Bone scans have high sensitivity, but poor specificity. Increase in activity is noted secondary to the increased bone metabolism. Some experts do not recommend a bone scan for the diagnosis because of the test's low specificity.
- Sympathetic blockade is the primary method of diagnosis. If a complete sympathetic blockade does not relieve the pain, the disorder is most likely not sympathetically derived.
  - ☐ This test is best performed using both saline as well as an α-blocker such as phentolamine. This blockade is short-acting and is used only for diagnostic purposes.
  - ☐ Other ways to obtain a sympathetic blockade include a spinal blockade to the lower extremity, epidural blockade, or a paravertebral blockade. An increase in skin temperature, due to vasodilation, indicates a successful symptomatic block.

TREATMENT

Early recognition and early treatment of CRPS are important for obtaining the best possible outcome. The goal of treatment is to recognize the condition before the late stages of the disease or the trophic changes occur. The longer the duration of untreated symptoms, the less likely a good outcome will be obtained. Important treatment modalities include physical therapy, various medications,

and disruption of the affected hyperactive sympathetic nerves. It is equally important to treat the patient's psyche. This condition often leads to severe frustration, depression, and lack of confidence, and it is more commonly found in neurotic patients.

Physical therapy is an important aspect of treatment. The ultimate goal is to regain full function to the leg and foot while preventing joint contractures. Good communication between the orthopaedist and the physical therapist is vital. Initial treatment focuses on desensitization treatment, which can include modalities such as transcutaneous electrical nerve stimulation, ultrasound, and gentle massage. Patients should be taught both active and active-assisted range-of-motion exercises. Passive exercises should be avoided because they may worsen the patient's symptoms. Equally important are attempts to decrease the edema with leg elevation and compression. Support stockings help if the patient can tolerate them. Biofeedback programs have also been described.

Many pharmacologic agents can be helpful. The use of topical dimethyl sulfoxide 50% (DMSO-50%) was found to be effective compared with placebo in providing relief. Bisphosphonates have been evaluated in two randomized control trials. This medication demonstrated efficacy in decreasing symptoms. Many pain specialists start with a program of a tricyclic antidepressant at bedtime (amitriptyline [Elavil] or nortriptyline [Pamelor]) combined with gabapentin (Neurontin) during the day. Although both can cause sedation, doses are generally increased until no additional benefit is noted or side effects develop. Many patients have fewer side effects with pregabalin than gabapentin. Patients who suffer from increased vasomotor response with a painful cold extremity, the use of α_1-adrenergic blockers or calcium channel blockers should be considered. Other medications that are frequently used include Topamax, selective serotonin reuptake inhibitors, clonidine, and mexiletine.

Sympathetic blockade can be accomplished in one of three options—pharmacologic spinal blockade, surgical sympathectomy, and intravenous regional chemical blockade.

- Pharmacologic spinal blockade is the most common of these options.
  - ☐ This treatment involves the injection of a long-acting anesthetic agent in the region of desired lumbar sympathetic chain.
  - ☐ Multiple blocks over a short period are often required.
- The use of radiofrequency denervation can be performed for a lumbar sympathetic nerve blockade if the use of local anesthetic, although effective, fails to provide long-lasting relief. Phenol has also been studied to create a long-lasting nerve blockade. However, this medication carries a risk of creating neuropathic pain; therefore it is not favored over radiofrequency.
  - ☐ Many centers use a spinal cord stimulator (SCS) before proceeding to surgical or chemical sympathectomy. The use of an SCS has proven to be clinically effective and cost-effective in the management of CRPS. Patients must be counseled that complications such as infection, dural injury, pain in the area of the stimulator, failure of the stimulator, or need for revision may occur 34% of the time.

☐ Occasionally, if only a single peripheral nerve is involved, a peripheral nerve stimulator can be tried. Although proven to be effective in reducing the pain for patients with CRPS type II, migration of the electrode occurs in 33% of patients, and infection has been reported in 15% of patients.

▨ Regional blockade is a relatively new treatment modality.
  ☐ Sympathetic blocking agents such as reserpine can be incorporated into a regional Bier block of the lower extremity.
  ☐ It is important to continue physical therapy throughout the treatment program. The earlier the clinician initiates physical therapy with the patient, the more favorable the outcome in this challenging disorder.

SUGGESTED READING

Akermark C, Crone H, Saartok T, et al. Plantar versus dorsal incision in the treatment of primary intermetatarsal Morton's neuroma. Foot Ankle Int 2008;29(2):136–141.

Aldea PA, Shaw WW. Management of acute lower extremity nerve injuries. Foot Ankle 1986;7:82–94.

Beskin JL. Nerve entrapment syndromes of the foot and ankle. J Am Acad Orthop Surg 1997;5:261–269.

Chiodo CP, Miller SD. Surgical treatment of superficial peroneal neuroma. Foot Ankle Int 2004;25(10):689–694.

Cimino WR. Tarsal tunnel syndrome: review of the literature. Foot Ankle 1990;11:47–52.

Dellon AL. Deep peroneal nerve entrapment on the dorsum of the foot. Foot Ankle 1990;11:73–80.

Espinosa N, Seybold J, Jankauskas L, et al. Alcohol sclerosing therapy is not an effective treatment for interdigital neuroma. Foot Ankle Int 2011;32(6):576–580.

Fabre T, Montero C, Gaugard E, et al. Chronic calf pain in athletes due to sural nerve entrapment. A report of 18 cases. Am J Sports Med 2000;28:679–682.

Gondring WH, Shields BS, Wegner S. An outcomes analysis of surgical treatment of tarsal tunnel release. Foot Ankle Int 2003;24(7):545–550.

Haddad SL. Compressive neuropathies of the foot and ankle. In: Myerson MS, ed. Foot and ankle disorders. Philadelphia: WB Saunders, 2000:808–833.

Johnston EC, Howell SJ. Tension neuropathy of the superficial peroneal nerve: associated conditions and results of release. Foot Ankle Int 1999;20(9):576–582.

Kim DH, Cho YJ, Ryu S, et al. Surgical management and results of 135 tibial nerve lesions at the Louisiana state university health sciences center. Neurosurgery 2003;53:1114–1125.

Lee KT, Lee YK, Young KW, et al. Results of operative treatment of double Morton's neuroma in the same foot. J Orthop Sci 2009;14:574–578.

Liu Z, Zhou J, Zhao L. Anterior tarsal tunnel syndrome. J Bone Joint Surg Br 1991;73(3):470–473.

Lusskin R, Battisat A, Lenzo S, et al. Surgical management of late post-traumatic and ischemic neuropathies involving the lower extremities: classification and results of therapy. Foot Ankle 1986;7:95–104.

Mann RA. Disease of the nerves. In: Coughlin MJ, ed. Surgery of the adult foot and ankle. St. Louis: Mosby–Year Book, 1993:507.

Mann RA, Reynolds JC. Interdigital neuroma: a critical clinical analysis. Foot Ankle 1983;3:238.

Nunley JA, Gabel GT. Tibial nerve grafting for restoration of plantar sensation. Foot Ankle 1993;14:489–492.

Pfeiffer W, Cracchiolo A. Clinical results after tarsal tunnel decompression. J Bone Joint Surg Am 1994;76:1222–1230.

Schon LC, Baxter DE. Neuropathies of the foot and ankle in athletes. Clin Sports Med 1990;9:489–509.

Thordarson DB, Estess A. Burial of sural neuroma: technique tip. Foot Ankle Int 2010;31(4):351–353.

Van Eijs F, Stanton-Hicks M, Van Zundert J, et al. Evidence based medicine—complex regional pain syndrome. Pain Pract 2011;11(1):70–87.

THE DIABETIC FOOT

DAVID E. OJI
LEW C. SCHON

INTRODUCTION

Far from being just a foot problem, the patient with diabetes mellitus requires an integrated multidisciplinary approach to address every problem that can arise from the many systemic manifestations. Management requires treatment from many providers such as orthotists, nurse educators, dietitians, and physical therapists as well as expertise from other disciplines such as vascular surgery, endocrinology, infectious diseases, and neurology. The foot is a complex target of this multisystem disease, with disastrous consequences if the labor-intensive treatments do not adequately resolve its manifestations and complications in the lower extremity. The spectrum of clinical manifestations can range from mild neuropathy to severe ulcerations, infections, vasculopathy, Charcot arthropathy, and neuropathic fractures.

PATHOGENESIS

Epidemiology

The number of individuals affected by diabetes and its cost to society are staggering. The Center for Disease Control estimates that 8.3% of the general population, or 25.8 million people in the United States, are affected by diabetes, costing the healthcare system close to $174 billion in direct and indirect costs. Amputations among patients with diabetes are the leading cause of nontraumatic amputations. In 2006 alone, close to 65,700 amputations were performed among patients with diabetes. Instituting a comprehensive foot care program comprising risk assessment, foot care education, preventative care, and referral to specialists is believed to be able to reduce amputation rates by 45% to 85%.[1] One study demonstrated an incidence of foot pathology among patients with diabetes in a medical clinic to be 68%, with manifestations ranging from callus formation, hammer toes, and peripheral and autonomic neuropathy.[2]

Pathophysiology
Neuropathy
The initiator of many foot complications in patients with diabetes is sensory neuropathy and to a lesser extent

autonomic and motor neuropathies. Neuropathic changes result in the loss of myelinated and nonmyelinated nerve fibers owing to poor regulation of microcirculation and delivery of oxygen. Moreover, hyperglycemia and the vascular changes have been shown to result in accumulation of sorbitol and advanced products of glycosylation in the nerves.[3] These changes are progressive and gradual and thought to cause slowed nerve conduction.[4] Enzymic blocking of aldose reductase conversion to sorbitol has been developed to slow the accumulation of sorbitol; however, the efficacy is still unknown.[5] Even though the exact cause of diabetic neuropathy is still unknown, poor glucose control, along with age and height, has been shown to increase the risk.[6]

Of the neuropathic consequences seen in patients with diabetes, sensory neuropathy, combined with excessive mechanical stress, is the primary initiating event in foot ulcerations and infections.[7] Sensory changes occur in the usual stocking glove fashion, affecting the distal aspect of the extremities first and progressing proximally. Diminished light touch sensation, proprioception, temperature awareness, and pain perception all combine to make the patient more susceptible to tissue failure from repetitive microtrauma. However, the loss of sensation itself does not result in foot complications. Brand,[8] in his review, emphasized that inflammation and tissues breakdown are the result of repetitive stress of a certain magnitude to a specific area with sensory deprivation. Ulcerations are the result of this combination of pressure or shearing forces from the ground, shoe, or even an adjacent toe to a given area, usually accentuated by a bony prominence that lacks the usual sensory protective mechanism.

Autonomic and motor neuropathies also play an important role in the pathogenesis of the diabetic foot. Autonomic dysfunction has been linked to foot ulcerations in patients with diabetes.[9] Neuropathy of the autonomic nervous system results in loss of normal regulation of perspiration, skin temperature control, and vascular flow. These changes result in the loss of pliability of local tissues, forming thick callus that is more prone to fissuring and cracking. Moreover, loss of normal perspiration prevents rehydration of the area, causing further tissue destruction and making the area more susceptible to bacterial seeding of the deep tissue.[4]

Motor neuropathy also plays a role because of contractures of the intrinsic foot muscles, which result in the classic claw toe deformity. Hyperextension of the metatarsophalangeal (MTP) joint has been shown to increase pressure directly under the metatarsal (MT) heads, thereby making the area more susceptible to ulcerations.[10] The flexed proximal interphalangeal joint leads to increased risk of dorsal ulcerations over the prominent knuckle and at the plantar tip of the toe.

Vascular Disease

Vasculopathy is common in patients with diabetes and affects the prognosis for all diabetic foot conditions and their treatments. In general, peripheral vascular diseases involving both large and small vessels are more extensive in patients with diabetes and can progressive more aggressively. Changes in basement membrane causing increased capillary pressure and decreased flow have been documented. The role of vascular disease leading to soft tissue breakdown is less compared to recurrent repetitive trauma combined with sensory neuropathy.[3]

DIAGNOSIS

Physical Examination and History

Clinical Features

A thorough examination of the lower extremities up to the level of the knee should be done on both sides; it should be conducted at least once a year and more frequently for high-risk individuals. Important features are as follows:

- Gait abnormalities should be documented.
- Footwear should be inspected for wear pattern and for foreign objects that may be protruding into the shoe.
- Pulses, hair growth, warmth, and capillary refill should be examined for vascular disease.
- Foot and heel abnormalities such as claw toes, hammer toes, bunions, skin breaks, ulcers, heel position (varus/valgus), or changes in foot shape, should all be documented thoroughly.
- If ulcers are present, the location, size, and whether erythema or drainage is present (Fig. 5.1) should be documented.
- The clinician should monitor for the presence of edema or signs of inflammation as early signs of neuroarthropathy or stress fractures.
- Instability of joints should be tested.
- Weakness in manual muscle testing may indicate tendon or neurologic dysfunctions.

In addition, a thorough neurologic examination should be done for reflexes, a motor examination, and a sensory examination, including the following:

- Qualitative sensory examinations such as light touch, two-point discrimination, pin prick, and proprioception.
- Quantitative sensory examination most commonly done using the Semmes–Weinstein monofilaments (Fig. 5.2). The monofilament is pressed onto the skin perpendicularly until it bends. The 5.07 monofilament is considered

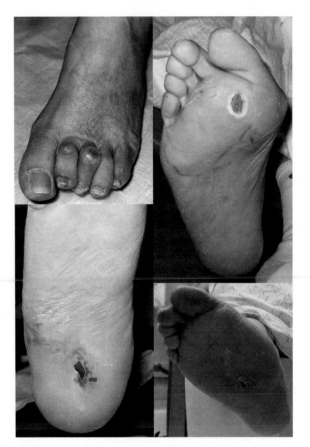

Figure 5.1 **A:** Dorsal toe ulcer; **B:** Plantar MT head ulcer; **C:** Heel ulcer; and **D:** midfoot ulcer secondary to rocker bottom deformity.

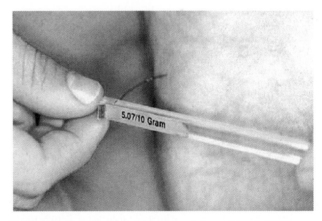

Figure 5.2 Examination of the patient's foot with a 5.07/10-g monofilament.

the standard for adequate sensation. However, it is important to keep in mind that 10% of patients who can feel the 5.07 monofilament can develop ulcerations.[7]

Vascular Studies. Noninvasive vascular studies can be done to supplement the clinical physical examination findings; the most common study is the arterial Doppler ultrasound. The data are expressed as absolute pressures or part of the ankle–brachial index. An ankle–brachial index of 0.45 was initially considered to be a minimum value for healing after amputations. However, the advent of toe pressure measurements has greatly improved the reliability of the ultrasound study. An absolute pressure of 40 mm Hg is considered the minimum toe pressure measurement needed for wound healing. However, falsely elevated values can be obtained in individuals with arteriosclerotic vessels.

Other tests for assessing vascularity include the determination of skin-perfusion pressures and transcutaneous oxygen pressures. The former is a test to determine the minimum pressure needed to prevent reddening of the skin after blanching. The latter can be used to determine healing potential also after amputation.[4] Pressures of less than 20 mm Hg have a high rate of wound infections, whereas readings higher than 30 mm Hg indicate adequate healing potential.

Laboratory Studies.   Glycolic control is very important in diabetic foot care. Poor metabolic control of diabetes has been linked to a higher risk of developing ulcers.[11,12] Elevated hemoglobin A1C levels are linked to increased ulcer healing times and recurrent ulcers.[13,14] These levels should be monitored because they are indicative of patient compliance and healing optimization.

In addition, total serum protein, serum albumin level, and total lymphocyte count should be evaluated. Minimum values for optimized tissue healing are as follows[15]:

- Total serum protein concentration greater than 6.2 g per dL
- Serum albumin level greater than 3.5 g per dL
- Total lymphocyte count greater than 1,500 per mm^3

Radiographic Features

Radiographs.   Radiographs should be obtained as a first line diagnostic workup to assess for changes that can result from a diabetic foot. These changes include stress fractures, fractures, osteolysis/bone destruction, dislocations, subluxations, and any change in the alignment of the foot and ankle bone structure. Specific changes seen in the Charcot foot will be discussed later in the chapter.

Computed Tomography.   The use of computed tomography provides improved detail of osseous anatomy compared with conventional radiographs and magnetic resonance imaging (MRI). Computed tomography is the preferred method for evaluating cortical details and changes, as in assessing postoperative bone healing of fractures or fusions. Moreover, computed tomography can also be used to evaluate soft tissue disease such as an abscess. However, MRI is favored for this type of analysis because of its ability to differentiate many types of tissues and their processes.

Magnetic Resonance Imaging.   MRI is very sensitive in detecting both soft tissue and bone changes resulting from various causes, changes such as stress fractures, abscess, osteomyelitis, or neuropathic arthropathy. However, the difficulty arises in differentiating between Charcot joint versus osteomyelitis. Both pathologies will result in increased bone marrow edema and erosions, as will be discussed more at length in later sections.

Bone Scans and Labeled White Blood Cell Scans. Nuclear technetium-99m (^{99}mTc) bone scans have been found to be more sensitive in detecting Charcot joint and osteomyelitis than conventional radiographs. However, when compared with MRI, bone scans has been found to be less sensitive.[4] Even though a negative study is a good indicator that osteomyelitis or a neuropathic joint is not present, a positive study is highly nonspecific. Uptake on all three phases of a bone scan is suggestive of infection as well as Charcot. Although cellulitis and soft tissue inflammation can be seen on the second phase of the study, a positive scan in the third phase indicative of inflammation in the bone cannot in itself distinguish between Charcot joint and osteomyelitis.[16]

A gallium-67 scan can be helpful for soft tissue infection and for detecting osteomyelitis, especially a chronic process. The specificity is improved compared with a ^{99}mTc study. However, when compared with a labeled white blood cell scan, the specificity is lower, and its use is further limited by its long imaging time (>24 hours) and high radiation burden.[17]

Indium 111- (^{111}In) labeled white blood cell scans provide higher specificity and sensitivity for infection than technetium labeled bone scan alone, especially when combined with a ^{99}mTc study.[18,19] Theoretically, ^{111}In-labeled scans help in evaluating for osteomyelitis and distinguish the area of interest from soft tissue infection or Charcot arthropathy. However, clinically it may be difficult to distinguish between the two. The counts produced by indium are low compared with technetium, and recognizing spatial patterns may be difficult. Moreover, bone marrow activation can be observed in chronic Charcot arthropathy, leading to a fasle-positive scan. The clinician should be aware that if there is an ulcer with an overlying dressing, the indium pool can be misleading. Overall, if the ^{111}In and ^{99}mTc scans are positive in a clinically suspicious area, the likelihood of osteomyelitis is high.

ULCERATONS

INTRODUCTION

Ulcerations in the diabetic foot result from continued pressure in the setting of neuropathy. The long-term cost of ulceration care is high owing to the patient's need for home care and social services in the setting of recurrent lesions and the need for new amputations.[20] Often ulcers are the precursor to subsequent infections, and therefore, they should be treated aggressively.

PATHOGENSIS

Epidemiology

The average annual incidence of new diabetic foot ulcerations was found to be 2.2%.[21] Risk factors for the development of diabetic ulcerations are prior or current ulcerations; abnormal neuropathy disability score comprising changes in vibratory, temperature, and pin prick perceptions; abnormal Achilles reflex; previous podiatric attendance; insensitivity to 10 g monofilament; reduced pulses; foot deformities; increased age; and abnormal ankle reflexes. Of these risk factors, prior or current ulcers, abnormal neuropathy disability score, and prior podiatric attendance were found to be highest risk factors for new foot ulcers. A combination of 10 g monofilament, neuropathy disability score, and palpation of foot pulses were recommended as a screening tool in general practice.[21]

Pathophysiology

The pathophysiology of foot ulcerations results from a combination of sensory neuropathy, autonomic changes causing the local tissue to be more prone to fissuring, and continued pressure, usually over bony prominences in the unprotected areas.

Classification

Meggitt[21a] and Wagner[15,21b] described six grades of lesions that are seen in diabetic foot lesions (Table 5.1). Another commonly used classification is the depth–ischemia classification[22]—a modification of the original Meggitt-Wagner classification separating evaluation of the foot lesion and vascular perfusions (Table 5.2 and Figs. 5.3 to 5.6).

DIAGNOSIS

Physical Examination and History

Clinical Features

Most diabetic foot ulcerations occur in the forefoot followed by the heel and midfoot. Treatment of all foot ulcerations must focus on the ulcer depth and vascularity, and

TABLE 5.1 WAGNER CLASSIFICATION FOR DIABETIC FOOT ULCERS

Grade	Definition	Description
0	Foot at risk	Thick callus, no break in skin, prominent bony lesion
1	Superficial ulcer	Total destruction full thickness of skin
2	Deep ulcer	Penetrates through skin, fat, and ligaments but not through bone
3	Abscessed deep ulcer	Localized osteomyelitis or abscess
4	Limited gangrene	Limited necrosis in toes or foot
5	Extensive gangrene	Necrosis of complete foot, with systemic effects

TABLE 5.2 DEPTH/ISCHEMIA CLASSIFICATION FOR ULCERS DEVELOPED BY WAGNER AND MODIFIED BY BRODSKY

Grade	Description
Depth Classification	
0	At risk foot, no ulcer (Fig. 5.3)
1	Superficial ulcer, not infected (Fig. 5.4)
2	Deep ulceration exposing tendon or joint, with or without superficial infection (Fig. 5.5)
3	Extensive ulceration with exposed bone and deep infection (Fig. 5.6)
Ischemia Classification	
A	Not ischemic
B	Ischemia without gangrene
C	Partial (forefoot) gangrene of the foot
D	Complete gangrene of the foot

whether infection is present. These factors, along with the location of the ulcer and foot deformities, such as claw toes, should be carefully documented. The ulcer depth will determine whether surgical treatment is needed, and the vascularity will help assess whether adequate healing will occur. If there is concern for a vascular pathology, such as decreased pulses and lack of hair growth on the dorsum of the toes, a vascular consultation should be sought. It is

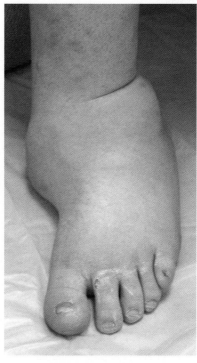

Figure 5.3 Grade 0 ulcer: foot at risk for ulceration.

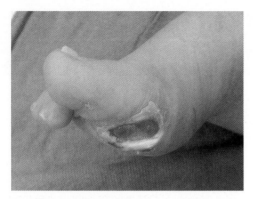

Figure 5.4   Grade 1 lesion: superficial uninfected ulceration.

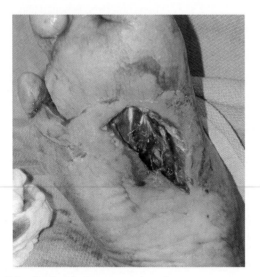

Figure 5.5   Grade 2 lesion: exposed tendon.

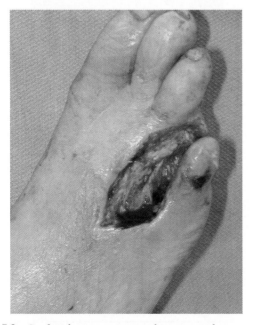

Figure 5.6   Grade 3 lesion: extensive ulceration with exposed bone and deep infection or abscess.

important to determine infection because surrounding erythema or purulent drainage with an ulcer will usually require inpatient hospital admission for intravenous antibiotics and surgical debridement.

TREATMENT

Grade 0 lesions with the foot at risk can be treated by shoe modifications, molded inserts or extra depth shoe, patient education, and regular examinations. Once skin breakdown occurs, it must be treated aggressively to prevent progression of the lesion. Options for external pressure relief of grade 1 lesions are postoperative shoes, ankle foot orthosis, prefabricated walking braces, and total contact casts. Of these options, the total contact cast was found to have both a higher rate of and shorter time to healing.[23] Healing rates of 90% were found at a mean of 5.5 weeks in grades 1 and 2 lesions. Of recurrent ulcers, 81% healed after 2 weeks in a second cast.[24]

In addition to proper offloading of pressure areas, appropriate wound care of the ulcer is necessary to prevent tissue dehydration cell death, and to help accelerate wound healing. The correct dressing will help absorb exudates from the ulcer, act as a barrier to further contamination, prevent wound desiccation, and is easily removed.[25] An array of products is available to help with ulcer management that have different properties, including maintaining moisture, decreasing fluids/maceration, protection from pressure and shearing, absorbance of exudates, debridement of tissues, delivery of antibiotics, controlling odor, contouring to the appendage's wound, and application of compression.

Furthermore, if the ulcer is recalcitrant to treatment or if vascular compromise is suspected, additional evaluation by vascular surgery should be sought. Vascular stents or reconstruction by the surgeon might be needed to allow optimal perfusion for tissue healing.

Surgical indications are when pressure modification fails or when higher-grade lesions are diagnosed. Grade 2 and 3 lesions require surgical intervention, with grade 3 lesions requiring antibiotics and possible amputation. Compared with ulcers in other areas, hindfoot ulcers are more likely to require surgical intervention because of the difficulty in unloading the tissues and the decreased perfusion in the area.

Techniques used in operative treatment comprise ulcer debridement, resection of bony prominences, and realignment of foot and ankle deformities. Correction of claw toes and hammer toes might also be considered to decrease occurrence or the recurrence of dorsal forefoot ulcers. Moreover, an Achilles tendon lengthening might also be considered to decrease forefoot or midfoot plantar pressures. One study found the recurrence of plantar ulcers decreased by 75% at 7 months and by 52% at 2 years in patients who underwent total contact cast with an Achilles tendon lengthening compared with patients with total contact cast alone.[26]

Complications

Total contact cast application can result in new ulcerations over bony prominences, especially the malleoli, fifth MT tuberosity, toes, and skin overlying the anterior tibia. To reduce these complications, a well-fitting cast covering the toes should be applied and checked regularly for loosening, which could lead to pistoning-induced rubbing. Moreover, placing the cast with the ankle in neutral will help to prevent increased pressure along the anterior tibia.[7]

Nonhealing ulcers after surgical debridement and resection of high pressure areas can be secondary to avascularity, inadequate relief of pressure, residual infection, or poor nutrition.[7] Although limb salvage is often preferred, amputation is a treatment option. Risk of amputation is considerably increased with a history of ulcerations. Five-year amputation rates in diabetic patients with ulcerations were found to be 19%.[27] Therefore, aggressive ulcer treatment is pivotal.

Achilles lengthening can also have complications. Holstein et al.[28] found increased transfer lesions to the heel in patients with complete anesthesia of the area and with placement of the ankle in extreme dorsiflexion postoperatively. They was against Achilles lengthening in individuals with complete anesthesia of the heel pad and suggested that the procedure should be done in a setting where complications can be identified and treated. If a lengthening were performed, the patient had to be protected with splinting, bracing, or casting in neutral or plantar flexion.

INFECTIONS

PATHOGENESIS

Epidemiology

Diabetic foot infections are commonly polymicrobial, with various combinations of organisms, although single-source infection can occur. Common organisms include Gram-positive cocci such as staphylococci, group B streptococci, and enterococci; Gram-negative aerobic rods (*Escherichia coli, Enterobacter, Proteus, Pseudomonas*); and anaerobes (*Bacteroides fragilis, Clostridium, Bacteroides*). Of the organisms listed, the most common is *Staphylococcus aureus, Streptococcus* species, and *Enterococcus* species. However, it is important to remember that one-third of diabetic foot infections test positive for anaerobes in addition to other organisms.[4,7]

Pathophysiology

Patients with diabetes are prone to infections from various factors. Autonomic dysfunction makes them more susceptible to skin fissures and cracks that introduce organisms into the body. Fibroblast function decreases, resulting in less collagen production, and reduces soft tissue strength, making the patient more susceptible to soft tissue breakdown.[4] Leukocytes respond less effectively because of altered chemotaxis.[29] Furthermore, hyperglycemia, decreased oxygen tension, and malnutrition all contribute

to soft tissue edema, increased acidity, hypertonicity, and inefficient anaerobic metabolisms. These changes result in an environment favorable for bacterial growth and impaired leukocyte function.[7] Moreover, vascular compromise can lead to decreased antibiotic delivery, which in turn leads to ineffective bacterial eradication.

DIAGNOSIS

Physical Examination and History

Clinical Features

Diagnostic cultures should be obtained to adjust antibiotics to specific organisms and their susceptibilities. As a result, proper culture technique is very important. Superficial swabs from the ulcers, sinus tracts, or outside layers from deep wounds have a poor correlation with organisms causing the deep tissue infection.[30–32] The most reliable method is to obtain surgical deep tissue biopsies and bone biopsy if osteomyelitis is suspected. In the outpatient setting, curettage of the base ulcer will have better correlation with deep cultures than with superficial swabs. Specimens should be sent for aerobic and anaerobic cultures, as well as for pathologic examination, to document signs of inflammation in the tissues and bone. In situations where the patient was already on antibiotics, negative culture results can occur. It is reasonable to stop antibiotics for several days before the procedure to aid in obtaining positive surgical cultures.[7]

Radiographic Features

In addition to basic radiographs, MRI should be obtained to localize infections, assess areas of fluid collection and abscess, and to evaluate the extent and planes of infection. The role of MRI in evaluating infection has been found to be highly sensitive and specific.[25] On MRI, infections will show as increased T2 signal intensity. In osteomyelitis, infected bone marrow with increased T2 signal might be observed compared with normal areas. Although not required for every infection, MRI imaging when done early in the hospital course can be cost-effective by leading to quick and proper diagnosis.[33] However, it is important to remember that MRI does not distinguish Charcot arthropathy from osteomyelitis.

TREATMENT

General Considerations

Grossly infected wounds or any wound with an abscess should be aggressively debrided down to viable bleeding tissue; debridement should not be limited to the superficial dermal layer. However, a balance between stability and removal of infectious foci must be reached. When draining abscesses, longitudinal linear incisions should be made to provide increased flexibility and better healing potential.[7] Established areas of osteomyelitis should also be debrided as much as possible while balancing foot stability with the removal of infectious foci. In addition to operative management, hospital admission for intravenous antibiotics is often required for grossly infected wounds. The duration of therapy and choice of antibiotics will be based on culture data, extent of infection, and clinical response to treatment. Infectious disease consultation should also be considered.

Surgical Treatment for Osteomyelitis

Forefoot Osteomyelitis. Osteomyelitis of the toes must be treated by an ablative surgery that transects or disarticulates all or part of the toe. Because the infection can track along the flexor and extensor tendons, squeezing the forefoot after toe removal and observing for purulent material around the proximal remaining tendon is important. Regardless of the level of amputation, preservation of adequate skin and subcutaneous tissue to provide primary closure of the wound is critical. A common complication after complete toe amputation is the drifting of the adjacent toes owing to lack of support from the adjacent toes and pressure from footwear.

Osteomyelitis of the Metatarsals. The most common site for osteomyelitis is the MT heads because of the high frequency of ulcers in these bony prominences. If infection involves the level of the first MTP head, partial or complete first ray resection is usually needed. However, the infected MTP head can be resected if the infection is isolated to that area. It is important to remember that there is a high incidence of transfer lesions requiring further MTP head resections. If the corresponding toe is viable, attempts can be made to preserve the toe to prevent migration of adjacent toes. If local resection is not possible, then single or multiple ray resections might be warranted. This option is more favorable than trans-MT amputations because it allows better footwear fit after surgery.

Osteomyelitis of the Midfoot, Hindfoot, and Ankle. Midfoot osteomyelitis is usually the result of varus deformity of the hindfoot and subsequent ulcer and osteomyelitis of the base of the fifth MT. After aggressive debridement, the deformity can be worsened if the peroneus brevis tendon is resected or not reattached. If reattachment is not possible, then future triple arthrodeisis may be needed to treat the deformity.

Hindfoot osteomyelitis can be treated by partial or total calcanectomy. Typically, these are performed through longitudinal posterior and plantar incisions. However, published series demonstrate a high failure rate in partial calcanectomies.[33a,33b] Negative pressure dressings can assist in achieving closure. Failure of calcanectomies are treated with a below-the-knee amputation.

Ankle osteomyelitis usually results from deformity secondary to Charcot arthropathy. If conservation management with casts, removable boots, or custom ankle foot orthosis fails, local debridement followed by realigning arthrodeisis should be considered. When osteomyelitis is the result of venous or arterial insufficiency or pressure ulcers, vascular intervention and resection of osteomyelitis are undertaken. The more challenging cases may ultimately require amputation.

CHARCOT ARTHROPATHY

INTRODUCTION

Charcot neuroarthropathy is a progressive disease associated with deterioration of weight-bearing joints that occurs most commonly in the foot and ankle. Charcot arthropathy was first described by Jean Martin Charcot[34] in 1868. Initially associated with tabes dorsalis infection, Jordan[35] recognized the association between Charcot and diabetes mellitus in 1936. In 1958, Jacobs[36] recognized that early and frequent radiographs are needed to follow the pathology closely in patients with diabetes, especially in those with concurrent ulcers. Currently, diabetes mellitus is the leading cause of the neuroarthropathy.

PATHOGENSIS

Epidemiology

The incidence of Charcot arthropathy has been estimated to be 1% to 37% among the diabetic population. A retrospective review of 456 patients with diabetes in 1997 noted radiographic changes of Charcot joint in 1.4% of patients.[36a] However, it is important to note that the rate of Charcot arthropathy has been increasing compared with older studies, which could be attributed either to an actual increase in the incidence of the disease or to increased awareness among treating physicians. Rates among men and women are similar. Approximately 30% of patients have bilateral involvement.[7]

Pathophysiology

The exact mechanism of Charcot neuroarthropathy has not been elucidated. Two major theories have been proposed, although the pathogenesis is likely multifactorial. The first is the neurotraumatic theory, attributing bony destruction to repetitive mechanical trauma or a single traumatic event secondary to loss of pain sensation and proprioception. The abnormal sensory function prevents proper offloading of the area by the patient, thereby allowing continued stress and tissue failure. Animal models have supported this theory by showing the development of Charcot denervation and mechanical trauma. Some doubt has been cast on this theory by clinicians who observe Charcot changes in non–weight-bearing joints.

The second theory is the neurovascular theory. This theory proposes that bone resorption and weakening occurs secondary to autonomic dysfunction, leading to increased blood flow to the area. In turn, repetitive minor trauma results in bone fragmentations and instability. Markers of bone turnover and resorption have been found to be elevated in acute Charcot arthropathy, indicating possible increased osteoclastic activity. Moreover, bone density studies have indicated osteopenia and the increased risk for neuropathic fractures.

More recently, the increased role of inflammatory cytokines such as tumor necrosis factor and interleukin-1 have been implicated. The increased expression of inflammatory cytokines has been proposed to stimulate osteoclast formation. Immunologic staining has confirmed the increased presence of the inflammatory markers along with elevated osteoclasts in pathologic specimens taken from patients with Charcot neuroarthropathy.[37]

The severity of the diabetic neuropathy does not necessarily correlate with the development of Charcot arthropathy. Severe Charcot neuroarthropathy can occur in patients with only mild type II diabetes.

Classification

The Eichenholtz classification describes the progression of Charcot arthropathy:

- Stage 0: The foot is at risk with loss of protective sensation, erythema, and clinical instability with normal radiographs. Soft tissue swelling may be observed on radiographs.
- Stage I: Fragmentation and acute stage, in which radiographs demonstrate fracture, joint subluxation, osteopenia, and periarticular fragmentation. Clinically, there is continued increased warmth, erythema, swelling, and increased ligamentous laxity.
- Stage II: Coalescence stage, with signs of healing and absorption, early fusion, and sclerosis seen on radiographs. Clinically, there is decreased warmth and swelling. Radiographically, new periosteal new bone formation, healing fractures, moderate joint destruction, osteopenia, and sclerosis may be seen.
- Stage III: Reconstruction and chronic stage, in which radiographs demonstrate joint arthrosis, osteophytes, subchondral sclerosis, multiple healing fractures, and

advanced deformity. Clinically, there is absence of erythema or warmth with radiographic evidence of bone consolidation.

The Brodsky classification describes the pattern of collapse based on anatomic location:

- Type 1: Involves the midfoot in the tarsometatarsal joints. This is the most common location of Charcot arthropathy, accounting for approximately 60% of cases.[38] Collapse may lead to a fixed rocker bottom deformity with valgus angulation. These patients also tend to develop bony exostosis increasing their risk for ulcerations.
- Type 2: Collapse affects the subtalar and Chopart joints. This type accounts for approximately 10% of cases.
- Type 3A: Collapse affects the ankle joint affecting 20% of cases. Deformities may lead to severe valgus or varus collapse with increased risk for recurrent ulcerations and osteomyelitis.
- Type 3B: Involves fracture of the calcaneal tuberosity. Late deformities may lead to more distal foot changes or proximal migration of the tuberosity.

Trepman et al.[39] later modified the classification by adding types 4 and 5:

- Type 4: Combination of areas affected concurrently or sequentially.
- Type 5: Collapse and deformities occur in the forefoot predominantly.

Schon et al.[38,40–42] described a more precise classification system with high reliability and reproducibility to clarify the anatomic location and severity of collapse in the midfoot clinically and radiographically (Figs. 5.7 to 5.11):

- Type I: Deformity occurs through the Lisfranc joint; Plantar prominence begins medially and progresses in stage C (severe) to plantarlaterally; most of these feet are abducted.

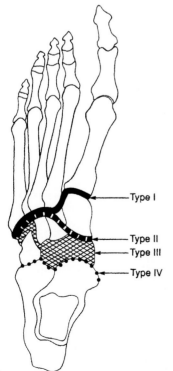

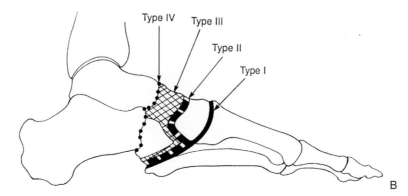

Figure 5.7 Graphic illustration of the types of chronic Charcot rocker bottom: (**A**) anteroposterior (AP) and (**B**) lateral views. (From Schon LC, Weinfeld SB, Horton GA, et al. Acquired midfoot tarsus. Foot Ankle Int 1998;19: 394–404.)

Type I

Type II
Type III
Type IV

Type IV Type III

Type II

Type I

A

B

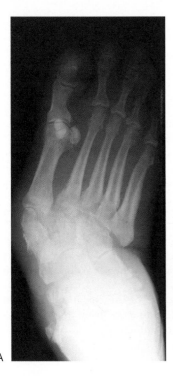

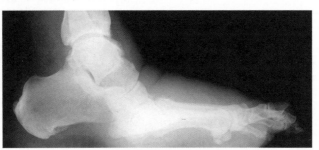

Figure 5.8 Schon type I moderate to severe deformity: (**A**) AP and (**B**) lateral views. (From Schon LC, Easley ME, Cohen I, et al. The acquired midtarsus deformity classification system: interobserver reliability and intraobserver reproducibility. Foot Ankle Int 2002;23:30–36.)

A   B

- Type II: Deformity occurs at the medial cuneiform–navicular joint, extending laterally to the fourth and fifth MT-cuboid joints. A lateral rocker bottom deformity can occur, leading to subsequent lateral ulcerations.
- Type III: Perinavicular pattern caused by fragmentation, fracture, or osteonecrosis of the navicular. There is an associated shortening of the medial column with supination and adduction of the foot, whereas the lateral

arch height decreases. The medial arch is maintained even at advanced stages. Ulcerations occur along the lateral aspect under the cuboid or fifth MT as the foot supinates and adducts.
- Type IV: Transverse tarsal pattern occurs between the talonavicular and calcaneocuboid joints. The deformity is caused by lateral subluxation of the navicular on the talus and abduction of the foot with a valgus calcaneus. Eventually, the calcaneal pitch decreases, and a central

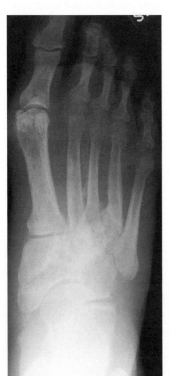

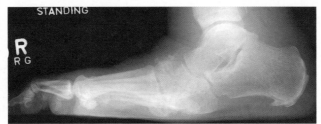

Figure 5.9 Schon type II moderate to severe deformity: (**A**) AP and (**B**) lateral views. (From Schon LC, Easley ME, Cohen I, et al. The acquired midtarsus deformity classification system: interobserver reliability and intraobserver reproducibility. Foot Ankle Int 2002;23:30–36.)

A   B

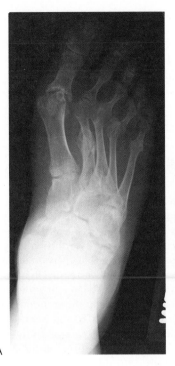

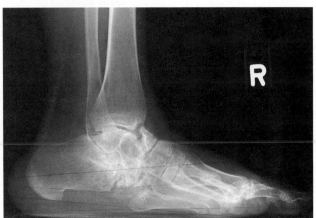

A   B

Figure 5.10 Schon type III moderate to severe deformity: (**A**) AP and (**B**) lateral views. (From Schon LC, Easley ME, Cohen I, et al. The acquired midtarsus deformity classification system: interobserver reliability and intraobserver reproducibility. Foot Ankle Int 2002;23:30–36.)

rocker bottom deformity develops at the calcaneocuboid joint. Later stages result in the talus being completely dislocated from the navicular and ulcerations developing along the calcaneocuboid interval. All four patterns may eventually progress to a rocker bottom deformity and chronic ulcerations.

The Schon classification severity scale (Figs. 5.12 and 5.13) is as follows:

■ Stage A: Patient with a low arch, and the foot is at low risk for ulcerations.

■ Stage B: Collapse of the arch; it is in the same plane as the MT heads and calcaneus.
■ Stage C: The arch is below the plane of the calcaneus and the MT heads. Stage C has a poor prognosis and a high risk of chronic ulcers and osteomyelitis

The Schon classification radiographic severity scale (Figs. 5.14 to 5.16) is as follows:

■ *Alpha*—better prognosis, less likely to require aggressive long-term surgical or nonsurgical intervention. Lower risk of ulceration, infection, or osteomyelitis. All of following criteria must be met:
  a) AP talo-first MT less than 35°
  b) Lateral talo-first MT less than 30°
  c) Lateral calcaneo-fifth MT greater than 0°
  d) No dislocation.
■ *Beta*—worse prognosis, more likely to require aggressive long-term care. Higher risk of ulceration, infection, and

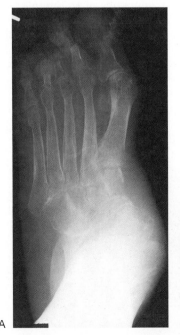

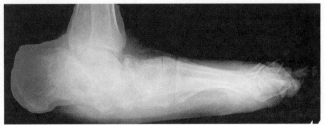

A   B

Figure 5.11 Schon type IV moderate to severe deformity: (**A**) AP and (**B**) lateral views. (From Schon LC, Easley ME, Cohen I, et al. The acquired midtarsus deformity classification system: interobserver reliability and intraobserver reproducibility. Foot Ankle Int 2002;23:30–36.)

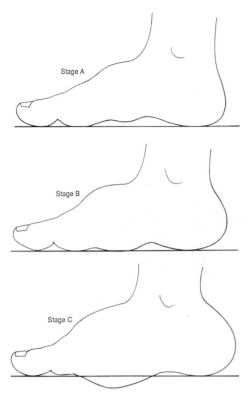

Figure 5.12 Classification of staging of chronic Charcot rocker bottom. (From Schon LC, Weinfeld SB, Horton GA, et al. Acquired midfoot tarsus. Foot Ankle Int 1998;19:394–404.)

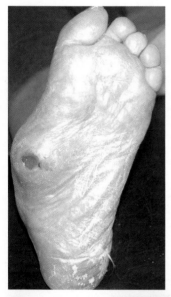

osteomyelitis. Any one of the following criteria establishes this stage:

a) AP talo-first MT greater than 35°
b) Lateral talo-first MT greater than 30°
c) Lateral calcaneo-fifth MT less than 0°
d) Dislocation.

DIAGNOSIS

Physical Examination and History

Clinical Features

Charcot arthropathy on physical examination depends on the stage of the neuroarthropathy. In the acute phase, the joint will have signs of inflammation such as swelling, erythema, and increased warmth. The difficulty will arise when attempting to differentiate between infectious etiology such as cellulitis, abscess, and osteomyelitis from Charcot arthropathy because both will appear clinically similar. The limb elevation test can help differentiate cellulitis and Charcot arthropathy. In the Charcot joint, limb elevation will result in decreased swelling and erythema, whereas the rubor will not dissipate with cellulitis. MRI can also help when attempting to differentiate cellulitis and abscess from Charcot arthropathy.

Contrary to acute Charcot arthropathy, subacute and chronic Charcot are characterized by disruption of the foot structure at a single joint or multiple joints. The structural changes seen are a widened foot, increased bony prominence on the plantar or medial and lateral aspects of the foot, longitudinal collapse of the foot, and loss of calcaneal pitch of the heel.

Ulcer formation in patients with diagnosed Charcot arthropathy can be as high as 35%.[43] Thus, a thorough foot and ankle examination for signs of skin breakdown is critical and can aid in the diagnosis of osteomyelitis. Osteomyelitis in the absence of soft tissue breakdown is rare in the patient with diabetes. The signs of systemic inflammation such as fever, elevated inflammatory laboratory markers (i.e., erythrocyte sedimentation rate, C-reactive protein), and leukocytosis can also help to differentiate between the two diagnoses.

When distinguishing between osteomyelitis and Charcot arthropathy is not possible clinically, a biopsied specimen of

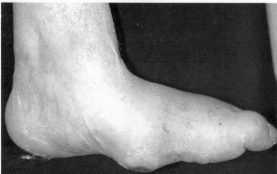

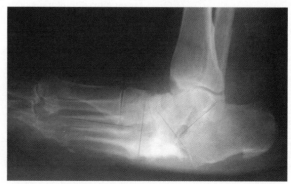

Figure 5.13 A,B: Clinical views of a rocker bottom deformity with ulcer. C: Preoperative lateral radiograph showing osteomyelitis and rocker bottom deformity.

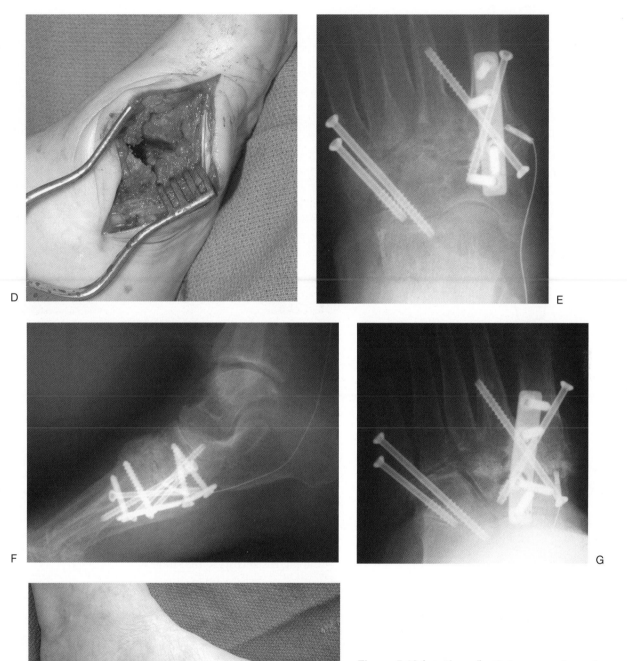

Figure 5.13 (continued)   **D:** Intraoperative wedge osteotomy through a medial approach. **E,F:** Oblique and lateral postoperative radiographs show fixation with plate and two oblique screws at the fourth to fifth MT and cuboid joints. Note an internal bone stimulator wire medially. **G:** AP view at 6 months after surgery. **H:** Clinical photograph of foot after wedge osteotomy and fixation with plate.

the area in question can be sent to be evaluated for signs of acute and chronic inflammation with possible associated osteonecrosis and fibrosis.

Radiographic Features

Initial radiographic evaluations should consist of weight-bearing three-view films of the foot and ankle. Radiographic disruptions of the foot can be observed once the disease has progressed to advanced stages with structural changes.

However, radiographic findings early in the disease process may be negative. When changes are observed in Charcot arthropathy, these radiographic findings may be seen (Fig. 5.17):

- New bony projections
- Fractures and dislocations
- Bone compressions
- Bone disintegrations

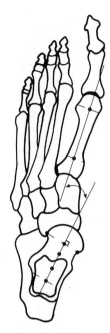

Figure 5.14 AP talo-first MT angle used to determine the degree of abduction/adduction.

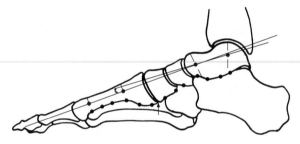

Figure 5.15 Lateral talo-first MT angle to measure medial column deformity.

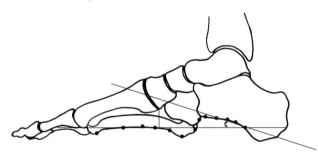

Figure 5.16 Lateral calcaneo-fifth MT angle to measure lateral column deformity.

- Fluffy new bone formation
- Increased diastasis between bones
- Gross alterations in skeletal anatomy.

More advanced imaging can be obtained if initial radiographs are negative or if there is suspicion for osteomyelitis or abscess. MRI can be obtained to rule out a fluid collection or signs of soft tissue inflammation consistent with cellulitis. However, MRI will not aid in distinguishing between osteomyelitis and Charcot arthropathy considering both pathologies will result in T2 enhancement and erosive changes seen in bone.

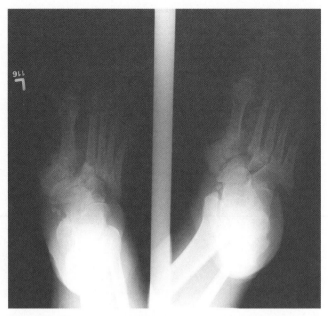

Figure 5.17 Radiographs of classic Charcot arthropathy showing bony projections, fractures, and dislocations, done disintegration, new bone formation, increased diastasis between MT bases, and gross alteration in skeletal anatomy.

Bone scans with ^{99}mTc-and ^{111}In-labeled white blood scans can be done in conjunction to aid in distinguishing between osteomyelitis and Charcot joint. If the indium scan is positive in the same spatial pattern in soft tissue and within the bone compared with the ^{99}mTc study, infection is likely present in bone. As indicated in earlier sections, the results from an ^{111}In scan must interpreted with caution owing to a false-positive study seen with bone marrow activation in the hematopoietic state. A third agent consisting of sulfur colloid can be added to rule out an area of activated bone marrow. However, this adds complexity and increased costs to the studies.

TREATMENT

A treatment algorithm has been developed based on the Eichenholz and Schon deformity types (Table 5.3).

Nonoperative Management

Most Charcot neuroarthropathy should be treated conservatively. Surgical fixation does not speed the healing of the disease. On the contrary, surgery can temporarily delay the healing of the affected area by creating new areas of instability or fractures around hardware fixation.

Treatment goals of Charcot arthropathy comprise the following:

1. Achieve Eichenholtz stage III of bone healing.
2. Minimize soft tissue breakdown and ulcerations.
3. Maintain normal ambulation.

Initial treatment for acute Charcot arthropathy comprises strict elevation, no weight-bearing, immobilization—preferably with a total contact cast, and frequent cast

TABLE 5.3 TREATMENT ALGORITHM BASED ON EICHENHOLTZ AND SCHON DEFORMITY TYPES

Category	Management Modalities
Eichenholtz I (any type, any stage)	Elevation, restricted weight-bearing, cast or brace
Eichenholtz II (any type, any stage)	Walking cast, brace, custom-molded ankle-foot orthosis, restricted activities
Eichenholtz III or nonneuroarthropathic:	
Types I-IV (asymptomatic), Stages A, B, and C	Extra-depth shoes, accommodative orthotic devices, occasionally custom-molded ankle-foot orthosis
Types I-IV (symptomatic or recurrent ulcer despite bracing, casts, or extra-depth shoes with accommodative orthosis)	Fusion (see Table 5.5)
Types I-IV (if osteomyelitis)	Excision of osteomyelitis bone, realignment of foot, external fixation

changes. To prevent increased pressure to the skin, closed reduction should not be attempted. Casts are preferred because of their ability to provide an intimate fit for swelling reduction and to prevent the patient from removing it. Removable devices, such as a controlled ankle movement boot, have a role in Charcot management, but in the acute phase, its limitation of not providing a custom fit can result in pressure sores and noncompliance use by the patient. When applying a total contact cast, the initial cast needs to be changed in 1 week owing to substantial swelling reduction achieved with the initial immobilization. An ill-fitting cast can result in friction ulcerations. Casting is continued until the patient reaches the chronic stage, which can take up to 6 months in the forefoot and 24 months in the hindfoot and ankle.

Pharmacologic trials of bisphosphonates have been undertaken to reverse the osteopenia seen in Charcot arthropathy. Short-terms studies have demonstrated a decrease in bone turnover markers with pamidronate or alendronate use.[44,45] However, additional studies are needed to determine long-term effects. Patients receiving calcitonin daily have shown a decrease in bone turnover markers, but no statistical difference was found at 6 months.[46]

Nonoperative management is successful in more than 70% of cases. The success rates are less for Charcot arthropathy in the hindfoot and ankle. Significant deformity might persist in the final stage of neuroarthropathy that might require the patient to continually wear a foot orthosis, such as a posterior shell ankle foot orthosis, hindfoot brace, or special footwear, to minimize future ulcerations.

Operative Management

Surgical Indications/Contraindications

Surgical options for Charcot arthropathy comprise ostectomy versus arthrodesis and osteotomy using either rigid internal fixation or external fixation to establish a broad bony surface to allow proper healing. Although seldom required, operative indications for patients in acute neuroarthropathy are as follows:

- Imminent or recurrent skin breakdown despite casting
- Acute reducible dislocation of hindfoot or midfoot
- Marked instability or nonplantigrade foot after inflammation is controlled
- Pre-Charcot neuropathic patients with displaced fractures (i.e., talus, calcaneus, or ankle)
- Open fractures or open dislocations
- Charcot associated with deep infection (i.e., osteomyelitis and septic joints).

Surgical indications for patients with chronic neuroarthropathy are as follows:

- Severe deformity and malalignment preventing proper use of a brace or custom shoe (i.e., Schon C or beta)
- Recurrent ulcerations
- Overlying infection
- Instability
- Pain and deformity preventing return to activities of daily living.

It is important to note that Bevan and Tomlinson[47] demonstrated significant association between feet classified as beta and the development of midfoot ulcerations. They concluded that patients with a beta foot should be treated aggressively with correction and fusion to prevent ulcerations that may lead to amputations.

Relative contraindications are as follows:

- Stages I, II, or III disease with clinical symptoms of inflammation
- Medical comorbidities requiring further workup
- Vascular insufficiency
- Draining ulcers or infection requiring a 2-stage procedure with initial debridement and intravenous antibiotics
- Poor bone stock—consider external fixation to maintain reduction.

Treatment for Charcot Arthropathy with Ulcerations or Osteomyelitis

Patients with Charcot arthropathy and draining ulcers must be treated differently from individuals with simple ulcerations. The risk of continued infection after internal fixation requires the use of external fixation to provide stability after deformity correction (Table 5.4).

Specific Operative Techniques

Ostectomy. Ostectomy is a procedure of resecting a bony prominence secondary to fracture and fragmentation that has consolidated to a stable deformity in the chronic stage. The cuboid is most often involved. Indications for an ostectomy are continuous ulcerations from bony prominences refractory to casting or bracing, and initial

TABLE 5.4 TREATMENT OPTIONS FOR PATIENTS WITH DEFORMITY AND ULCERS

Grade	Description
Deformity with no ulceration or history of ulcer	Deformity correction with plantar plate, screws, and possible external fixator.
Deformity with superficial nondraining ulceration	Single stage debridement and deformity correction with plantar plates, screws, and possible external fixator.
Deformity with draining ulceration not tracking to bone	Intravenous antibiotics and two-stage procedure with initial debridement followed by deformity correction using plates and screws once healthier tissue is obtained.
Ulceration with drainage tracking to bone in the setting of foot deformity	Intravenous antibiotics, two-stage surgical treatment with ulcer debridement, and delayed deformity correction with external fixator, percutaneous screws, and Kirschner wire augmentation. Avoid plantar plate and screw fixation.

TABLE 5.5 FUSION TECHNIQUES FOR SCHON DEFORMITY TYPES

Deformity Type	Method
Midfoot	
IA	Fuse involved metatarsocuneiform joints using screws or plantar plate.
IB	Fuse involved metatarsocuneiform joints medially with plantar plate. If lateral fourth or fifth metatarsocuboid collapse, fuse and apply lateral plantar plate.
IC	Fuse entire tarsometatarsal complex with plantar closing wedge osteotomy and apply medial and lateral plantar plates.
IIA	Fuse naviculocuneiform joint with plantar plate or screws.
IIB	Fuse naviculocuneiform joint and fourth and fifth metatarsocuboid joint if collapsed with plantar lateral plate or screws.
IIC	Fuse metatarsonaviculocuneiform joints and fourth and fifth metatarsocuboid joints with plantar-based closing wedge osteotomy and medial and lateral plantar plates.
IIIA	Fuse talonavicular and/or naviculocuneiform joints.
IIIB	Fuse talonavicular and/or naviculocuneiform joints and fourth and fifth metatarsocuboid joints with plantar plate if collapsed.
IIIC	Fuse entire involved midtarsus medially and laterally with closing wedge osteotomy and medial and lateral plantar plates.
IVA	Triple arthrodesis.
IVB	Triple arthrodesis.
IVC	Triple arthrodesis; may require plantar closing wedge osteotomy and medial and lateral plantar plates.
Ankle	
Avascular necrosis with no osteomyelitis	Tibiocalcaneal fusion, rod, blade plate, or frame.
Arthritis, no osteomyelitis	Tibitotalocalcaneal fusion, screws, rod, or frame.
Osteomyelitis or open ulcer	Tibiotalocalcaneal fusion or tibiocalcaneal fusion with frame.

treatment for ulcerations to allow the soft tissues to heal before definitive correction and fusion. A contraindication is an unstable deformity where resection can lead to further destabilization. The technique involves a lateral incision for the cuboid, a medial incision for the navicular or cuneiforms, and a plantar incision for a central bony mass. The bony prominence is resected. If an ulcer or infection is present, the area is debrided. The wound can then be left open, treated with a negative pressure dressing, or closed using a retention suture. That patient should be evaluated to determine whether a tendo-Achilles lengthening or a gastrocnemius recession procedure is needed.

Arthrodesis/Osteotomy. Corrective osteotomy and fusion should be considered in patients with recurrent ulcers, deformity preventing appropriate brace or footwear, severe malalignment or instability, and pain limiting function (Table 5.5 and Fig. 5.13).[42]

In severe deformities, a fusion of the first through fifth tarsometarsal fusion is required and has been shown to be effective and necessary. Based on the location of the deformity, fusions of the naviculocuneiform, talonavicular, and calcaneocuboid joints may also be necessary. Lateral column collapse has been shown to be quite destructive in individuals with severe rocker bottom deformity. As a result, additional fusion of the lateral column might be considered. Raikin and Schon[48] demonstrated improved pain and American Orthopedic Foot and Ankle Society midfoot scores in patients treated with a lateral column fusion.

Surgical fixation should consist of plantar plates (Fig. 5.13) and interfragmentary screws when possible.

Plantar plates have been shown to be biomechanically stronger than screw fixation constructs because the fixation is done on the tension side of the deformity.[49] However, deep ulcerations that extend down to bone are a contraindication for plate fixation. In individuals with poor bone stock and osteomyelitis, external fixation should

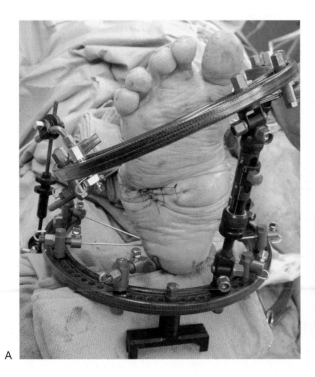

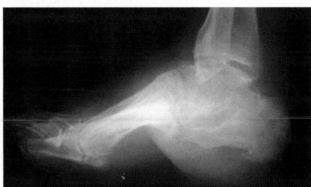

Figure 5.18 *A*: Plantar view of foot with frame intraoperatively. *B*: Postoperative lateral radiograph after wedge osteotomy and external frame fixation.

A

B

be considered (Fig. 5.18). Axially placed interfragmentary screws that are perpendicular to the joint have been shown to provide better fixation. Kann et al.[50] in a biomechanical study demonstrated significantly higher stiffness and maximum load to failure using axially placed screws in the arthrodesis of the calcaneocuboid joint compared with obliquely placed screws. Furthermore, a tendo-Achilles lengthening or Strayer procedure might be considered to improve any equines deformity that might be present.

Postoperative care consists of prolonged immobilization with a cast or brace for 6 months for disease affecting the midfoot and 9 to 12 months for arthropathy at the tibiotalar joint. Weight-bearing should be restricted until warmth and swelling decreases. Even after the immobilization period, chronic use of ankle foot orthosis or protective footwear will typically be needed.

Outcomes.
- Limb salvage rates reached 89% with ostectomies although revision surgeries were required in 38% of patients.[51] Brodsky[52] reported in his series that only 1 of his 12 patients had a recurrence after undergoing exostectomy for intractable ulcerations.
- A high rate of limb salvage can be obtained with surgical correction.[53,54]
- External fixation has demonstrated limb salvage rates as high as 90% with minimal recurrent ulcerations.[55–57]
- Schon et al. in an unpublished series of 250 patients with rocker bottom deformity who underwent aggressive surgical correction, demonstrated improved function, improved ability to wear footwear, and easier foot maintenance compared with nonoperative measures.

Complications
Complications associated with Charcot midfoot reconstruction include infection, ulceration, recurrence of deformity, nonunion, patient noncompliance with

restrictions, hardware failure and prominence, and amputation. Reported postoperative infection rates range from 0% to 10%, with nonunion rates ranging from 0% to 50%.[38,58–63] Hardware failure rates of 0% to 32% have been reported, with higher occurrences seen with intramedullary screw fixation.[38,60–62] Hardware prominence, which can lead to additional surgery, is reported to be as high as 27%.[61] Loss of correction has been reported to range from 0% to 19%.[38,62,63] Wound complication rates range from 0% to 29%;[38,58,60–63] many can be treated with local wound care and antibiotics. Amputation in the setting of uncontrollable infection has been reported to range from 0% to 10%.[38,58–63] Charcot arthropathy alone was not found to have a higher risk for amputation compared with patients with diabetes alone. However, Charcot patients with ulcerations were found to have a rate 12 times higher for amputation compared with patients without ulcerations.[27]

ACUTE ANKLE FRACTURE IN THE PATIENT WITH DIABETES

INTRODUCTION

Acute ankle fractures occurring in the patient with diabetes, especially those with complicated diabetes, pose increased risks compared with nondiabetics. These patients have increased length of stay, higher in-hospital mortality rate, and increased rate of complications. Moreover, these patients are more prone to fracture, malunion, hardware failure, Charcot arthropathy, infection, and wound breakdown, regardless of whether the fracture was treated nonoperatively or with surgical fixation.

PATHOGENESIS

Epidemiology

The rate of diabetes in patients sustaining an ankle fracture has been estimated to be nearly 6%.[64] More important, the rate of complications among patients with diabetes, such as fracture displacement, infections, hardware failure, in-hospital mortality, length of stay, or neuropathic arthropathy, is considerably higher in patients with diabetes compared with nondiabetics.[64–67] Factors that correlated with increased risk for complications after ankle fractures in patients with diabetes were other known comorbidities, such as Charcot arthropathy and end-organ damage, comprising peripheral vascular disease, peripheral neuropathy, and nephropathy, longer duration of diabetes, and insulin dependency.[66–69] Known comorbidities also had increased rate of continued brace use. A history of Charcot arthropathy had a significantly increased risk for infection.[66]

PATHOPHYSIOLOGY

Many factors contribute to the higher complication rate in patients with diabetes sustaining an acute fracture. Hyperglycemia has been shown to result in accumulation of sorbitol and advanced products of glycosylation. These products can result in the impairment of collagen, basement membranes, inflammatory cell receptors, and fibroblast function.[70] Moreover, hyperglycemia has been linked to vascular disease and local soft tissue ischemia. Wound collagen deposition has been shown to be directly proportional to soft tissue perfusion. As a result, the hypoxic environment severely impairs local collagen production and ultimately soft tissue healing.[71,72]

The delay in fracture healing in patients with diabetes is well known, although the specific cause is not clear. Several mechanisms have been proposed. One of them is the reduction in early cellular proliferation during endochondral ossification. Another is abnormal and decreased collagen synthesis. Ultimately, there is both a delay in endochondral ossification and decreased mechanical strength of the fracture callus.[70,73–75]

DIAGNOSIS

Physical Examination and History

Clinical Features

A thorough history and physical examination should be obtained so that the clinician is aware of the mechanism of injury and pertinent medical history, such as history of Charcot arthropathy, neuropathy, retinopathy, vascular disease, insulin dependency, previous ulcerations, and previous fracture complications. The amount of soft tissue swelling should be assessed. In addition, neurologic status should be evaluated using a 5.07 Semmes–Weinstein monofilament along with a thorough motor examination.

Another vital part of the physical examination is the vascular examination, evaluating for dorsalis pedis and posterior tibial pulse, hair growth in the toes, and capillary refill. If there is concern for vascular disease, noninvasive studies such as ankle–brachial index and transcutaneous oxygen pressures should be done to evaluate the severity of the disease and potential for soft tissue healing if surgery is needed. If vascular disease is suspected, a vascular surgery consult should be obtained.

Radiographic Features

A thorough radiographic evaluation of the foot, hindfoot, and ankle should be obtained at the time of presentation to assess not only the fracture but also to rule out a Charcot process. A stress radiograph of the ankle can be obtained to determine the instability of the fracture pattern.

TREATMENT

The treatment goal, regardless of whether surgery is done, is to achieve a stable and congruent joint, restore function, and prevent complications that can lead to amputations. The initial step is to reduce the fracture, place the patient in a well-padded splint, and elevate the foot for soft tissue rest. A multidisciplinary treatment plan should be made to treat the patient's metabolic dysfunction, optimize glucose control, and evaluate for the presence of vascular disease.

Nonoperative Management

Indications

Indications for nonoperative management are nondisplaced fractures with a stable joint or a patient with severe comorbidities who cannot undergo operative treatment. Treatment involves immobilization with non–weight-bearing restrictions two to three times the usual duration and with frequent office visits. If loss of fracture reduction is seen in subsequent office visits, operative management should be considered when soft tissues permit open surgery. Furthermore, an additional 2 to 3 months of protected weight-bearing in a total contact cast or brace is recommended even after fracture union.

Contraindication

Contraindications for nonoperative management are fractures that are displaced with unstable patterns and joint incongruency or loss of reduction at subsequent follow-up visits.

Outcomes

McCormack and Leith[76] reported on 26 ankle fractures in patients with diabetes with a nonsurgical group of 7 patients. They reported that 5 of the 7 patients developed an asymptomatic malunion, with a functional lower limb, whereas the other 2 cases healed uneventfully. The operative group had a 42.3% complication rate comprising infection, wound necrosis, and malunion, with 2 patients developing fulminant infection leading to amputation and death. The authors concluded that nonoperative management may be preferable even in displaced fractures in an older low-demand patient because of the high complication rate in the operative group. However, they did not report on the degree of fracture severity or the functional level of patients with malunion in the nonoperative group.

Furthermore, Schon et al.[38] reported on 28 neuropathic ankle fractures in patients with diabetes whose 15 nondisplaced and 13 displaced fractures were treated without surgery. Treatment consisted of no weight-bearing immobilization for 3 to 9 months. All patients in the nondisplaced group healed without evidence of Charcot arthropathy or infection. However, displaced fractures treated nonoperatively resulted in nonunion or malunion, with 3 fractures needing an ankle fusion. Schon et al.[38] concluded that nondisplaced fractures can heal uneventfully and nonoperatively. However, they recommended operative fixation for displaced fractures.

Poor results also been reported for nonoperative treatment of minimally displaced ankle fractures. Connolly and Csencsitz[77] reported on six ankle fractures treated with cast immobilization. One resulted in necrotizing fasciitis, requiring a below-the-knee amputation; two required ankle fusions; one had continued injury progression that ultimately required a calcaneal–tibial arthrodesis with a partial talectomy; and two developed Charcot arthropathy. They concluded that severe complications can still occur from nonoperative management and that early surgical stabilization is preferable in patients with diabetes with ankle fractures.

Regardless of whether nonoperative or surgical treatment is considered, the duration of immobilization needs to be prolonged two to three times the usual duration. Furthermore, it is important to remember that serious complications can still occur with nonsurgical management and that these patients should be followed closely.

Operative Management

Surgical Indications/Contraindications

Surgical indications are any ankle fractures with joint incongruency, fracture displacement, or unstable fracture patterns. Treatment involves stabilizing the fracture with a rigid internal construct to prevent Charcot progression. Postoperatively, the patient should be immobilized for two to three times the usual duration with no weight-bearing for at least 8 weeks, followed by protected weight-bearing in a brace or cast for an additional 8 to 12 weeks even if fracture callus is present.

Before the definitive open reduction and internal fixation, a staged protocol should be followed, consisting of 10 to 14 days of soft-tissue rest to minimize infection and surgical site wound breakdown. The presence of skin wrinkles indicates a favorable indicator to proceed with operative fixation. If severe soft tissue injury is present, an external fixator, with or without limited internal fixation, may be considered as a temporizing measure. The importance of proper soft tissue stabilization and delayed staged surgical intervention can be found in the trauma literature with pilon fractures. Wyrsch et al.[78] serendipitously demonstrated the effect of surgical timing and wound

complications in pilon fractures. Patients who underwent a delayed surgical procedure had significantly less infection, less wound breakdown, and lower amputation rate. Sirkin et al.[79] using the staged protocol reported low wound complication rates of 5.3% in all fractures and 2.9% in closed pilon fractures.

Contraindications for open reduction and internal fixation are patients medically unstable for surgery or those with severe soft tissue injury or swelling that requires delayed internal fixation.

Surgical Techniques

In nonosteoporotic patients with mild peripheral neuropathy, standard small fragment fixation with a lag screw and neutralization plate and cancellous screws for the medial malleolus fragment can be done. A stable operative construct can maintain joint congruity and prevent progression to a Charcot joint.[38,80] Intraoperatively, the surgeon should use bone reduction clamps carefully to avoid fragmenting the fracture. Moreover, the soft tissues should be handled carefully by avoiding instruments that can compress the skin and minimizing periosteal dissections to use full thickness skin flaps with wide skin bridges if two incisions are to be used.[81]

Individuals with peripheral neuropathy or severe osteopenia require more rigid fixation, thereby increasing the biomechanical strength of the construct and minimizing complications.[38,67,70,80,82,83] Poor outcome has been reported with inadequate fixation.[38] A stable construct can be achieved through the use of longer or larger plates, such as the 4.5-mm dynamic compression plate with multiple syndesmotic screw fixation advocated by Perry et al.,[84] supplementary Kirschner wires in the plated fibula, multiple syndesmotic fixation, and transcalcaneal–talar–tibial screw or Steinmann pin fixation, as advocated by Jani et al.[83] Locked plate fixation can also be considered for fractures with severe bone loss or severe comminution.

Perry et al.[84] reported that all six of their patients who underwent the salvage procedure with the 4.5-mm dynamic compression plate and multiple syndesmotic screws after failing traditional fixation achieved satisfactory outcomes and avoided amputation.

Koval et al.[85] reported a 100% union rate with Kirschner wire intramedullary supplemental fixation with no loss of reduction. This construct was noted to be superior to standard fixation, with 81% greater resistance to bending and twice the torsional resistance to motion.

Advocated by Schon et al.,[81] multiple tetracortical screw fixation has been shown to provide significant structural stiffness in resisting axial and external rotation loads compared with Kirschner intramedullary supplemental fixation.[86]

In patients with severely unstable ankle fractures or those who sustained fracture dislocations with concurrent loss of protective sensation, a retrograde transcalcaneal–talar–tibial fixation with large Steinmann pins or screws can be done to improve the rigidity of the standard open reduction internal fixation construct. The intramedullary implants were removed at 12 to 16 weeks. Jani et al.[83] reported a 25% complication rate in a case series of 16 patients using this technique. Of the 16 patients, four had deep infections, and two of those patients required a transtibial amputation. The authors reported stable ankle fixation in 13 of 15 patients and no deaths or Charcot malunions. In comparison, Blotter et al.[65] reported a 43% complication rate in a series of 21 diabetic patients treated operatively for an isolated ankle fracture using conventional techniques, with complications including deep or superficial infections, loss of fixation, and the need for additional procedures such as an amputation.

Another technique for pin fixation has been described through the use of extra-articular ankle pin fixation to avoid complications found with disruptions through the sole of the foot or crossing the tibiotalar articular surface. Pins are placed from the anterior distal tibia to the posterolateral aspect of the calcaneus tuberosity and from the distal medial tibial metaphysis to the dorsal navicular passing anterior and dorsal to the ankle and talonavicular joint, respectively. League et al.[87] reported no difference in stiffness of the construct compared with transarticular fixation in a biomechanical study.

Fixed angle screws through the use of locked plates can also be done to minimize individual screw loosening and localized construct failure. Fixation with locked plates was found to be independent of bone mineral density compared with conventional plating.[88] As a result, locked plates may be advantageous in osteoporotic patients with distal fibular fractures.

If soft tissue injury is a concern, percutaneous fibula fixation may be considered. The plate is inserted retrograde through a small distal incision and fixed to bone using percutaneous cortical screws along with multiple syndesmotic screws to increase rigidity. Furthermore, external fixation, such as a ring fixator, can be used in patients with soft tissue concerns to provide a more stable construct in conjunction with internal hardware or by itself without internal fixation as the definitive treatment.[67,82]

Outcomes

Schon et al.[38] reported on nine patients with diabetes with a displaced ankle fracture treated operatively. Seven of the patients were immobilized for a total of 3 to 6 months with 8 to 12 weeks of initial non–weight-bearing restrictions. Two of the patients were treated with a shortened immobilization protocol of 6 weeks of non–weight-bearing followed by 6 weeks of bracing. The shortened protocol resulted in an infected nonunion in one case and a malunion requiring an ankle arthrodesis in the other. Prolonged immobilization healed uneventfully in six of the seven patients. One of the patients in that group had fixation with rush rods and malleolar screws, resulting in a talar avascular necrosis requiring eventual tibiotalar–calcaneal arthrodesis.

Costigan et al.[68] reported on 84 patients undergoing open reduction and internal fixation for unstable ankle fractures in the diabetic population. Most of the patients healed uneventfully and without complications. However, patients with peripheral neuropathy or lack of pedal pulses were found to be at increased risk for infection, Charcot arthropathy, amputation, nonunion, and malunions.

Egol et al.[89] evaluated the predictors of short-term functional outcome in patients who underwent operative management for ankle fractures. In that level I prognostic study, they found that absence of diabetes along with younger age, male sex, and lower American Society of Anesthesia classification were predictive of improved functional recovery. At 1 year, 71% of patients with diabetes versus 92% of nondiabetics regained more than 90% of their baseline function.

Complications rates for the different methods of surgical fixation were compared in a study by Wukich et al.[67] Patients treated with supplemental fixation comprising either tetracortical screws or transarticular pins in addition to the usual internal fixation had significantly fewer overall complications compared to those treated with standard fixation alone or with external fixation with or without limited internal fixation. The highest overall complications rates were found in those treated with external fixation or external fixation with limited internal fixation. The authors attributed this finding to higher rates of open fractures and less optimal soft tissue envelope in those treated with external fixation. They were careful to not condemn the use of external fixation in the patient with diabetes and recommended its use in those with severe soft tissue compromise and in those who cannot comply with prolonged non–weight-bearing restrictions. They noted that patients in the latter group might benefit from a neutral circular ring fixator with limited internal fixation to minimize potential problems from premature weight-bearing.

Complications

Although surgical complications can be minimized by recognizing the importance of soft tissue stabilization and providing extra rigid fixation, it is clear that patients with diabetes, especially those with comorbidities such as peripheral neuropathy and peripheral vascular disease, have a significantly higher complication rate compared with nondiabetics.[67,68,82,89,90] SooHoo et al.[90] reported increased short-term risk of wound infection and breakdown, revision open reduction internal fixation, amputation, and mortality among patients with diabetes, especially those with complicated diabetes, peripheral vascular disease, or open fractures. Those with complicated diabetes were also strong predictors of reoperation with ankle fusion or replacement.

Rates of deep infections and loss of fixation has been noted to be 43% in patients with diabetes compared with 15.5% in nondiabetics.[65] An infection rate as high as 30% has been reported.[91] McCormack et al.[76] reported six major complications in his surgically treated group of 19 diabetic patients with ankle fractures versus no complications in the nondiabetic group. The serious complications included malunions, deep infections resulting in sepsis, severe necrosis requiring a flap or amputation, and death.[76]

REFERENCES

1. Centers for Disease Control and Prevention. National diabetes fact sheet: national estimates and general information on diabetes and prediabetes in the United States 2011. http://www.cdc.gov/diabetes/pubs/factsheet11.htm. Accessed June 5, 2011.
2. Holewski JJ, Moss KM, Stess RM, et al. Prevalence of foot pathology and lower extremity complications in a diabetic outpatient clinic. J Rehabil Res Dev 1989;26(3):35–44.

3. Guyton GP, Saltzman CL. The diabetic foot: basic mechanisms of disease. Instr Course Lect 2002;51:169–181.

4. Laughlin RT, Calhoun JH, Mader JT. The diabetic foot. J Am Acad Orthop Surg 1995;3(4):218–225.

5. Asbury AK. Understanding diabetic neuropathy. N Engl J Med 1988;319(9):577–578.

6. Adler AI, Boyko EJ, Ahroni JH, et al. Risk factors for diabetic peripheral sensory neuropathy. Results of the Seattle Prospective Diabetic Foot Study. Diabetes Care 1997;20(7):1162–1167.

7. Brodsky JW. The diabetic foot. In: Coughlin MJ, Mann RA, Saltzman CL, eds. Surgery of the foot and ankle, 8th ed. Philadelphia: Mosby Elsevier, 2007:1281–1368.

8. Brand PW. Tenderizing the foot. Foot Ankle Int 2003;24(6):457–461.

9. Gilmore JE, Allen JA, Hayes JR. Autonomic function in neuropathic diabetic patients with foot ulceration. Diabetes Care 1993;16(1):61–67.

10. Fernando DJ, Masson EA, Veves A, et al. Relationship of limited joint mobility to abnormal foot pressures and diabetic foot ulceration. Diabetes Care 1991;14(1):8–11.

11. Lavery LA, Armstrong DG, Vela SA, et al. Practical criteria for screening patients at high risk for diabetic foot ulceration. Arch Intern Med 1998;158(2):157–162.

12. Singh N, Armstrong DG, Lipsky BA. Preventing foot ulcers in patients with diabetes. JAMA 2005;293(2):217–228.

13. Markuson M, Hanson D, Anderson J, et al. The relationship between hemoglobin A(1c) values and healing time for lower extremity ulcers in individuals with diabetes. Adv Skin Wound Care 2009;22(8):365–372.

14. Mantey I, Foster AV, Spencer S, et al. Why do foot ulcers recur in diabetic patients? Diabet Med 1999;16(3):245–249.

15. Wagner FW Jr. A classification and treatment program for diabetic, neuropathic, and dysvascular foot problems. American Academy of Orthopaedic Surgeons. Instr Course Lect 1979;28:143–165.

16. Jay PR, Michelson JD, Mizel MS, et al. Efficacy of three-phase bone scans in evaluating diabetic foot ulcers. Foot Ankle Int 1999;20(6):347–355.

17. El-Maghraby TA, Moustafa HM, Pauwels EK. Nuclear medicine methods for evaluation of skeletal infection among other diagnostic modalities. Q J Nucl Med Mol Imaging 2006;50(3):167–192.

18. Schauwecker DS, Park HM, Burt RW, et al. Combined bone scintigraphy and indium-111 leukocyte scans in neuropathic foot disease. J Nucl Med 1988;29(10):1651–1655.

19. Johnson JE, Kennedy EJ, Shereff MJ, et al. Prospective study of bone, indium-111-labeled white blood cell, and gallium-67 scanning for the evaluation of osteomyelitis in the diabetic foot. Foot Ankle Int 1996;17(1):10–16.

20. Apelqvist J, Ragnarson-Tennvall G, Larsson J, et al. Long-term costs for foot ulcers in diabetic patients in a multidisciplinary setting. Foot Ankle Int 1995;16(7):388–394.

21. Abbott CA, Carrington AL, Ashe H, et al. The north-west diabetes foot care study: incidence of, and risk factors for, new diabetic foot ulceration in a community-based patient cohort. Diabet Med 2002;19(5):377–384.

21a. Meggitt B. Surgical management of the diabetic foot. Br J Hosp Med 1976;16:227–332.

21b. Wagner FW. The dysvascular foot: a system for diagnosis and treatment. Foot Ankle 1981;2(2):64–122.

22. Brodsky JW. Outpatient diagnosis and management of the diabetic foot. Instr Course Lect 1993;42:121–139.

23. Armstrong DG, Nguyen HC, Lavery LA, et al. Off-loading the diabetic foot wound: a randomized clinical trial. Diabetes Care 2001;24(6):1019–1022.

24. Myerson M, Papa J, Eaton K, et al. The total-contact cast for management of neuropathic plantar ulceration of the foot. J Bone Joint Surg Am 1992;74(2):261–269.

25. Philbin T. The diabetic foot. In: Pinzur M, ed. OKU, orthopaedic knowledge update. Foot and ankle 4. Rosemont: American Academy of Orthopaedic Surgeons, 2008:273–290.

26. Mueller MJ, Sinacore DR, Hastings MK, et al. Effect of Achilles tendon lengthening on neuropathic plantar ulcers. A randomized clinical trial. J Bone Joint Surg Am 2003;85-A(8):1436–1445.

27. Sohn MW, Stuck RM, Pinzur M, et al. Lower-extremity amputation risk after Charcot arthropathy and diabetic foot ulcer. Diabetes Care 2010;33(1):98–100.

28. Holstein P, Lohmann M, Bitsch M, et al. Achilles tendon lengthening, the panacea for plantar forefoot ulceration? Diabetes Metab Res Rev 2004;20(suppl 1):S37–S40.

29. Bagdade JD, Root RK, Bulger RJ. Impaired leukocyte function in patients with poorly controlled diabetes. Diabetes 1974;23(1):9–15.

30. Sapico FL, Canawati HN, Witte JL, et al. Quantitative aerobic and anaerobic bacteriology of infected diabetic feet. J Clin Microbiol 1980;12(3):413–420.

31. Sapico FL, Witte JL, Canawati HN, et al. The infected foot of the diabetic patient: quantitative microbiology and analysis of clinical features. Rev Infect Dis 1984;6(suppl 1):S171–S176.

32. Sharp CS, Bessman AN, Wagner FW Jr, et al. Microbiology of deep tissue in diabetic gangrene. Diabetes Care 1978;1(5):289–292.

33. Morrison WB, Schweitzer ME, Wapner KL, et al. Osteomyelitis in feet of diabetics: clinical accuracy, surgical utility, and cost-effectiveness of MR imaging. Radiology 1995;196(2):557–564.

33a. Crandall RC, Wagner FW Jr. Partial and total calcanectomy: a review of thirty-one consecutive cases over a ten-year period. J Bone Joint Surg Am 1981;63(1):152–155.

33b. Smith WJ, Jacobs RL, Fuchs MD. Salvage of the diabetic foot with exposed os calcis. Clin Orthop Related Res 1993;296:71–77.

34. Charcot JM Leçons sur les Maladies du Système Nervoux. Faites a la Salpetriere. Paris, Victor Coupy, 1872–1873.

35. Jordan WR. Neuritic Manifestations in diabetes mellitus. Arch Intn Med 1936;57:307–366.

36. Jacobs JE. Observations of neuropathic (Charcot) joints occurring in diabetes mellitus. J Bone Joint Surg Am 1958;40-A(5):1043–1057.

36a. Smith DG, Barnes BC, Sands AK, Boyko EJ, Ahroni JH. Prevalence of radiographic foot abnormalities in patients with diabetes. Foot Ankle Int 1997;18(6):342–346.

37. Baumhauer JF, O'Keefe RJ, Schon LC, et al. Cytokine-induced osteoclastic bone resorption in Charcot arthropathy: an immunohistochemical study. Foot Ankle Int 2006;27(10):797–800.

38. Schon LC, Easley ME, Weinfeld SB. Charcot neuroarthropathy of the foot and ankle. Clin Orthop Relat Res 1998;(349):116–131.

39. Trepman E, Nihal A, Pinzur MS. Current topics review: Charcot neuroarthropathy of the foot and ankle. Foot Ankle Int 2005;26(1):46–63.

40. Schon LC, Easley ME, Cohen I, et al. The acquired midtarsus deformity classification system—interobserver reliability and intraobserver reproducibility. Foot Ankle Int 2002;23(1):30–36.

41. Schon LC, Weinfeld SB, Horton GA, et al. Radiographic and clinical classification of acquired midtarsus deformities. Foot Ankle Int 1998;19(6):394–404.

42. Schon LC, Cohen I, Horton GA. Treatment of the diabetic neuropathic flatfoot. Techniq Orthop 2000;15(3):277–289.

43. Sohn MW, Lee TA, Stuck RM, et al. Mortality risk of Charcot arthropathy compared with that of diabetic foot ulcer and diabetes alone. Diabetes Care 2009;32(5):816–821.

44. Jude EB, Selby PL, Burgess J, et al. Bisphosphonates in the treatment of Charcot neuroarthropathy: a double-blind randomised controlled trial. Diabetologia 2001;44(11):2032–2037.

45. Pitocco D, Ruotolo V, Caputo S, et al. Six-month treatment with alendronate in acute Charcot neuroarthropathy: a randomized controlled trial. Diabetes Care 2005;28(5):1214–1215.

46. Bem R, Jirkovská A, Fejfarová V, et al. Intranasal calcitonin in the treatment of acute Charcot neuroosteoarthropathy: a randomized controlled trial. Diabetes Care 2006;29(6):1392–1394.

47. Bevan WP, Tomlinson MP. Radiographic measures as a predictor of ulcer formation in diabetic Charcot midfoot. Foot Ankle Int 2008;29(6):568–573.

48. Raikin SM, Schon LC. Arthrodesis of the fourth and fifth tarsometatarsal joints of the midfoot. Foot Ankle Int 2003;24(8):584–590.

49. Marks RM, Parks BG, Schon LC. Midfoot fusion technique for neuroarthropathic feet: biomechanical analysis and rationale. Foot Ankle Int 1998;19(8):507–510.

50. Kann JN, Parks BG, Schon LC, Biomechanical evaluation of two different screw positions for fusion of the calcaneocuboid joint. Foot Ankle Int 1999;20(1):33–36.

51. Rosenblum BI, Giurini JM, Miller LB, et al. Neuropathic ulcerations plantar to the lateral column in patients with Charcot foot deformity: a flexible approach to limb salvage. J Foot Ankle Surg 1997;36(5):360–363.

52. Brodsky JW, Rouse AM. Exostectomy for symptomatic bony prominences in diabetic Charcot feet. Clin Orthop Relat Res 1993;(296):21–26.

53. Dalla Paola L, Volpe A, Varotto D, et al. Use of a retrograde nail for ankle arthrodesis in Charcot neuroarthropathy: a limb salvage procedure. Foot Ankle Int 2007;28(9):967–970.

54. Stone NC, Daniels TR. Midfoot and hindfoot arthrodeses in diabetic Charcot arthropathy. Can J Surg 2000;43(6):449–455.

55. Cooper PS. Application of external fixators for management of Charcot deformities of the foot and ankle. Foot Ankle Clin 2002;7(1):207–254.

56. Conway JD. Charcot salvage of the foot and ankle using external fixation. Foot Ankle Clin 2008;13(1):157–173, vii.

57. Pinzur MS. Neutral ring fixation for high-risk nonplantigrade Charcot midfoot deformity. Foot Ankle Int 2007;28(9):961–966.

58. Assal M, Stern R. Realignment and extended fusion with use of a medial column screw for midfoot deformities secondary to diabetic neuropathy. J Bone Joint Surg Am 2009;91(4):812–820.

59. Early JS, Hansen ST. Surgical reconstruction of the diabetic foot: a salvage approach for midfoot collapse. Foot Ankle Int 1996;17(6):325–330.

60. Sammarco GJ, Conti SF. Surgical treatment of neuroarthropathic foot deformity. Foot Ankle Int 1998;19(2):102–109.

61. Sammarco VJ, Sammarco GJ, Walker EW Jr, et al. Midtarsal arthrodesis in the treatment of Charcot midfoot arthropathy. J Bone Joint Surg Am 2009;91(1):80–91.

62. Simon SR, Tejwani SG, Wilson DL, et al. Arthrodesis as an early alternative to nonoperative management of Charcot arthropathy of the diabetic foot. J Bone Joint Surg Am 2000;82-A(7):939–950.

63. Thompson RC Jr, Clohisy DR. Deformity following fracture in diabetic neuropathic osteoarthropathy. Operative management of adults who have type-I diabetes. J Bone Joint Surg Am 1993;75(12):1765–1773.

64. Ganesh SP, Pietrobon R, Cecílio WA, et al. The impact of diabetes on patient outcomes after ankle fracture. J Bone Joint Surg Am 2005;87(8):1712–1718.

65. Blotter RH, Connolly E, Wasan A, et al. Acute complications in the operative treatment of isolated ankle fractures in patients with diabetes mellitus. Foot Ankle Int 1999;20(11):687–694.

66. Jones KB, Maiers-Yelden KA, Marsh JL, et al. Ankle fractures in patients with diabetes mellitus. J Bone Joint Surg Br 2005;87(4):489–495.

67. Wukich DK, Joseph A, Ryan M, et al. Outcomes of ankle fractures in patients with uncomplicated versus complicated diabetes. Foot Ankle Int 2011;32(2):120–130.

68. Costigan W, Thordarson DB, Debnath UK. Operative management of ankle fractures in patients with diabetes mellitus. Foot Ankle Int 2007;28(1):32–37.

69. Flynn JM, Rodriguez-del Rio F, Pizá PA. Closed ankle fractures in the diabetic patient with. Foot Ankle Int 2000;21(4):311–319.

70. Chaudhary SB, Liporace FA, Gandhi A, et al. Complications of ankle fracture in patients with diabetes. J Am Acad Orthop Surg 2008;16(3):159–170.

71. Hunt TK, Linsey M, Sonne M, et al. Oxygen tension and wound infection. Surg Forum 1972;23(0):47–49.

72. Jonsson K, Jensen JA, Goodson WH III, et al. Tissue oxygenation, anemia, and perfusion in relation to wound healing in surgical patients. Ann Surg 1991;214(5):605–613.

73. Lu H, Kraut D, Gerstenfeld LC, et al. Diabetes interferes with the bone formation by affecting the expression of transcription factors that regulate osteoblast differentiation. Endocrinology 2003;144(1):346–352.

74. Macey LR, Kana SM, Jingushi S, et al. Defects of early fracture-healing in experimental diabetes. J Bone Joint Surg Am 1989;71(5):722–733.

75. Shimoaka T, Kamekura S, Chikuda H, et al. Impairment of bone healing by insulin receptor substrate-1 deficiency. J Biol Chem 2004;279(15):15314–15322.

76. McCormack RG, Leith JM. Ankle fractures in diabetics. Complications of surgical management. J Bone Joint Surg Br 1998;80(4):689–692.

77. Connolly JF, Csencsitz TA. Limb threatening neuropathic complications from ankle fractures in patients with diabetes. Clin Orthop Relat Res 1998;(348):212–219.

78. Wyrsch B, McFerran MA, McAndrew M, et al. Operative treatment of fractures of the tibial plafond. A randomized, prospective study. J Bone Joint Surg Am 1996;78(11):1646–1657.

79. Sirkin M, Sanders R, DiPasquale T, et al. A staged protocol for soft tissue management in the treatment of complex pilon fractures. J Orthop Trauma 1999;13(2):78–84.

80. Lillmars SA, Meister BR. Acute trauma to the diabetic foot and ankle. Curr Opin Orthop 2001;12(2):100–105.

81. Schon LC, Marks RM. The management of neuroarthropathic fracture-dislocations in the diabetic patient. Orthop Clin North Am 1995;26(2):375–392.

82. Prisk VR, Wukich DK. Ankle fractures in diabetics. Foot Ankle Clin 2006;11(4):849–863.

83. Jani MM, Ricci WM, Borrelli J Jr, et al. A protocol for treatment of unstable ankle fractures using transarticular fixation in patients with diabetes mellitus and loss of protective sensibility. Foot Ankle Int 2003;24(11):838–844.

84. Perry MD, Taranow WS, Manoli A II, et al. Salvage of failed neuropathic ankle fractures: use of large-fragment fibular plating and multiple syndesmotic screws. J Surg Orthop Adv 2005;14(2):85–91.

85. Koval KJ, Petraco DM, Kummer FJ, et al. A new technique for complex fibula fracture fixation in the elderly: a clinical and biomechanical evaluation. J Orthop Trauma 1997;11(1):28–33.

86. Dunn WR, Easley ME, Parks BG, et al. An augmented fixation method for distal fibular fractures in elderly patients: a biomechanical evaluation. Foot Ankle Int 2004;25(3):128–131.

87. League AC, Parks BG, Oznur A, et al. Transarticular versus extraarticular ankle pin fixation: a biomechanical study. Foot Ankle Int 2008;29(1):62–65.

88. Kim T, Ayturk UM, Haskell A, et al. Fixation of osteoporotic distal fibula fractures: a biomechanical comparison of locking versus conventional plates. J Foot Ankle Surg 2007;46(1):2–6.

89. Egol KA, Tejwani NC, Walsh MG, et al. Predictors of short-term functional outcome following ankle fracture surgery. J Bone Joint Surg Am 2006;88(5):974–979.

90. SooHoo NF, Krenek L, Eagan MJ, et al. Complication rates following open reduction and internal fixation of ankle fractures. J Bone Joint Surg Am 2009;91(5):1042–1049.

91. Kristiansen B. Results of surgical treatment of malleolar fractures in patients with diabetes mellitus. Dan Med Bull 1983;30(4):272–274.

HALLUX VALGUS, HALLUX VARUS, AND SESAMOID DISORDERS

JEFFREY A. MANN

INTRODUCTION

Hallux valgus deformity refers to a lateral deviation of the great toe at the first metatarsophalangeal (MTP) joint. Although this description sounds relatively simple, hallux valgus is a complicated anatomic deformity and is challenging to treat. The term *bunion* refers to the prominent medial eminence that is present in a hallux valgus deformity, but in general these terms are used interchangeably. It is important to note that although clinically a bunion may appear to be an exostosis, it is actually the misaligned first metatarsal head that is prominent. Hallux valgus is the most common pathologic condition affecting the great toe. It most likely occurs as a combination of genetic predisposition and prolonged wearing of shoes that place abnormal pressure on the first toe.

Despite its common occurrence, there is little consensus as to the best treatment method of hallux valgus. Dozens of surgical procedures have been described to correct the deformity. When evaluating a patient with hallux valgus, it is essential to determine the primary complaint and expectations of treatment, such as whether the patient desires relief of pain or the ability to wear certain shoes. When surgery is contemplated, it is critical to carefully evaluate the patient's foot clinically as well as radiographically to determine the best procedure(s) to correct the deformity. This chapter focuses on the evaluation of bunion deformities and the decision-making process for selecting the appropriate surgical procedure to correct a bunion deformity. Juvenile bunions differ substantially from adult hallux valgus and therefore a separate section on this entity is included.

Hallux varus deformity is uncommonly encountered and is most often a result of failed bunion surgery. The etiology of hallux varus as it relates to bunion surgery, and its treatment options are discussed in this chapter.

The third section in this chapter reviews sesamoid disorders of the hallux. These disorders fall into the categories of acute fractures, osteonecrosis, sesamoiditis, painful subluxation, and degenerative changes. Diagnosis and treatment for these sesamoid disorders are discussed.

HALLUX VALGUS

PATHOGENESIS

Etiology

Bunion deformities are 15 times more prevalent in populations where shoes are worn than in populations where they are not. Footwear that constricts the forefoot appears to be the primary causative factor for development of a hallux valgus deformity. However, because bunions do not develop in all people who wear such shoes, there must be other predisposing factors.

Heredity appears to play a role in development of a bunion, especially the juvenile form; a positive family history has been reported in many studies. Metatarsus primus varus, medial angulation of the first metatarsal at the metatarsocuneiform joint, may also be a predisposing factor for development of a bunion, especially in juvenile bunions as observed in a high percentage of patients. Bunions are also more common in patients with systemic arthritides, such as rheumatoid arthritis, wherein the synovial inflammation causes attenuation of the MTP joint capsule and leads to the hallux valgus deformity.

The association of bunions in patients with flat feet and in those with Achilles tendon contractures has been hypothesized. Patients with severe flat feet as a result of generalized ligament laxity are more susceptible to bunions because of the lack of ligament stability. However, most patients with mild-to-moderate flat feet do not have a higher incidence of bunion deformities.

Hypermobility of the first metatarsocuneiform joint may play a role in the development of bunions in a small percentage (probably <5%) of patients. This concept is controversial because the obliquity of this joint makes it difficult to measure its motion by any standard means. Some authors attribute a majority of bunion deformities to hypermobility of the first metatarsocuneiform, but there is a paucity of data to support this hypothesis.

Anatomy and Pathophysiology

Normal Anatomy of the First Metatarsophalangeal Joint

The pathophysiology of hallux valgus deformity is a function of the unique anatomic relationships of the first MTP articulation. Even though no muscle inserts onto the metatarsal head, it lies in a sling of muscles and tendons. Its position is related to the position of the proximal phalanx, which has multiple muscle and tendon attachments. To understand how a bunion deformity develops and how best to treat it, a thorough understanding of the first MTP joint anatomy is necessary.

On the plantar aspect of the first MTP joint lies the plantar plate complex. The plantar plate comprises the joint capsule, the tendons of the flexor hallucis brevis, the plantar portions of the abductor and adductor hallucis tendons, and portions of the medial and lateral collateral ligaments (Fig. 6.1). The sesamoids lie within the tendons of the flexor hallucis brevis and articulate with facets on the plantar surface of the metatarsal head, which are separated by a ridge or crista. The plantar plate and sesamoid complex are attached to the base of the proximal phalanx. The flexor hallucis longus tendon runs on the plantar aspect of this sesamoid complex and inserts onto the distal phalanx.

The medial aspect of the first MTP joint is stabilized by the fan-shaped medial collateral ligament, which runs from the medial epicondyle of the metatarsal head to the proximal phalanx and the medial sesamoid. The stout abductor hallucis tendon also attaches to the medial sesamoid and plantar aspect of the base of the proximal phalanx. Similarly, the lateral aspect of the MTP joint is stabilized by the lateral collateral ligament and the two heads of the adductor hallucis tendon, which attach to the base of the proximal phalanx, the plantar plate, and the lateral sesamoid.

On the dorsal aspect of the first MTP lies the extensor hood, which attaches the extensor hallucis longus (EHL)

to the sides of the base of the proximal phalanx. The extensor hallucis brevis (EHB) lies beneath the hood ligament and attaches to the base of the proximal phalanx as well.

Pathophysiology of Bunion Deformity

Before discussing the pathophysiology of bunions, a few important concepts about the first MTP joint must be emphasized.

- The shape of the first metatarsal head articular surface is variable and therefore has a bearing on the development of a bunion deformity. A round head is less stable than a flat head and therefore more prone to develop angulation.
- The distal metatarsal articular angle (DMAA), which measures the relationship of the articular surface to the long axis of the first metatarsal, is also variable and may greatly influence a bunion deformity (Fig. 6.2).
- Joint congruence measures the relationship between the articular surface of the first metatarsal head and the articular surface of the proximal phalanx
  - □ In a congruent joint, the two articular surfaces are parallel to one another (Fig. 6.3).
  - □ In an incongruent or subluxed joint, the two articular surfaces are not parallel.

Although bunions can be classified in numerous ways, it is helpful from the standpoint of pathophysiology to classify bunions into progressive and nonprogressive deformities. A progressive bunion deformity usually starts as a normal or minimally angulated MTP joint that is unstable as a result of a round articular surface. Prolonged exposure to valgus force on the first toe, such as it occurs with the use of tight shoes, begins to cause a slight angulation of the toe. Alternatively, a genetic predisposition to valgus angulation may influence the unstable joint. Once established, the valgus angulation tends to worsen with time because of the

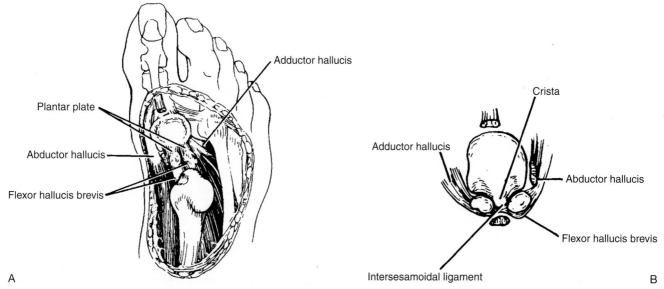

Figure 6.1 **A:** Dorsal view of first MTP joint and plantar plate anatomy with toe in plantarflexion. **B:** Cross section through MTP joint demonstrates relation of sesamoids and tendons to first metatarsal head. (From Coughlin MJ, Mann RA. Surgery of the foot and ankle, 7th ed. St. Louis: Mosby, 1999.)

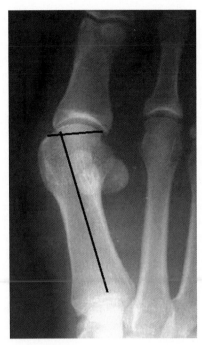

Figure 6.2 The DMAA measures the relationship of the articular surface of the metatarsal head to the long axis of the first metatarsal. The angle is the deviation from a right angle.

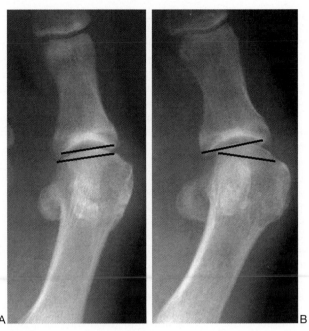

Figure 6.3 Congruent joint versus incongruent joint. A congruent joint is one in which the articular surfaces are parallel to each other (**A**). An incongruent joint is one in which the articular surfaces are not parallel or subluxed (**B**).

muscular pull of the EHL and adductor hallucis tendons on the proximal phalanx and a valgus stress during the toe-off phase of gait. Any valgus force on the proximal phalanx causes a resultant medially directed force on the metatarsal head. This contributes to a varus angulation of the first metatarsal shaft (metatarsus primus varus). Over time, the medial joint capsule becomes elongated, and the lateral joint capsule becomes contracted.

As the metatarsal head deviates medially, the sesamoid sling is held in place by strong attachments of the transverse metatarsal ligament and adductor hallucis muscle leading to lateral subluxation of the sesamoids under the metatarsal head (Fig. 6.4). On the medial aspect of the joint, attenuation of the capsular complex occurs just dorsal to the abductor hallucis tendon because this region is the weakest portion of the medial capsule. Therefore, as the

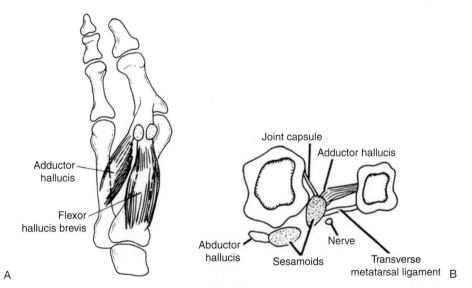

Figure 6.4 **A:** Dorsal view of hallux valgus pathology with lateral subluxation of the sesamoids. **B:** Transverse view through the metatarsal head, showing lateral subluxation of the sesamoids, contracture of the medial joint capsule, and position of abductor hallucis tendon under the metatarsal head. (From Coughlin MJ, Mann RA. Surgery of the foot and ankle, 7th ed. St. Louis, MO: Mosby, 1999.)

metatarsal head deviates medially and the proximal phalanx deviates laterally, the abductor hallucis tendon slides underneath the metatarsal head. The attachment of the abductor hallucis tendon on the proximal phalanx causes the entire first toe to rotate around its axis into pronation. As the proximal phalanx is rotated around the metatarsal head, an incongruent or subluxed joint is created.

The mechanism whereby bunions occur in nonprogressive joints is different. These deformities usually occur in congruent joints because of to anatomic features. Occasionally, an enlarged medial eminence may be present that exerts pressure on the medial side of the foot, causing a painful bursa or impingement on the cutaneous nerves. In other cases, patients have lateral deviation to the articular surface of their metatarsal head (an increased DMAA). A large enough deformity of this type causes a prominent medial eminence and varus tilting of the first metatarsal shaft. This deformity is more stable and less likely to progress because of a congruent MTP joint, but it may still be painful if the deformity is severe.

Hallux valgus interphalangeus is defined as a valgus deformity of the great toe due to valgus angulation of more than 10° of the proximal or distal articular surface of the proximal phalanx in relation to the long axis of the proximal phalanx (Fig. 6.5). Hallux valgus interphalangeus tends to be a nonprogressive deformity.

DIAGNOSIS

History

Although a diagnosis of a bunion deformity is usually straightforward, the history yields important information about the etiology of the patient's symptoms and expectations. The chief complaint is usually pain. Pain can be located diffusely around the MTP joint, or it may be more localized over the medial eminence, dorsal MTP joint, beneath the sesamoids, or along the cutaneous nerves. Pain may also occur from lesser toe deformities or from transfer metatarsalgia lesions underneath the lesser metatarsal heads. Other concerns include inability to wear certain shoes, limitation of physical activities, and the appearance of the foot.

Other important factors include a history of surgery on the foot or ankle and general medical problems, including a history of gout, osteoarthritis, rheumatoid arthritis, diabetes, or peripheral vascular disease. Occupational demands are important, especially the amount of time a patient spends on his or her feet and whether heavy labor is performed. Activities that exacerbate pain, such as walking, jogging or running, and hill or stair climbing, should be noted. Noting whether the pain is worsened by wearing certain types of shoes or going barefoot and noting what footwear modifications have been made are important.

A critical issue when obtaining a history is the patient's expectations of the treatment. Expectations should include decreasing pain and increasing activity, but patients should not have unrealistic footwear expectations. Some physical activities may be limited after bunion surgery, including long-distance running, aggressive pivoting sports, and ballet dancing; forewarning patients of possible limitations is important.

Physical Examination

Clinical Features

- The physical examination begins with the patient standing to assess the degree of hallux valgus, lesser toe deformities, and posture of the longitudinal arch.
- With the patient seated, a comprehensive examination of the hindfoot and forefoot is performed.
- The medial eminence is observed for its degree of prominence and presence of a callus or painful bursa (Fig. 6.6).

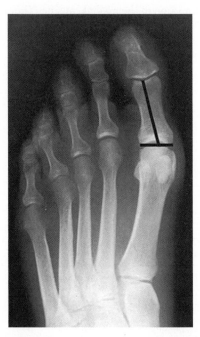

Figure 6.5   Hallux valgus interphalangeus resulting from abnormal lateral tilting of the articular surface at the base of the proximal phalanx. (From Coughlin MJ, Mann RA. Surgery of the foot and ankle, 7th ed. St. Louis, MO: Mosby, 1999.)

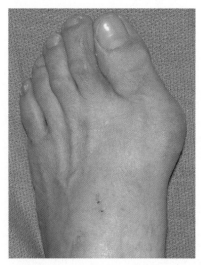

Figure 6.6   Clinical appearance of typical bunion deformity.

- The first MTP joint is evaluated for the range of motion, swelling, and the presence of dorsal bone spurs.
- Joint range of motion is compared with that of the opposite foot.
  - □ If motion is limited and exostoses are present, this indicates that some degree of osteoarthritis is present.
- The MTP joint should be palpated for tenderness dorsally, medially, and on the plantar surface.
- On the plantar surface, localized sesamoid pain (which tends to be located proximal to the joint with the MTP joint held in neutral) should be noted.
- Neuritic pain should be elicited from the dorsal or plantar cutaneous nerves, especially when there is a complaint of numbness or tingling in the hallux.
- The mobility of the first metatarsocuneiform joint is determined by grasping the foot proximal to this joint and then moving the first metatarsal and comparing it with the opposite foot with the ankle in neutral position. More than 7° to 10° of motion indicates hypermobility at this joint.
- As a simple test to assess joint congruity and flexibility of the deformity, one can manually straighten the hallux valgus deformity and move the MTP joint.
  - □ This test can help to determine the amount of correction that can be obtained at surgery without compromising motion at the MTP joint.
  - □ If the patient has a congruent bunion deformity, straightening the toe at the MTP joint makes it incongruent and therefore limits motion.
  - □ This test is less reliable with a severe bunion deformity in which significant soft-tissue contractures are present at the MTP joint.
- The lesser toes should be evaluated for hammer toes, MTP joint instability or dislocation, and plantar pain or callosities, especially underneath the second metatarsal head.
- Evaluation of the neurovascular status is important.
  - □ Overall perfusion of the foot is determined by capillary refill of the digits and palpation of pulses.
  - □ If there is a question about the vascular status, appropriate diagnostic studies should be carried out.
  - □ Careful neurologic examination helps to determine whether there is preexisting peripheral or cutaneous nerve damage that may be contributing to the patient's symptoms.

Radiologic Features

Weight-bearing radiographs are essential for accurate evaluation of hallux valgus deformity. Several features need to be assessed on these radiographs:

- Hallux valgus angle: The angle between lines bisecting the first metatarsal and proximal phalanx: normally less than 15° (Fig. 6.7).
- Intermetatarsal angle: The angle between lines bisecting the shafts of first and second metatarsals: normally less than 9° (Fig. 6.8).
- DMAA: Measure of the articular surface of the first metatarsal head, as it relates to the long axis of first metatarsal (Fig. 6.2): normally less than 10° of lateral deviation of the articular surface of the metatarsal head.

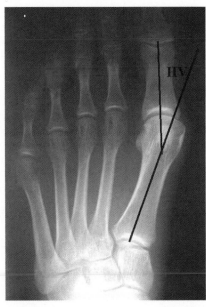

Figure 6.7 The hallux valgus (*HV*) angle measures the angle between the first metatarsal and the proximal phalanx.

- Joint congruity: Assesses whether the joint surfaces of the metatarsal head and proximal phalanx are subluxated: if the joint margins are offset, the joint is incongruent (Fig. 6.3).
- Interphalangeal angle: Angle between lines bisecting the proximal and distal phalanges of the first toe: normal, less than 10°.
- Joint arthrosis: Severity noted.
- Sesamoid position: Some degree of subluxation of the sesamoids from beneath the meatatarsal head is inevitable. Although it is not usually considered preoperatively, its correction intraoperativly is essential.

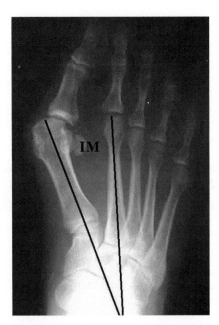

Figure 6.8 The intermetatarsal (*IM*) angle measures the angle between the first and the second metatarsals.

Bunions Are Classified by Their Severity

◼ Mild bunion: Hallux valgus angle less than 30°, intermetatarsal angle less than 13°. The joint is usually congruent, and the deformity may be due to a hallux valgus interphalangeus.

◼ Moderate bunion: Hallux valgus angle between 30° and 40°, intermetatarsal angle between 13° and 20°. MTP joint usually incongruent (subluxed); hallux is pronated and often presses against the second toe.

◼ Severe bunion: More than 40° hallux valgus angle, intermetatarsal 20° or more. Hallux is pronated and often overlapping or underlapping the second toe; MTP joint incongruent; frequently painful transfer lesion underneath the second metatarsal head; possible arthritic changes.

TREATMENT

Conservative Treatment

The cornerstone of conservative treatment is footwear modification. If the primary problem is a painful medial eminence caused by an advanced bunion, then wearing shoes with a wide toe box or open-toed shoes can minimize rubbing over the medial eminence. Bunion pads, night splints, and toe spacers may provide temporary relief, but tend to be of little help in the long term. Similarly, custom orthotics do not usually provide lasting pain relief. However, if the symptoms are primarily pain underneath the sesamoids or transfer lesions underneath the lesser metatarsal heads, soft pads can be placed in the shoes just proximal to these prominences to alleviate pressure from the painful areas. If lesser-toe deformities are the chief complaint, these can also be addressed with wide or open-toed shoes, or commercially available toe sleeves. Contraindications to surgical treatment are considered in Box 6.1.

Surgical Treatment

If conservative measures have failed to relieve symptoms from a hallux valgus deformity, surgical correction of the bunion can be offered. The anatomic deformity and other factors considered are as follows:

◼ The patient's main complaint, profession, and athletic pursuits.

◼ The physical examination findings, including the severity of deformity, the area of maximum tenderness, and associated lesser toe deformities.

BOX 6.1 CONTRAINDICATIONS TO SURGICAL TREATMENT OF HALLUX VALGUS

Absolute
■ Active infection of the MTP joint
■ Poor vascularity
■ Unreliable
■ Unable to participate in the postoperative regimen of dressing changes

Relative
■ Mild arthritis or arthrofibrosis
■ Unrealistic expectations

◼ Radiographic evaluation, including the parameters discussed previously.

◼ The neurovascular status of the foot.

◼ The patient's expectations of the operative procedure.

Not all professional or high-level athletes can return to full function after bunion surgery because of limited motion, diminished strength, or residual discomfort. If a patient's complaint is lesser-toe deformities or transfer lesions, correction of the bunion may be the only way to alleviate the problem by restoring proper weight bearing to the first ray and by providing room to straighten out the lesser toes especially the second toe.

Patients must be made fully aware about the time necessary to return to work or athletics after surgery. Furthermore, patients must be warned of the possible postoperative appearance of their foot. Mild residual deformity resulting from anatomic factors (e.g., mild hallux valgus interphalangeus), incomplete correction at surgery, or mild postoperative recurrence of the bunion may be present.

Decision-Making Algorithm

A single surgical procedure cannot be used to correct the different types of bunions. Radiographs guide the decision-making algorithm. If the MTP joint is congruent, any surgical procedure that is contemplated must not change the relationship of this articulation. With an incongruent joint, soft tissues require rebalancing, which rotates the proximal phalanx back onto the metatarsal head, recreating a congruent joint.

When starting with a congruent joint, the next step is to measure the DMAA. If the DMAA is less than 10°, three procedures result in correction of the deformity without altering the relationship between the phalanx and the metatarsal head. These include a chevron procedure, an isolated distal soft-tissue procedure, and an Akin procedure with an excision of the medial eminence (Algorithm 6.1). If only a hallux valgus interphalangeus is present, then an isolated Akin procedure can be used.

With a congruent joint and a DMAA greater than 10°, the distal articular surface must be realigned. A biplanar (medial closing wedge) chevron procedure can correct

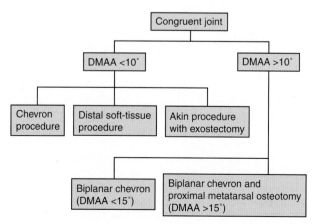

Algorithm 6.1 Decision-making flowchart for patients with a congruent joint.

up to 15° of DMAA. If the DMAA is greater than 15° or if there is an increased intermetatarsal angle, a proximal metatarsal osteotomy is required as well. These procedures are most commonly necessary in the juvenile type of hallux valgus rather than in hallux valgus associated with older patients.

In the patient with an incongruent MTP joint, numerous procedures can be performed to regain joint congruity. In general, the procedure that is indicated depends on the severity of the deformity (Algorithm 6.2). Various operative procedures have greater "power" to correct a deformity. For example, a chevron procedure can reliably correct a mild deformity, but cannot correct a severe deformity.

- A *mild* hallux valgus deformity with an incongruent joint can be treated with a chevron procedure, a Mitchell procedure, or a distal soft-tissue procedure with or without a proximal osteotomy. A proximal metatarsal osteotomy is indicated if the intermetatarsal angle is greater than 13°, although some surgeons use it for 9° to 13° deformities.
- A *moderate* deformity can be corrected with a distal soft-tissue procedure with a proximal osteotomy or a Mitchell procedure. As a general rule, the chevron procedure does not result in a satisfactory correction of this degree of deformity.
- A *severe* deformity requires a distal soft-tissue procedure with some type of proximal metatarsal osteotomy. This

procedure can usually correct deformities with up to 50° of hallux valgus and a 25° intermetatarsal angle. When the proximal phalanx is subluxed more than 50% of the metatarsal head and the soft tissues are contracted, an MTP joint arthrodesis is considered.

As indicated in Algorithm 6.2, many types of proximal metatarsal osteotomies are used for bunion surgery, and the one selected is the surgeon's choice. The ones most commonly performed include the crescentic osteotomy, chevron osteotomy, proximal oblique osteotomy (Ludloff), opening wedge osteotomy, and the Scarf (Z-shaped) osteotomy. The basic principle is that if the intermetatarsal angle is not corrected by some type of osteotomy, then the distal soft-tissue procedure will fail.

Specific Circumstances

- When moderate to severe arthrosis is present with a bunion deformity, an arthrodesis or resection arthroplasty (Keller procedure) is recommended. Attempting to correct the hallux valgus, even if the joint is left in its preoperative alignment, will most likely worsen the pain and stiffness in the joint.
- In the case of hypermobility of the first metatarsocuneiform joint, it may be necessary to carry out an arthrodesis of the first metatarsocuneiform joint (Lapidus procedure), along with a distal soft-tissue procedure. Of

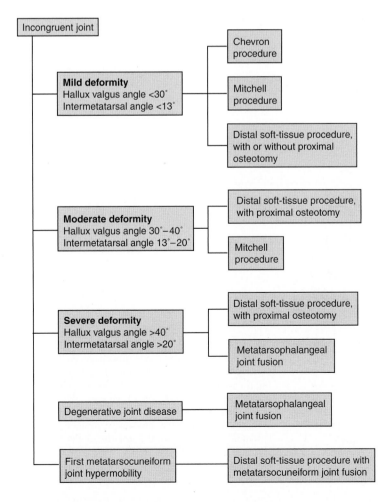

Algorithm 6.2 Decision-making flowchart for patients with an incongruent joint. DMAA, distal metatarsal articular angle.

note, a Lapidus procedure is often used by its advocates for bunion correction in the absence of hypermobility.

■ A Keller resection arthroplasty is an alternative for a severe bunion deformity when poor soft tissues may preclude bone and ligament healing. This procedure can eliminate bony prominences and crossover toes, relieve arthritic pain, and allow for some deformity correction. The sacrifice is loss of push-off strength and stability of the first toe. This procedure is generally used only in elderly, inactive persons.

■ Joint implants are seldom indicated for the treatment of bunion deformities. In a low-demand patient with degenerative changes in the MTP joint, an implant can be considered, but there is a high rate of postoperative complications, including stiffness, synovitis, transfer metatarsalgia, loosening, and implant breakage. Joint implants are contraindicated in active individuals.

Specific Surgical Procedures

Distal Soft-Tissue Procedure.   This procedure, also commonly known as the modified McBride procedure, is indicated for mild hallux valgus deformity; it can be combined with a proximal metatarsal osteotomy to correct moderate to severe deformities. The distal soft-tissue procedure corrects the anatomic deformities that lead to the hallux valgus.

■ An incision is made in the first web space to approach the lateral aspect of the MTP joint.
■ The contracted lateral structures are released, including the joint capsule, adductor hallucis tendon, and transverse metatarsal ligament (Fig. 6.9).
■ A medial longitudinal approach and capsulotomy are made to expose the medial eminence.
■ The medial eminence is removed in line with the medial aspect of the metatarsal shaft.

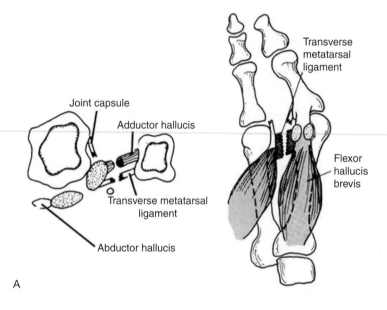
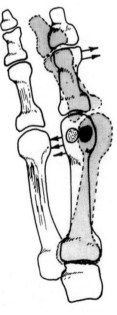
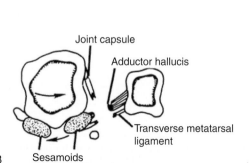

Figure 6.9   Distal soft-tissue procedure. **A:** The contracted lateral structures are released, including the joint capsule, adductor hallucis tendon, and transverse metatarsal ligament. **B:** The valgus pull on the proximal phalanx is released, allowing the metatarsal and proximal phalanx to straighten. The sesamoids can be reduced under the metatarsal head. (From Coughlin MJ, Mann RA. Surgery of the foot and ankle, 7th ed. St. Louis, MO: Mosby, 1999.)

■ The medial joint capsule and abductor hallucis tendon are plicated to hold the toe in correct alignment.

■ Postoperatively, dressing is changed weekly for a total of 8 weeks, making sure that the toe remains in alignment during this period.

■ Ambulation is permitted in a postoperative shoe.

Distal Soft-Tissue Procedure with Proximal Metatarsal Osteotomy

■ The distal soft-tissue procedure is performed as described above.

■ The metatarsal osteotomy is carried out through a third incision over the dorsal base of the first metatarsal.

■ A common type of proximal osteotomy is crescent shaped, with the concavity directed proximally.

■ Once the crescentic osteotomy is made, the surgeon rotates the metatarsal head laterally as the metatarsocuneiform joint is pushed medially. This creates approximately 2 to 3 mm of lateral displacement of the osteotomy site.

■ Care is taken not to allow the metatarsal head to dorsiflex or plantarflex.

■ Stabilization is carried out with a screw placed from distal to proximal across the osteotomy site (Fig. 6.10).

■ In osteoporotic bone or when a severe deformity is corrected, a low-profile L-shaped plate may be used to stabilize the osteotomy.

■ Other types of osteotomies have been used to realign the first metatarsal, including proximal oblique (Ludloff), chevron-shaped, Z-shaped (Scarf), and opening-wedge osteotomies (Fig. 6.11). A Lapidus procedure (first metatarsal–cuneiform joint fusion) can also be used to realign the first metatarsal.

■ Postoperatively, the treatment is the same as for the distal soft-tissue procedure.

Chevron Procedure

■ The joint is approached surgically through a midline medial incision, the capsule opened, and the medial eminence removed.

■ A chevron-shaped (sideways V) cut is made, with the apex pointing distally.

■ The metatarsal head is translated laterally approximately 3 to 4 mm on the proximal aspect of the metatarsal (Fig. 6.12).

■ The medial bony prominence created by the shifting the metatarsal head is excised and the medial joint capsule plicated.

■ The osteotomy site can be fixed with a pin or a screw.

■ If the chevron procedure is being used to correct a bunion with a DMAA of between 10° and 15°, a biplanar chevron cut should be made.

■ This type of osteotomy removes more bone medially at the osteotomy site, thereby reorienting the distal metatarsal head, decreasing the DMAA.

■ Postoperatively, weekly dressing changes are performed for 6 to 8 weeks.

■ If a percutaneous pin has been used for fixation, it is removed after 4 weeks.

Akin Procedure

■ Using a straight medial approach, the base of the proximal phalanx is exposed and a small (usually 2 to 3 mm) medially based wedge of bone is removed.

■ The osteotomy is closed down manually and then stabilized at the osteotomy site with sutures, K-wire, a staple, or minifragment screw.

■ The medial joint capsule is then plicated.

■ An Akin procedure is usually combined with a chevron osteotomy or simple removal of the medial eminence.

■ Dressings are applied for 6 to 8 weeks postoperatively.

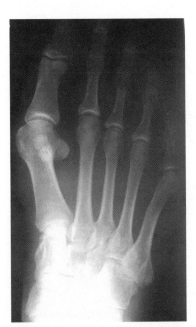 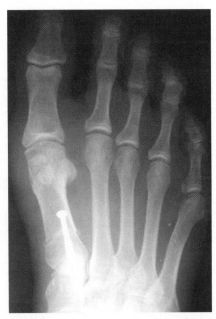

A   B

Figure 6.10 Proximal crescentic osteotomy. **A:** Preoperative radiograph. **B:** Postoperative radiograph following proximal crescent-shaped osteotomy with the concavity directed proximally.

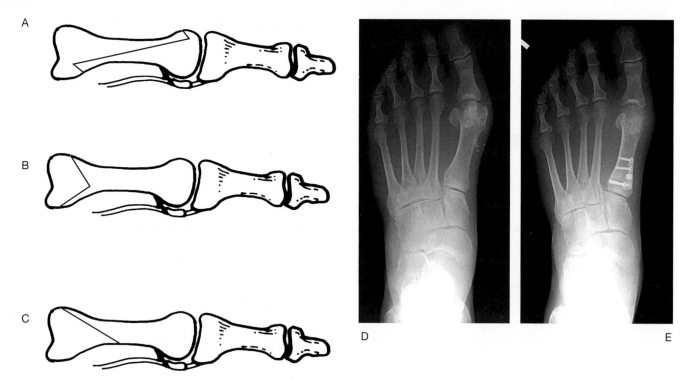

Figure 6.11. Various osteotomies that have been used to realign the first metatarsal including (**A**) proximal oblique (Ludloff), (**B**) chevron-shaped, and (**C**) Z-shaped (Scarf) osteotomies. **D:** Preoperative photo of bunion deformity. **E:** Postoperative photo after treatment with opening-wedge metatarsal osteotomy.

Mitchell Procedure

- The Mitchell procedure is a step-cut osteotomy, performed proximal to the metatarsal head.
- The distal fragment is translated laterally a variable amount, depending on the degree of deformity that needs to be corrected.

- The head can be rotated as well to correct a mild increase in the DMAA and plantarflexed to compensate for any shortening.
- Osteotomy is stabilized with heavy suture, wire, or a K-wire (Fig. 6.13).
- The medial eminence is removed.

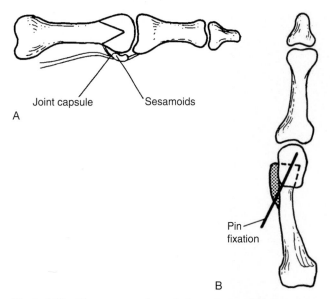

Figure 6.12 Chevron procedure. **A:** Lateral view of chevron osteotomy with the apex pointing distally. **B:** Dorsal view of chevron osteotomy after lateral translation of metatarsal head and pin fixation. (From Coughlin MJ, Mann RA. Surgery of the foot and ankle, 7th ed. St. Louis, MO: Mosby, 1999.)

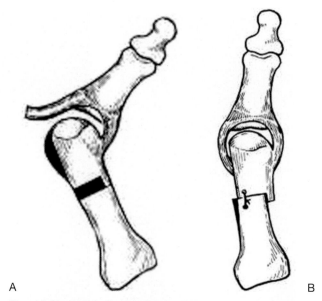

Figure 6.13 Mitchell procedure. **A:** The step-cut osteotomy is performed and the medial eminence removed. **B:** The distal fragment is reduced to the proximal fragment, and the osteotomy is stabilized. (From Coughlin MJ, Mann RA. Surgery of the foot and ankle, 7th ed. St. Louis, MO: Mosby, 1999.)

■ The Mitchell procedure can lead to significant shortening of the metatarsal and therefore should be avoided in patients with a short first metatarsal. It is generally less commonly performed today than in the past.

■ The patient is kept non–weight bearing for 3 weeks after surgery, and dressings are changed for 8 weeks.

Keller Procedure

■ The Keller procedure or resection arthroplasty consists of removal of approximately one-third of the proximal phalanx, which decompresses the MTP joint (Fig. 6.14).

■ The plantar plate and medial capsular structures are reapproximated to the remaining base of the proximal phalanx.

■ The medial eminence is also excised, and longitudinal pins are used to stabilize the operative site for 4 to 6 weeks.

■ Postoperatively, the patient is permitted to ambulate in a postoperative shoe, and dressings are changed for approximately 6 weeks to maintain alignment.

Results

Following proximal metatarsal osteotomy and distal soft-tissue release, 90% to 95% patient satisfaction has been reported with all previously mentioned techniques of proximal osteotomy. In addition to good correction of the bunion deformity, pain from the medial eminence is eliminated in most patients, and second metatarsal head pain is reduced or eliminated. MTP joint motion is usually maintained, and most patients can perform at the same or higher activity level following surgery. Preoperatively, approximately one-third of patients can wear any shoe, and postoperatively this increases to two-thirds of patients. Seventy-five percent of patients have correction of their joint to the normal range of hallux valgus angle, that is, less than 15°.

Following a chevron procedure, 80% of patients rate their result as good or excellent. The main cause for dissatisfaction is recurrence of the deformity or incomplete correction. This occurs when trying to "overextend" the indications for a chevron procedure.

Complications

The most common complication following bunion surgery is recurrence of the hallux valgus deformity. This may be a result of incorrect procedure selection, such as using a less "powerful" procedure to correct a more severe deformity or if congruency of the joint was not recognized or considered before surgery. Another common cause of recurrence is malposition of the osteotomy site. Taking care during the surgical procedure to align and fixate the osteotomy correctly can help minimize this problem.

The complication of hallux varus following bunion surgery may occur from various causes, including overplication of the medial joint capsule, excessive medial eminence resection, or overcorrection at the metatarsal osteotomy site (Fig. 6.15). It is a less common complication than hallux valgus recurrence, but often more symptomatic and more difficult to correct. Mild hallux varus deformity of up to 7° to 10° is usually painless unless the joint is also hyperextended.

Excessive shortening of the first metatarsal is an uncommon complication following bunion surgery, although minor shortening usually follows any metatarsal osteotomy. In the chevron or proximal crescentic osteotomy, approximately 2 mm of shortening occurs. A greater degree of shortening occurs following MTP fusion, Lapidus procedure, or Mitchell procedure. If there is excessive shortening, the first metatarsal head may not adequately support weight during ambulation, resulting in painful transfer lesions under the lesser metatarsal heads. Usually 6 mm or more of shortening is required before transfer metatarsalgia occurs.

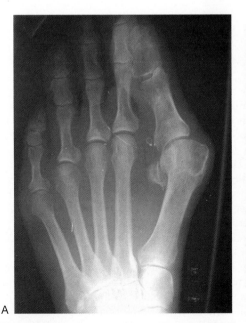 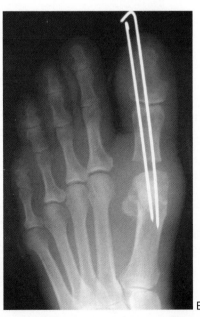

A   B

Figure 6.14   Keller procedure. **A:** Preoperative photo of severe bunion deformity with arthritis. **B:** Postoperative photo after Keller procedure. The base of the proximal phalanx has been resected along with the medial eminence.

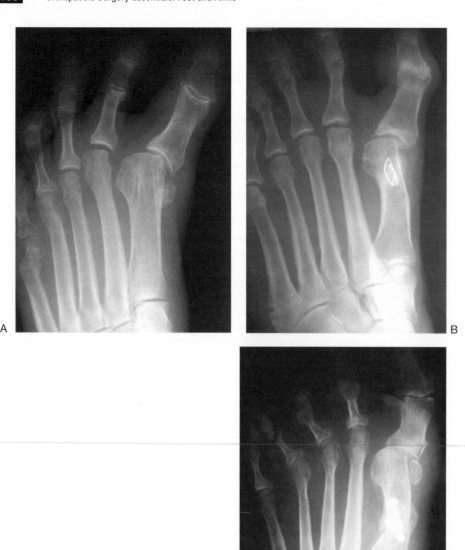

Figure 6.15 Hallux varus owing to various causes. **A:** Overplication following a bunion procedure. **B:** Excessive medial eminence resection. **C:** Lateral translation of the metatarsal head.

Malposition can occur following an osteotomy or arthrodesis procedure, leading to symptomatic sequelae. Dorsiflexion of the first metatarsal can lead to transfer metatarsalgia under the lesser metatarsal heads. Plantarflexion can lead to pain under the first metatarsal head, because more weight is borne by the first metatarsal. Varus malposition of the metatarsal can lead to recurrence of the bunion deformity, whereas valgus malposition can cause a hallux varus deformity.

Infections can occur following any procedure but are uncommon. Nonunion or delayed unions of osteotomy sites occur infrequently and are rarely symptomatic when they do occur. Arthrofibrosis of the joint can take place following surgery, especially if one has created an incongruent joint. Entrapment of the dorsal or plantar cutaneous nerves can occur, resulting in

neuritic symptoms. However, this is uncommon when care is taken to use a midline approach as described in the technique section.

Distal Soft-Tissue Procedure. The most common complication following an isolated distal soft-tissue procedure is recurrence of the deformity, usually because the deformity was too severe to be corrected by this procedure alone. In these cases, revision of the bunion surgery with a metatarsal osteotomy added to the distal soft-tissue procedure corrects the problem.

Hallux varus can occur in approximately 5% to 7% of cases. In the past, hallux varus occurred more frequently as a result of excision of the fibular sesamoid, which caused joint instability and asymmetric pull on the proximal phalanx by the medial flexor hallucis brevis.

Distal Soft-Tissue Procedure with Proximal Metatarsal Osteotomy.   The addition of the osteotomy to the soft-tissue procedure adds the increased risks associated with malposition of the osteotomy site. Dorsiflexion of the osteotomy site may occur in up to 30% of cases, but it is usually not clinically significant. Delayed union of the osteotomy site (more than 4 to 6 months) occurs in up to 10% of cases, but nonunion of the osteotomy develops in less than 1% of cases. Hallux varus deformity can occur as a result of excessive lateral displacement of the metatarsal head.

Chevron Procedure.   The most serious complication following a chevron procedure is avascular necrosis of the metatarsal head, which is probably the result of extensive stripping of the soft tissue surrounding the head. Avascular necrosis occurs in 1% to 2% of cases. As with any type of osteotomy, the distal fragment can be placed or can migrate either too far laterally or too far medially, resulting in a hallux varus or recurrent valgus deformity. Furthermore, the distal fragment can infrequently dorsiflex or plantarflex, which can lead to symptoms of metatarsalgia.

Akin Procedure.   The primary complication that occurs following an Akin osteotomy is undercorrection or overcorrection of the deformity. Nonunion occasionally occurs, but is usually not symptomatic.

Keller Procedure.   Because the base of the proximal phalanx has been removed, instability and loss of weight bearing by the first MTP joint occurs following a Keller procedure with resultant loss of foot function and is the prime reason for its use in elderly, low demand patients. A transfer lesion often develops underneath the second metatarsal head. The great toe may drift into dorsiflexion and varus or valgus.

Mitchell Procedure.   The main complication following the Mitchell procedure is shortening of the metatarsal and subsequent transfer lesion. To counteract this, the metatarsal must be plantarflexed slightly when creating the osteotomy. Furthermore, because the osteotomy is somewhat unstable, displacement into dorsiflexion can occur. For these reasons, it is used less commonly today.

JUVENILE HALLUX VALGUS

PATHOGENESIS

Juvenile hallux valgus starts in the preteen or teenage years. Approximately half of bunions fall into this category, although less than 10% of bunion procedures are actually performed on juveniles.

The typical juvenile bunion differs from adult hallux valgus in several ways. Most juvenile deformities have congruent MTP joints with an increased DMAA and often have only mildly increased hallux valgus and intermetatarsal angles. Conversely, most adult deformities have incongruent joints and tend to have greater increases in hallux valgus and intermetatarsal angles. There is a higher incidence of hypermobility of the metatarsocuneiform joint in juveniles. The juvenile form is primarily an inherited condition in contrast to adult-onset hallux valgus. Care must be taken when performing a proximal metatarsal osteotomy in younger patients to avoid growth plate damage.

TREATMENT

Despite the differences between adult and juvenile bunions, the treatment principles and decision-making process are the same. Nonoperative treatment is attempted initially. Most surgeons discourage surgery until the growth plates are closed to avoid inadvertent growth plate injury and subsequent shortening or angulation of the first metatarsal.

When surgery is planned, one must determine whether the joint is congruent. A congruent joint, even in a fairly advanced deformity, must be treated with a procedure that maintains joint congruency. Mild deformities can be treated with chevron osteotomy. If the deformity is more severe, it usually means that the DMAA is greater, which requires a biplanar chevron or a proximal and distal metatarsal osteotomy (double osteotomy). Occasionally, an Akin procedure is necessary as well if the DMAA is quite advanced.

In the case of an incongruent joint, a mild deformity can be treated with a distal soft-tissue procedure, Chevron, or Mitchell procedure. A deformity with an increased intermetatarsal angle requires a proximal metatarsal osteotomy or opening wedge medial cuneiform osteotomy.

Results

There are few published series of the results of surgical correction of juvenile bunions. However, a slightly higher rate of recurrence after surgery is noted than in the adult population; therefore, patients must be warned about this fact.

HALLUX VARUS

Hallux varus deformity is medial deviation of the proximal phalanx on the metatarsal head (Fig. 6.15). It occurs most commonly as a complication of hallux valgus surgery, but occasionally is a posttraumatic or congenital deformity. The treatment of hallux varus depends on the severity of the deformity and the level of symptoms. This section focuses exclusively on hallux varus that occurs as a result of hallux valgus surgery.

PATHOGENESIS

Hallux varus most commonly occurs after a distal soft-tissue procedure (with or without a metatarsal osteotomy) but can occur following any bunion procedure. Several factors contribute to development of a hallux varus deformity as follows:

- Removal of the fibular sesamoid
- Excessive resection of the medial eminence
- Overplication of the medial capsular structures
- Malalignment of the osteotomy site
- Overcorrection with the postoperative bunion dressing

In the past, hallux varus was associated with a distal soft-tissue procedure when the fibular sesamoid was removed, a practice no longer advised. Sesamoid removal leads to muscle imbalance because the adductor tendon and the lateral head of the flexor hallucis brevis are detached, resulting in the unopposed pull of the abductor hallucis and the medial flexor hallucis brevis, leading to a varus deformity. Furthermore, the metatarsal head may "buttonhole" through the defect left after sesamoid removal. The MTP joint may become hyperextended with interphalangeal joint flexion (a cockup deformity). Even without removal of the fibular sesamoid, however, the distal soft-tissue procedure is at risk of developing a hallux varus deformity because all of the lateral capsular structures are released during the course of the procedure. If the medial capsule is over-tightened or the toe is pulled into varus during dressing changes, there is minimal opposing force from the lateral joint, and a progressive varus may occur.

When performing the distal soft-tissue procedure, the medial eminence should be resected in line with the medial border of the metatarsal shaft. If an excessive amount of the medial eminence is removed, a hallux varus can develop because the MTP joint may no longer be stable with the toe in the corrected position (see Fig. 6.15B).

If a metatarsal osteotomy is overcorrected and the metatarsal head is translated too far laterally, the MTP joint is destabilized, which increases the risk of developing hallux varus. This situation most commonly occurs with a less stable proximal osteotomy such as a crescentic osteotomy (see Fig. 6.15C).

DIAGNOSIS AND TREATMENT

The diagnosis of a hallux varus deformity is obvious clinically, and the etiology usually becomes clear with radiographs. Identifying a foot at risk for developing hallux varus in the early postoperative period may allow for a simpler solution. If there is a mild varus, then frequent dressing changes that pull the toe into valgus may successfully reestablish alignment of the MTP joint. If dressing changes do not correct the deformity, then a medial capsular release can be performed, followed by a careful follow-up and dressing changes.

For a more long-standing deformity, the treatment of hallux varus depends on the degree of deformity and level of symptoms. A mild varus deformity of 7° to 10° is usually flexible and painless and is not clinically significant. However, more severe varus or a stiffer deformity is usually not well tolerated because the medial side of the great toe pushes against the shoe. Furthermore, once a hallux varus becomes fixed, a simple soft-tissue release is not adequate treatment. Common corrective procedures are as follows:

- EHL or EHB transfer—indicated if there is no evidence of degenerative joint disease, preserves motion.
- First MTP fusion—for degenerative changes at the MTP joint, guarantees proper alignment of the joint, but motion is sacrificed.

If the hallux varus has been caused by excessive lateral translation of the metatarsal head from an osteotomy, one must evaluate whether a soft-tissue correction alone will be adequate. A corrective osteotomy may be necessary to translate enough of the metatarsal head into position to prevent recurrence of the varus. Similarly, if the hallux varus is a result of excessive resection of the medial eminence, a tendon transfer may lead to recurrence, even with a corrective osteotomy. In this circumstance, a fusion may be necessary.

Extensor Hallucis Longus Transfer

- The medial joint capsule is released using a long oblique incision until the MTP joint can be passively reduced, taking care to release the abductor hallucis tendon.
- If the interphalangeal joint has a flexion contracture greater than 15°, the interphalangeal joint should be fused.
- The lateral two-thirds of the extensor hallucis tendon is detached from the distal phalanx and split from the medial one-third.
- This tendon slip is then routed deep to the transverse metatarsal ligament in the first web space and passed lateral to medial through a transverse drill hole in the base of the proximal phalanx.
- The tendon is pulled taut and sutured to the periosteum over the medial aspect of the phalanx, holding the toe in 10° to 15° of valgus (Fig. 6.16). Some surgeons advise placement of a K-wire temporarily to help protect the repair.
- Weekly dressing changes are performed for 8 weeks.

Approximately 80% of the time this procedure is effective in correcting the hallux varus. Generally, there is some residual stiffness in the MTP joint, but adequate range of motion remains for normal function.

Extensor Hallucis Brevis Tendon Transfer

- The first two steps are identical to EHL tendon transfer.
- The EHB tendon is identified, left attached to the base of the proximal phalanx, and released as proximally as possible, near the base of the first metatarsal. It is usually necessary to make several small incisions to follow the tendon proximally.
- The EHB tendon is routed deep to the transverse metatarsal ligament in the first web space.
- The EHB tendon is then passed through a drill hole in the neck of the first metatarsal from lateral to medial, pulled taut and sutured to the periosteum over the medial aspect of the metatarsal, holding the toe in 10° to 15° of valgus.

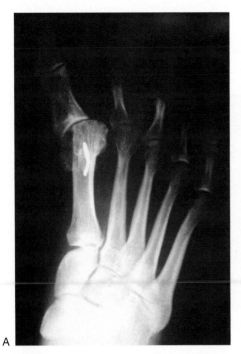 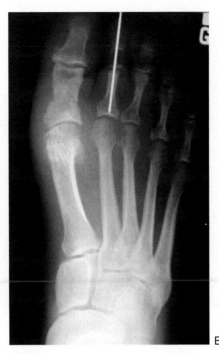

A   B

Figure 6.16 **A:** Hallux varus deformity. **B:** Correction of hallux varus deformity with tendon transfer.

SESAMOID DISORDERS OF THE HALLUX

The two sesamoids of the first MTP joint are contained within the tendons of the flexor hallucis brevis (see Fig. 6.1). Their functions include proper weight bearing of the first ray, increasing the mechanical advantage of the flexor hallucis brevis to make it a stronger plantarflexor, and stabilizing the first ray. Fractures, osteonecrosis, arthritis, sesamoiditis, and subluxation can affect these structures.

PATHOGENESIS

The anatomy of the plantar plate and sesamoid complex is detailed in the section on hallux valgus. The etiology of sesamoid pain can be obvious, as in the case of an acute fracture or stress fracture. On occasion, the sesamoids may also become painful as a result of a bunion deformity. As the metatarsal head subluxes off of the sesamoid sling, the medial sesamoid may become prominent directly under the metatarsal head, thereby causing pain (see Figs. 6.4 and 6.17).

Often, sesamoid pain is insidious in onset without a clear causative factor such as in osteonecrosis and sesamoiditis. Loss of blood supply leading to osteonecrosis frequently occurs without known trauma to the foot, implicating the tenuous blood supply to the sesamoids as the etiology. Sesamoiditis is a painful condition affecting a sesamoid, which usually occurs without known trauma to the foot. Evidence points to abnormalities of the sesamoid cartilage, similar to that found in chondromalacia patella,

as the likely etiology of sesamoiditis. Inflammation of the sesamoid bursa or peritendinous structures has been noted in cases of sesamoiditis.

The medial sesamoid is located more directly under the weight-bearing surface of the first MTP joint and is more commonly symptomatic in conditions where weight bearing is a causative factor.

DIAGNOSIS

History

Pain is usually localized on the plantar aspect of the first metatarsal head. It is worse with weight-bearing activities, especially during the toe-off portion of gait when the majority of weight is on the sesamoid–metatarsal head articulation. The level of pain also tends to be affected by the amount of padding found in the shoes. Walking barefoot is frequently very painful.

The onset of symptoms can be helpful in determining the cause of sesamoid pain. A single episode of trauma or repetitive trauma is most likely to cause a fracture or stress fracture, respectively, or a plantar plate disruption. Insidious onset of pain is found with osteonecrosis or sesamoiditis. A history of prior foot surgery or a hallux valgus deformity may indicate metatarsal malalignment as the cause of sesamoid pain.

Physical Examination

Clinical Features

Careful evaluation is necessary to identify the most painful area. The medial and lateral sesamoids are palpated

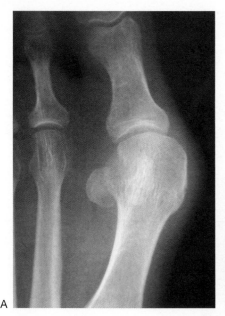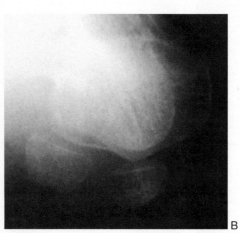

A   B

Figure 6.17   **A:** Anteroposterior radiograph of sesamoid subluxation. **B:** Axial radiograph of sesamoid subluxation.

separately, as are the plantar plate and MTP joint. Swelling or callus formation under the sesamoids is noted. If a bunion is present, a prominent medial sesamoid may be the source of pain.

Range of motion and strength of the first MTP joint should be noted. Foot posture such as a cavovarus foot may place excessive pressure under the first metatarsal head and therefore the sesamoids.

Radiologic Features

Standard anteroposterior and lateral radiographs of the foot are obtained. An axial tangential, sesamoid view of the sesamoids may show subluxation of the sesamoids or joint space narrowing and may help detect fractures (Figs. 6.17 and 6.18). Medial and lateral oblique views to evaluate the sesamoids with minimal overlay from the metatarsal head may also be helpful. Fragmentation of

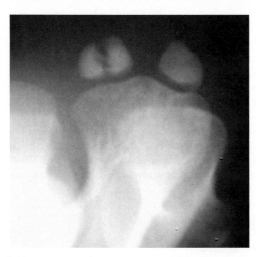

Figure 6.18   Axial radiograph of sesamoid fracture.

the sesamoid, or focal areas of lysis or sclerosis, may be seen on any of the radiographs. Displaced fractures are easy to diagnose, but nondisplaced fractures may be difficult to distinguish from a bipartite sesamoid, which is a normal finding. A bone scan may be helpful to distinguish an acute fracture from a nonfractured bipartite sesamoid. If a plantar plate injury is suspected, getting an anteroposterior radiograph of the opposite side will help to determine whether there is proximal migration of the sesamoids, indicative of complete disruption of the plantar plate. In the case of normal radiographs, a bone scan may help make diagnoses of osteonecrosis or sesamoiditis. A magnetic resonance imaging (MRI) scan is occasionally indicated for sesamoid disorders, particularly to evaluate the integrity of the plantar plate.

TREATMENT

In the case of a displaced sesamoid fracture or avulsion of the sesamoid–plantar plate complex off the proximal phalanx, acute surgical repair of the sesamoids is indicated (Fig. 6.19). Most other sesamoid disorders are treated nonoperatively initially. Placing a soft pad in the shoe just proximal to the sesamoids to take the pressure off the affected area is the first step. Taping the hallux into neutral or slight plantarflexion is often helpful to immobilize the sesamoids. If these modalities do not relieve pain, a stiff-soled shoe, steel shank, or short leg-walking cast for 6 to 8 weeks is used for more complete immobilization.

Sesamoidectomy

Surgical excision of a sesamoid is indicated if conservative treatment for 6 months or longer does not alleviate the symptoms. Removal of a single sesamoid usually does not affect strength or stability of the toe, although occasionally

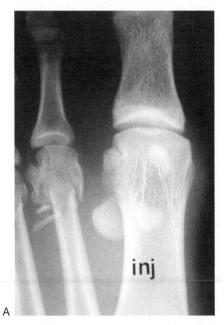
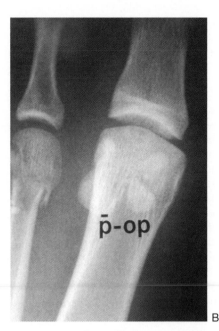

Figure 6.19   **A:** Displaced sesamoid fractures. **B:** Postoperative radiograph after sesamoid fracture repair.

a mild dorsiflexion deformity occurs. Removal of both sesamoids causes a significant cocking up of the toe because the flexor hallucis brevis tendons are detached, leading to poor function of the toe. Therefore removal of both sesamoids is avoided if possible.

Excision of the medial sesamoid is performed through a medial approach, with care taken to avoid damaging the plantar cutaneous nerve.

■ The joint capsule is incised along the dorsal edge of the sesamoid, which is retracted plantarward, allowing visualization of the articular surface.
■ The sesamoid is resected in its entirety, with care taken to perform a subperiosteal dissection and avoid damage to surrounding structures. Some authors have advocated transferring the abductor hallucis tendon into the defect area to try to avoid postoperative hallux valgus.
■ The flexor hallucis longus is vulnerable in the depth of the wound.
■ An attempt is made to close the defect in the brevis tendon with sutures.
■ A soft dressing is placed and weight bearing is allowed in 2 weeks in a stiff-soled shoe.
■ Dressings are applied, keeping the toe taped in neutral or slight plantar flexion for 4 to 6 weeks.

Excision of the fibular sesamoid is performed through a dorsal incision in the first web space. Although a plantar approach can be used, there is a risk of a painful scar developing; therefore, a dorsal approach is recommended.

■ A self-retaining retractor is placed between the metatarsal heads, and the adductor hallucis tendon is identified.
■ The adductor tendon and transverse metatarsal ligament are dissected off the lateral side of the sesamoid.
■ The sesamoid is grasped with a clamp or a threaded K-wire that is drilled into the sesamoid.

■ The remaining attachments of the sesamoid are carefully divided, including the intersesamoid ligament, avoiding damage to the flexor hallucis longus tendon.
■ The postoperative care is identical to tibial sesamoid removal.

Fractures

Fractures of nonbipartite sesamoids occur infrequently. Significant trauma is necessary to fracture a sesamoid, such as a fall or a crush injury to the forefoot, or forced dorsiflexion of the first toe. Focal swelling and pain are present over the sesamoid, and dorsiflexion of the MTP joint worsens the pain. Radiographs demonstrate an acute fracture line and possibly comminution or displacement of the fracture (see Figs. 6.18 and 6.19).

A fracture through a bipartite sesamoid is not uncommon and may occur with less significant trauma. Bipartite sesamoids are frequent, usually bilateral, and 80% occur in the tibial sesamoid. Distinguishing an acute fracture of the sesamoid from a painful bipartite sesamoid or a fracture through a bipartite sesamoid is often difficult.

Treatment of a nondisplaced or minimally displaced sesamoid fracture consists of a non–weight-bearing cast for 6 to 8 weeks, followed by another 4 weeks in a postoperative shoe or with secure tape immobilization. A persistently painful sesamoid may indicate that the sesamoid has not healed, and a computed tomography scan should be obtained. A painful nonunited sesamoid is generally treated with surgical excision. Some surgeons have advocated resecting only the smaller portion of the sesamoid. Bone grafting of a tibial sesamoid fracture nonunion may be attempted if the articular cartilage is noted to be intact at the time of surgical exploration.

Surgical repair of a displaced sesamoid fracture is technically difficult, but should be attempted in an active individual with greater than 2 mm of displacement. If there is significant displacement, this usually indicates that both sesamoids are fractured, or there is disruption of the plantar plate ligaments.

Plantar Plate Disruption

Plantar plate injury, commonly known as "turf toe," occurs with a forced dorsiflexion injury to the first MTP joint. The plantar plate, or phalangeal–sesamoid ligament, can become disrupted at the base of the proximal phalanx, from the distal end of the sesamoids or in the midsubstance of the ligament. If the injury affects only one of the sesamoids, or if there is radiographic evidence that the sesamoids have not displaced, the injury can be treated with a non–weight-bearing cast for 6 to 8 weeks and careful observation. If there is radiographic evidence of proximal migration of the sesamoids, or MRI evidence of complete disruption of the plantar plate mechanism, surgical repair of the plantar plate is indicated. This is performed through a plantar approach to the sesamoid complex. The area of the tear is identified and repaired with heavy suture through the affected ligament and periosteum of the sesamoid, or by using suture anchors if the plantar plate has been avulsed from the proximal phalanx.

Osteonecrosis

Osteonecrosis of the sesamoids is one of the more common causes of sesamoid pain. It most frequently occurs in women in their teens or 20s, but can be found in either gender at any age. Also known as osteochondritis, this condition can be seen after a single episode of trauma to the foot or with repetitive trauma such as running or dancing. Frequently there is no history of trauma.

Physical examination reveals pain under the affected sesamoid. Radiographs may show a spectrum of abnormalities. In the initial phase, X-rays may be normal. Later, fragmentation with areas of lysis and sclerosis are noted. Over time, the sesamoid may become flattened and elongated, although occasionally the sesamoid regains its normal appearance.

In general, with conservative modalities and patience, as the acute phase of osteonecrosis subsides, the reparative phase takes over, and symptoms gradually disappear over 6 to 12 months in the absence of fragmentation. If pain persists for more than 12 months, the affected sesamoid may require removal, which is more common with fragmentation.

Arthritis

Arthritis may occur at the sesamoid-–metatarsal head articulation. It may be associated with degenerative arthritis of the first MTP joint, rheumatoid arthritis, or as a result of trauma, chronic dislocation of the sesamoids, or osteonecrosis. Examination shows localized tenderness under the sesamoid. First MTP joint motion is limited in the case of rheumatoid or degenerative arthritis. Radiographs demonstrate osteophytes and often distortion of the sesamoid. Narrowing of the joint space is noted on axial view.

Conservative treatment of sesamoid arthritis is aimed at unweighting the sesamoid and limiting MTP joint motion. Surgery is indicated if these modalities fail. If only one

sesamoid is affected, it is removed. If both sesamoids are affected, removal of both is contraindicated because a cockup deformity will result. Instead, an MTP joint fusion or Keller procedure is recommended where the sesamoids can be removed.

Sesamoiditis

Sesamoiditis is a painful affliction of the sesamoids not attributable to other sources making it a diagnosis of exclusion. It most commonly occurs in teenagers and young adults and may or may not be associated with trauma to the forefoot. Pain occurs while weight bearing with localized tenderness over the affected sesamoid. Radiographs are normal, but should be followed closely to distinguish sesamoiditis from early states of osteonecrosis. Although the treatment is essentially the same, the prognosis differs for these two abnormalities.

Nonoperative modalities usually relieve the symptoms over time, but surgical excision of the affected sesamoid is occasionally necessary.

Subluxation

Subluxation of the sesamoids from underneath the metatarsal head occurs in a hallux valgus deformity. The magnitude of the subluxation varies from mild to complete dislocation of the sesamoids. Technically, the sesamoids remain in the same location relative to the second metatarsal, although the first metatarsal head displaces into varus. The medial sesamoid is no longer located in its groove on the plantar medial aspect of the first metatarsal. Instead, it comes to lie underneath the crista or ridge, which makes it more prominent on the undersurface of the metatarsal and potentially painful (see Fig. 6.17). Not infrequently, patients with a hallux valgus deformity seek treatment for the pain from a prominent sesamoid. Therefore, it is important to examine the sesamoids for pain when evaluating a patient with a bunion.

Nonoperative treatment of a painful subluxed sesamoid consists of padding the affected area to take pressure off the sesamoid. If this does not relieve the symptoms, a bunion correction is performed, with special care given to realigning the sesamoids in their proper positions.

SUGGESTED READING

Alvarez R, Haddad RJ, Gould N, et al. The simple bunion: anatomy at the first metatarsophalangeal joint of the great toe. Foot Ankle 1984;4:229–240.

Anderson RB, McBryde AM Jr. Autogenous bone grafting of hallux sesamoid nonunions. Foot Ankle Int 1997;18:293–296.

Bednarz PA, Manoli A II. Modified Lapidus procedure for the treatment of hypermobile hallux valgus. Foot Ankle Int 2000;21(10):816–821.

Coughlin MJ. 1. Juvenile hallux valgus. 2. Sesamoids and accessory bones of the foot. In: Coughlin MJ, Mann RA, eds. Surgery of the foot and ankle, 7th ed. St. Louis: Mosby, 1999.

Coughlin MJ, Jones CP. Hallux valgus: demographics, etiology, and radiographic assessment. Foot Ankle Int 2007;28:759–777.

Coughlin MJ, Mann RA. Hallux valgus. In: Coughlin MJ, Mann RA, Saltzman CL, eds. Surgery of the foot and ankle, 8th ed. Philadelphia: Mosby, 2007.

Donley BG. Acquired hallux varus. Foot Ankle Int 1997;18:586–592.

Dreeben S, Mann RA. Advanced hallux valgus deformity: long-term results utilizing the distal soft tissue procedure and proximal metatarsal osteotomy. Foot Ankle Int 1996;17:142–144.

Easley ME, Trnka HJ. Current concepts review: hallux valgus part I: pathomechanics, clinical assessment, and nonoperative management. Foot Ankle Int 2007;28:654–659.

Easley ME, Trnka HJ. Current concepts review: hallux valgus part II: operative treatment. Foot Ankle Int 2007;28:748–758.

Kristen KH, Berger S, Stelzig S, et al. The SCARF osteotomy for the correction of hallux valgus deformities. Foot Ankle Int 2001;23:221–229.

Mann RA, Donatto KC. The chevron osteotomy: a clinical and radiographic analysis. Foot Ankle Int 1997;18:255–261.

Myerson MS, Komenda GA. Results of hallux varus correction using an extensor hallucis brevis tenodesis. Foot Ankle Int 1996;17:21–27.

Richardson EG. Hallucal sesamoid pain: causes and surgical treatment. J Am Acad Orthop Surg 1999;7:270–278.

Richardson EG. Keller resection arthroplasty. Orthopaedics 1990;13:1049–1053.

Shurnas PS, Watson TS, Crislip TW. Proximal first metatarsal opening wedge osteotomy with a low profile plate. Foot Ankle Int 2009;30:865–872.

Thordarson DB, Rudicel SA, Ebramzadeh E, et al. Outcome study of hallux valgus surgery—an AOFAS multi-center study. Foot Ankle Int 2001;22:956–959.

7 LESSER TOE DEFORMITIES AND BUNIONETTES

MARK E. EASLEY
UMUR AYDOGAN

Lesser toe deformities may occur in isolation or may be associated with other forefoot disorders. Although some lesser toe deformities are attributable to traumatic, neuromuscular, degenerative, or congenital etiologies, the majority probably result from inappropriate footwear. This chapter addresses the nonoperative and surgical management of lesser toe deformities. To enhance the understanding of lesser toe deformities, functional anatomy and pathogenesis of the various disorders are highlighted. Selected lesser toe disorders include claw toe, hammer toe, mallet toe, metatarsophalangeal (MTP) joint instability, Freiberg infraction, bunionette, intractable plantar keratosis (IPK), and corns.

DEFINITIONS AND ETIOLOGY

Often, lesser toe and forefoot disease are conveniently termed *hammer toe* and *metatarsalgia*, respectively; however, metatarsalgia is not a diagnosis, but a general term for plantar forefoot pain. To direct appropriate management, the treating physician must distinguish between the various lesser toe deformities and be familiar with their typical etiologies. Deformities involving the lesser toe joints are classified as follows:

- Flexible: passively correctable, usually short to intermediate duration.
- Fixed: not passively correctable, long-standing.

Hammer Toe

The hammer toe is the most commonly treated lesser toe deformity. Hammer toe deformity is defined by extended MTP and distal interphalangeal (DIP) joints and flexed proximal interphalangeal (PIP) joint posture (Fig. 7.1). Typically, the hammer toe is acquired secondary to direct pressure from inappropriately tight or short footwear. It can be flexible or rigid depending on the passive correctibility to a neutral position.

Claw Toe

The MTP joint in a claw toe deformity is in extension and the PIP and DIP joints are in flexion (Fig. 7.2). Similar to a claw deformity of the hand, a claw toe deformity is considered an intrinsic minus deformity with weakness or loss of function of the intrinsic muscles of the foot (Fig. 7.3). Tight footwear may contribute to the claw toe deformity, but intrinsic muscle weakness leads to an imbalance between the extrinsic and intrinsic muscles. Occasionally, in bilateral disease, claw toes are secondary to a neurologic condition (and an associated cavus foot) or inflammatory arthritis such as rheumatoid arthritis. Although the terms *hammer toe* and *claw toe* are often used interchangeably, these two entities should be distinguished because their treatments may vary.

Mallet Toe

The mallet toe is defined by neutral MTP and PIP joints' position with DIP joint flexion (Fig. 7.4). Trauma to the DIP joint or extensor mechanism may produce a mallet toe, but tight footwear can be a contributing factor.

Metatarsophalangeal Joint Instability

MTP joint instability may occur in any of the lesser toes, but is most prevalent in the second, followed by third and fourth MTP joints. A single traumatic event or, more commonly, repetitive stress or cumulative trauma leads to MTP joint synovitis and eventual subluxation or even dislocation of the second MTP joint (Fig. 7.5). MTP joint imbalance results from weakening of the passive joint restraints. The extrinsic and intrinsic muscles act on the joint without the physiologic resistance of the ligaments. Isolated coronal plane instability is secondary to collateral ligament attenuation and causes toe deviation; isolated plantar plate disruption leads to subluxation and dislocation in the sagittal plane.

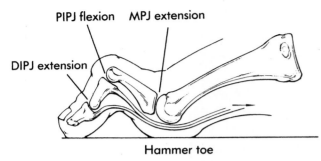

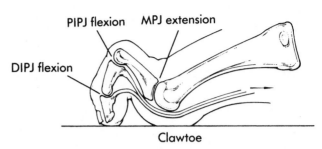

Figure 7.1 Illustration of hammer toe deformity with mild metatarsophalangeal dorsiflexion, PIP joint flexion, and DIP joint extension. There is also a callus over the prominent PIP joint. (Reproduced with permission from McGlamry ED, Jimenez AL, Green DR. Lesser ray deformities. Part 1: deformities of the intermediate digits and the metatarsophalangeal joint. In: Banks AS, Downey MS, Martin DE, et al., eds. McGlamry's comprehensive textbook of foot and ankle surgery, 3rd ed, vol 1. Philadelphia: Lippincott Williams & Wilkins, 2001:263.)

Figure 7.2 Claw toe deformity showing hyperextended MTP joint and flexed PIP and DIP joints. (Reproduced with permission from McGlamry ED, Jimenez AL, Green DR. Lesser ray deformities. Part 1: deformities of the intermediate digits and the metatarsophalangeal joint. In: Banks AS, Downey MS, Martin DE, et al., eds. McGlamry's comprehensive textbook of foot and ankle surgery, 3rd ed, vol 1. Philadelphia: Lippincott Williams & Wilkins, 2001:263.)

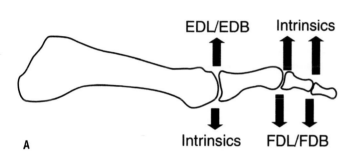

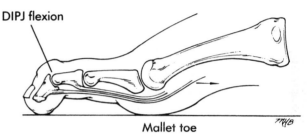

Figure 7.4 Mallet toe with neutral MTP and PIP joints and flexed DIP joint. (Reproduced with permission from McGlamry ED, Jimenez AL, Green DR. Lesser ray deformities. Part 1: deformities of the intermediate digits and the metatarsophalangeal joint. In: Banks AS, Downey MS, Martin DE, et al, eds. McGlamry's comprehensive textbook of foot and ankle surgery, 3rd ed, vol 1. Philadelphia: Lippincott Williams & Wilkins, 2001:263.)

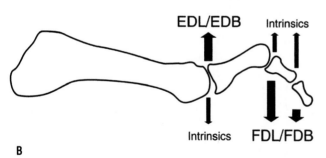

Figure 7.3 (A) Physiologic balance of extrinsic and intrinsic muscles. (B) Imbalance of extrinsic and intrinsic muscles: claw toe secondary to extrinsics overpowering weak intrinsics creating proximal and DIP flexion. (Reproduced with permission from Watson AD, Anderson RB, Davis WH. Lesser toe deformities. In: Kelikian AS, ed. Operative treatment of the foot and ankle. Stamford: Appleton & Lange, 1999:101.)

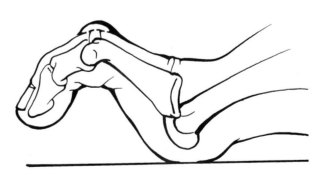

Figure 7.5 End-stage MTP joint instability with dislocation. Note the associated hammer toe deformity.

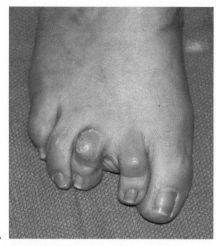
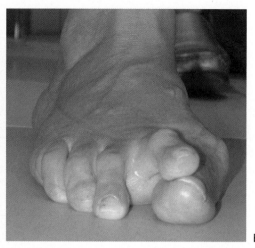

A   B

Figure 7.6 (A) Deviated deformity—the result of isolated weakness or rupture of the lateral ligaments or capsule. (B) Multiplanar instability of the MTP joint causes a crossover toe deformity.

A combination of plantar plate and collateral ligament weakening may result in multiplanar instability, termed a *crossover toe*, with the unstable toe displacing over the adjacent toe (Fig. 7.6). A relatively common mechanism for the crossover toe is a patient with hallux valgus and overload of the second MTP joint. Mechanical stress on the second MTP joint eventually leads to the second toe crossing over the hallux. Other factors that may create greater than physiologic stresses to the MTP joint, leading to instability, include the following:

- Long second or third metatarsal
- Congenital or iatrogenic shortening of the first metatarsal
- Poorly fitting shoes with a tight toe box

Bunionette (Tailors Bunion)

A painful lateral bony prominence of the fifth metatarsal head is termed a *bunionette* and can be thought of as hallux valgus of the fifth ray. Traditionally, tailors sat in a cross-legged position, creating chronic irritation on the lateral fifth metatarsal head, hence the expression *tailor's bunion*. Although chronic pressure on the fifth metatarsal head can produce symptoms without deformity, an increase in the intermetatarsal and MTP joint angle is associated with symptoms. Physiologically, the 4-5 intermetatarsal and MTP-5 angles average 6.2° and 10.2°, respectively (Fig. 7.7). On the basis of radiologic appearance, three types of bunionettes have been defined:

- Type I is a simple enlargement of the fifth metatarsal head with lateral prominence, without increase in the intermetatarsal or MTP joint angles.
- Type II bunionette deformity is characterized by a congenital lateral bowing of the fifth metatarsal shaft that creates a symptomatic increase in the MTP-5 angle.
- Type III deformity is defined by a greater than physiologic 4-5 intermetatarsal angle (Fig. 7.8).

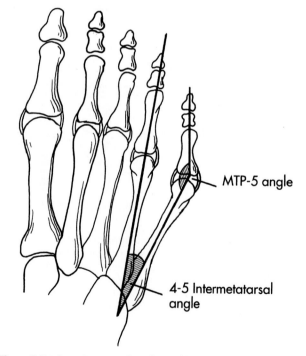

Figure 7.7 The MTP-5 angle is formed by the axis of the proximal phalanx and the fifth metatarsal. The 4-5 intermetatarsal angle is formed by the axis of the fourth and the fifth metatarsals. (Reproduced with permission from Mann RA, Coughlin MJ. Keratotic disorders of the plantar skin. In: Coughlin MJ, Mann RA, eds. Surgery of the foot and ankle, 7th ed, vol 1. St. Louis: Mosby, 1999:417.)

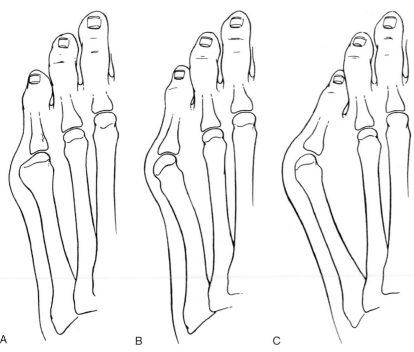

Figure 7.8 Three types of bunionette deformity. (**A**) Type I deformity with enlarged fifth metatarsal head. (**B**) Type II deformity with lateral bowing of the fifth metatarsal. (**C**) Type III deformity with increased 4-5 intermetatarsal angle. (Reproduced with permission from Cooper PS. Disorders and deformities of the lesser toes. In: Myerson MS, ed. Foot and ankle disorders, vol 1. Philadelphia: WB Saunders, 2000:336.)

Freiberg Infraction

Freiberg infraction (*not* infarction) is an osteochondrosis of the lesser metatarsal heads, most commonly recognized in the second metatarsal head. Although the exact etiology remains unknown, current theory suggests that repetitive stress or cumulative trauma results in microfractures and avascular necrosis of the metatarsal subchondral bone. Initial synovitis may progress to articular degeneration. The prevalence of Freiberg infraction appears to be greatest in healthy, adolescent females, but these avascular changes are not isolated to that patient population (Fig. 7.9).

Corns

Hyperkeratotic tissue may form over bony prominences with chronic external pressure; in the toes, these areas of hyperkeratosis are called *corns*. Purely hyperkeratotic lesions are hard corns, whereas macerated hyperkeratotic lesions are soft corns. Hard corns most commonly occur on the dorsal or lateral aspect of a toe where a prominent condyle contacts the shoe (Fig. 7.10). Soft corns develop between toes in response to contact of adjacent prominent phalangeal exostoses or condyles; the maceration is a result of the web space location (Fig. 7.11). Whereas hard corns are most common on the lateral fifth toe, soft corns are typically found in the fourth web space. Factors that may contribute to formation of corns include tight shoe toebox and relatively long toes.

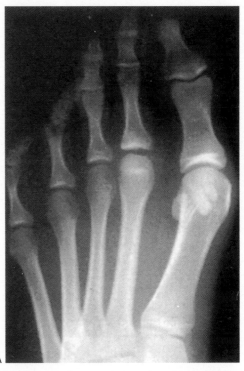

Figure 7.9 Radiographic appearance of Freiberg infraction. (**A**) Early stage with osteolysis and central collapse.

(continued on next page)

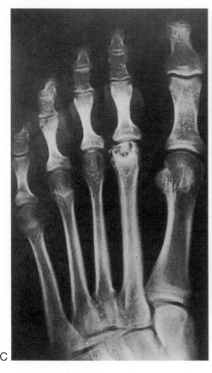
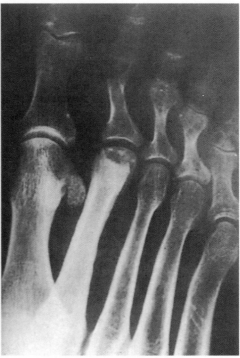

B,C

Figure 7.9 (*continued*) (B,C) Late stage with significant collapse and degeneration with new bone formation. (Reproduced with permission from Mann RA, Coughlin MJ. Keratotic disorders of the plantar skin. In: Coughlin MJ, Mann RA, eds. Surgery of the foot and ankle, 7th ed, vol 1. St. Louis: Mosby, 1999:414–415.)

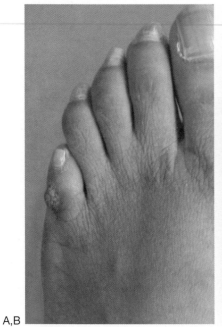
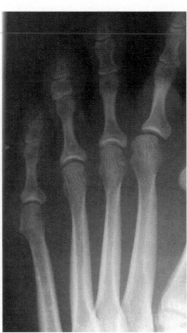

A,B

Figure 7.10 (A) Hard corns are typically found over the superolateral aspect of the fifth toe. (B) The cause is usually a prominent fibular condyle of the distal phalanx.

is highly vascular, and if shaved, punctate bleeding can be identified instead of a seed of hard tissue. The diffuse IPK affects more than one metatarsal and is usually a result of a substantial mechanical imbalance of the forefoot, such as a short first metatarsal (congenital or iatrogenic) or cavus foot. The IPK develops diffusely as the primary weight-bearing area is transferred to the lesser metatarsal heads.

FUNCTIONAL ANATOMY

The lesser toes increase the forefoot weight-bearing area during the stance phase of gait. Proper balance of the extrinsic and intrinsic musculatures and passive ligamentous or capsular restraints allows physiologic propulsion during pushoff and a physiologic resting position of 20° of dorsiflexion relative to the metatarsals.

Physiologic lesser toe balance and function rely on intact passive and dynamic stabilizers. The primary passive MTP joint stabilizers are the plantar fascia, plantar plate, and collateral ligaments. The plantar fascia augments the stabilizing effect of the plantar plate; these two structures have a combined 30% role in preventing the dorsal dislocation of the MTP joint. Although greater tensile strength of the plantar plate will be advantageous for joint stability, it will be deleterious to effective joint dorsiflexion during gait. The collateral ligaments are the more powerful static MTP joint stabilizers, contributing 50% of the resistance to dorsal dislocation and the majority of medial and lateral stability. The remainder of the stability is derived from the dynamic stabilizers.

Lesser toe extensor and flexor anatomy is complex. The extensor digitorum longus (EDL) branches into three slips over the proximal phalanx. The central slip inserts onto the dorsal base of the middle phalanx, and the two lateral slips converge distally and insert onto the dorsal base of

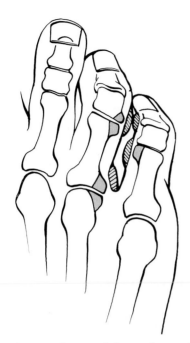

Figure 7.11 Schematic drawing of the usual sites of prominent condyles causing soft corns in the fourth web space.

Intractable Plantar Keratosis

IPKs are symptomatic proliferations of hyperkeratotic tissue occurring on a plantar area subjected to greater than physiologic stress, generally under the metatarsal heads. IPKs may be focal or diffuse (Fig. 7.12). The focal IPK comprises a rigid core of avascular tissue and generally develops under the fibular condyle (plantar lateral aspect of the metatarsal head). Often, an IPK is confused with a plantar wart. In contrast, a plantar wart

Figure 7.12 (**A**) Focal IPK plantar to the second metatarsal head. (**B**) Bilateral diffuse IPK involving more than one area on the plantar surface.

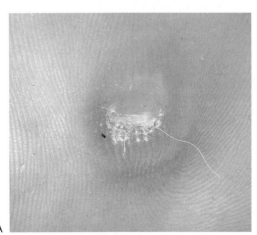

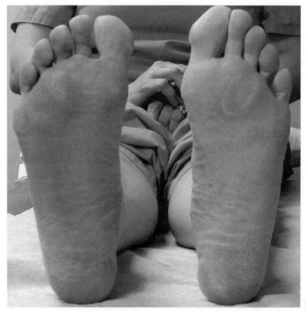

A   B

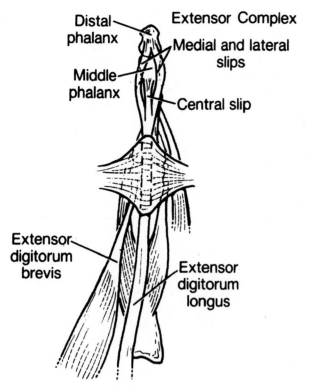

Figure 7.13 Extensor mechanism of the lesser toes from dorsal view. (Reproduced with permission from McGlamry ED, Jimenez AL, Green DR. Lesser ray deformities. Part 1: deformities of the intermediate digits and the metatarsophalangeal joint. In: Banks AS, Downey MS, Martin DE, et al., eds. McGlamry's comprehensive textbook of foot and ankle surgery, 3rd ed, vol 1. Philadelphia: Lippincott Williams & Wilkins, 2001:255.)

the distal phalanx (Fig. 7.13). Although the EDL has no direct connection to the proximal phalanx, it has indirect attachments through a fibroaponeurotic sling. The three EDL slips and fibroaponeurotic sling form the extensor hood. The EDL dorsiflexes the toe most effectively with the MTP joint in plantarflexion or neutral position; this explains why EDL function is neutralized by extension of the proximal phalanx in a hammer toe deformity. The extensor digitorum brevis (EDB) inserts into the lateral part of the extension hood of the second, third, and fourth proximal phalanges, enhancing toe dorsiflexion.

The flexor group of muscles comprise the flexor digitorum longus (FDL), flexor digitorum brevis (FDB), and intrinsic muscles. The FDL inserts onto the distal phalanx base to flex the DIP joint; the two slips of the FDB attach at the base of the middle phalanx base to flex the PIP joint. The intrinsic muscles comprise seven interosseus and four lumbrical muscles. The interossei originate from the metatarsals, course plantar to the metatarsal head axis, and attach at the proximal phalangeal bases and plantar plate. The lumbricals take origin from the FDL tendons, pass plantar to the transverse intermetatarsal ligament, and insert onto the medial proximal phalanx and extensor hood. Because there is no lumbrical laterally, attenuation of the lateral collateral ligament may be exacerbated by the effects of the lumbrical anatomy. Under physiologic conditions, however, the interossei contribute balanced dynamic plantarflexion and transverse axis MTP stabilizing forces. In addition to plantarflexing the MTP joints, the lumbricals extend the interphalangeal joints (Fig. 7.14).

PATHOPHYSIOLOGY

Trauma, congenital deformity, neuromuscular disease, and inflammatory arthropathy may induce lesser toe deformities, but the commonest factor leading to acquired lesser toe malalignment remains improper footwear. Consistent use of unaccommodating narrow shoes with tight toeboxes creates external forces on the MTP and interphalangeal joints that over time may disrupt the delicate static and dynamic balance responsible for maintaining anatomic toe alignment (Fig. 7.15). Initial synovitis evolves into ligament (static restraint) attenuation and eventual eccentric forces from the dynamic stabilizers (intrinsic and extrinsic muscles). Furthermore, unaccommodative footwear may promote the development of hallux valgus, leading to second toe impingement and further eccentric second toe joint stresses.

Imbalance between the extrinsic and intrinsic muscles, either from neuromuscular disease (i.e., Charcot–Marie–Tooth, peripheral neuropathy) or from consistent external pressure (tight footwear) may lead to shortening of the intrinsic musculotendinous units. Without the physiologic stabilizing effect of the intrinsics, the MTP joint assumes an extended posture and the interphalangeal joint a flexed posture. Ultimately, this imbalance may evolve into hammer toes, claw toes, or MTP joint instability.

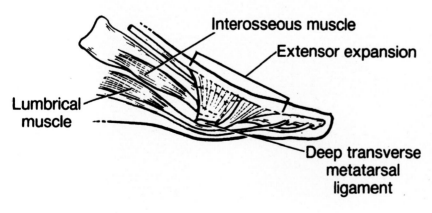

Figure 7.14 Lateral view of a lesser toe showing the anatomy and orientation of the intrinsic and extrinsic muscles. Note that the intrinsics are part of the extensor complex. (Reproduced with permission from McGlamry ED, Jimenez AL, Green DR. Lesser ray deformities. Part 1: deformities of the intermediate digits and the metatarsophalangeal joint. In: Banks AS, Downey MS, Martin DE, et al., eds. McGlamry's comprehensive textbook of foot and ankle surgery, 3rd ed, vol 1. Philadelphia: Lippincott Williams & Wilkins, 2001:254.)

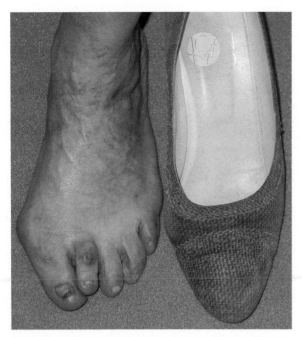

Figure 7.15 A narrow toebox shoe can cause significant crowding of the toes, which can lead to deformities.

Cumulative trauma or repetitive stress and inflammatory arthropathies may create MTP joint synovitis that contributes to attenuation of the static restraints (MTP joint capsule, collateral ligament, and plantar plate). Eventually, MTP joint subluxation and even dislocation may occur. In the second toe, development of deformity may be accentuated by a relatively long second metatarsal or concomitant hallux valgus. Moreover, if the lateral collateral ligament weakens, the medial pull of the unopposed lumbrical may further disrupt the balance. With loss of both the transverse and the sagittal restraints, instability may evolve into a claw toe that crosses over the hallux (see Fig. 7.6B).

DIAGNOSIS

History

The patient may have difficulty in identifying the focus of pain, but the pain is typically isolated to the forefoot. Occasionally, the symptoms are easy to localize, if they are confined to the dorsum of the affected toes. Hammer and claw toes may impinge on the toe box of tighter shoes; the pain is typically relieved when the patient is barefooted. Likewise, a mallet toe is usually symptomatic at the tip of the toe only. With synovitis and attenuation of the MTP joints, patients typically report pain on the plantar forefoot, but may not be able to identify the exact location of pain. Freiberg infraction may have a similar but vaguer presentation. In contrast, IPKs, particularly focal IPKs, are simple to isolate on the plantar foot. Bunionettes are also easy for the patient to localize because the pain is uniformly over the fifth metatarsal head—laterally or plantarward.

Occasionally, forefoot pain involving the lesser toes may have a systemic etiology. Given that forefoot pain may have a neurogenic component, the patient should be questioned about diabetic neuropathy and lower back pain with radiating symptoms. If symptoms persist despite non–weight-bearing and rest, peripheral neuropathy may be contributing to the generation of pain. Typically, these symptoms are burning in nature. Neuralgia may also be focal, as with a Morton neuroma; patients may describe a vague lateral forefoot discomfort interrupted by occasional sharp, shooting pains. If symptoms continue or even worsen with elevation, consideration should be given to peripheral vascular disease. Forefoot symptoms may also be secondary to an inflammatory arthritis, and the patient should be questioned about a possible rheumatologic condition.

The history should help focus the diagnosis. Although metatarsalgia is relatively nondescript, some patients may have atrophic fat pads. These individuals often feel pain relief in shoes and cannot ambulate comfortably barefooted.

Physical Examination

Although the diagnosis may appear obvious, the physician should resist the temptation to focus the examination to the affected toe. For example, a tight heel cord may be contributing to forefoot overload and should be treated in conjunction with correction of the toe deformity. Similarly, a relatively obvious claw toe deformity may be associated with hallux valgus, and treatment of the lesser toe without addressing the great toe malalignment leads to early recurrence of the lesser toe deformity.

A brief examination of the lower back with a straight leg raise test can rule out a radiculopathy. Checking pulses and sensation should identify peripheral vascular disease and neuropathy, respectively. An equinus contracture or cavus foot alignment may lead to forefoot overload. Percussion and compression over the tibial nerve to elicit a Tinel sign should rule out a compressive plantar neuralgia.

A thorough forefoot examination should avert missing associated forefoot pathology. Whereas tenderness with direct dorsal palpation of the metatarsals is suggestive of a stress fracture, tenderness between the metatarsals is indicative of an interdigital neuralgia (compressive neuropathy from perineural fibrosis of the common digital nerve, i.e., "Morton neuroma").

Lesser toe deformities frequently occur in association with disorders of the great toe. Hallux valgus may contribute to second toe disease, with chronic impingement. in combination with tight footwear, second toe hammering, clawing, or instability in particular may occur (see Fig. 7.15). Hallux rigidus or stiffness of the great toe MTP joint may lead to compensatory overload of the lesser metatarsal heads; likewise, a congenitally or iatrogenically short first metatarsal may have a similar effect.

Lesser toe MTP joint instability evolves from synovitis and capsulitis. Tenderness directly over the joint with dorsal and plantar pressure indicates articular disease. With metatarsalgia and IPKs, the tenderness is isolated to the plantar aspect of the metatarsal heads. As synovitis and repetitive trauma to the involved joint progresses, plantar

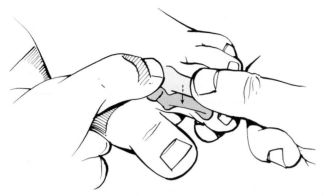

Figure 7.16 Lachman test to demonstrate instability of the MTP joint. The examiner grabs the toe with one hand and attempts to dorsally sublux the joint while stabilizing the metatarsal bone with the other hand. The test is positive if the joint subluxes and reproduces the patient's symptoms. The examiner should avoid pressing on the joint because it can cause false-positive results.

plate and collateral ligament insufficiency can be demonstrated with a toe Lachman test (Fig. 7.16). Toe deviation, subluxation, or dislocations become clinically apparent with more advanced disease.

It is difficult to distinguish MTP joint synovitis from interdigital neuralgia, especially the second MTP joint instability from a second web space interdigital neuroma. If no deformity is noted, no instability is demonstrated, and there is some difficulty in distinguishing MTP joint disease from interdigital neuralgia, then a diagnostic (and possibly therapeutic) injection may be diagnostic. The injection can be performed into the joint, the web space, or both, but in a staged

fashion. With advancing MTP joint instability, deformity progresses. The proximal phalanx may be subluxed or dislocated on the lesser metatarsal head. The joint and prominent metatarsal head are tender. The MTP joint may be reducible if the deformity is flexible. With associated collateral ligament attenuation, toe deviation is noted. Occasionally, the deformity is not apparent when the patient is non–weight-bearing, but becomes obvious with the patient standing. A common example of this is a crossover second toe in a patient with hallux valgus. Deviation is apparent, but the crossover may not occur until the patient stands (Fig. 7.17).

The clinical examination should document whether the deformity is flexible or fixed because this finding dictates the surgical treatment. *Metatarsalgia* is an inexact term meaning pain beneath the metatarsal heads. With atrophy of the fat pads (typically in older patients) or in patients with claw toe deformities (where the fat pads are displaced distally), tenderness is directly over the metatarsal heads. IPKs also produce tenderness on the plantar aspect of the metatarsal heads but with thickened skin. A focal plantar keratosis is located under a specific metatarsal head and a diffuse IPK is under multiple heads. The diffuse form is typically associated with hallux disorders, typically shortening of the first metatarsal. To distinguish a focal IPK from a plantar wart, the callused area should be trimmed. With paring of the lesion, the IPK has a deep keratotic area, whereas the plantar wart reveals punctate bleeding. Furthermore, an IPK is most tender with direct pressure, whereas a plantar wart is most tender with side-to-side "pinching" of the lesion.

A bunionette is tender on the lateral fifth metatarsal head; occasionally, tenderness is also present on the plantar aspect of the fifth metatarsal head. Although the problem may be isolated to the fifth MTP joint, typically widening of the forefoot

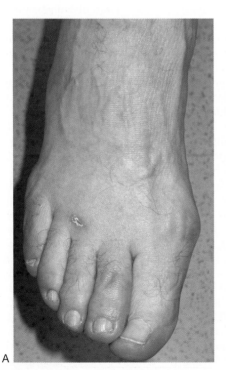
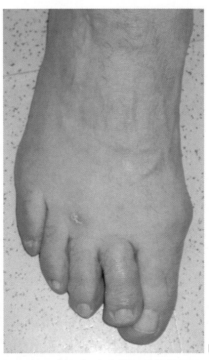

A   B

Figure 7.17 Patients should also be examined in non–weight-bearing (**A**) and weight-bearing (**B**) positions to see the dynamic nature of the deformity.

is evident. The examination should not only identify widening of the 4-5 intermetatarsal angle, but also include an evaluation of the hallux and 1-2 intermetatarsal angle because occasionally to effectively relieve lateral symptoms, the first ray may need to be addressed. Coexisting hindfoot varus and fifth toe clawing need to be identified because these may be responsible for lateral and plantar fifth metatarsal overload, respectively.

Finally, we also evaluate the midfoot, hindfoot, and ankle with the patient standing. Limited active or passive ankle or transverse tarsal joint (talonavicular and calcaneocuboid) dorsiflexion and/or cavus foot posture may contribute to forefoot overload or deformity. Limited active or passive hindfoot eversion or varus hindfoot position may contribute lateral forefoot overload. Although the problem and patient's complaints may be isolated to the forefoot, we recommend examining the entire foot and ankle to identify associated pathology.

Imaging Studies

A standard set of standing foot radiographs (anteroposterior [AP], lateral, and oblique) generally suffices to evaluate lesser toe deformities. It is important to obtain weight-bearing X-rays, which provide a better appreciation for the extent of deformity. The hindfoot and midfoot are also inspected to ensure that there is no deformity that may contribute to forefoot disease. First ray deformities (e.g., hallux valgus, hallux rigidus, short first metatarsal) should be noted. Radiographs usually rule out stress fractures and arthritic change. Furthermore, relative length discrepancies, such as a long second metatarsal, can be confirmed (Fig. 7.18). AP and particularly oblique X-rays may reveal evidence for Freiberg infraction (subchondral collapse of the metatarsal head) or inflammatory arthropathy (periarticular erosions); in our opinion, Freiberg infraction is best visualized on the oblique foot radiograph. All three views help define hammer toe, claw toe, and MTP instability. The hammer toe and claw toe deformities are evident on the lateral view, with the affected phalanges visualized in profile, dorsal to the other toes. On the AP

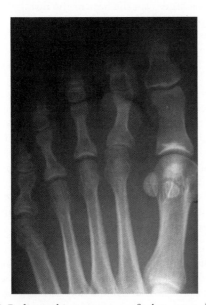

Figure 7.18 Radiographic appearance of a long second metatarsal.

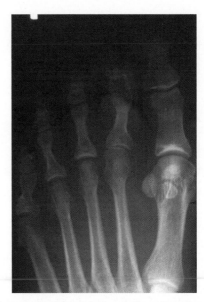

Figure 7.19 Radiographic appearance of gun barrel sign on the third MTP joint. Note the end-on appearance of the proximal phalanx, which superimposes over the condyle.

view with severe hammering, clawing, or MTP joint dislocation, the proximal phalanx may be seen axially, giving a "gun barrel sign" (Fig. 7.19).

Weight-bearing AP views are critical to determine the extent of malalignment: MTP joint instability with deviation can be defined, the hallux deformity is revealed, and the extent of bunionette deformity is noted. The bunionette classification is based on the radiographs. Furthermore, the extent of fifth MTP joint deviation can be documented.

Plain radiographs of the toes are often difficult to interpret, but close-up views provide greater detail. Prominent condyles, joint deformity, or exostoses may correlate with pressure areas or corns noted on physical exam.

MRI and Bone Scan

Plain radiographs generally suffice in the evaluation of lesser toe deformities. If forefoot inflammation is difficult to confirm clinically, a bone scan may be supportive, but nonspecific. A bone scan of the foot is most useful in confirming that a stress fracture exists—before plain radiographic confirmation. MRI can also confirm a subtle stress fracture and has the advantage of providing soft tissue detail. With continued advances in MRI technology, the forefoot capsular tissues, ligaments, and even digital nerves can be evaluated with great detail. The disadvantage is that often MRI also reveals surrounding edema that may lead to overinterpretation of disease. MRI can also be useful in defining the extent of avascular disease in Freiberg infraction, which typically affects the dorsal one-third to one-half of the metatarsal head.

TREATMENT

Nonoperative Treatment

Many symptoms related to lesser toe diseases can effectively be managed nonoperatively. Although deformity

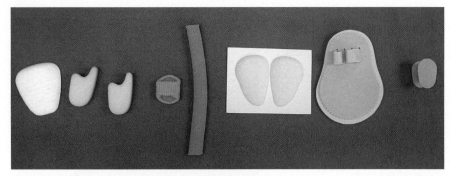

Figure 7.20 Pedorthic devices such as toe straps and spacers or metatarsal bars can be used in the conservative treatment of the lesser toe deformities.

may not be corrected, pressure relief is accomplished with shoe modifications, orthotics, or simple pads and spacers (Fig. 7.20). Dorsal pressure on hammer, claw, and crossover toes is relieved with extra depth shoes that have a deeper toebox. Wider toebox shoes relieve transverse pressure, particularly when a bunion or bunionette deformity is symptomatic. Moreover, pressure between phalanges is also diminished. Toe spacers, silicone sleeves, and lamb's wool between toes can limit the formation of corns. With flexible hammer and claw toe deformities, hammer toe slings or taping may be beneficial; even if they fail to provide a permanent solution, they may have some diagnostic purpose to determine the effect that realignment has in relieving symptoms. Distal toe pressure in mallet toe deformity can be relieved with a toe crest that bears load on the proximal and middle phalanges to unload the distal phalanx. With plantar pain, a stiffer-soled shoe with a slight rocker bottom may diminish metatarsal head pressure and plantar plate stress during the pushoff phase of gait.

Shoe modifications alone are generally inadequate in relieving metatarsal pain in advanced MTP joint deformity, in particular with MTP joint dislocation. In addition to extradepth shoe modifications, metatarsal support should be added. Full-length, custom orthotics may not be warranted; often, simple metatarsal pads or soft, cushioned, over-the-counter orthotics are helpful. Metatarsal supports accept the load directly under the metatarsals, thereby unloading the metatarsal heads. If the pads are ineffective, then more expensive custom orthotics can be considered. Seldom is casting necessary in the management of lesser toe problems. A walking boot (i.e., cam walker), stiffer-soled shoes, and temporary heel weight-bearing are adequate for unloading of metatarsal stress fractures and acute symptoms related to Freiberg infraction.

Nonoperative treatment is effective for management of acute symptoms and pressure relief; however, conservative measures fail to correct deformity. Patients with a deformity, especially a fixed deformity, may need surgical management.

Operative Treatment

With failed conservative measures, surgical intervention of lesser toe deformities may relieve symptoms. Despite correction with proper surgical technique, realigned lesser toes develop some degree of MTP or PIP joint stiffness or recurrence of deformity; therefore patients should be counseled appropriately. Furthermore, no surgical intervention should be undertaken unless digital perfusion is known to be adequate. Correction of several lesser toe deformities is similar. Despite similarities, surgical techniques are described by individual lesser toe problems.

Hammer Toe

Flexible. A flexible hammer toe deformity can generally be corrected with a flexor-to-extensor tendon transfer (Fig. 7.21).

- The FDL tendon is transferred from its distal phalangeal insertion to the dorsum of the proximal phalanx. Given that the deformity is flexible, the transfer rebalances the MTP and DIP hyperextension and PIP hyperflexion.
- With this technique, a plantar incision is made in the proximal plantar crease of the involved toe to expose the FDL tendon.
- The FDL is brought into this incision after incising the flexor sheath and put under tension while the distal FDL is released from the base of the distal phalanx with a distal percutaneous release.
- The slips of the FDL are brought into the proximal plantar wound and are gently separated.
- A short longitudinal dorsal incision is created over the proximal aspect of the proximal phalanx.
- The FDL slips are passed from plantar to dorsal, one on each side of and directly adjacent to the proximal phalanx.
  - ☐ It is important to ensure that the neurovascular bundles are not entrapped between the transferred tendon slip and the phalanx.
- The FDL tendon slips are sewn to one another and the surrounding extensor hood, with the toe and ankle held in slight plantarflexion and neutral position, respectively.
- For additional temporary support, the toe can be taped or pinned for several weeks.

Occasionally, the MTP joint has mild extension contractures, despite a flexible PIP joint (or a PIP joint that can easily be corrected with simple manipulation). Hammer toe correction is then performed in conjunction with Z-lengthening of the extensor tendons and an MTP joint dorsal capsulotomy.

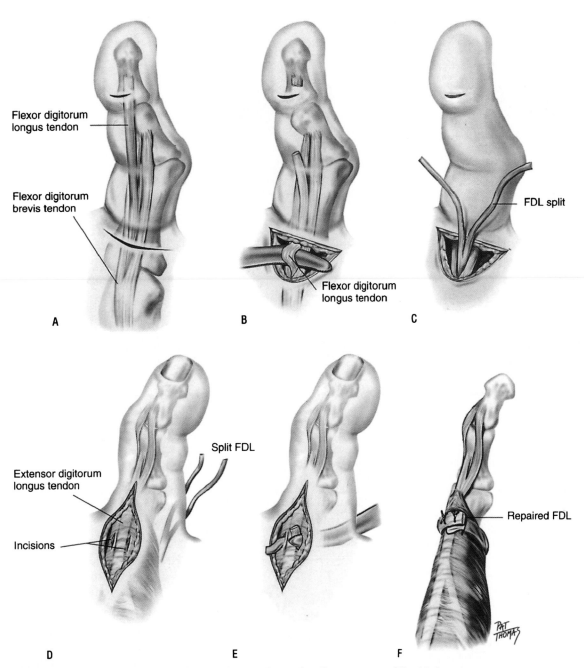

Figure 7.21 (A–F) Girdlestone–Taylor procedure can be used in the treatment of flexible hammer toe deformity. See page 141 for procedure details. (Reproduced with permission from Watson AD, Anderson RB, Davis WH. Lesser toe deformities. In: Kelikian AS, ed. Operative treatment of the foot and ankle. Stamford: Appleton & Lange, 1999:105.)

Fixed. A hammer toe with a fixed PIP joint contracture cannot be effectively managed with soft-tissue procedures alone.

- The fixed PIP joint is approached through a dorsal incision and the capsule, and collateral ligaments are released.
- The proximal phalangeal condyles are exposed and resected while protecting the neurovascular structures.

- At this point, the decision is made whether to perform a DuVries resection arthroplasty or a PIP joint arthrodesis (Fig. 7.22).
  - □ No further bony work is required for the DuVries procedure.
- For the PIP joint arthrodesis, the cartilage of the middle phalanx is resected.
- Next, the PIP joint is reduced and the toe is pinned from distal across the MPT joint with the toe in slight plantarflexion.

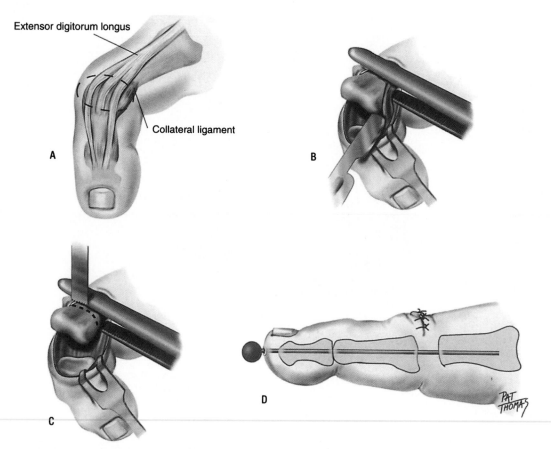

Figure 7.22 DuVries PIP joint resection arthroplasty is the commonest method for the treatment of fixed hammer toe deformity. (**A**) Make an elliptical or longitudinal incision through the skin, extensor tendon, and capsule. (**B**) Release the collateral ligaments, capsule, and plantar plate to expose the distal head of the proximal phalanx. (**C**) Cut the head at the level of the neck with the help of a saw or rongeur. (**D**) Reduce the PIP joint and advance a 0.045-in to 0.062-in Kirschner wire from distal across the MTP joint in slight plantarflexion. (Reproduced with permission from Watson AD, Anderson RB, Davis WH. Lesser toe deformities. In: Kelikian AS, ed. Operative treatment of the foot and ankle. Stamford: Appleton & Lange, 1999:107.)

Occasionally, decompression of the joints is inadequate to allow for complete correction; therefore, a percutaneous distal FDL release from the distal phalanx is necessary.

With an associated contracture of the MTP joint, the extensor tendons require Z-lengthening in combination with MTP joint dorsal capsulotomy and collateral ligament release.

Occasionally, the MTP joint is so severely subluxated that a metatarsal shortening osteotomy is warranted in addition to the PIP procedure. Toe pinning is facilitated with exposure of the PIP joints, MTP joints, or both. The pin can be driven antegrade from the residual PIP joint distally and then reversed in a retrograde fashion across the PIP and MTP joints. With residual deformity despite PIP joint resection arthroplasty or arthrodesis or MTP degeneration, partial proximal phalangectomy with partial syndactylization has been described, but most surgeons favor the adjunctive procedures of the MTP joint described earlier.

Claw Toe

Flexible.   Flexible claw toe correction is similar to that of a flexible hammer toe deformity. However, the need to add soft-tissue releases to the MTP joint is generally greater. Occasionally, the FDL tendon needs to undergo percutaneous lengthening to correct the DIP joint flexion deformity.

Rigid.   Similarly, the treatment of a rigid claw toe mimics that of a rigid hammer toe deformity, but the need for MTP joint soft-tissue releases and metatarsal shortening tends to be greater than for hammer toe correction. Traditionally, the problem of MTP joint reduction has been solved with PIP joint resection and MTP joint release. With more advanced contractures, subluxation, or dislocation, a DuVries resection arthroplasty of the MTP joint (different from the PIP joint procedure) has been performed (Fig. 7.23). This involves resection of the distal 3 to 4 mm and plantar 2 to 3 mm of the metatarsal head

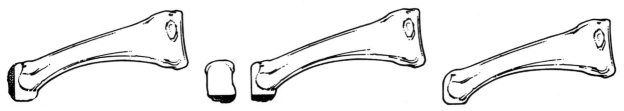

Figure 7.23 DuVries metatarsal head arthroplasty. See text for procedure details. (Reproduced with permission from McGlamry ED, Jimenez AL, Green DR. Lesser ray deformities. Part 1: deformities of the intermediate digits and the metatarsophalangeal joint. In: Banks AS, Downey MS, Martin DE, et al., eds. McGlamry's comprehensive textbook of foot and ankle surgery, 3rd ed, vol 1. Philadelphia: Lippincott Williams & Wilkins, 2001:301.)

to decompress or reduce the MTP joint and possibly create some plantar plate adhesion for maintaining MTP joint reduction. Although this procedure is effective, particularly with associated arthrosis, it destroys the joint. Currently, the favored bony procedure to reduce the MTP joint is the Weil metatarsal oblique shortening osteotomy (Fig. 7.24), particularly when radiographs suggest a relatively long metatarsal of the involved claw toe.

- Initially, the same soft-tissue releases are performed for the MTP joint.
- Through a dorsal incision, the extensor tendons are Z-lengthened, a dorsal capsulotomy is performed, and the collateral ligaments are released.
- In theory, the collateral ligaments may be left intact because the metatarsal will be shortened, but no adverse effects have been reported when collateral ligament release is performed in conjunction with metatarsal shortening.
- The metatarsal head is exposed by plantarflexing the proximal phalanx.
- Retractors are used to protect the adjacent soft tissues.
- An oblique osteotomy is performed in the distal metatarsal, parallel to the plantar aspect of the foot, and incorporating the dorsal 5% of the articular surface. Given the physiologic position of the metatarsal relative to the plantar foot, osteotomy is performed at approximately 20° relative to the metatarsal. Care must be taken to avoid directing the osteotomy too far plantarward because plantar displacement of the metatarsal head may lead to an overload phenomenon despite metatarsal shortening.
- Once the osteotomy is completed, the metatarsal head spontaneously translates a few millimeters proximally, but may need to be forced proximally a few more mil-

limeters to achieve reduction. The goal is to shorten the involved metatarsal without disrupting the natural metatarsal cascade from the second to fifth metatarsal.
- The osteotomy is secured with a small screw. Care is taken to avoid penetration of the plantar metatarsal head with the screw.
- Finally, the excess bone is resected from the proximal aspect of the osteotomy, and the wound is closed.
- Despite screw placement, a percutaneous pin may be placed across the MTP joint with the toe in slight plantarflexion.
  - □ This pin should be placed first antegrade through the toe and then retrograde across the MTP joint while avoiding the screw in the metatarsal head.
  - □ The pin should engage the metatarsal proximal to the osteotomy to ensure that stress is not placed directly on the repositioned metatarsal head that may lead to displacement.
  - □ If a Weil osteotomy is performed simultaneously with a PIP joint procedure, the pin can be placed through the PIP joint and then driven across the MTP joint.

The Weil osteotomy is effective in decompressing and reducing the subluxed or dislocated MTP joint. It is not designed to treat metatarsal head overload or metatarsalgia. However, if the osteotomy is performed with a double-cut, wedge resection, or stacked blades that allow for greater resection at the osteotomy site, some elevation of the metatarsal head can be achieved. The goal of metatarsal head elevation is to maintain the optimal center of rotation for the metatarsal head and proper axis for the lesser toe flexor tendons. If the head is simply shifted proximally, the flexor tendons may shift dorsal to the axis of rotation, effectively being converted into an MTP joint extensor. However, if a wedge resection is incorporated into the osteotomy, then

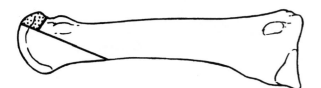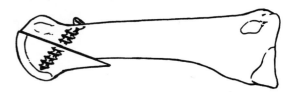

Figure 7.24 Weil metatarsal head shortening osteotomy. (Reproduced with permission from Cooper PS. Disorders and deformities of the lesser toes. In: Myerson MS, ed. Foot and ankle disorders, vol 1. Philadelphia: WB Saunders, 2000:370.)

the flexor tendons are more likely to remain plantar to the axis of rotation and thus continue to function as flexors of the MTP joint.

Mallet Toe

Flexible.   A flexible mallet toe can be treated with a percutaneous FDL release. The percutaneous procedure is performed in the distal plantar flexion crease with a dorsiflexion force on the distal phalanx. Care is taken to avoid medial or lateral excursion of the blade that may damage the adjacent neurovascular structures.

Rigid.   With a fixed mallet toe, resection arthroplasty or DIP joint arthrodesis is usually effective. The procedure mimics the PIP joint procedures described for hammer and claw toes. Occasionally, DIP joint resection arthroplasty or arthrodesis fails to relieve the FDL contracture adequately, warranting percutaneous FDL release. The DIP joint is temporarily stabilized with a pin or taping. Pinning is performed as for the PIP joint, first antegrade distally followed by retrograde pinning across the DIP joint (Fig. 7.25).

Metatarsophalangeal Joint Instability

MTP joint instability varies in severity; not all stages of this disease need to be treated with surgical intervention. When surgical correction is performed, other predisposing factors should be addressed simultaneously. A common example is second MTP joint instability associated with hallux valgus.

Even when the first ray is asymptomatic, the hallux valgus and second MTP joint should be surgically corrected to ensure that persistent hallux deformity does not promote recurrence of the second MTP joint pathology.

Synovitis.   When second MTP joint synovitis without deformity or instability is refractory to nonoperative measures, joint debridement may be beneficial. Through a dorsal capsulotomy, a synovectomy can be performed. Generally, deformity and instability accompany synovitis by the time this problem is considered for surgery.

Mild or Moderate Subluxation.   Even without evidence for lesser MTP joint subluxation on static examination, dynamic instability may be identified with a toe "Lachman test" (see Fig. 7.16). The main problem for pure dorsal lesser MTP joint instability is an attenuated plantar plate (Fig. 7.26). Currently, techniques for plantar plate reconstruction have not been universally adopted, and indirect MTP joint stabilization/realignment procedures are recommended. Similar to MTP joint management in hammer or claw toe deformity, soft-tissue releases and tendon transfers are performed as needed. Through a dorsal approach, contracted structures are released in a sequential manner. The contracted extensor tendons are Z-lengthened, whereas the contracted dorsal capsule and collateral ligaments are released and inflamed synovial tissue is debrided. With associated medial or lateral MTP joint instability, collateral ligament rebalancing should be performed. Ideally, the

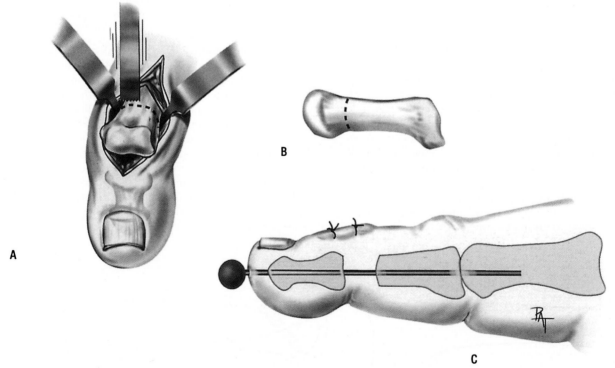

Figure 7.25 (A–C) DIP resection arthroplasty is the treatment of choice in rigid mallet toe deformities. Technique is similar to PIP resection arthroplasty. (Reproduced with permission from Watson AD, Anderson RB, Davis WH. Lesser toe deformities. In: Kelikian AS, ed. Operative treatment of the foot and ankle. Stamford: Appleton & Lange, 1999:104.)

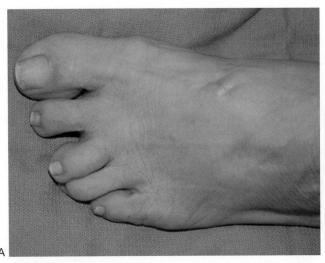
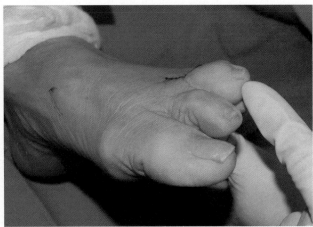

A   B

Figure 7.26 Clinical views of a third MTP joint instability. (**A**) Valgus deviation. (**B**) Claw toe deformity.

contracted collateral ligament is released and the attenuated collateral ligament is reefed by means of capsular or collateral imbrication. If instability is evident after the aforementioned releases, a flexor-to-extensor tendon transfer (as described for hammer and claw toe deformities) indirectly reestablishes MTP joint stability (see Fig. 7.21)

Severe Subluxation or Dislocation.   With increasing severity of lesser toe MTP joint subluxation or dislocation, the same sequential releases described for mild to moderate MTP joint subluxation are followed. Typically, however, soft-tissue procedures alone are inadequate to correct a more severe deformity, particularly when the affected metatarsal is relatively long compared with the adjacent metatarsals. Joint decompression

is accomplished by metatarsal shortening. Currently, the Weil metatarsal shortening osteotomy (described for claw toe correction) is favored (Fig. 7.27). Because there is some risk of recurrence of severe deformity, consideration should be given to simultaneous flexor-to-extensor tendon transfer. One advantage of the DuVries MTP joint resection arthroplasty is that a plantar metatarsal head cancellous surface may allow for scarring and stabilization of the plantar plate and plantar capsular tissues; however, the procedure does not preserve the articular cartilage (see Fig. 7.23). Basilar hemiphalangectomy has also been described, but persistent instability and a proposed simultaneous syndactylization to the adjacent toe as a solution appear less effective than the Weil metatarsal osteotomy with or without flexor-to-extensor tendon transfer

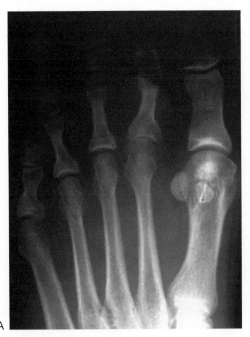
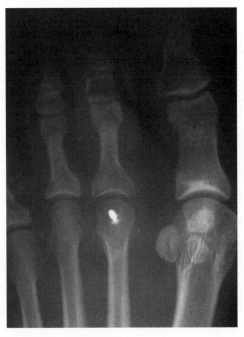

A   B

Figure 7.27 Fifty-year-old patient with second MTP instability (**A**) treated with Weil metatarsal-shortening osteotomy (**B**).

(Figs. 7.28 to 7.31). Rarely, severe deformity and risk of vascular compromise to the involved toe warrants complete metatarsal head resection, as described for inflammatory arthropathies. The risk with resection of an isolated metatarsal head is development of an adjacent transfer metatarsalgia.

Crossover Toe. Crossover toe deformity is similar to MTP joint subluxation or dislocation but with associated collateral ligament attenuation. Generally, the crossover toe occurs in the presence of a hallux valgus deformity. Unless the hallux is corrected, the second toe deformity tends to recur. In addition to the soft-tissue releases and bony joint decompression procedures described earlier for MTP joint instability, the collateral ligament and capsular abnormalities need to be addressed. In crossover toe deformity associated with hallux valgus, the medial collateral ligament, medial capsule, and medial intrinsic muscles are contracted, whereas the lateral soft tissues are attenuated along with the plantar tissues. Furthermore, as with MTP joint instability, the second metatarsal may be

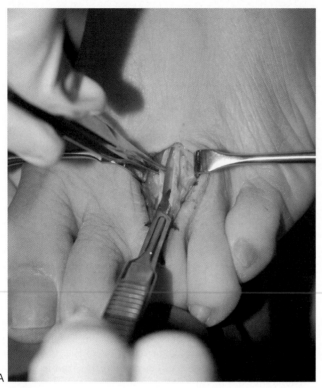
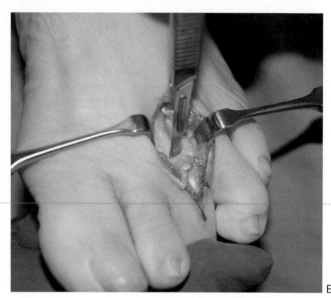

A   B

Figure 7.28 Soft-tissue releases for valgus deviation and claw toe deformity.
(**A**) Z-lengthening of the extensor tendon. (**B**) Dorsal and lateral capsular release.

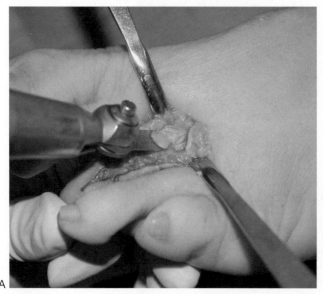
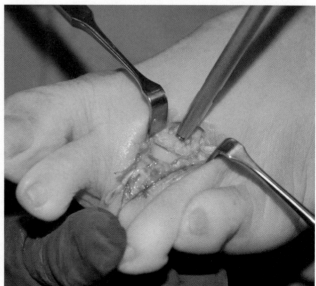

A   B

Figure 7.29 Weil metatarsal shortening osteotomy for third toe with valgus deviation and clawing. (**A**) Transverse intra-articular osteotomy. (**B**) Fixation after metatarsal shortening.

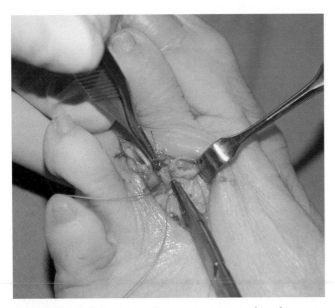

Figure 7.30 Medial capsular plication to correct valgus deviation.

relatively long.

Surgical management of the crossover toe deformity is modified from that of MTP joint instability by incorporating management of the contracted, attenuated capsular, or collateral ligaments in the coronal plane (Figs. 7.32 to 7.35).

- Although the EDL is Z-lengthened in standard fashion, the EDB is transected about 4 to 5 cm proximal to the joint and tagged proximally and distally.
- The capsulotomy is extended from dorsal to include the medial capsule, resulting in a complete dorsal and medial capsular release.

- Laterally, however, the residual attenuated tissues are carefully inspected.
- Typically, these structures are particularly attenuated at their distal aspect.
- Through the thickest portion of the residual lateral structures, the tissues are divided.
- If the metatarsal is relatively long, a Weil metatarsal shortening osteotomy is performed (as described earlier). However, with medial deviation, the distal aspect of the Weil osteotomy can be shifted medially to assist in realignment of the second MTP joint (similar to correction of hallux valgus deformity in which the metatarsal head is shifted in conjunction with the distal soft-tissue procedure; see Fig. 7.24).
  - With residual bony deformity, a lateral wedge resection may be considered for the proximal phalanx (Fig. 7.36), sometimes referred to as an Akinette osteotomy.
  - It is accomplished with dorsal to plantar drilling of the lateral cortex of the proximal phalanx and impaction.
- Soft-tissue rebalancing is the final step.
  - The lateral capsule and collateral ligament are imbricated.
  - If necessary, the tissues can be anchored to the lateral metatarsal head with a minisuture anchor, but this should probably be reserved for cases where no metatarsal osteotomy has been performed.
  - To augment the lateral stability and further combat the plantar instability, the EDB transfer is completed.
  - The EDB tendon is rerouted under the transverse intermetatarsal ligament in the second web space and then reattached to its proximal limb to create a dynamic transfer.
  - With severe instability and crossover, a flexor-to-extensor tendon transfer can be performed instead of the EDB transfer.

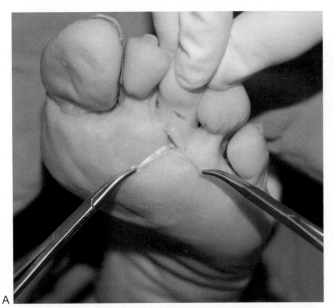 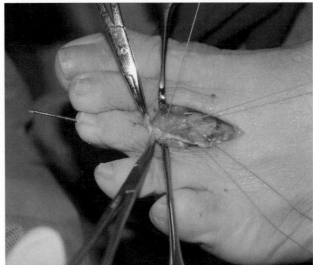

Figure 7.31 Flexor-to-extensor tendon transfer. (**A**) Flexor digitorum longus release on plantar aspect of toe with split through tendon raphe. (**B**) Securing tendon transfer on dorsum of proximal phalanx after tendon slips transferred to dorsum of toe, immediately adjacent to bone.

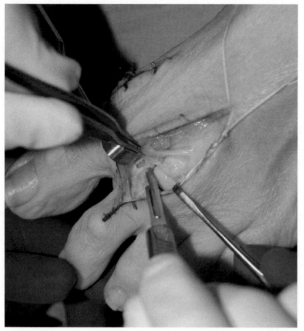

Figure 7.32 Dorsal and medial capsular release for second claw toe deformity associated with medial deviation.

□ The toe can be pinned or taped temporarily to maintain alignment during healing.
□ Pinning is best performed antegrade through the toe from the proximal phalanx and then retrograde across the MTP joint (in slight valgus and plantarflexion).
□ In practice, it may be easier to pin the toe before performing the tendon transfer procedures to ensure that the delicate tendon repairs are not compromised during pinning.
□ The pin should be left in place only for 3 weeks to prevent excessive MTP joint stiffness.

Bunionette. As for hallux valgus, there exists an algorithm for the surgical correction of bunionette deformities. The specific deformity (types I, II, and III) needs to be identified to direct proper treatment. Occasionally, plantar overload is present in addition to lateral metatarsal head pressure. If some of the plantar or lateral overload is secondary to hindfoot varus deformity, then forefoot correction alone will probably be insufficient and hindfoot realignment may be necessary.

Type I. Surgical management of a type I deformity in which there is a prominent or enlarged fifth metatarsal head (without bowing of the fifth metatarsal or increase

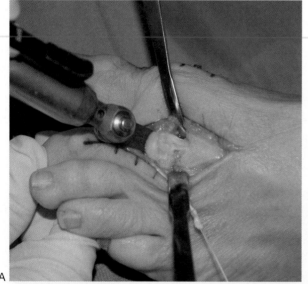

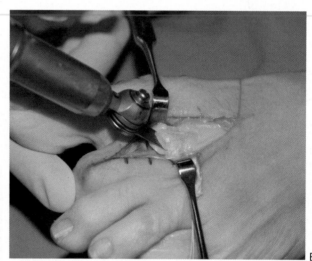

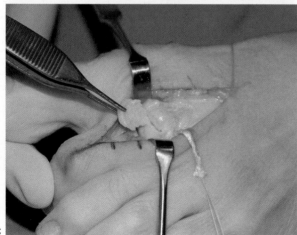

Figure 7.33 Weil metatarsal shortening osteotomy.
(**A**) Transverse intra-articular osteotomy. (**B**) Wedge resection to elevate metatarsal head in an effort to maintain the plantar orientation of the flexor tendons. Without wedge resection metatarsal shortening may lead to the flexor tendon reorienting above the midaxis of the metatarsal head and potentially promoting postoperative toe elevation. (**C**) Wedge extraction.

in the 4-5 intermetatarsal angle) consists of lateral fifth metatarsal head exostectomy (Fig. 7.37). If performed as the sole procedure in patients with increased 4-5 intermetatarsal angle or lateral bowing of the fifth metatarsal, persistent pain is common.

Through a lateral incision over the fifth MTP joint, the procedure mimics several steps of hallux valgus correction: (1) capsulotomy, (2) lateral eminence excision (Fig. 7.38), and (3) capsular repair (with the fifth MTP joint slightly overcorrected). If an osteotomy is performed, fixation with a pin or small screw may be necessary for initial stability. The amount of medial shift of the metatarsal head is limited by the narrow width of the metatarsal neck (Figs. 7.39 and 7.40). Because there is no increased 4-5 intermetatarsal angle, an osteotomy is seldom indicated for type I deformity. Postoperatively, the toe is strapped in slight valgus for several weeks to maintain alignment and immediate weight-bearing is permitted in a postoperative shoe.

If the exostectomy or osteotomy fails to provide pain relief, the fifth metatarsal alignment should be reviewed.

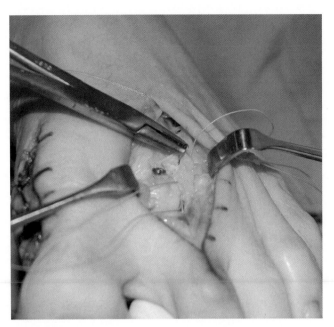

Figure 7.34 Lateral capsular plication to rebalance MTP joint. Note fixation screw for metatarsal shortening osteotomy.

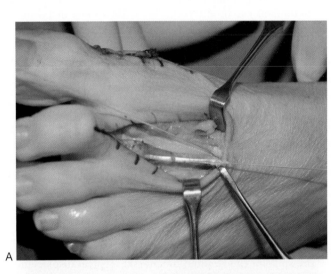

A

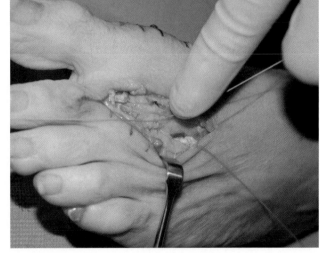

B

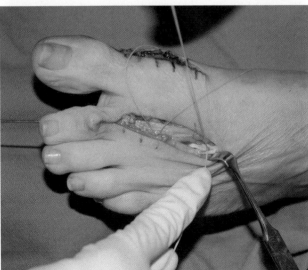

C

Figure 7.35 EDB transfer. (**A**) Distal aspect of EDB to second toe, still attached to second toe, after being divided near its proximal musculotendinous junction. (**B**) Completion of lateral capsular plication; note distal slip of EDB exiting from under transverse intermetatarsal ligament. (**C**) Reapproximation of EDB tendon after distal slip is passed deep to transverse intermetatarsal ligament; note that toe is pinned in slight valgus overcorrection.

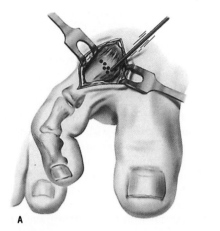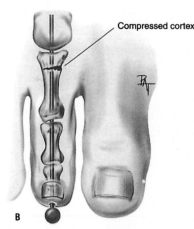

Figure 7.36 Closing wedge osteotomy of the base of the proximal phalanx (Akinette procedure). (**A**) Multiple perforations of the cortex are performed on the preferred side. (**B**) Osteotomy is closed and deformity is corrected with osteoclasis. (Reproduced with permission from Watson AD, Anderson RB, Davis WH. Lesser toe deformities. In: Kelikian AS, ed. Operative treatment of the foot and ankle. Stamford: Appleton & Lange, 1999:111.)

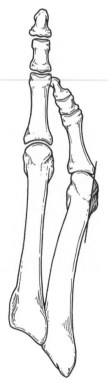

Figure 7.37 Treatment of type I bunionette deformity is lateral condylectomy (fifth metatarsal exostectomy). (Reproduced with permission from Crawford ME. Lesser ray deformities. Part 4: deformities of the fifth metatarsal. In: Banks AS, Downey MS, Martin DE, et al., eds. McGlamry's comprehensive textbook of foot and ankle surgery, 3rd ed, vol 1. Philadelphia: Lippincott Williams & Wilkins, 2001:345.)

Type II. The lateral fifth metatarsal bow, characteristic of a type II deformity, should be addressed with fifth metatarsal realignment. Reestablishment of a physiologic 4-5 intermetatarsal angle in type II deformity can be accomplished with either distal (see Fig. 7.38A, B) or midshaft metatarsal osteotomy (see Fig. 7.38C). The distal metatarsal osteotomy does not correct the deformity at its apex but helps narrow the 4-5 intermetatarsal angle. As noted for type I deformity, the narrow fifth metatarsal neck limits the amount of correction possible. A 1-mm medial shift of the metatarsal head corresponds to 1° correction of the 4-5 intermetatarsal angle. Techniques of fifth distal metatarsal osteotomies include chevron and oblique methods. Both are performed through a lateral approach centered over the fifth MTP joint and a lateral capsulotomy. The distal chevron osteotomy mimics the procedure performed for hallux valgus correction, and fixation with a small diameter screw or pin may be necessary. A distal oblique osteotomy has also been described. The oblique orientation of the osteotomy allows for medial and proximal translation of the metatarsal head to correct the deformity. Fixation is achieved by impaling the metatarsal head on the spike of the residual metatarsal. Typical displacement is 3 to 5 mm for either osteotomy.

To correct the lateral bowing of the fifth metatarsal at the apex of the deformity, a midshaft oblique osteotomy has been developed. This technique mirrors that described for the proximal oblique osteotomy for hallux valgus correction and is discussed next for type III deformity.

Type III. Mild to moderate increases in the 4-5 intermetatarsal angle can be corrected with the distal metatarsal osteotomies described for type II deformity. More severe 4-5 intermetatarsal angles should be corrected with a midshaft oblique osteotomy. Although the procedure is similar to the proximal oblique osteotomy described for hallux valgus correction, the fifth metatarsal procedure must avoid the poorly vascularized proximal aspect of the fifth metatarsal. The metatarsal osteotomy is typically combined with a lateral fifth metatarsal head exostectomy and fifth MTP joint soft-tissue rebalancing. (Figs. 7.41 to 7.46)

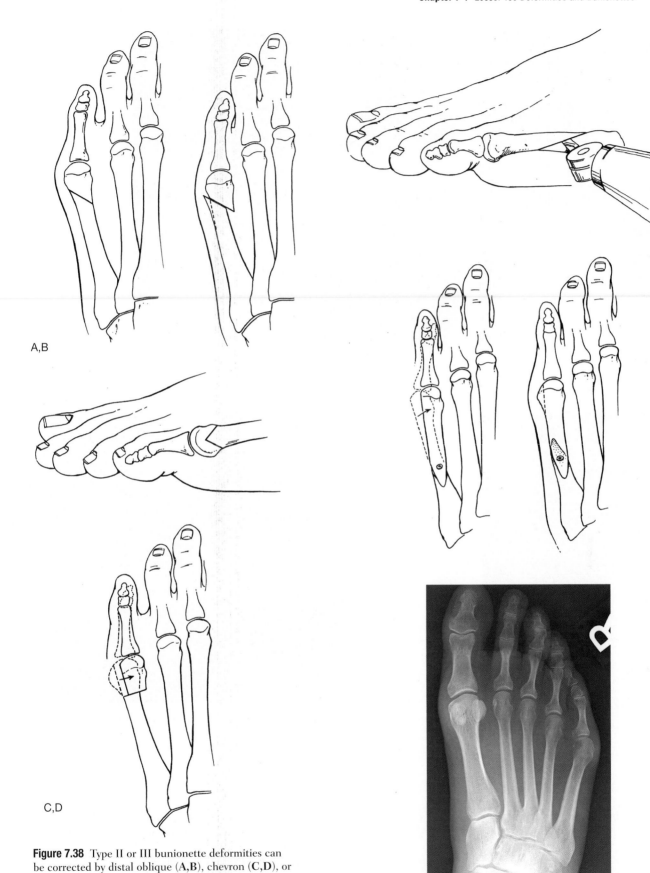

A,B

C,D

E-G

Figure 7.38 Type II or III bunionette deformities can be corrected by distal oblique (**A,B**), chevron (**C,D**), or midshaft oblique (**E–G**) osteotomy. (Reproduced with permission from Cooper PS. Disorders and deformities of the lesser toes. In: Myerson MS, ed. Foot and ankle disorders, vol 1. Philadelphia: WB Saunders, 2000:339–340.)

Figure 7.39 Preoperative AP radiograph of Type I bunionette deformity.

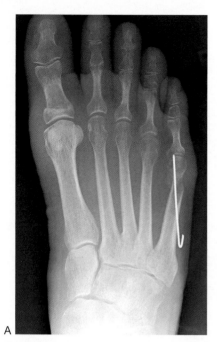

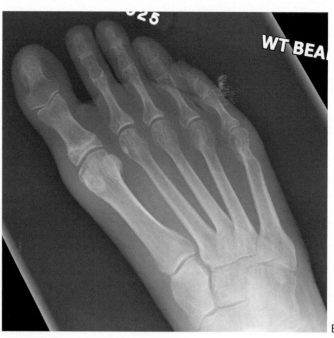

A   B

Figure 7.40 Postoperative AP radiographs following distal fifth metatarsal head osteotomy. (**A**) Osteotomy secured with K-wire. (**B**) Longer follow-up.

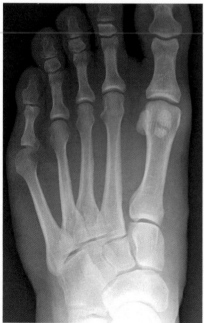

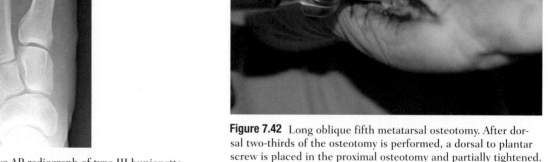

Figure 7.42 Long oblique fifth metatarsal osteotomy. After dorsal two-thirds of the osteotomy is performed, a dorsal to plantar screw is placed in the proximal osteotomy and partially tightened.

Figure 7.41 Preoperative AP radiograph of type III bunionette deformity.

- A lateral incision is performed from the fifth MTP joint along the fifth metatarsal while protecting the sural nerve.
- A capsulotomy and lateral metatarsal head exostectomy are performed.
- Care must be taken to avoid an aggressive lateral head resection because the intermetatarsal angle will be narrowed.

- With minimal periosteal stripping, an oblique midshaft osteotomy is outlined on the metatarsal and scored with the oscillating saw.
- The dorsal two-thirds is completed.
- Next, a mini or small fragment screw is placed in compression across the proximal aspect of the osteotomy without full compression.
- The distal aspect of the osteotomy is completed.

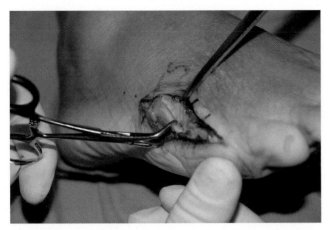

Figure 7.43 Long oblique fifth metatarsal osteotomy completed and distal fragment rotated to decrease 4-5 intermetatarsal angle.

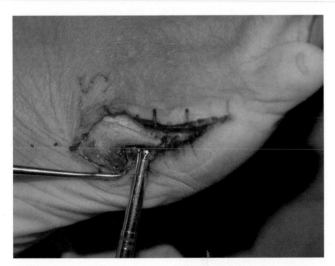

Figure 7.44 Osteotomy secured with distal plantar-to-dorsal screw after deformity correction.

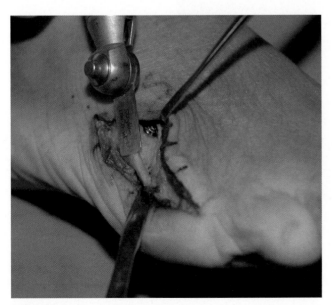

Figure 7.45 Lateral eminence resection.

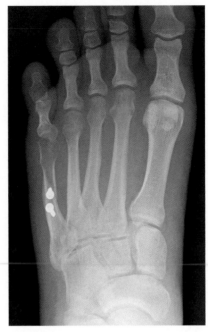

Figure 7.46 Follow-up AP weight-bearing radiograph.

▪ The osteotomy is rotated and correction is confirmed fluoroscopically.
▪ A second screw are placed distally across the osteotomy.
▪ Both screws are tightened in compression, and prominent bone is resected. The capsulotomy is repaired.

If there is associated plantar overload of the fifth metatarsal, the angle of the oblique osteotomy may be altered. By directing the saw blade from plantar lateral to dorsal medial, the metatarsal head is elevated while the intermetatarsal angle is narrowed. This simple alteration to the osteotomy is effective, but persistent hindfoot varus leads to persistent fifth metatarsal head overload unless corrected.

Freiberg Infraction

Freiberg infraction may respond to nonoperative treatment with immobilization and unloading. Temporary use of a surgical shoe, CAM walker, or cast may provide symptomatic relief. Symptoms may remain limited by gradual return to activities with an orthotic, metatarsal support, and even a slight rocker bottom modification to the shoe. However, these conservative measures do not alter the avascular and degenerative changes to the involved metatarsal head.

Surgical management of Freiberg infraction depends on the stage of disease. In the early stage of synovitis and minimal degenerative changes, joint debridement and synovectomy may be beneficial. With advancing degenerative changes, a dorsal cheilectomy (like that described for hallux rigidus) and drilling of the metatarsal head through eburnated bone may relieve mechanical symptoms related to impingement. Commonly, joint exploration reveals that the disease process selectively affects the dorsal aspect of the metatarsal while sparing the plantar aspect. For this situation, a dorsiflexion osteotomy of the metatarsal head and neck junction may be beneficial (Fig. 7.47). This osteotomy decompresses the joint

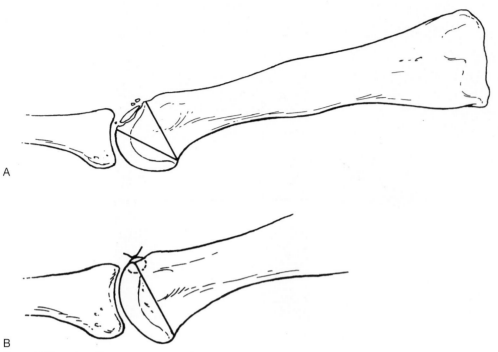

Figure 7.47 A dorsiflexion osteotomy of the metatarsal neck (**A**) brings the normal articular cartilage in contact with the proximal phalanx (**B**).

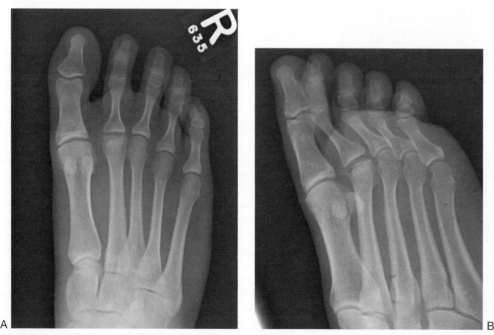

Figure 7.48 Preoperative imaging studies of a 17-year-old adolescent girl with second metatarsal head Freiberg infraction. (**A**) AP radiograph. (**B**) oblique radiograph.

and permits the healthier plantar cartilage to articulate with the phalanx. Moreover, this osteotomy elevates the second metatarsal head slightly to unload the metatarsal head. The procedure is performed through a dorsal approach with a longitudinal capsulotomy. (Figs. 7.48 to 7.54)

In patients with diffuse metatarsal head osteonecrosis and advanced degenerative changes or when the previously described surgical treatments fail, salvage with a DuVries resection arthroplasty or metatarsal head excision may improve symptoms. Preservation of some of the metatarsal head typically preserves toe alignment and limits transfer overload to adjacent metatarsals; however, postoperative orthotic use or metatarsal support is often warranted.

Corns

Recalcitrant hard and soft corns are managed with condylectomy. If possible, indirect approaches to the condyles are favored. Performing an incision directly over a corn in the intertriginous areas between two toes or on the lateral aspect of the fifth toe may lead to persistent irritation

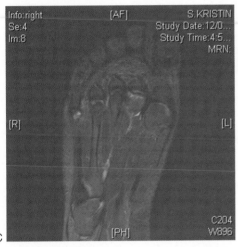
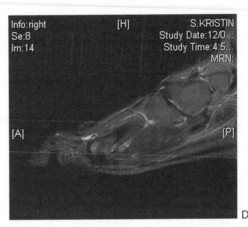

Figure 7.48 (*continued*)   (**C**) T2-weighted MRI coronal view. (**D**) T2-weighted MRI sagittal view.

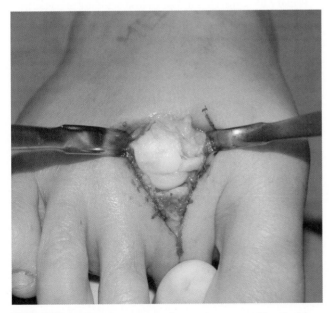

Figure 7.49 Intraoperative view of second metatarsal head with deformity secondary to Freiberg infraction.

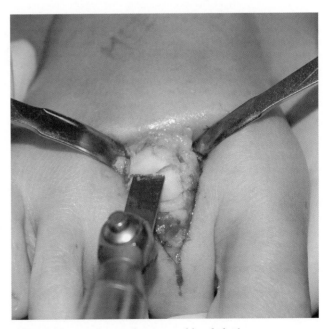

Figure 7.50 Dorsal second metatarsal head cheilectomy.

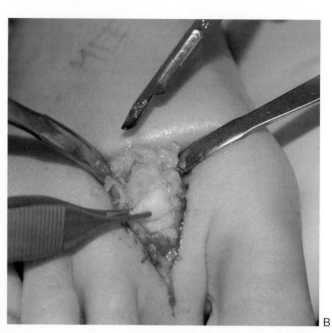

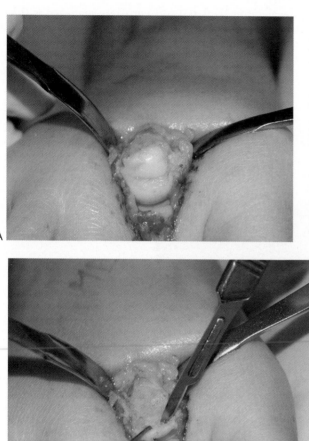

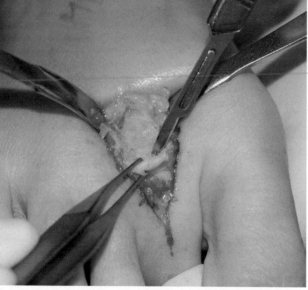

Figure 7.51 Unstable cartilage (dorsal one-third of metatarsal). (**A**) Photo of unstable cartilage on dorsal one-third of second metatarsal head. (**B**) Careful elevation of unstable cartilage so as not to damage stable, more plantar residual healthy cartilage. (**C**) Unstable cartilage removed.

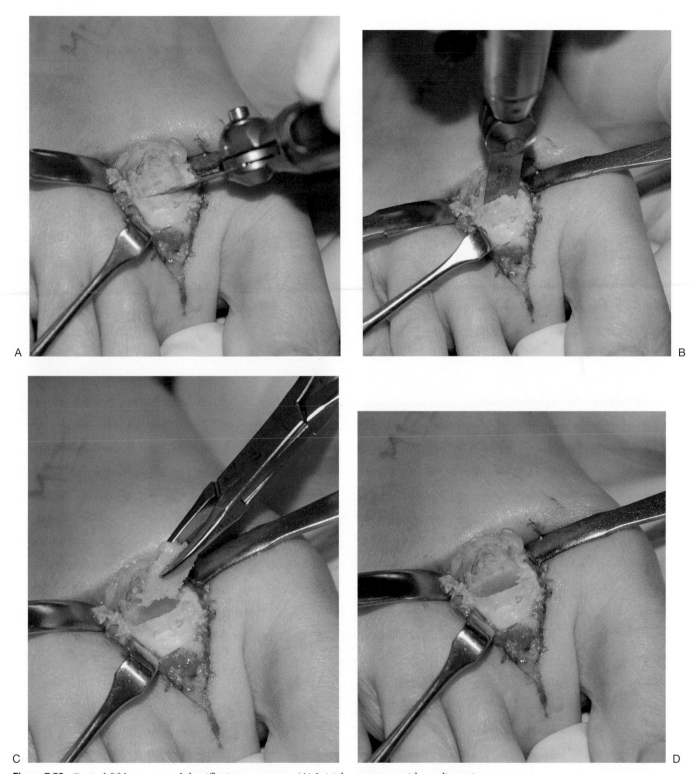

Figure 7.52 Capital fifth metatarsal dorsiflexion osteotomy. (**A**) Initial osteotomy, without disruption of plantar cortex. (**B**) Second osteotomy to connect with initial cut. (**C**) Wedge resection. (**D**) Residual bone with stability between metatarsal shaft and residual head (plantar cortex left intact).

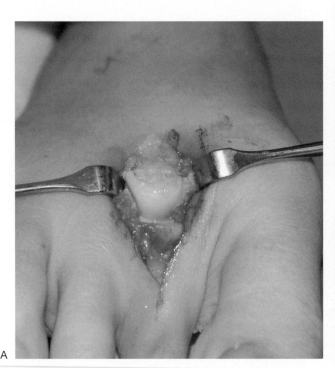
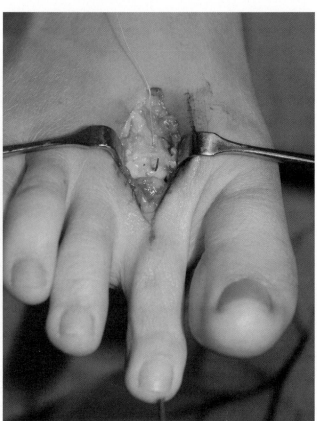

A B

Figure 7.53 Reducing residual metatarsal head and cartilage to metatarsal shaft. (**A**) After wedge resection, osteotomy is closed. (**B**) Fixation with longitudinal pin and dorsal suture.

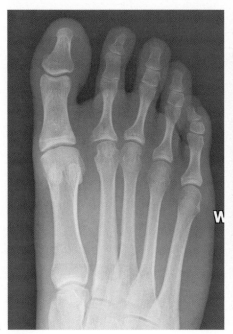
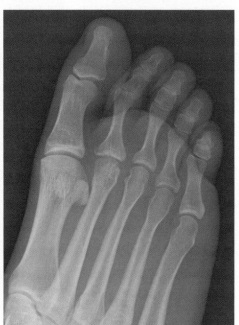

A B

Figure 7.54 Follow-up radiographs 2 years after dorsiflexion osteotomy; mild joint space narrowing noted that may be secondary to reorientation of metatarsal head (patient with minimal symptoms and with well-preserved range of motion of second MTP joint. Also, mild symptoms related to transfer metatarsalgia to third metatarsal head). (**A**) Weight-bearing AP view. (**B**) Oblique view.

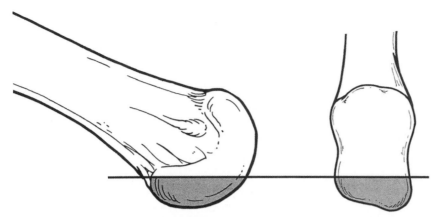

Figure 7.55 DuVries plantar condylectomy performed to resect more of the fibular side. The modification removes 20% to 30% of the condyle while preserving the distal part of the metatarsal head. (Reproduced with permission from Jimenez AL, Fishco WD. Lesser ray deformities. Part 3: central metatarsals. In: Banks AS, Downey MS, Martin DE, et al., eds. McGlamry's comprehensive textbook of foot and ankle surgery, 3rd ed, vol 1. Philadelphia: Lippincott Williams & Wilkins, 2001:327.)

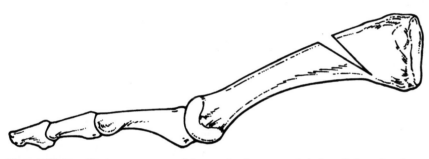

Figure 7.56 Dorsiflexion osteotomy of the proximal metatarsal. A dorsally based wedge is removed from the proximal metaphysis to correct the deformity. (Reproduced with permission from Jimenez AL, Fishco WD. Lesser ray deformities. Part 3: central metatarsals. In: Banks AS, Downey MS, Martin DE, et al., eds. McGlamry's comprehensive textbook of foot and ankle surgery, 3rd ed, vol 1. Philadelphia: Lippincott Williams & Wilkins, 2001:326.)

due to subsequent scar formation. Following excision of a soft corn, the wound needs to be kept dry to improve wound healing.

Intractable Plantar Keratosis

Focal. If an IPK fails nonoperative treatment, surgical management can relieve symptoms. Focusing only on the IPK and ignoring associated foot pathology generally lead to persistent symptoms. For example, performing a simple second metatarsal head plantar condylectomy without addressing an associated hallux valgus leaves the forefoot unbalanced.

- The modified DuVries plantar condylectomy (Fig. 7.55) is performed through a dorsal incision.
- Following the dorsal capsulotomy, the proximal phalanx is plantarflexed to expose the plantar aspect of the metatarsal head. Often, the metatarsal head has a lateral plantar process that is more prominent than the medial plantar aspect of the metatarsal head.

- With an osteotome or narrow microsagittal saw, the plantar quarter of the metatarsal head is removed.
- Postoperatively, the toe and MTP joint are protected until adequate wound healing is noted. Progressive weight-bearing on the forefoot is then initiated.

Alternatively, a dorsiflexion osteotomy of the proximal metatarsal may be performed (Fig. 7.56).

- Over the proximal aspect of the involved metatarsal, a longitudinal incision is made.
- While protecting the extensor tendons and neurovascular structures, the periosteum is elevated over the proximal metatarsal.
- A "greenstick" osteotomy is performed, in which the plantar aspect of the osteotomy is not violated.
- After removal of the dorsal wedge, gentle plantar pressure on the metatarsal head closes the osteotomy, thereby elevating the metatarsal head.

■ Care must be taken to ensure that the correction is not excessive because a transfer metatarsalgia may develop.

■ The osteotomy may be fixed with Kirschner wires or a small staple. Weight-bearing is gradually advanced after wound healing.

Diffuse. Diffuse IPK is difficult to manage surgically. Generally, nonoperative management is favored. It is important to address any associated pathology, such as hallux valgus or equinus contracture. Dorsiflexion osteotomies, as described for focal IPK earlier, may be considered, but with multiple metatarsal osteotomies, rebalancing of the forefoot may be challenging.

SUGGESTED READING

Bhatia D, Myerson MS, Curtis MJ, et al. Anatomical restraints to dislocation of the second metatarsophalangeal joint and assessment of a repair technique. J Bone Joint Surg Am 1994;76:1371–1375.

Barbari SG, Brevig K. Correction of clawtoes by the Girdlestone–Taylor flexor–extensor transfer procedure. Foot Ankle 1984;5:67–73.

Barouk P, Bohay DR, Trnka HJ, et al. Lesser metatarsal surgery. Foot Ankle Spec 2010;3(6):356–360.

Boyer ML, DeOrio JK. Transfer of the flexor digitorum longus for the correction of lesser-toe deformities. Foot Ankle Int 2007;28(4):422–430.

Coughlin MJ. Crossover second toe deformity. Foot Ankle 1987;8:29–39.

Coughlin MJ. Lesser toe abnormalities. Instr Course Lect 2003;52:421–444.

Coughlin MJ. Treatment of bunionnette deformity with longitudinal diaphyseal osteotomy with distal soft tissue repair. Foot Ankle 1991;11:195–203.

Coughlin MJ. Operative repair of the mallet toe deformity. Foot Ankle Int 1995;16:109–116.

Coughlin MJ, Dorris J, Polk E. Operative repair of the fixed hammertoe deformity. Foot Ankle Int 2000;21:94–104.

Coughlin MJ, Kennedy MP. Operative repair of fourth and fifth toe corns. Foot Ankle Int 2003;24(2):147–157.

Deland JT, Lee KT, Sobel M, et al. Anatomy of the plantar plate and its attachments in the lesser metatarsophalangeal joint. Foot Ankle Int 1995;16:480–486.

Deland JT, Sobel M, Arnoczky SP, et al. Collateral ligament reconstruction of the unstable metatarsophalangeal joint: an in vitro study. Foot Ankle Int 1992;13:391–395.

Deland JT, Sung IH. The medial crossover toe: a cadaveric dissection. Foot Ankle Int 2000;21(5):375–378.

Edwards WH, Beischer AD. Interpahlangeal joint arthrodesis of the lesser toes. Foot Ankle Clin 2002;7(1):43–48.

Freiberg AA, Freiberg RA. Core decompression as a novel treatment for early Freiberg's infraction of the second metatarsal head. Orthopedics 1995;18(12):1177–1178.

Haddad SL, Sabbagh RC, Resch S, et al. Correcting and stabilizing the cross-over second toe: a comparison of the medium term results of flexor to extensor tendon transfer and of extensor tendon transfer. Foot Ankle Int 1998;19:503.

Kitaoka HB, Holiday AD Jr, Campbell DC II. Distal chevron metatarsal osteotomy for bunionette. Foot Ankle Int 1991;12:80–85.

Mann RA, Mizel MS. Monoarticular nontraumatic synovitis of the metatarsophalangeal joint: a new diagnosis. Foot Ankle Int 1985;6:18–21.

Migues A, Slullitel G, Bilbao F, et al. Floating-toe deformity as a complication of the Weil osteotomy. Foot Ankle Int 2004;25:609–613.

Myerson MS, Shereff MJ. The pathological anatomy of claw and hammer toes. J Bone Joint Surg Am 1989;71:45–49.

Shirzad K, Kiesau CD, DeOrio JK, et al. Lesser toe deformities. J Am Acad Orthop Surg 2011;19(8):505–514.

Smillie IS. Treatment of Freiberg's infraction. Proc R Soc Med 1967;60(1):29–31.

Smith BW, Coughlin MJ. Disorders of the lesser toes. Sports Med Arthrosc 2009;17(3):167–174.

Thompson FM, Deland JT. Flexor tendon transfer for metatarsophalangeal instability of the second toe. Foot Ankle 1993;14:385–388.

Trnka HJ, Nyska M, Parks BG, et al. Dorsiflexion contracture after the Weil Osteotomy: results of cadaver study and three-dimensional analysis. Foot Ankle Int 2001;22(1):47–50.

Vandeputte G, Dereymaeker G, Steenwerckx A, et al. The Weil osteotomy of the lesser metatarsals: a clinical and pedobargraphic follow-up study. Foot Ankle Int 2000;21(5):370–374.

TENDON DISORDERS

SHELDON S. LIN
ERIC BREITBART
CONSTANTINE A. DEMETRACOPOULOS
JONATHAN T. DELAND

ACUTE ACHILLES TENDON RUPTURE

The incidence of acute Achilles tendon rupture has increased over the past 50 years. A primary reason for the increase is the growing interest and participation in sports-related activities. More than 75% of all tendon ruptures occur during sports-related activities in patients between 30 and 50 years of age.

PATHOGENESIS

Etiology and Epidemiology

A sedentary lifestyle with weekend recreational athletics leads to an increased incidence of acute Achilles tendon rupture. The annual number ranges from 2 to 10 cases per 100,000 people in industrialized nations, but it is extremely rare in other parts of the world. Achilles tendon ruptures occur in younger patients (mean age 36 years) than those with other ruptured tendons (mean age greater than 60 years). Male predominance is seen in every series of Achilles tendon ruptures with a male-to-female ratio varying from 2:1 to 19:1. An increased incidence in white-collar workers or professionals with a more sedentary lifestyle has been noted. An increased incidence during the warmer months of May through August has been thought to result from the increased sporting activity during the "play season." Achilles tendinopathy is the most common running-associated tendinopathy, and veteran runners (>10 years) have an increased risk of Achilles tendinopathy.

Less common causes of Achilles tendon rupture include the following:

- Use of corticosteroids (local injection or systemic use leading to collagen necrosis)
- Use of anabolic steroids causing collagen dysplasia and reduced tensile strength
- Use of quinolone antibiotics
- Gout, hyperthyroidism, renal insufficiency, and arteriosclerosis

Other predisposing factors include the following:

- Prior Achilles tendon injury or tendinopathy
- Infection, systemic inflammatory disease, and ochronosis
- Hypertension and obesity

Pathophysiology

Several theories (degenerative, impaired healing, mechanical overload, etc.) have been proposed for the pathogenesis of Achilles tendon rupture. The "degenerative" theory describes a sequence of events with a sedentary lifestyle leading to a decrease in tendon vascularity. Subsequent microtrauma in a tendon with an impaired healing process leads to diffuse tendon degeneration and injury. Eventually, the impaired tendon undergoes a catastrophic failure (rupture) at a critical load.

The posterior tibial artery supplies blood to the proximal and distal parts of the tendon with the middle part supplied by the peroneal artery. In an anatomic study, the midsection of the tendon tends to be hypovascular, which may explain the high incidence of midsection tendon ruptures, especially in patients with compromised blood supply.

Several studies analyzing angiographic and histologic data support the concept of tendon degeneration. More than 15% of the patients with an acute Achilles rupture report prior symptoms. Histologic analysis of acute ruptured tendons reveals degenerative and necrotic tendon changes with hypoxic degeneration, mucoid degeneration, and calcifying tendinopathy resulting in increased water content and decreased collagen content. There is also an increase in denatured and damaged collagen in Achilles tendinopathy indicating an increased collagen turnover rate.

Structural changes of the Achilles tendon occur as a part of normal aging. These changes include decreased cell density, decreased collagen fibril diameter and density, and loss of fiber waviness, which may explain the increased prevalence of ruptures in older patients.

175

DIAGNOSIS

Physical Examination and History

- Classically, an acute Achilles tendon rupture is diagnosed by the patient's history.
- Most patients describe feeling a direct blow localized to the posterior aspect of the ankle or hearing a "pop."
- It most commonly occurs during an explosive gastrocsoleus eccentric contraction.
- Twenty-five percent of diagnoses are missed in the emergency department because of presence of active plantarflexion when non–weight bearing and swelling over the Achilles tendon, which makes palpation of the defect difficult.
- A history of steroid or flouroquinolone usage.
- A history of endocrine disorders or systemic inflammatory conditions.
- A positive Thompson squeeze test (0.96 sensitivity and 0.93 specificity).
- A palpable defect (0.73 sensitivity and 0.83 specificity).

Clinical Features

- Difficulty with ambulation and weakness on attempted pushoff is noted.
- Physical examination demonstrates an indentation of the posterior aspect of the tendon initially. With the onset of soft-tissue swelling, these findings are frequently masked.
- Ecchymosis and swelling commonly develop along the posterior aspect of the ankle (Fig. 8.1).
- The calf squeeze test (Thompson sign) is the simplest and most reliable test to evaluate the continuity of the gastrocnemius–soleus complex. Absence of plantarflexion of the foot against gravity on squeezing of the calf with the patient in a prone position confirms a ruptured Achilles tendon.
- Another finding is the "hyperdorsiflexion sign," which results in a relatively dorsiflexed position compared with the intact contralateral side; however, this sign may be difficult to elicit following an acute injury, secondary to pain inhibition until sufficient time has elapsed after injury.

Radiographic Features

- Plain radiographs are of limited value for an acute Achilles tendon rupture.

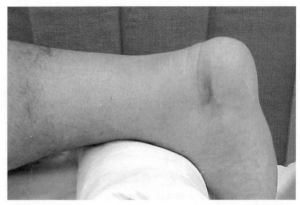

Figure 8.1 Clinical appearance of acute Achilles rupture. (Courtesy of Stewart Fisher, MD.)

- □ Rarely, an acute avulsion of the Achilles insertion with proximal migration of bony fragments can be seen.
- □ Definitive treatment of this rare condition requires an advancement of the Achilles tendon and internal fixation of the bone–tendon complex (Fig. 8.2).
- Magnetic resonance imaging (MRI) demonstrates an Achilles tendon rupture, but is not necessary for diagnosis or treatment (Fig. 8.3).
  - □ MRI is superior to other imaging technique for diagnosing partial ruptures of the Achilles tendon.
- Ultrasound (US) can be used to assess the gap between the tendon ends. With the foot held in plantarflexion, the presence or absence of a gap between the tendon ends can help determine the success of nonoperative management of Achilles tendon rupture.
  - □ Serial US studies can be used to determine the proximal migration of the tendon tear and its potential for healing.

TREATMENT

Nonsurgical Treatment

Nonoperative treatment is associated is higher risk of rerupture compared with the risk associated with operative treatment (1.7% to 10%); however, it has significantly lower risk of impaired wound healing, wound infection, and nerve damage.

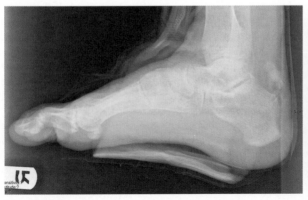
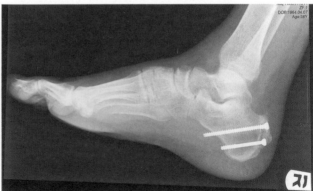

Figure 8.2 A: Lateral X-ray of right foot demonstrating avulsion of superior calcaneal tuberosity. B: Postoperative reduction with internal fixation of superior calcaneal fragment.

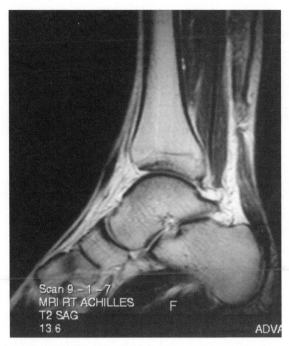

Figure 8.3 T2-weighted MRI of the ankle demonstrating acute Achilles tendon rupture.

The use of serial casting or a solid removable boot in plantarflexion helps to join the ends of the ruptured tendon. It should be noted that immobilization in a cast or boot in neutral ankle position is inadequate care.

Surgical Indications

Recently, advances in surgical technique have led to superior results in most series compared with nonoperative management. Aggressive postoperative protocols have demonstrated the benefits of functional rehabilitation with improved function, increased patient satisfaction, acceptable complication rate, and avoidance of cast immobilization disease (muscle atrophy, loss of muscle or tendon strength, and stiffness). Currently, surgical repair with functional rehabilitation has gained increasing acceptance. Nonoperative management should be used for patients with significant medical issues or limited functional gains and expectation.

The AAOS *Guideline* has a consensus recommendation that surgical management should be approached with caution in a patient with the following conditions:

- diabetes
- neuropathy
- history of tobacco use
- obesity
- a sedentary lifestyle
- peripheral vascular disease
- local or systemic
- age more than 65 years dermatologic disorder
- immunocompromised state

The basic concept of surgical repair of an acute Achilles tendon rupture is to durably restore the continuity of the ruptured tendon, such that healing occurs in a physiologic position, allowing for restoration of the normal muscle function. This goal may be technically challenging when the ends of the degenerative Achilles tendon are frayed.

Several suture and repair techniques have been advocated to achieve this goal. The first end-to-end suture technique for ruptured tendon was popularized by Bunnell and Kessler. Currently, more popular techniques include the six-strand suture technique, suture weave, Krackow stitch, and three-bundle technique. New percutaneous techniques have been described, with less initial pain and a smaller scar, but concerns exist regarding potential complications including sural nerve injury and possibly rerupture.

In addition to these various suture constructs, several augmentation techniques have been described, using either a gastrocnemius turndown flap or the plantaris tendon. Although these constructs do augment the soft tissues and theoretically may improve the strength of the repair, their routine use and benefit have not been confirmed in an acute Achilles repair.

Surgical Technique

Surgery can be performed either before significant swelling or after soft-tissue injury resolution.

- The patient is placed in the prone position. Both feet can be prepped into the operative field to allow for side-to-side comparison of the resting dynamic tension of the repaired tendon.
- An incision is made over the rupture from medial to the posterior midline of the Achilles tendon to avoid injury to the sural nerve; the paratenon is split longitudinally and can be tagged with suture on the medial and lateral aspects to facilitate closure at the end of the operation (Figs. 8.4 and 8.5).
- The ragged ends of the proximal and distal Achilles tendon are trimmed and repaired with a large (no. 3) nonabsorbable suture using a modified whip (Bunnell, Kessler, or Krackow) stitch. Depending on the size of

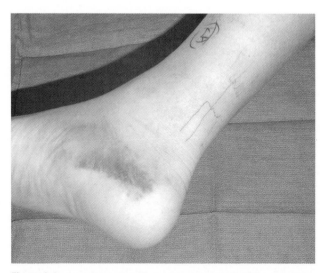

Figure 8.4 Intraoperative photo prior to acute Achilles repair.

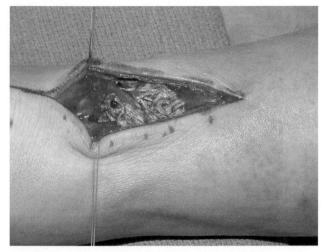

Figure 8.5 Intraoperative photo of acute Achilles rupture with "mop-like" fibers.

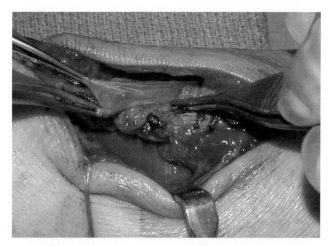

Figure 8.7 Intraoperative photo of Achilles tendon repair with plantaris augmentation fanned over nonabsorbable suture.

the tendon, one or two strands of suture can be used at each end (Fig. 8.6).
- One critical step is to accurately assess the dynamic resting tension of the Achilles tendon.
  - □ The goal is to approximate the two ends of ruptured tendon together with the appropriate tension to achieve a comparable foot position similar to the opposite foot.
  - □ Subtle adjustments to the suture tension can be made to achieve appropriate tension of the tendon.
- Once the ends are tied, the suture knots should be secured in the anterior position to minimize soft-tissue irritation and adhesions.
- A circumferential 3-0 absorbable running suture can be used to reinforce the repair.
  - □ Another technique to reinforce the repair and minimize the soft-tissue adhesion is to release the plantaris tendon (absent in 15% of the patients) and fan it over the repair site (Fig. 8.7). This step may improve the outcome by preventing adhesions and reinforcing the surgical repair.

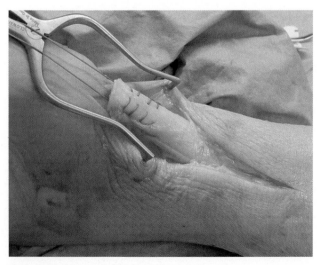

Figure 8.6 Photo of whipstitch for Achilles repair.

- Subsequently, the paratenon is approximated with absorbable suture. The soft tissue is closed in the standard fashion, and a standard posterior splint is applied in mild plantar flexion.

Postoperative Management

Prolonged cast immobilization leads to "cast disease," with muscle atrophy, joint stiffness, adhesions, and cartilage atrophy. Both nonoperative and operative techniques for Achilles repair have demonstrated significant permanent functional deficits (based on Cybex testing) following prolonged cast immobilization.

The basic concept of functional rehabilitation protocols is to avoid the morbidity of cast immobilization with an acceptable complication rate to facilitate the remodeling and maturation phase of tendon repair. Early limb and joint mobilization minimizes muscle atrophy and joint stiffness. During the remodeling phase, the functional activity may assist in the organization of the collagen fibers along their proper orientation to ideally resist the tensile forces. Subsequently, during the maturation phase, the rehabilitation protocol stimulates the intrinsic tendon healing processes with increasing collagen cross-linking, which leads to increased strength.

Functional Rehabilitation Protocol
- Patients should be immobilized for 10 to 14 days for the incision to heal.
- Once the sutures are removed (by day 14), weight bearing is initiated with a hinged range-of-motion (ROM) boot, removable splint, or ankle–foot orthosis (AFO) that permits ankle motion. Early functional weight-bearing and ROM exercise have superior outcomes compared with early immobilization.
- Rehabilitation of the Achilles tendon begins with progressive ROM exercises and accelerated weight bearing.
- Close attention for any symptoms of overuse during the retraining phase is necessary.
  - □ If excessive pain or swelling occurs, the rehabilitation protocol may be slowed down.

- Initially, the patient is encouraged to perform progressive ROM exercises and increase their weight-bearing status to full weight by 4 weeks.
- Isometric exercises are useful during the initial phase of rehabilitation. Active plantarflexion with passive dorsiflexion (stretching with a strap or towel) is encouraged, and pushoff strengthening can be started with a stair-climbing device.
- By 10 to 12 weeks, single heel rise, increasing pushoff activities, and jogging exercise are started.

Complications

Acute Achilles tendon ruptures may be missed during the initial evaluation in as many as 25% of the patients, leading to misdiagnosis, unsuccessful management, or rerupture. If the diagnosis is uncertain, advanced imaging studies such as MRI or US may confirm the diagnosis, but these are generally unnecessary.

Complications exist for both the nonoperative and operative management of acute Achilles tendon rupture. For these reasons, there has been little consensus regarding their ideal management. The major complication of nonoperative management with cast immobilization is the incomplete return to function as a result of the loss of functional continuity of the tendon with appropriate dynamic resting length. Tendon reruptures are three to four times more common after nonoperative treatment.

The most serious operative complications include infection, adhesions, nerve injury, and wound dehiscence (Fig. 8.8). Soft-tissue dehiscence with infection can be disastrous as a result of the limited soft-tissue coverage options. Percutaneous surgery is associated with sural nerve damage, but overall it has reduced risk of complications. Postoperative thromboembolic events, such as deep vein thrombosis, are common in patients who receive an Achilles tendon rupture repair. Initial treatment comprises early weight-bearing and ROM exercises, oral antibiotics, and wound debridement. Adjunct treatments include local topical antibiotics (silver sulfadiazine) or exogenous growth factors (e.g., Regranex, Ortho-McNeil, Raritan, New Jersey) that may facilitate the granulation process. For large wound

defects, a conservative approach may be attempted with local wound care or a wound suction device (Wound VAC, KCI, San Antonio, Texas). In rare instances, a free flap is required.

Results and Outcomes

Recently, improved outcomes and a trend toward fewer complications have been reported. A meta-analysis, published in 2005, of 12 trials involving 800 patients concluded that open operative treatment (3.5%) of acute Achilles tendon ruptures significantly reduces the risk of rerupture compared with nonoperative treatment (12.6%), but operative treatment is associated with a significantly higher risk (26.1%) of other complications. Operative risks may be reduced by performing surgery percutaneously (8.3% risk of complications). Postoperative splinting with use of a functional brace reduces the overall complication rate.

CHRONIC RUPTURES OF ACHILLES TENDON

Many patients have significant delay in diagnosis of an acute Achilles tendon rupture. Even though the patient is able to walk or function to some extent, compromised pushoff strength limits activities, such as sporting activities and climbing stairs. This delay in treatment leads to much more complex reconstructive options.

PATHOGENESIS

A delay greater than 4 to 6 weeks is considered a "chronic Achilles tendon rupture." The tendon sheath becomes thickened, whereas repair tissue fills the gap. Any delay beyond 2 weeks allows the gap to fill with fibrous scar tissue in a disorganized pattern. Over time, the disorganized scar tissue can stretch and elongate, exacerbating proximal muscle tendon retraction.

DIAGNOSIS

Physical Examination and History

Clinical Features
- The diagnosis of chronic Achilles rupture may be difficult to confirm on physical examination.
- The physical examination may demonstrate a significant soft-tissue deficit, but often scar tissue fills the area resulting in loss of functional continuity.
- One test, the *hyperdorsiflexion sign (Matles test)*, demonstrates greater maximum passive dorsiflexion on the injured side than on the uninjured side when the patient is prone.
  - ☐ This loss of symmetry usually indicates a compromised Achilles tendon complex.

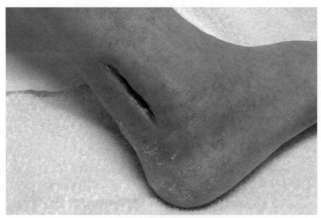

Figure 8.8 Clinical photo of wound complication treated by wet-to-dry dressing changes.

- Decreased plantarflexion strength helps confirm the presence of a compromised Achilles tendon.
  - □ Manual testing may be performed, but is often difficult because of the secondary recruitment of other ankle plantarflexors.
  - □ Clawing of the toes and an increase in the medial arch of the foot may result from the accommodation by the flexor digitorum longus (FDL) muscle for the functional loss of the gastrocnemius and soleus muscles.
  - □ Although a patient may be able to perform a single heel rise, repetitive heel rises are too difficult.
- The *calf squeeze test (Thompson test)* has a positive finding if the plantarflexion on the affected side is less than the unaffected side.
- For equivocal cases and high-level professional athletes, objective testing can be used to determine the exact isokinetic strength and power.
  - □ Cybex motor testing can be performed through the motion of ankle dorsiflexion and plantarflexion and analyzed as a percentage deficit of the contralateral normal side.
- A careful history regarding general daily activities, athletic interests, work issues, and treatment expectations is important.
- Even though the patient is able to walk or function to some extent, significant compromised pushoff strength exists.
- Activities such as single or repetitive heel rise or activities involving stairs often are not possible.

Radiologic Features

- Plain radiographs usually do not demonstrate any significant osseous findings after a chronic Achilles rupture.
- A subtle soft-tissue finding is the presence of increased density consistent with the calcification of the proximal or distal Achilles tendon end (Fig. 8.9).

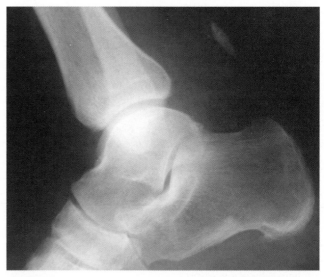

Figure 8.9 Lateral X-ray of ankle demonstrating proximal calcified density consistent with retracted chronic ruptured Achilles tendon.

- One critical parameter is the size of the gap defect between the tendon ends. In many patients with chronic Achilles rupture, a palpable gap exists.
  - □ MRI or US can be used to confirm the diagnosis and determine the extent of retraction of the proximal tendon and length of the defect (Fig. 8.10).
  - □ Increased signal intensity on a T2-weighted image is present in the tissue at the gap deficit.
- Some surgeons think an MRI study may be of limited value for the patient who has a chronic Achilles rupture because the patient will require surgical intervention; an intraoperative evaluation may be most useful to determine the type of Achilles reconstruction technique.

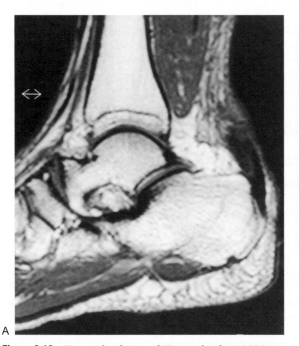
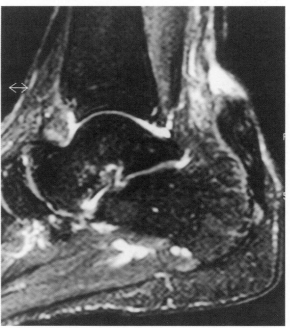

Figure 8.10 T1-weighted (A) and T2-weighted (B) MRI images of chronic Achilles tendon rupture.

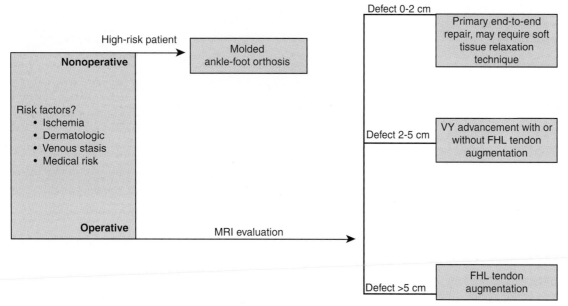

Algorithm 8.1 Diagnostic workup for chronic rupture of the Achilles tendon. FHL, flexor hallucis longus; MRI, magnetic resonance imaging.

Diagnostic Workup

See Algorithm 8.1 for the diagnostic workup of chronic rupture of the Achilles tendon.

TREATMENT

Surgical Indications and Contraindications

The surgical reconstruction of chronic Achilles rupture requires significant soft-tissue dissection. Ideally, the clinical scenario is optimized by minimizing the various risk factors for wound compromise, such as having the patient quit smoking or discontinue the use of certain medications (e.g., immunosuppressant anti-inflammatory medications) as well as accomplish the appropriate workup for chronic swelling, venous stasis, or lower limb ischemia. Certain patients may not be surgical candidates for reconstruction if chronic dermatologic or arterial/venous problems are significant.

For patients with local surgical contraindications (chronic venous stasis ulcer, lower extremity ischemia) or significant medical contraindication, brace management is a nonsurgical alternative. The standard brace option includes a molded polypropylene AFO with or without spring-loaded hinge. The standard AFO permits passive dorsiflexion with resistance. The spring-loaded component may provide a significant amount of torque and strength. Even though this alternative may improve some functional deficits, most active patients who are candidates for surgical reconstruction will not tolerate a brace long term and desire surgical reconstruction.

Surgical Concepts

Several concepts must be considered regarding chronic Achilles tendon reconstruction. Ideally, the repaired gastrocnemius–soleus complex will heal with appropriate muscle tension and absence of muscle atrophy. End-to-end contiguous tendon repair is usually not obtainable because

there is significant gap secondary to the proximal tendon retraction. The first concept consists of vascularity of the repair site. The blood supply to the Achilles tendon plays a critical role in the healing process. The blood supply arises from the paratenon, the musculotendinous junction, and the distal tendon insertion. Local scarred soft tissue often demonstrates suboptimal local vascularity, which can compromise the healing process. Several techniques involving autologous soft-tissue augmentation (i.e., strips of fascia lata, proximal Achilles turndown, and plantaris tendon weave) are avascular free tendon grafts. Even the V–Y tendon advancement involves significant soft-tissue dissection and comprises mainly of avascular tissue transfer. Even so, tendon healing does occur after a tendon advancement technique with resumption of strength and activities.

Another concept is the type of tendon transfer for augmentation of a deficient Achilles tendon. Flexor tendons, such as peroneus brevis, FDL, and flexor hallucis longus (FHL) have been proposed for the augmentation of the chronic Achilles tendon rupture. The selection of a donor tendon requires consideration of its phase, its relative strength, and the donor morbidity with regard to the loss of function. Theoretically, the FHL tendon transfer has the benefit of in-phase transfer, increased relative strength compared with the FDL, and minimal effect upon hallux function; therefore, it is currently the most commonly used technique. In addition, the transfer of the FHL most closely reproduces the axial contractile forces of the Achilles tendon and provides a local contiguous muscle for revascularization of the scarred tendon bed.

Most surgeons base their Achilles tendon reconstruction technique on the length of the gap deficit of the Achilles tendon, although other factors such as the length of delay, the age and athletic expectations of the patient, and muscle quality of the gastrocnemius–soleus complex may be important. The gap deficit is a key determining factor because certain techniques may be performed only with minimal soft-tissue defect. One may be able to palpate the deficit and determine its length or it may be estimated preoperatively with MRI or US.

Surgical Technique

Defects 0 to 2 cm Long

For a minimal defect, it is possible to achieve a primary end-to-end repair without any additional augmentation or reconstruction. The muscle can usually be mobilized after the primary repair in a similar protocol to an acute rupture, with the foot held initially in minimal plantarflexion. For a defect of 1 to 2 cm, gradual soft-tissue relaxation stretching technique is used. After the sutures are placed in the proximal tendon, 10 to 15 lb of traction is applied manually or with a weight for 10 minutes to stretch and relax the contracted gastrocnemius–soleus complex. This technique should easily gain up to 2 cm in length and allow an end-to-end repair without significant foot equinus contracture. Occasionally, the scar completely fills the gap, but the tendon has "healed" in a lengthened fashion. One can consider Z-shortening tenotomy (opposite of Z-lengthening) with appropriate tensioning and repair with resection of the redundant tendon.

- A standard posteromedial approach is used, similar to the repair of an acute Achilles rupture. This approach avoids the sural nerve and allows the use of the plantaris tendon, if necessary.
- The paratenon should be carefully split and preserved for later repair.
- The bulbous ends are identified, and both the distal and the proximal ends are resected to remove the disorganized fibrous scar tissue.
- The end-to-end tendon repair is performed with no. 3 nonabsorbable suture using a standard technique (whip stitch or modified Krakow).
- The paratenon and soft tissue are closed in a sequential fashion.
- The postoperative protocol is similar to an acute Achilles tendon repair.

Defects 2 to 5 cm Long

For a larger defect, several options exist, including V–Y advancement with or without FHL tendon transfer augmentation. The V–Y advancement avoids sacrifice of a normal muscle tendon unit. This procedure relies on a functional muscle and theoretically may not work if significant scarring or severe atrophy exists within the gastrocnemius–soleus complex. Often, an atrophied gastrocnemius soleus muscle can still be mobilized and rehabilitated with sufficient function. The V–Y advancement technique has been reported in several series with restoration of plantarflexion strength and with minimal complications of soft tissue compromise and sural neuritis.

- Advancement of the proximal Achilles tendon in a V–Y fashion has been described as an augmentation technique for chronic Achilles rupture (Fig. 8.11).
- Using a longitudinal posterior incision, an inverted V-shaped incision is made in the muscle tendon junction of the gastrocsoleus aponeurosis. Care must be taken

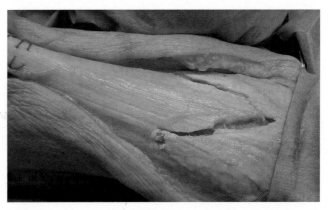

Figure 8.11   V–Y advancement for chronic Achilles repair.

not to violate the underlying gastrocnemius muscle, which is attached to the anterior paratenon.
- The arms (approximately 12 to 18 cm in length depending on the size of the defect) of the V must be at least one-and-a-half times the length of the gap deficit to allow for the appropriate proximal limb closure of the Y (Fig. 8.12).
- The critical aspect is adequate soft-tissue dissection with preservation of the posterior muscle in continuity and advancement of the proximal soft tissue for tendon coverage.
- An end-to-end repair is performed using the standard suture technique described earlier, and the limbs of the Y are closed with no. 2 nonabsorbable suture (Fig. 8.13).
- Postoperative rehabilitation is as described earlier.

Defects Longer Than 5 cm

For a defect longer than 5 cm, few options exist. One option is to perform a turndown flap, but criticisms exist regarding the bulk of the tendon at the point of the turndown. Surgical options include the use of a flexor tendon transfer (FHL or FDL) alone or in combination with the V–Y advancement technique described earlier.

- The procedure is performed with the patient in the supine position with contralateral hip bump. A thigh tourniquet is used.
- Attention is first directed to the medial border of the foot, where the FHL is harvested.

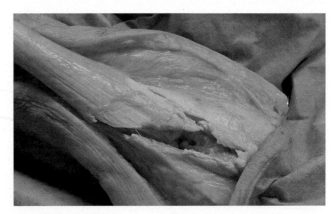

Figure 8.12   The V portion of limb should be double the length of the distance to be repaired.

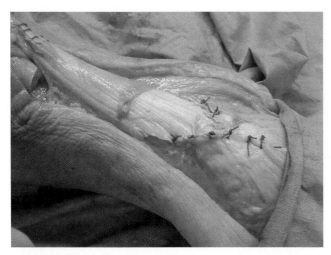

Figure 8.13 Limbs of the Y are closed with no. 2 nonabsorbable suture.

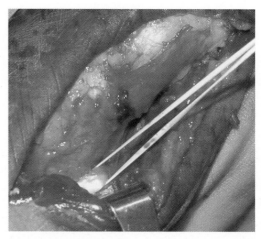

Figure 8.15 Intraoperative photo of vessel loop around flexor hallucis longus in midfoot.

- A longitudinal incision is made along the medial border of the midfoot just above the abductor muscle, from the navicular to the head of the first metatarsal (Fig. 8.14).
- The skin and subcutaneous tissue are sharply reflected down to the fascia.
- The abductor with the flexor hallucis brevis muscle is reflected plantar, exposing the deep midfoot.
- The FHL and FDL are identified within the substance of the midfoot.
- The FHL is divided as far as possible, allowing the distal stump adequate length for transfer to the FDL (Fig. 8.15). The proximal portion is tagged with a suture.
- The distal limb of the FHL is sewn into the FDL with the toes held in neutral position.
- A second longitudinal incision is made along posteromedial aspect of the Achilles, starting from the level of its musculotendinous junction to 1 in below its insertion on the calcaneus (Fig. 8.16).
- The paratenon of the tendon is opened longitudinally, and the substance of the tendon is evaluated (Fig. 8.17).

- Care is taken to dissect deep to the paratenon to create full-thickness skin flaps and avoid any skin sloughs.
- The deep fascia over the posterior compartment of the leg is incised longitudinally, and the FHL is identified.
- The tendon is retracted from the midfoot into the posterior incision.
- A transverse drill hole is made approximately 1.0 to 1.5 cm distal and anterior to the superior calcaneal process perpendicular to the calcaneus.
- A lateral incision is made over the drill hole with care to avoid damaging the sural nerve. A curette is used to smooth the sharp edges.
- A suture passer is placed through the bone tunnel from lateral to medial. The tagged suture is passed through the tunnel, drawing the FHL tendon through the drill hole.
- A blunt hemostat is subcutaneously passed from the medial incision to the lateral incision, and the newly transferred FHL is passed proximal and medial.
- The FHL is then woven from distal to proximal through the Achilles tendon with a tendon weaver, using the full length of the harvested tendon (Fig. 8.18).
- Some surgeons advocate harvesting the FHL through the posterior incision as far distal along the medial calcaneus as possible. It is then anchored to the calcaneus just deep to the Achilles insertion with an interference screw.
- Care is taken to maintain the foot in 10° of plantar flexion.

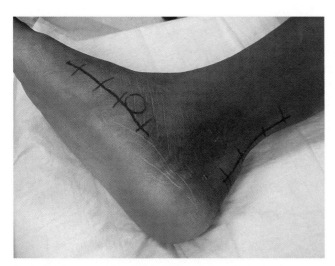

Figure 8.14 Surgical technique of chronic Achilles tendon repair using flexor hallucis longus.

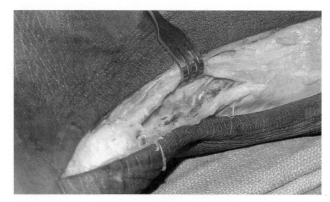

Figure 8.16 Intraoperative photo demonstrating significant gap deficit.

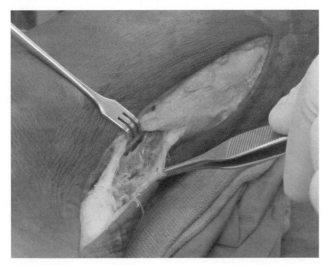

Figure 8.17 Intraoperative photo of paratenon opened demonstrating absence of Achilles tendon.

Complications

- Rerupture: Higher incidence in patients with inflammatory disorders or on drugs such as steroids.
- Ankle stiffness: Avoid extreme plantarflexion position of the foot, proper tension of repair.

- Wound necrosis: Minimize with soft-tissue handling, full-thickness flap, and appropriate immobilization.
- Infections: Potentially devastating, treat with wound care, possible skin graft or flap.

Results and Outcomes

In general, the surgical treatment of chronic Achilles tendon ruptures with some type of gastrocsoleus repair and FHL transfer has yielded good results.

NONINSERTIONAL ACHILLES TENDINOSIS

Renewed interest in sports activities and increased duration and training intensity have led to a significant increase in overuse injuries of the Achilles tendon. Noninsertional Achilles tendinosis comprises a wide spectrum of clinical presentations, with the most common subset of patients being the high-level athlete who presents with an inflamed Achilles tendon 2 to 6 cm above its insertion. Another subset of patients comprises the older, sedentary patient who presents with an inflamed heel consistent with insertional Achilles tendonitis (discussed elsewhere). A third subset

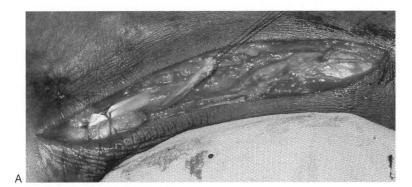

A

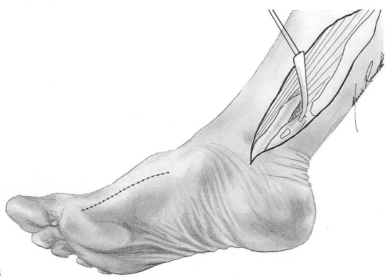

B

Figure 8.18 Intraoperative photo (**A**) and artist's rendering (**B**) of flexor hallucis longus repair of chronic Achilles rupture.

comprises young males with seronegative arthropathy who present with an Achilles insertional enthesopathy.

PATHOGENESIS

Etiology

The development of Achilles tendinosis has been attributed to an overuse phenomenon, especially running activities, leading to excessive forces on the Achilles tendon. Forces on the Achilles tendon approximate 10 times the body weight during running. A significant correlation between the incidence of Achilles tendinosis and the intensity of training or excessive training has been found.

Classically, the overuse phenomenon occurs in a high-end athlete who subjects his or her tendons to repetitive stresses beyond its ability to heal. Patients commonly report a change in training pattern or activity with the subsequent development of symptoms. Changes, such as increased duration, type of activity, or frequency of sports activities, are commonly noted findings. More subtle changes include alterations in athletic shoewear or local changes in the running environment. Whether the patient is a high-end athlete or mainly sedentary, alterations in training patterns or environment may lead to Achilles tendinosis.

Overuse injuries of the Achilles tendon are increasing and occur in 6.5% to 18% of all runners and in one study was diagnosed in 56% of elite middle-aged runners. A relatively high number of cases of noninsertional Achilles tendinosis occurs in other athletic activities, including those who dance ballet or play soccer, basketball, tennis, or racquetball. Repetitive overuse with increased biomechanical stress placed upon the Achilles tendon is a contributing factor in all of these activities.

Pathophysiology

The blood supply of the Achilles arises from the osseous insertion, musculotendinous junction, and ventral mesotenal vessels. Injection studies have shown that the ventral vessels are fewest 2 to 6 cm proximal to the Achilles tendon insertion, correlating to the area of reduced vascularity and the site of pathology. Neovascularization of the tendon is considered an important etiologic factor and a pain generator in Achilles tendinopathy. Doppler ultrasound has been used to demonstrate neovascularization in Achilles tendons with tendinopathy. Abnormal vessels have been found in the ventral aspect of the tendon adjacent to Kager triangle. These vessels are accompanied by proliferating nerves that are hypothesized to be integral in pain transmission.

Classification

A histopathologic classification system has been developed for noninsertional tendinosis with three distinct subgroups (Table 8.1).

DIAGNOSIS

Physical Examination and History

Clinical Features

- The triad of symptoms of Achilles tendonitis are pain, swelling localized 2 to 6 cm above the Achilles tendon insertion, and impaired performance.
- Increased pain during exercise progresses to constant pain, independent of physical activities.
- In acute paratenonitis, the tendon appears acutely swollen, edematous, and tender.
  - Gentle compression of the tendon at the swollen foci reproduces the symptoms.
  - Often crepitation is noted during ankle ROM.
  - For ambiguous cases, an MRI scan may differentiate whether tendinosis is present along with the finding of slight thickening of the paratenon (Fig. 8.19).
- Paratenonitis with tendinosis has increased symptoms with maximum point tenderness and irregularity within the tendon substance.
  - The pain is more severe and reproducible with palpation of the diffusely thickened tendon.
  - Isolated tendinosis comprises an area of localized irregularity, swelling, and pain with significant weakness in pushoff strength.
  - Increased dorsiflexion motion may exist secondary to elongation.

TABLE 8.1 CLASSIFICATION OF NONINSERTIONAL ACHILLES TENDONITIS

Type	Description
Paratenonitis	Inflammation and thickening of the paratenon, formation of adhesions, fibrosis, myxomatous degeneration, round cell inflammatory infiltrate, proliferation of fibrovascular connective tissue
Paratenonitis with tendinosis	Greater paratenon inflammation, intratendinous degeneration, paratenon thickening, edema, proliferation of fibroblasts, new connective tissue, proliferation of blood vessels
Tendinosis	Noninflammatory intratendinosis degeneration owing to aging, microtrauma, or vascular compromise

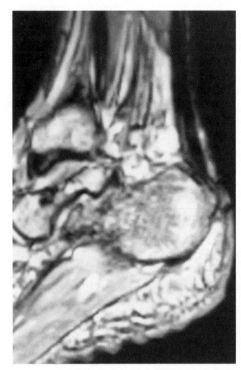

Figure 8.19   T2-weighted MRI study of Achilles, sagittal view, demonstrating increased signal within the paratenon consistent with Achilles paratenonitis.

Radiologic Features

◼ Plain radiographs are generally not useful in evaluating and diagnosing noninsertional Achilles tendinopathy, but they may demonstrate intratendinous calcifications that are suggestive of tendinosis.

◼ Even though MRI is not necessary for diagnosis, its application can be especially useful for planning the surgical treatment of patients who have failed nonoperative management or in ambiguous clinical situations. The MRI is accurate in assessing the extent of the disease process and localizing the extent of diseased paratenon or the presence of tendinosis.
   ☐ For paratenonitis, MRI findings consist of increased T2 signal in the paratenon with no signal changes in the tendon, which is relatively uncommon (see Fig. 8.19).
   ☐ For paratenonitis with tendinosis, MRI findings comprise T2 increased signal changes in the paratenon and tendon (Fig. 8.20).
   ☐ For tendinosis, the MRI appearance comprises fusiform thickening with longitudinal linear signal change within the Achilles tendon (Figs. 8.20 and 8.21).

◼ US evaluation has recently gained popularity in its use for diagnosing tendinopathies because of its cost-effectiveness and portability to be performed in one's office, and it can be performed dynamically. Although the use of US is operator dependent, it has the advantage of better delineation of neovascularization associated with tendinopathy using Doppler techniques. Diseased tendons demonstrate hypoechogenic areas owing to irregular tendon structure and changes in the patterns of fibrillar collagen and increased cross-sectional and anterior–posterior tendon diameter.

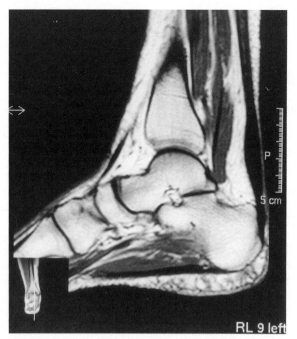

Figure 8.20   T1/T2-weighted MRI study, sagittal view, demonstrating paratenonitis with Achilles tendinosis.

Abnormal echogenicity of Kager fat pad, thickening of the paratenon, and subtle microtears are also indicative of Achilles tendinopathy.

Diagnostic Workup

See Algorithm 8.2 for the diagnostic workup of noninsertional Achilles tendinosis.

TREATMENT

Nonoperative Treatment

◼ The initial treatment of acute paratenonitis or paratenonitis with tendinosis comprises heel lift, ice, and nonsteroidal anti-inflammatory treatment. Once the acute phase has resolved (in approximately 2 weeks), a rehabilitation protocol of physical therapy can commence with local anti-inflammatory modalities and stretching and strengthening of the Achilles tendon with eccentric exercises as outlined below. Upon successful resolution of symptoms, an orthotic support may be useful for patients with excessive pronation. Most patients should be counseled regarding a protocol of activity modification and shoewear changes.

◼ For the high-end athlete, initial management consists of cross-training and decreasing weekly mileage, avoidance of hill running, and interval training. Before any athletic activity, an Achilles tendon stretching program should be initiated. Later, the clinician needs to emphasize preventive measures such as cross-training exercise (swimming, bicycling) and the avoidance of overtraining.

◼ Eccentric strengthening exercises, a technique of elongating a tendon during a simultaneous voluntary muscle contracture, has become a widely used treatment

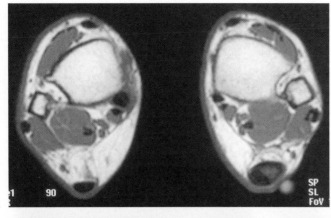

Figure 8.21 **A:** T2-weighted MRI study, axial view of contralateral uninvolved side versus Achilles tendinosis. T1-weighted (**B**) and T2-weighted (**C**) MRI scans, sagittal views demonstrating Achilles tendinosis.

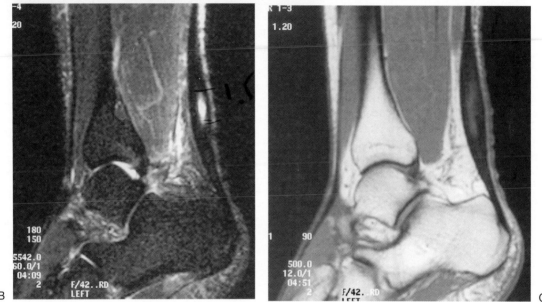

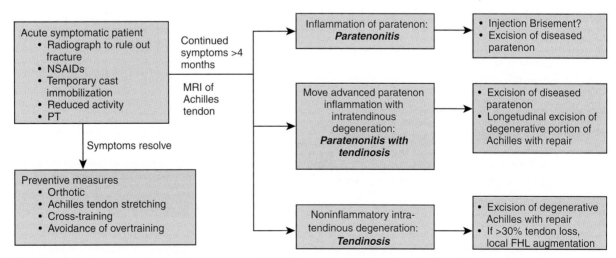

Algorithm 8.2 Diagnostic workup for noninsertional Achilles tendonitis. FHL, flexor hallucis longus; MRI, magnetic resonance imaging; NSAIDs, nonsteroidal anti-inflammatory drugs; PT, physical therapy.

for Achilles tendinopathy. Although the mechanism of action is unknown, it is theorized that eccentric exercise decreases neovascularization within a symptomatic tendon. The tensile force generated within the tendon during the exercise temporarily ceases blood flow through the newly formed vessels. With repetition over time, these vessels are obliterated, along with their associated pain receptors leading to the resolution of symptoms.

- Other noninvasive therapies that are currently used to treat Achilles tendinopathy include US, low-level laser therapy, and shockwave therapy. These therapies do not have high-level evidence to support their routine use, but small studies with levels I and II evidence have shown their efficacy.
- Invasive nonsurgical therapies include various injections into the affected site. Corticosteroids have shown effectiveness in short-term relief of pain, but are contraindicated because of their catabolic effect and increased risk of tendon rupture. Injection of platelet rich plasma has also demonstrated potential in its clinical use in treating Achilles tendinopathy by delivering superphysiologic doses of cytokines to the tendon, promoting healing.
- A key distinction must be noted between patients who present with an acute and chronic Achilles paratenonitis. More than 90% of cases with acute symptoms resolve without surgical intervention. In contrast, the prognosis for those patients with chronic process treated by nonoperative protocol is less certain, with only about half being successful. For those patients who fail conservative management, surgical intervention may be indicated.

Surgical Treatment

Paratenonitis

For patients who have chronic Achilles paratenonitis, clinical series have reported limited success with a nonoperative approach. Symptoms usually resolve with an excision of the diseased and thickened paratenon.

- A 4-cm incision is made medially over the area of maximum tenderness (Fig. 8.22).
- The thickened inflamed paratenon is identified, with the release of all adhesions.
- The posterior two-thirds of the paratenon is removed at this level, preserving the anterior blood supply.
- Closure comprises subcutaneous suture approximation with nonabsorbable skin closure.
- The limb is held immobilized with a short leg cast for 1 week followed by early weight bearing and rehabilitation.

Chronic Tendinosis

Analysis of the preoperative MRI scan usually provides the location and the extent of the diseased tendon. The surgeon must consider debridement of the inflamed paratenon as well as resection of the degenerative mucoid portion of Achilles tendon.

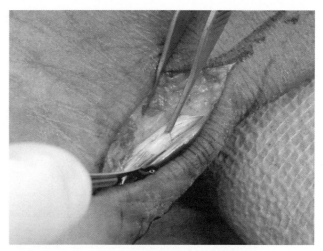

Figure 8.22 Intraoperative photo of surgical debridement of paratenonitis.

- For mild-to-moderate symptoms, percutaneous longitudinal tenotomies can be made to the affected area to stimulate regeneration and tendon healing. This can be performed with or without minimally invasive stripping of the tendon with a large diameter suture. Success rates between 67% and 97% have been reported with good results in athletic patients, and worse outcomes have been shown in patients with extensive tendinopathies, multinodular tendons, and paratendinopathies.
- In an open procedure, the diseased paratenon is first debrided, and the tendon is carefully evaluated. The goal of the surgical debridement is to eliminate the degenerative tendon. Often it is difficult to determine the true extent of degeneration.
- The gross clinical examination may reveal a centralized area of mucoid degeneration.
- The central degenerative portion of the Achilles tendon is excised through a longitudinal approach.
- Small longitudinal incisions (5 to 10 mm in length) can then be placed in the remaining portion of the Achilles tendon to stimulate revascularization and the healing process.
- The defect is closed with nonabsorbable 2-0 or 3-0 sutures.
- For a larger defect with severe tendon compromise involving greater than one-third of the normal tendon width or significant risk of rupture, local tissue augmentation is indicated.
  - An FHL tendon transfer can be undertaken as described previously for chronic Achilles tendon rupture.

Postoperative Management

The postoperative course includes short leg cast immobilization for a minimum of 3 weeks (longer for patients undergoing FHL tendon transfer; see Chronic Rupture of Achilles Tendon), followed by a protocol of partial weight bearing for 3 weeks. Patients are gradually increased to full weight bearing. Recovery is slower and less reliable than acute Achilles rupture with repair. Patients should be counseled regarding a rehabilitation period of up to 6 months.

Results and Outcome

For patients with paratenonitis, surgical excision of the inflamed paratenon has led to painless clinical recovery in 90% or more of the patients. When tendinosis accompanies the paratenonitis, a lower rate of success and longer rehabilitation period may be anticipated.

ANTERIOR TIBIALIS TENDON RUPTURE

PATHOGENESIS

Etiology and Pathophysiology

The anterior tibialis tendon is the primary dorsiflexor of the ankle. Rupture of this tendon may be traumatic (open or closed) or nontraumatic. Open traumatic ruptures most often occur as the result of a sharp object being dropped on the foot. Closed traumatic ruptures usually arise during athletics. The mechanism may be either a direct blow or a forced plantarflexion–eversion moment on a dorsiflexed ankle. The tendon may tear in its midsubstance or avulse off its insertion at the medial cuneiform and the first metatarsal bone.

Nontraumatic ruptures occur in degenerative tendons where tendinosis causes a gradual attenuation and rupture of the tendon. This type of rupture generally occurs between the superior and the inferior extensor retinaculum, a relatively avascular region.

Epidemiology

Nontraumatic anterior tibialis tendon rupture is rare, and primarily occurs in men 50 to 70 years of age. Common comorbidities include diabetes mellitus, rheumatoid arthritis, and gout. Patients with a history of steroid injection or prior surgery in the area have an increased likelihood of nontraumatic rupture.

Closed traumatic anterior tibialis tendon rupture occurs in a younger and more active population.

DIAGNOSIS

Physical Examination and History

Clinical Features

- Patients with open traumatic ruptures present with a painful laceration on the dorsum of their foot and weak dorsiflexion of their ankle because a sharp object (e.g., kitchen knife or piece of glass) has been dropped on the foot.
  - The laceration may be deceptively small, which may lead to a delay in diagnosis.
  - On physical examination, the patient is usually able to dorsiflex the ankle, but it is weaker than the contralateral side, and a palpable defect or lack of tension in the tendon is present. They cannot stand on their heel on the injured side.
  - The patient may hyperdorsiflex the toes while dorsiflexing the ankle in an effort to recruit the toe extensors to dorsiflex the ankle.
  - Patients ambulate with a slapping, steppage gait.
- Closed traumatic ruptures present with a history of a direct blow to the anterior ankle or an injury involving forced plantarflexion to a dorsiflexed ankle.
  - Aside from the absence of a laceration, the remainder of the history and physical examination is similar to that for patients with open traumatic ruptures.
- Nontraumatic rupture of the anterior tibialis tendon usually presents in elderly patients often with systemic disease or steroid use.
  - These patients do not recall a discrete traumatic incident and initially fail to notice their problem because of its insidious onset.
  - Patients usually do not complain of pain, but do complain of an alteration in their gait pattern.
  - The condition may be mistaken for peroneal motor neuropathy, especially in diabetics.
  - The thickened tendon and mass of fibrous tissue enveloping it in the anterior ankle may be misdiagnosed as a neoplasm.

Radiologic Features

- Plain radiographs can be used to rule out the presence of a foreign body with an open traumatic rupture or to visualize a bony fragment with an avulsed tendinous insertion, but most often they are noncontributory.
- A midsubstance rupture may be confirmed on MRI, but this is usually not necessary.
- US imaging can also be used to confirm a rupture.

Diagnostic Workup

Algorithm 8.3 covers the diagnostic workup for anterior tibialis tendon rupture.

TREATMENT

Surgical Indications and Contraindications

Surgical indications depend on the type and age of the rupture as well as the age and activity level of the patient. Open lacerations and closed traumatic ruptures should be repaired if detected acutely. Chronic ruptures and nontraumatic ruptures should be reconstructed in active patients with a significant functional deficit. Less active patients should be treated nonoperatively such as with a molded AFO.

Contraindications to surgery include a compromised soft-tissue envelope and the presence of severe systemic disease or peripheral vascular disease.

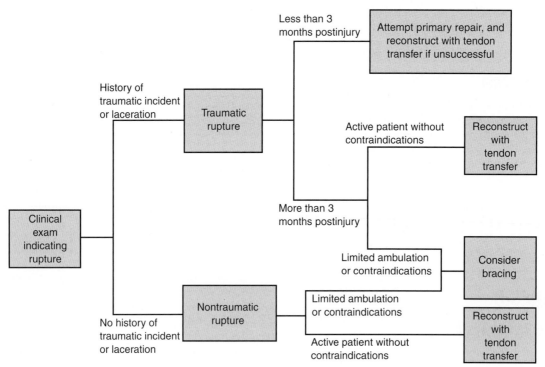

Algorithm 8.3   Diagnostic workup for anterior tibialis tendon rupture.

Surgical Technique

- An incision is made along the course of the tendon over the site of the rupture.
- An acute traumatic rupture should be repaired end- to end with nonabsorbable suture, with repair of the extensor retinaculum over the tendon to prevent bowstringing.
- A nontraumatic or chronic rupture may be reconstructed with an extensor hallucis longus (EHL) or extensor digitorum longus tendon transfer.
- A delayed diagnosis often requires tendon transfer or augmentation.
- The distal stump of the transferred tendon should be tenodesed to its corresponding brevis tendon to minimize donor site morbidity.
- In the presence of a tight gastrocnemius muscle, a gastrocnemius recession can be used to treat an associated contracture and weaken plantarflexion to help restore muscle balance between dorsiflexion and plantarflexion. This can protect the repair against avulsion and recurrent tendon degeneration.
- The wound is closed in layers, and a splint is applied with the ankle in neutral dorsiflexion.

Postoperative Management

The patient should follow up 10 to 14 days after surgery for suture removal and application of a short leg cast. Four weeks after surgery, the cast is changed to a controlled active motion (CAM) walker boot, and the patient begins weight-bearing and active dorsiflexion ROM exercises. Ambulation in a sneaker and strengthening exercises begin 2 months postoperatively.

Results and Outcome

The American Orthopedic Foot and Ankle Society/AOFAS Ankle–Hindfoot scale and isokinetic strength testing can be used to evaluate improvement postoperatively. Subjective results show a high level of patient satisfaction with anterior tibial tendon repair and reconstruction. Objective results also show a significant improvement postoperatively compared with the preoperative evaluation of the affected limb. However, there remains a significant difference in dorsiflexion and inversion strength between the affected and the uninvolved limb. Other possible complications include recurrent rupture, infection, neuroma, bowstringing, and deformity or weakness of toes at the donor site.

EXTENSOR HALLUCIS LONGUS TENDON RUPTURE

PATHOGENESIS

Etiology and Pathophysiology

EHL injuries fall into one of two categories depending on the nature of the injury: open laceration or closed rupture of the tendon. Open lacerations, classified as either total or partial tendon injuries, often occur.

Open lacerations of the EHL tendon may also be classified as total or partial tendon injuries. Open lacerations often result from dropping a sharp object onto the ankle, tibial fracture, and lawn-mowing accidents. Partial tendon injuries, where 40% to 50% of the tendon substance is involved, may impinge on the synovial sheath and result in triggering.

Closed EHL rupture, although rare, may be caused by a forced active extension of the joint against resistance, hypovascularity from consistent external compression around the ankle, and attrition induced by osteophytes and steroid injections. After the initial rupture or laceration, the EHL tendon may retract a significant distance such that a tendon transfer or grafting becomes necessary.

Epidemiology

There are few reports of EHL ruptures in the literature; however, from the available published studies, these ruptures occur most commonly in men between the ages of 21 and 49 years. Injuries proximal to the MTP joint are most commonly seen, whereas lacerations and ruptures distal to the MTP joint are scarce and associated with injury to the extensor hallucis brevis tendon. Injuries that occur proximal to the extensor retinaculum are generally related to injuries to the extensor digitorum longus and anterior tibialis muscles.

DIAGNOSIS

Physical Examination and History

Clinical Features

- Rupture of the EHL tendon results primarily in the loss of extensor function in the great toe.
- EHL tendon rupture leads to weakened dorsiflexion and decreased inversion of the foot.
- These consequences can result in tripping during the swing phase of the gait cycle when barefoot.
- Closed and spontaneous EHL tendon ruptures are associated with a history of diabetes mellitus, rheumatoid arthritis, and steroid injections.
- Chronic EHL ruptures result in fixed flexion contractures of the hallux at the interphalangeal joint, warranting hallux IP joint arthrodesis.

Radiologic Features

- Plain radiographs have limited use in the diagnosis of EHL ruptures. MRI may be used to confirm the diagnosis prior to surgical intervention.

TREATMENT

Surgical Indications and Contraindications

In determining the appropriate treatment of a ruptured EHL tendon, the site of injury is an important factor. If the injury site is distal to the extensor expansion, conservative therapy may be an appropriate first line treatment. Although most studies elucidate successful outcomes of EHL repair operations, other studies agree that an unrepaired EHL tendon is minimally inconvenient to patients, especially while wearing shoes.

If the injury site is proximal to the extensor expansion, primary repair is recommended. Acute ruptures are repaired primarily. Delayed diagnosis, especially of more than 3 months, usually precludes an end-to-end repair. A late diagnosis or repetitive movement of the injured ankle may cause the tendon to retract, and over time, gaps may reach 5 cm or more. These cases may require tendon transfer or tendon grafting procedures as opposed to exclusive end-to-end repair. A side-to-side tenodesis (tendon transfer) with the distal end of the EHL to the extensor hallucis brevis tendon, or to an adjacent extensor digitorum longus tendon, may be required. Some authors also transfer the distal EHL tendon to the peronous tertius tendon.

In cases of degenerated EHL tendon at sites of insertion and origin or chronic conditions when tendon ends cannot be reapproximated, tendon grafts are generally used. Some authors have used autografts from the extensor hallucis brevis, semitendinous, palmaris longus, and gracilis tendons. Zielaskowski et al. used allograft tensor fascia lata for repair.

Surgical Technique

- Begin by immobilizing the foot by inserting two Kirschner (K-)wires:
  - □ IP joint of the hallux: This maintains the joint in a position of extension.
  - □ MTP joint: This maintains the joint in a position of slight hyperextension.
- Irrigate wound and identify the two ends of the ruptured EHL tendon.
- In primary repair, rejoin the ends of the tendon via one of the following recommended suturing techniques:
  - □ Kessler–Tajima.
  - □ Bunnell.
  - □ Locking Loop.
- In cases of a retracted tendon where primary repair is no longer possible, tendon graft or tendon transfer procedures are preferred using the extensor hallucis brevis tendon or peronous tertius tendon. Autografts from the extensor hallucis brevis, semitendinous, palmaris longus, and gracilis tendons can be used to repair EHL ruptures.
- Position of the tendon after repair should be neutral so that it is not under excess tension after completion of the procedure, and the ankle should be positioned neutrally so as to free the EHL tendon of any strain or pressure.
- Proceed with standard wound closure and discharge patient with a short leg walking cast.

Postoperative Management

- During the first 3 weeks following surgery, the treated area should be strictly immobilized.

- Most studies recommend 6 weeks of short leg walking cast application with the ankle and big toe in neutral position. The shape of the cast blocks plantarflexion of big, toe and by removing the section of cast over the dorsum of the toe, it eliminates the opportunity of extension of the big toe with resistance. Specifically, some authors use K-wires to maintain big toe hyperextension to protect the repair after surgery.
- Three weeks after surgery, dynamic splinting and limited ROM exercises can be started.
- To avoid reinjuring the tendon, patients should not practice full ROM exercises for at least 1 month post-operatively.

Results and Outcome

The literature suggests minimal disadvantages and complications of primary repair of the EHL tendon. However, scarring and adhesion formation may occur posttreatment, causing a loss of motion in the great toe and being a potential source of continuous pain. These effects may be minimized by the use of dynamic splinting. Furthermore, surrounding muscle strands may lose varying degrees of power if the healing EHL tendon is subjected to excessive stress. Patients generally recover active extension of the big toe and can resume work without persistent pain; however, a full active range of motion may not be reached after surgery.

POSTERIOR ANKLE IMPINGEMENT AND FLEXOR HALLUCIS LONGUS TENDONITIS

PATHOGENESIS

Posterior ankle impingement is characterized by pain in the posterior aspect of the ankle with maximum plantarflexion. It is most often seen as a result of overuse and commonly occurs in dancers, runners, and soccer players. The talus has a prominent posteromedial process with discrete posteromedial and posterolateral projections. Failure of the posterolateral projection to fuse with the talus results in an ossicle termed the *os trigonum*. This is present in approximately 14% of the population and present bilaterally in 50% of affected patients. Activities that require repetitive plantarflexion can place added stress on the os trigonum and its synchondrosis, thus resulting in pain.

The flexor hallucis longus tendon runs between the posteromedial and the posterolateral projections of the posterior process of the talus. Therefore, FHL tendonitis will often present as posteromedial ankle pain. Patients who have soft-tissue impingement of the FHL tendon at the master knot of Henry will present with arch pain.

Distinguishing between FHL tendinosis and posterior ankle impingement is important, especially because they may be coexistent. Therefore, careful evaluation is warranted. The differential diagnosis of posterior ankle pain includes other bony injuries such as posterior tibial avulsion, posteromedial talar process fracture, osteochondral lesions of the posterior portion of the talus, or subtalar pathology.

DIAGNOSIS

Physical Examination and History

Clinical Features

- Patients with posterior impingement complain of pain in the posterior ankle or along the Achilles tendon region.
- Patients with FHL tenosynovitis complain of posteromedial ankle pain with pain possibly radiating toward the arch. There can be a "clicking" or locking sensation of the great toe, especially when pointing the toe in maximal flexion.
- Distinguishing between posterior impingement and FHL tendinosis is a significant clinical challenge because of their close anatomic proximity.
  - In patients with posterior impingement, there may be a remote history of trauma to the ankle. The forced hyperplantarflexion test may be used to reproduce the patient's symptoms. With the knee flexed at 90°, the examiner applies a repetitive hyperflexion force to the ankle with the leg both internally and externally rotated. Pain will occur as the os trigonum or the trigonal process contacts the tibia and calcaneus.
  - A selective diagnostic lidocaine injection with or without sonographic guidance into the posterior ankle may confirm the diagnosis.
  - In patients with FHL tenosynovitis, pain occurs along the posteromedial aspect of the ankle adjacent to the sustentaculum tali.
  - Symptoms of tendinosis may be reproduced with passive motion of the hallux.
  - An audible "popping" may be present with active contraction of the FHL tendon, especially with the foot pointed.

Radiologic Features

- Plain radiographs will often demonstrate a large posterior process of the talus or an os trigonum (Fig. 8.23).
- A lateral radiograph of the foot in maximal plantarflexion demonstrates abutment between the calcaneus and the tibia.
- A bone scan can be used to confirm this diagnosis because there is increased radionuclide uptake in this region.
- MRI may demonstrate the presence of an os trigonum with bone marrow edema and inflammation in the surrounding soft tissue as a result of posterior impingement (Fig. 8.24). Thickening of the posterior capsule may also be present.

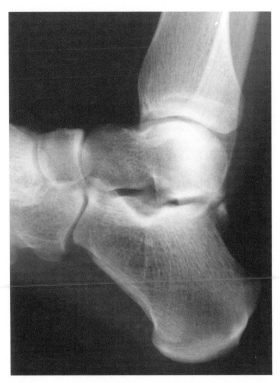

Figure 8.23 Lateral X-ray of foot of symptomatic dancer with pain upon ankle plantarflexion, demonstrating large os trigonum.

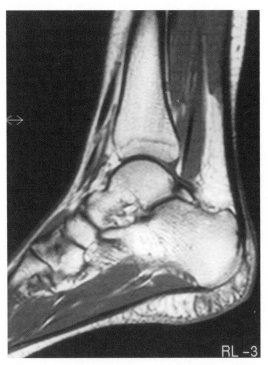

Figure 8.24 T1-weighted MRI scan of ankle. Sagittal view revealing os trigonum.

TREATMENT

Nonoperative Treatment

Nonoperative management comprises temporary reduction of all activities that aggravate the symptoms. A protocol of nonsteroidal anti-inflammatories and physical therapy may provide relief. A heel lift can produce symptomatic relief. For cases of posterior impingement, an injection with lidocaine and a steroid may be used for therapeutic purposes. Failure of nonoperative management may necessitate surgical intervention.

Surgical Treatment

Open Technique
Isolated Posterior Bony Impingement

- A posterior trigonal fragment may be accessed through a posterolateral approach to the ankle.
- With the patient prone, a 1.5- to 3-cm incision is made posterior to the peroneal tendons between the sural nerve and the peroneal tendon sheath interval.
- The ankle and subtalar joint are opened, and subperiosteal dissection is performed around the posterior aspect of the talus.
- The FHL tendon is identified and retracted medially.
- A rongeur or osteotome is used to remove the os trigonum fragment.
- The patient is immobilized with a splint or cast for 2 weeks.
- Subsequently, ROM exercises of the ankle and toes are initiated, followed by a gradual return to activities by 8 to 10 weeks.

Flexor Hallucis Longus Tendinosis

- A 5-cm posteromedial incision is made over the FDL and FHL tendons (Figs. 8.25 and 8.26).
- The FDL tendon is first identified.
- With manipulation of the hallux, the FHL tendon is palpated.
- After the tendon sheath of the FHL is identified, and the neurovascular bundle gently retracted posteriorly, the sheath is released from the posterior tubercle of the talus and extended distally until the patient is able to flex and extend the hallux without locking.
- The patient is immobilized in a splint for 1 week, and during this period, active and passive ROM exercises are initiated.
- The patient is advanced to full activities over 4 to 6 weeks.

Arthroscopic Technique

- The patient is positioned prone. A nonsterile tourniquet is placed on the upper thigh. A soft-tissue noninvasive distractor may be used as necessary.
- The anatomic landmarks for portal placement are the sole of the foot, the tip of the lateral malleolus, and the medial and lateral borders of the Achilles tendon. With the ankle at neutral, a line parallel to the sole of the foot is drawn from the tip of the lateral malleolus, directed posteriorly around the Achilles tendon (Fig. 8.27A).

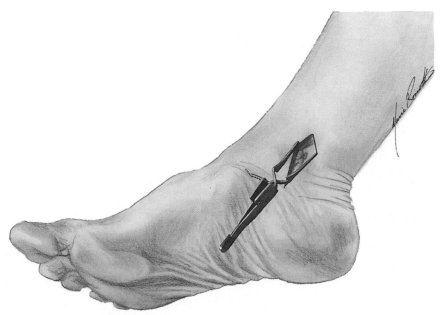

Figure 8.25 Surgical incision for flexor hallucis longus decompression.

- The posterolateral portal is located just proximal and 5 mm anterior to the intersection of the line drawn, and the lateral border of the Achilles tendon. The posteromedial portal is placed at the same level on the medial side of the Achilles (Fig. 8.27B).
- With the foot plantarflexed, a hemostat is placed in the posterolateral portal and directed anteriorly toward the first web space and toward the center of the posterior aspect of the talus. Blunt dissection is used until bone is palpated.
- The hemostat is exchanged for a 4.0-mm 30° arthroscope, which is directed in the same path as the hemostat. The scope should rest at the level of the posterior talar process superficial to the capsule.

- The hemostat is then placed in the posteromedial portal and directed perpendicular to the arthroscope. Once the arthroscope is palpated, the hemostat is tilted anteriorly, and allowed to slide anteriorly to the tip of the scope (Fig. 8.28).
- With the clamp, a small opening is created in the crural fascia, just lateral to the posterior talar process under direct visualization with the arthroscope.
- The hemostat is exchanged for a shaver, and the joint capsule and soft tissue are released.
- The flexor hallucis longus is an important landmark during the procedure, as the area lateral to the tendon is safe.
- If there is suspicion of FHL tendinosis, the flexor retinaculum can be released from the posterior talar

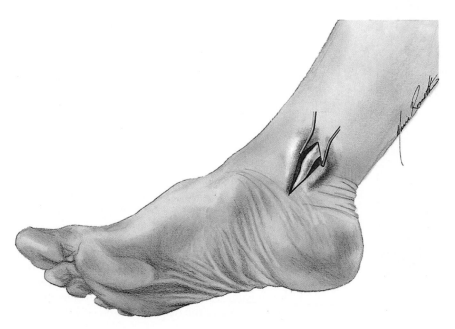

Figure 8.26 Artist's rendering of nodule within flexor hallucis longus.

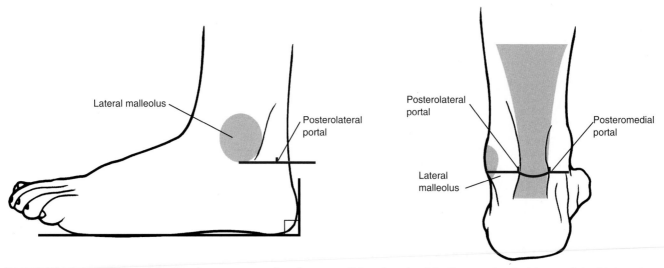

Figure 8.27 **A:** Lateral view of the foot demonstrating a line drawn parallel to the sole of the foot just distal to the tip of the fibula and directed posteriorly toward the Achilles tendon. **B:** Posterior view of the foot demonstrating the continuation of the line drawn across the Achilles tendon, ending just anterior to its medial border. The portal sites are located just proximal and 5 mm anterior to the intersection of the reference line and the Achilles tendon on either side.

process, and the tendon sheath may be opened taking care to stay on the lateral aspect of the tendon. From here, the tendon can be debrided as needed.

■ To remove a symptomatic os trigonum, the posterior talofibular ligament, the talocalcaneal ligament, and the flexor retinaculum must be released. After doing so, a small periosteal elevator can be used to detach the os trigonum, and it may be removed with a grasper.

■ A soft dressing is applied, and patients are allowed to bear weight after 4 days. Patients are instructed in ROM of the ankle to begin immediately after surgery. A gradual return to full activity is expected by 8 weeks.

PERONEAL TENDON DISORDERS

PATHOGENESIS

Etiology and Pathophysiology

The peroneus longus and peroneus brevis tendons are the primary evertors of the foot. Originating as muscle bellies in the lateral compartment of the leg, their tendons enter the hindfoot by traversing a fibroosseous tunnel posterior to the lateral malleolus. This tunnel is bordered anteriorly by the fibula and is confined posterolaterally by the superior peroneal retinaculum. Anatomic studies have shown that approximately 10% to 20% of individuals have a flat or convex-shaped fibular groove, which may predispose them to subluxation or dislocation events. The superior

peroneal retinaculum is the primary restraint to peroneal subluxation. It inserts into a fibrocartilaginous rim on the posterolateral fibula that serves to functionally deepen the retromalleolar groove. Laxity of the superior peroneal retinaculum has also been implicated in chronic peroneal tendon subluxation.

The peroneus longus tendon runs posterolateral to the peroneus brevis behind the fibula and follows an angular course before inserting on the plantar aspect of the first metatarsal base. The tendon turns sharply at the tip of the fibula, slants under the trochlear process on the lateral aspect of the calcaneus, and enters the plantar surface of the foot after turning over a groove in the cuboid. An os peroneum, or accessory ossicle adjacent to the plantar aspect of the cuboid, may be present in the tendon.

The peroneus brevis tendon, with its muscle belly projecting further distally than that of the longus, lies between the posterior fibula and the peroneus longus tendon in the fibroosseous tunnel before turning under the tip of the fibula to insert on the fifth metatarsal base. Because of its intimate relationship with the distal fibula, tears of the peroneus brevis are significantly more common than those of the peroneus longus and occur at the level of the distal tip of the fibula. An accessory muscle, the peroneus quartus, may accompany the other peroneal tendons in the tunnel.

The peroneal tendons receive their blood supply through contributions from the posterior peroneal artery and branches of the medial tarsal artery. Two avascular zones have been described, one located distal to the tip of the fibula affecting both the brevis and longus tendons, and one region affecting the longus tendon as it turns around the cuboid. These regions correspond with the most frequent locations of peroneal tendinopathy and are also the locations where stress risers can occur in the tendons as they traverse bony prominences and change direction.

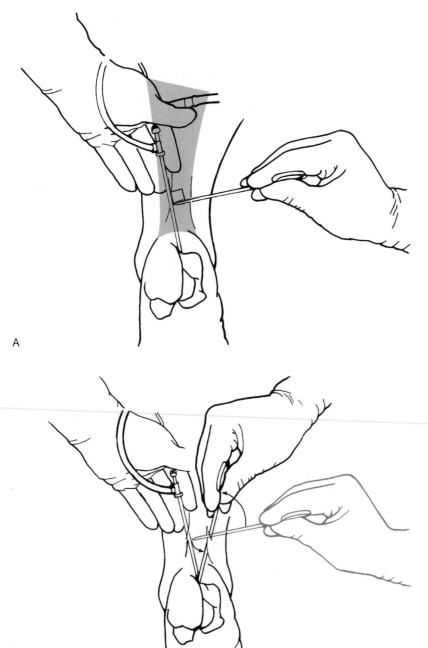

Figure 8.28 **A:** With the arthroscope held in place, a hemostat is introduced in the posteromedial portal directly perpendicular to its long axis. The hemostat is advanced until the arthroscope can be palpated. **B:** Once the arthroscope is palpated, rotate the hemostat so it is directed anteriorly down to bone. This maneuver should be repeated every time a new instrument is introduced into the posteromedial portal.

Acute peroneal dislocations are commonly associated with trauma during athletics such as skiing. The mechanism is controversial, with extreme dorsiflexion or eversion postulated as positions of the ankle at the time of injury. An eccentric contraction of the peroneal muscles coupled with external forces cause the tendons to avulse the superficial peroneal retinaculum from the fibula. The avulsed retinaculum may be accompanied by periosteum or cortical bone from the lateral aspect of the fibula, creating a "pseudopouch" in which the dislocated tendons reside.

Chronic peroneal subluxation may not be associated with a discrete traumatic event. The peroneal tendons subluxate laterally from behind the distal fibula to a variable degree, attenuating the superficial peroneal retinaculum and causing a peritendinitis. A longitudinal split of the peroneus brevis occurs by the tendon rubbing against the fibrocartilaginous rim. Seldom is a complete rupture found in long-standing cases. Individuals with flat or convex retromalleolar grooves may be predisposed to chronic subluxation of these tendons.

Peritendinitis of the peroneals may be a result of stenosis of the synovial sheath. This stenosing tenosynovitis usually occurs at a spot where the tendons change their course. The most common locations are posterior and at the tip of the lateral malleolus, at the trochlear process, and at the undersurface of the cuboid. The presence of a low-lying peroneus brevis muscle belly or peroneus quartus may decrease the available volume in the fibroosseous tunnel, resulting in inflammation of the synovial sheath. Peritendinitis may also occur following acute trauma. Up to 77% of patients with chronic lateral ankle instability have peroneal tendinitis and tenosynovitis.

Fibula fractures and calcaneal malunions may cause painful os peroneum syndrome (POPS), a disorder stemming from the accessory ossicle of the peroneus longus tendon. The POPS may have an acute or chronic etiology, and involves fracture of the ossicle or diastasis of a multipartite os peroneum, or attrition or rupture of the peroneus longus tendon adjacent to the ossicle.

Classification

Classification systems for acute peroneal dislocations, peroneus brevis tears, and POPS are listed in Tables 8.2 to 8.4, respectively.

DIAGNOSIS

Physical Examination and History

Clinical Features

Acute and chronic peroneal tendon instabilities differ in their clinical presentation.
- Acute dislocations usually occur during an athletic event such as snow skiing or playing football and are accompanied by a palpable or audible snap.
  - Activities may be limited by pain in the lateral aspect of the ankle.
  - Physical examination reveals a swollen, tender, and sometimes ecchymotic area in the retrofibular region.
  - The tendons may reduce spontaneously.

TABLE 8.2 CLASSIFICATION OF ACUTE PERONEAL DISLOCATIONS

Grade	Description
I	Retinaculum and periosteum are stripped away; pseudopouch contains the dislocated tendons
II	Fibrocartilaginous rim is avulsed with retinaculum and periosteum
III	Posterolateral cortex of the fibula is avulsed with the fibrocartilaginous rim and retinaculum

TABLE 8.3 CLASSIFICATION OF PERONEUS BREVIS TEARS

Grade	Description
1	Flattened tendon
2	Partial thickness tear <1 cm
3	Full thickness tear <2 cm
4	Full thickness tear >2 cm

TABLE 8.4 CLASSIFICATION OF PAINFUL OS PERONEUM SYNDROME

Type	Description
I	Acute os peroneum fracture or diastasis of a multipartite os peroneum
II	Healing of a type I with callus formation
III	Attrition or partial rupture of the peroneus longus tendon proximal or distal to the os peroneum
IV	Frank rupture of the peroneus longus
V	Large trochlear process on the calcaneus impinging on the ossicle or peroneus longus

  - This condition is often misdiagnosed as a routine ankle sprain.
  - Resisted active eversion of the affected foot with a dorsiflexed ankle is a provocative test for peroneal dislocation as well as being a mechanism of injury.
- Chronic subluxation of the peroneal tendon may not be associated with a discrete traumatic event.
  - Patients usually present with a painful snapping behind the lateral malleolus.
  - They may also complain of "giving way" of the ankle.
  - Peroneal subluxation may coexist with lateral ankle ligament instability.
  - Light pressure exerted on the tendons with the fingertips during provocative testing may reproduce pain and allow the examiner to assess the degree of subluxation.
- Peritendinitis presents with pain over the tendons that is usually reproduced with foot eversion.
  - The patient may give a history of prior bony trauma such as a calcaneus fracture.
  - It is most common that a peritendinitis coexists with tendinosis and tendon tears.
- Acute POPS is characterized by sudden onset of pain in the plantar-lateral aspect of the foot.
  - Tenderness is present along the course of the peroneus longus tendon at the cuboid tunnel.
  - Pain is reproduced with resisted eversion, resisted plantarflexion of the first ray, and when passively inverting the foot.
  - Sural nerve dysesthesia may occur secondary to the proximity of branches of the nerve in proximity to the tendons.
- Chronic POPS has a similar presentation, but is bothersome over a period of weeks or months. It may mimic a recurrent ankle sprain.

Radiologic Features
- Acute peroneal dislocation can be detected on plain radiographs by the presence of the "wafer sign," an avulsion of the posterolateral fibular cortex that is pathognomonic for this injury. This is best seen on the mortise view of the ankle, but it is present in less than 50% of cases.
- Radiographs do not significantly contribute to the diagnosis of chronic peroneal subluxation. They may be helpful in detecting bony malunion in a case of peritendinitis.

- POPS may be evident on radiographs as a fracture of the os peroneum, with or without callus.
  - ☐ A multipartite ossicle may show a diastasis between its parts.
  - ☐ An os peroneum that has migrated proximally is indicative of peroneal tendon rupture distal to the ossicle.
- Finally, an axial Harris heel view may detect the presence of an enlarged calcaneal trochlear process.
- Ultrasonography is gaining popularity, as it is less expensive than MRI and does not expose patients to ionizing radiation. Abnormalities such as peritendinous fluid, tendon thickening, and tendon tears can be identified with US evaluation. Real-time imaging may be used to confirm episodic subluxation of the peroneal tendons, with a reported positive predictive value of 100%. In addition, experienced ultrasonographers can identify peroneal tears with a high degree of sensitivity and specificity.
- MRI is the standard method for evaluating for peroneal tendon tears. However, it is usually not necessary for the diagnosis of acute peroneal dislocation. Occasionally, it may be used to confirm a dislocation with spontaneous reduction or in a patient whose ankle is too swollen or painful to perform an adequate examination.
  - ☐ Fluid in the tendon sheath is indicative of peroneal tendon injury (Fig. 8.29).
  - ☐ MRI has been shown to diagnose peroneus brevis tears with a sensitivity of 83% and a specificity of 75% to 80%. Peroneus longus tears are detected with a specificity of 100%, and tears of both tendons are detected with a specificity of 60%. Despite this, there is debate as to whether MRI overestimates or underestimates peroneal tendon pathology. Therefore, a careful history and physical examination are of paramount importance.
  - ☐ The cross-sectional fibular morphology may be examined for a flat or convex retromalleolar groove that may predispose a patient to subluxation. In addition, injuries to the superior peroneal retinaculum may be visualized.

Diagnostic Workup

The diagnostic workup of peroneal tendon disorders is considered in Algorithm 8.4.

TREATMENT

Surgical Indications and Contraindications

The treatment of acute peroneal tendon dislocations is controversial. Non–weight-bearing cast immobilization with the ankle positioned in slight plantarflexion and inversion for 6 weeks has been shown to be effective in more than 50% of cases. Proponents of this approach cite the avoidance of an unnecessary surgical procedure. Surgical treatment has also been advocated in the acute setting and may prevent recurrence in more than 95% of cases. It is particularly appropriate in the presence of a shallow fibular groove. Surgery for an acute injury is simpler than in the chronic setting. Contraindications to surgery include compromise of the soft-tissue envelope as well as the presence of severe systemic disease or peripheral vascular disease.

Chronic peroneal subluxation or dislocation should be treated surgically if symptomatic. Contraindications remain the same as in an acute injury.

Technique

Peritendinitis

- Peritendinitis of the peroneal tendons should initially be managed nonsurgically.
- Nonsteroidal anti-inflammatory drugs and immobilization followed by shoe modifications such as a lateral heel wedge may be effective at relieving pain.
- In recalcitrant cases, debridement of inflamed tenosynovium may be considered.

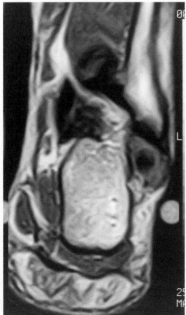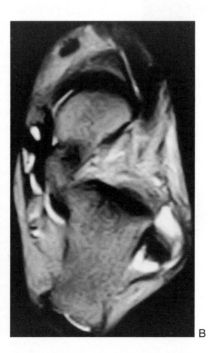

Figure 8.29 **A:** T1-weighted MRI scan of ankle, axial view, revealing significant fluid around the peroneal tendon tear. **B:** T2-weighted MRI scan of ankle, axial view, showing "tiger eye" with fluid around peroneal tendon.

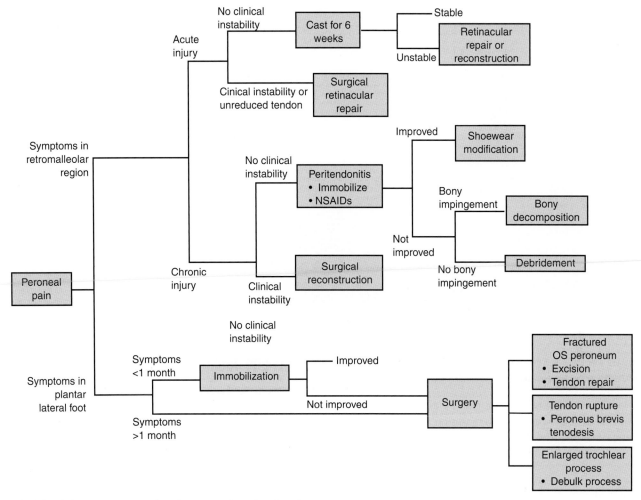

Algorithm 8.4 Diagnostic workup for peroneal tendon disorder.

■ Cases that are associated with impingement from a malunion should be treated by decompressing the tendons with resection of the offending bone.

Peroneal Subluxation/Dislocation

■ The approach for acute or chronic peroneal subluxation begins with a curved incision located posterior to the fibula.

■ The incision should follow the course of the tendons as they curve anteriorly under the tip of the lateral malleolus (Figs. 8.30 and 8.31). Care should be taken to avoid branches of the sural nerve.

■ Full-thickness flaps should be used to expose the superior peroneal retinaculum.

■ In an acute dislocation, the attenuated retinaculum is reattached to the fibula or incised and plicated after reducing the tendons into the retromalleolar groove.

□ If a cortical avulsion fracture is present, it is reduced and internally fixed back to the fibula, effectively reestablishing the length and function of the retinaculum.

■ Chronic peroneal subluxation may be treated with a number of procedures used singly or in combination.

□ Anatomic repair or plication of the retinaculum

□ Excision of a congenital anomaly (i.e., peroneus quartus, low-lying muscle belly), if present

□ Deepening the retromalleolar groove of the fibula to better accommodate the tendons

□ Osteotomy of the fibula to block displacement of the tendons

□ Reconstruction of the retinaculum using soft-tissue augmentation (i.e., a slip of Achilles tendon, periosteal flap, calcaneofibular ligament)

■ These procedures should be tailored to the anatomic variations and pathologic condition of the patient.

■ The peroneal tendons should be carefully inspected for longitudinal tears, and, if found, these should be debrided and repaired.

■ In cases of chronic dislocation with a shallow fibular groove, a groove deepening and retinacular repair is necessary.

■ The flattened peroneus brevis tendon should then be tubularized.

■ Primary repair and tubularization are indicated for tears involving less than 50% of the tendon; otherwise tenodesis should be considered.

■ The wound should be closed in layers and a splint applied with the ankle in slight plantarflexion.

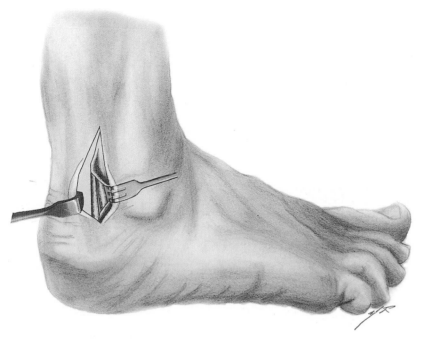

Figure 8.30   Peroneal tendon exposure.

Painful Os Peroneum Syndrome

- Acute POPS should be treated with immobilization.
- In a chronic case, when symptoms have been present for more than 1 month, surgical treatment is considered. Surgical treatment consists of excision of the os peroneum and repair of the peroneus longus tendon. Most often, repair is not possible and tenodesis to the peroneus brevis is indicated.
- If a hypertrophic peroneal tubercle exists, it should be debulked.

Postoperative Management

The patient should return for follow-up in 14 days for suture removal and application of a short leg cast. Patients should practice toe-touch weight bearing for 4 weeks, after which they may begin weight bearing in a CAM walker boot and active ROM exercises. Peroneal strengthening should begin at 8 weeks, and the patient may return to normal daily activities in 3 months. Athletics can begin at 4 to 6 months.

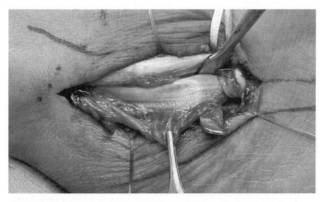

Figure 8.31   Intraoperative photo demonstrating low-lying muscle belly of peroneal brevis.

Results and Outcome

Surgical outcomes with peroneal tendon stabilization are generally favorable. Complications, which occur overall in less than 5% of cases, include recurrence, sural nerve neuroma, infection, and persistent swelling or pain. Hardware complications and graft resorption may occur with bone block procedures and osteotomies.

POSTERIOR TIBIAL TENDON DYSFUNCTION

Posterior tibial tendon dysfunction (PTTD), although identified by pathology in the posterior tibial tendon, is associated with various deformities in the foot and ankle. The pathology not only is confined to the posterior tibial tendon, but also involves the arch of the foot. Failure of the ligaments supporting the arch, which occurs before, during, or after the dysfunction of the tendon, produces the foot deformities. The deformity itself, particularly in its later stages, becomes painful and most debilitating for the patient.

PATHOGENESIS

Etiology and Epidemiology

No one specific factor has been identified as the cause of PTTD, also known as posterior tibial tendon insufficiency, or the adult acquired flatfoot. PTTD is not necessarily associated with a particular injury, but is usually a gradual degenerative process. A zone of hypovascularity in the posterior tibial tendon exists between the medial malleolus and

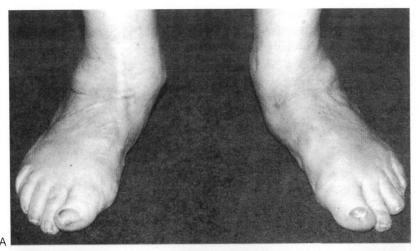

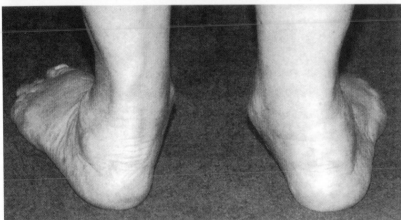

Figure 8.32 Views of a patient from the front (**A**) and behind (**B**). Forefoot abduction, heel valgus, and "too many toes sign" are seen. (Reproduced with permission from Lin SS, Lee TH, Chao W, et al. Nonoperative treatment of patients with posterior tibial tendinitis. Foot Ankle Clin 1996;1:261–277.)

the navicular tuberosity. Commonly, the condition occurs in patients who start out with a flatfoot, which would theoretically excessively stress the tendon and ligaments, and the tendon pathology and deformity progress from that starting point. The condition occurs more commonly in women. The average age of presentation is 50 to 60 years (Fig. 8.32).

The posterior tibial muscle and tendon are the second strongest of the lower limb and work with a short excursion. Therefore, when the tendon becomes degenerated and stretches, significant loss of function of this critical inverter (which locks the hindfoot during heel rise) occurs. Without good inverter function, the strain is more on the medial ligaments, including the adjacent spring ligament complex. The spring or calcaneonavicular ligament complex comprises primarily a medial portion directly adjacent to the posterior tibial tendon and a plantar portion at the plantar aspect of the talonavicular joint. Failure of the ligament with cyclic loading promotes a progressive flatfoot deformity. Conversely, when the spring ligament complex becomes injured or attenuated after repetitive stress, flatfoot deformity results placing a greater strain on the posterior tibial tendon.

Whichever comes first, when the deformity occurs, the heel goes into valgus and the Achilles becomes a less effective inverter. With enough heel valgus, the Achilles becomes a strong everter. This makes the most powerful muscle complex in the lower extremity a deforming force.

As the heel goes into valgus, the gastrocnemius–soleus complex frequently becomes contracted. Its tightness must be assessed because, if it is significantly contracted, it should be lengthened as part of the surgical correction. Ligament strain and failure can occur anywhere along the arch, including at the first tarsometatarsal joint and the naviculocuneiform joint.

Classification

PTTD is classified in four stages, as shown in Table 8.5.

DIAGNOSIS

Physical Examination and History

Clinical Features

- The diagnosis of PTTD can most often be made by physical examination.
- In stage I, and in most patients in stage II, patients present with a history of pain in the posteromedial hindfoot over the region of the posterior tibial tendon just distal and inferior to the medial malleolus.
- On physical examination, there is tenderness over the tendon.

TABLE 8.5 CLASSIFICATION OF POSTERIOR TIBIAL TENDON DYSFUNCTION

Stage	Description
I	Degeneration or tear of the tendon but no deformity. Patient often has preexisting flatfoot deformity
II	Tendon degeneration with a flexible deformity
A (early)	Heel valgus with mild-to-moderate flattening of the arch; >35% talonavicular uncoverage
B (late)	Considerable collapse of the arch most often involving abduction at the midfoot through the talonavicular joint; >35% talonavicular uncoverage
III	Fixed deformity of the triple joint complex, not passively correctible
IV	Above with valgus tilt of the talus within the ankle mortise; occurs from progressive failure of the deltoid ligament

- Patients have pain and/or difficulty with a single heel rise test.
- The single heel rise test is the most sensitive physical examination finding for diagnosing PTTD. When viewed from behind, one should note inversion during the single heel rise.
- Patients with PTTD may complain of pain or weakness, or they may be able to heel rise but most often with less inversion than normal or compared to the contralateral side.
- With progression of the disease and failure of the tendon, the medial pain and tenderness paradoxically usually resolves.
- The patient may have a period of relatively few symptoms, other than perhaps noticing weakness or that the arch does not feel as strong.
- As the deformity progresses, pain and tenderness develop laterally at the tip of the fibula and lateral subtalar joint where bony impingement occurs from the progressive deformity.
- These patients in late stage II or III have a more severe flatfoot deformity with considerable pronation of the arch. MRI can show tendinosis, a longitudinal split in the tendon, and, more rarely, complete rupture. An MRI scan is not necessary for diagnosis.
- As part of an evaluation of all patients with PTTD, tightness of the gastrocnemius–soleus complex must be assessed.
  - With the patient seated, the hindfoot is positioned in neutral position with the navicular reduced on the head of the talus and passive dorsiflexion assessed with the knee straight (assesses gastrocnemius and soleus tightness) and with the knee flexed (assesses soleus tightness).
  - Most patients with a contracture have isolated gastrocnemius tightness.
  - With gastrocnemius and soleus contracture, a percutaneous tendo-Achilles lengthening can be performed (benefit: quick, good cosmesis; downside: weakens gastrocnemius and soleus, and potential for overlengthening).
  - With an isolated gastrocnemius contracture, a gastrocnemius recession is the usual procedure.

TREATMENT

Stage I

Surgical Indications and Contraindications

Surgical indications for patients with stage I disease include tenosynovitis or a partial tear in the tendon with pain of more than 3 to 6 months' duration despite conservative treatment. The much more unusual complete tear is strongly considered for immediate surgical treatment. Conservative treatment consists of supporting the foot, most commonly in a removable boot with an orthotic (Fig. 8.33). These boots are generally used for 6 weeks but can be used longer to relieve discomfort. Patients are warned that they should monitor themselves and return for follow-up to make sure that a progressive deformity does not develop, even if the tenderness and pain in the tendon resolve. The consequences of allowing the deformity to progress must be explained to the patient, including the potential need for a larger surgery with a less functional end-result.

Patients who continue to have pain or progressive deformities are considered for operative treatment. These patients usually have continued tenderness over the tendon but often some inversion strength remains because there is most commonly a partial tear and elongation of the tendon. Surgery comprises FDL tendon transfer to either augment or replace the torn posterior tibial tendon. If the tendon has 50% or less degeneration in cross section, one option is to leave the tendon in continuity and the degenerative portion excised. If a tendon transfer is necessary, the FDL is transferred to the medial aspect of the navicular. It can be combined with a medial displacement calcaneal osteotomy to take the strain off the tendon transfer and prevent progressive deformity in the patient with significant hindfoot valgus deformity. The osteotomy helps statically by improving the alignment of the arch and dynamically by providing better inversion from the Achilles tendon by medializing its origin. Care must be taken to realign the heel directly under the long axis of the tibia and not overcorrect into varus.

When assessing patients with stage I disease, an MRI scan can be helpful to determine the degree of degeneration

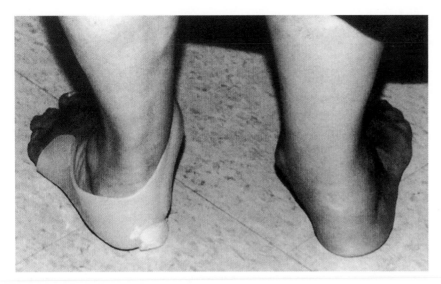

Figure 8.33 University of California Biomechanical Laboratory orthosis insert with medial posting for left stage II PTTD corrects the hindfoot valgus angulation to neutral alignment. In comparison, the right foot demonstrates rigid hindfoot valgus and forefoot abduction deformity. (Reproduced with permission from Lin SS, Lee TH, Chao W, et al. Nonoperative treatment of patients with posterior tibial tendinitis. Foot Ankle Clin 1996;1:261–277.)

of the tendon or identify unusual patients with tenosynovitis but no tear or degeneration of the tendon (Fig. 8.34). If there is just tenosynovitis, further conservative care is warranted, and if necessary, a tenosynovectomy can be performed later. Tenosynovectomy of the posterior tibial tendon is a rare operation because patients who fail conservative treatment almost invariably have degeneration or partial tear of the tendon.

Surgical Technique (Fig. 8.35)
◾ A medial incision is made directly over the posterior tibial tendon from the medial malleolus to the navicular.
◾ The tendon is exposed and carefully inspected on both its medial and lateral sides.

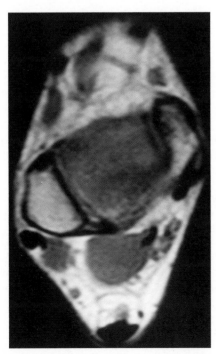

Figure 8.34 T1-weighted MRI scan of ankle, axial view, demonstrating posterior tibial tendon tear with fluid within the sheath.

◾ The tear or degeneration usually extends to the level of the medial malleolus. The incision should be made above the level of the medial malleolus and the tendon inspected proximally, most often leaving a 1- to 2-cm portion of the flexor retinaculum intact. The tendon is repaired if 50% or more of the cross-sectional area of the tendon is not degenerated.
◾ For the flexor transfer, the FDL is identified just inferior to the posterior tibialis tendon at the medial aspect of the talonavicular joint and is followed distally.
◾ Often, interconnections between the FOL and FHL tendon distally can be left intact, or, if necessary, the two tendons are tenodesed together distally and the tendon harvested at the level of the tarsometatarsal joint.
◾ The transfer is passed through a drill hole in the navicular from plantar to dorsal and fixed in the tunnel if the surgeon chooses to harvest the tendon proximal to the master knot of Henry. Alternatively, if the tendon is harvested more distally, it is tied to the dorsal soft-tissues.
◾ Careful tensioning of the transfer is performed with the foot halfway between the neutral and the inverted positions, allowing the foot to be brought back to neutral without excessive tension on the transfer.
◾ The medial slide calcaneal osteotomy is performed prior to tying down the tendon transfer through an oblique incision just posterior to the sural nerve over the posterior calcaneus.
◾ Care is taken not to extend this incision proximal to the level of the superior calcaneus but to use retraction so that branches of the sural nerve are not be sacrificed.
◾ Subperiosteal dissection is done and pins are placed to mark the level of the osteotomy. The pins can then be checked under fluoroscopy to assess the level of the osteotomy.
◾ The osteotomy is made with about 45° obliquity to the lateral border of the foot.
◾ Once the osteotomy is carefully completed on the medial aspect, a laminar spreader is used to distract the osteotomy site and to stretch the medial soft tissues to allow for easier slide of the osteotomy.

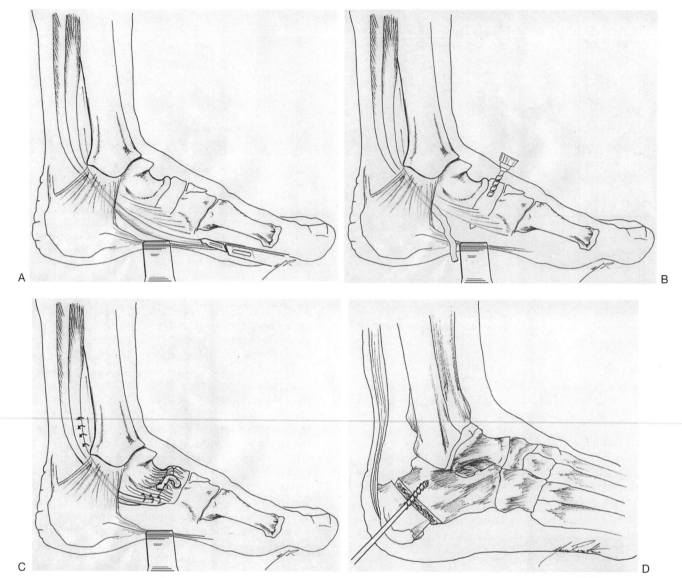

Figure 8.35   Posterior tibial tendon reconstruction with medial calcaneal slide. **A:** Knife releasing the FDL. **B:** Drilling into the navicular for FDL transfer. **C:** Transferring FDL into the navicular. **D:** Medial calcaneal slide with placement of internal fixation.

- The amount of slide is determined by the alignment of the foot. The goal is to place the calcaneus under the center of the ankle joint so that the calcaneus is in straight alignment underneath the tibia and out of excessive valgus, but in general, it is translated 8 to 12 mm.
- It is temporarily fixed with a K-wire or guide wire and assessed from anterior and posterior by lifting the leg up with the foot in neutral position and checking the alignment from a posterior view of the heel versus the lower leg and ankle.
- The osteotomy is then fixed with one or two cannulated screws or other devices, checking the lateral view and anteroposterior view of the foot to make certain that the screw is within the calcaneus anteriorly. Large cannulated cancellous screws can be used for fixation, but prominence of screw heads can be a problem.

- The lateral prominence and edge of the osteotomy is beveled because it will be prominent and uncomfortable after swelling subsides.

Postoperative Management

The patients are managed in a non–weight-bearing cast or boot for 4 to 6 weeks. By 6 weeks, they can progress to full weight bearing and, by 10 to 12 weeks, can progress to a shoe with an orthotic support. In the first 4 months, only gentle inversion strengthening is done, but after the tendon is fully healed, more aggressive strengthening can be done.

Results and Outcome

Patients with stage I disease can expect good relief of medial pain and, if good alignment of the foot is present, are not likely to develop progressive deformity. Some can return to sports that involve some running and develop good inversion power, especially if they participate in physical therapy after the tendon is adequately healed, 4 to 5 months after the surgery. Some cannot return to highly competitive sports that involve running and jumping because they do not consistently regain full strength. The tendon transfer can help balance the inversion pull against the peroneus brevis, although overall inversion strength is not as strong as the normal foot.

Complications

Possible complications include undercorrection or overcorrection of the osteotomy, which can be avoided by careful intraoperative assessment. Also avoidable is overtensioning or undertensioning the FDL transfer to the navicular. At the end of the operative procedure, it should be possible to bring the foot to neutral position and have good alignment. Bone graft from the calcaneal osteotomy may be placed within the tunnel in the navicular bone to encourage early healing of the tendon transfer.

Stage II

Surgical Indications and Contraindications

Patients with stage II disease (progressive flexible deformity with insufficiency of the posterior tibial tendon) are strongly considered for surgical treatment. Long-term bracing can be effective long-term therapy, but patients with significant deformity may still progress. The rate of progression of the deformity is variable and close follow-up is indicated. Surgical procedures for more progressive deformity become more complicated and often less satisfactory. Patients with medical contraindications to surgery or who do not wish to have surgery can be treated conservatively. An AFO is one option, although a hinged custom ankle brace with a longitudinal arch support (i.e., short-articulated AFO) is often better tolerated. A reinforced leather tie-up (i.e., Arizona) brace from above the level of the ankle to the midfoot limits motion, but is better tolerated by some patients. With these braces, patients should be instructed that progressive deformity can still develop, and therefore they should be monitored.

Surgical management of early stage II patients, with less than 30° to 40° of talonavicular uncoverage on a standing AP view of the foot, is controversial. A calcaneal osteotomy and tendon transfer can be sufficient if the patient has moderate pronation in the arch, mild or moderate heel valgus, and minimal lateral subluxation of the navicular on the talar head. Patients should be examined, however, for elevation of the first ray and Achilles contracture. If there is considerable instability of the first tarsometatarsal joint, a first tarsometatarsal fusion is considered. With less instability, an opening wedge osteotomy of the medial cuneiform (Cotton osteotomy) is performed.

For stage II patients with considerable abduction and talonavicular joint sag resulting in severe flattening of the arch and abduction on the standing AP view of the foot, treatment is more controversial. Many surgeons perform some type of lateral column lengthening of the calcaneus, whereas others may accept less correction or proceed to fusions involving the talonavicular or subtalar joint. The overall surgical goal is to correct the alignment of the foot while maintaining maximum function. Care is taken to adequately correct the deformity. Lateral column lengthening can either be performed just proximal to or through the calcaneocuboid joint. The lengthening performed through the calcaneus proximal to the calcaneocuboid joint (Evans procedure) heals more easily and has less incidence of nonunion. Moreover, patients who undergo an Evans procedure have less incidence of lateral column stiffness, and lateral plantar pain. It is important to maintain normal passive eversion in these patients. The concern for development of arthritis in the calcaneocuboid joint has led some surgeons to perform the distraction arthrodesis through the joint. However, in studies to date, few patients have required conversion to a fusion after an Evans procedure.

Surgical Technique

- The Evans procedure is performed through a longitudinal incision just above the peroneal tendons on the anterior calcaneus.
- Care is taken to retract the sural nerve plantarly and subperiosteally expose the anterior calcaneus and retract the peroneal tendons laterally and inferiorly.
- The osteotomy is made 1.5 cm proximal to the level of the joint and can be marked with a K-wire first and checked with fluoroscopy. It is made perpendicular to the plantar aspect of the foot. A good alternative may be a step-cut osteotomy.
- Care is taken to fatigue the medial side of the osteotomy. Pins are placed in the proximal and distal fragments, and a laminar spreader or Hintermann retractor is used to wedge open the osteotomy the desired amount.
- Overcorrection or undercorrection, as seen on an intraoperative anteroposterior view of the foot, should be avoided. In addition, stiffness of the lateral column must be assessed intraoperatively as the osteotomy is increasingly distracted. Using a graft that is too large may stiffen the lateral column and cause more lateral symptoms postoperatively.
- The size of the graft can vary between 5 and 10 mm, with grafts more commonly in the 6- to 8-mm range.
- Some surgeons perform the lateral column lengthening with a medial displacement osteotomy for more severe deformity.
  - □ If both osteotomies are used, it is especially important to avoid overcorrection.
  - □ The lateral column lengthening should be fixed first, and then the medial slide calcaneal osteotomy shifted as much as necessary to bring the calcaneus underneath the center of the ankle joint.
- A calcaneocuboid distraction fusion is performed by creating flat surfaces at the calcaneocuboid joint, inserting a well-fitting tricortical autograft or allograft and securing with internal fixation such as an H-plate under compression to avoid a nonunion.
- The risk of nonunion for lateral column lengthening has been shown in some studies to be greater with use of

allograft; therefore, we prefer the use of tricortical iliac crest autograft.

■ For cases of truly severe flexible deformity, additional procedures may be necessary. Release of the lateral talonavicular capsule will allow for better correction through the lateral column lengthening procedure. In addition, in cases of severe spring ligament attenuation, reconstruction with allograft in addition to lateral column lengthening can be used to correct alignment. Patients must have good triple joint motion to be candidates for this procedure. Finally, in cases of severe hindfoot valgus with a valgus tilt in the ankle mortise, deltoid reconstruction may be necessary to address deltoid insufficiency.

■ Other fusions are described in the section for treatment of stage III disease.

Postoperative Management

With the lateral column lengthening, performed as either an Evans procedure or fusion of the calcaneocuboid joint, the patient is non–weight bearing for 8 weeks. This time may be less in patient who undergo a step-cut calcaneal osteotomy.

After a calcaneal lengthening procedure, at 6 weeks the patient may come out of the cast and use a removable boot. With a calcaneocuboid distraction arthrodesis, the patient is left in the cast for longer with weight bearing started at 8 weeks. After cast removal, triple joint motion with inversion and gentle eversion are started, as is regaining power of the toes.

Results and Outcome

After surgery, patients with early stage II disease usually maintain good motion of the triple joint complex. Although they may not have full inversion strength, active inversion is present. Patients may notice slight stiffness and weakness in the foot and some discomfort medially or laterally, but these complaints are generally minor. Patients with late stage II disease tend to gain less motion and inversion strength, but it is usually acceptable as long as appropriate correction occurs and good inversion and eversion motions are maintained. Following a lateral column lengthening or fusion, patients can have some degree of lateral discomfort or stiffness that interferes with recreational sports that involve running. This can be minimized with careful selection of the size of the graft. Most can walk comfortably for exercise and have overall good function of the foot. The goal for them is to have minimal stiffness but adequate correction of alignment.

In addition to the complications mentioned for stage I disease, stage II disease has a greater incidence of undercorrection or overcorrection. Although nonunion is rare with the other procedures, it is more frequent with lengthening arthrodesis of the calcaneocuboid joint and can occur with an Evans type of lateral column lengthening. A calcaneocuboid fusion nonunion may be treated with further casting; however, graft collapse and loss of correction can occur. Although in general calcaneocuboid fusion does not restrict as much motion as a subtalar or talonavicular fusion, the loss of motion is greater than with an Evans calcaneal lengthening procedure.

Stage III

Surgical Indications and Contraindications

Patients with considerable deformity but not too much pain can be treated conservatively with a lace-up ankle brace. Many patients use an orthotic without such a brace, although this provides less support. Aside from medical contraindications, another contraindication to surgery is unrealistic expectations for the surgery. Patients who require fusion of the talonavicular or subtalar joint should not expect to return to a running sport and may have trouble walking for exercise. Uneven ground or prolonged walking can be uncomfortable after fusion of the talonavicular or triple joint complex. Fusions of these joints should be considered a salvage procedure to preserve the patient's ability to walk.

Surgical Technique

Patients with a true fixed deformity so that good inversion cannot be obtained even under anesthesia necessitate a capsular release and hindfoot fusion for deformity correction. The number of joints fused in the hindfoot depends on what is needed to correct alignment. The key joint to correcting alignment is the talonavicular joint because this joint determines in large part the position of the triple joint complex.

■ To perform a talonavicular fusion, an anterior medial incision is made over the talonavicular joint, and the joint is debrided with the curved nature of the joint surfaces preserved.

■ Even though an isolated talonavicular fusion could be performed, for additional stabilization without additional loss of motion, most often the calcaneocuboid joint is included. For this joint, a lateral incision is made longitudinally above the peroneal tendons, and the joint is debrided without shortening the lateral column significantly.

■ A lateral column lengthening through the calcaneocuboid joint usually does not need to be performed because positioning and shortening of the medial side can gain adequate alignment of these joints.

■ If the subtalar joint is not arthritic and is in good position after correction of the other two joints, it does not necessarily need to be fused. Adding the subtalar joint is often necessary in the most severe deformities.

■ Fusing the foot in a plantigrade position is critical.
  □ This means that, with the foot in neutral, the first ray is not elevated and the hindfoot is in a neutral position, directly beneath the tibia and ankle joint.
  □ The navicular should be well centered on the talar head without overcorrection into varus or undercorrection.

■ On occasion, with severe deformity the calcaneus can remain in valgus even after appropriate fusion of the subtalar as well as talonavicular and calcaneocuboid joints.

■ Further correction of the heel can be obtained during the same operative procedure by adding a medial slide calcaneal osteotomy as described earlier.

■ With this procedure, the triple arthrodesis is performed first and the amount of correction is assessed. If it is determined that the slide is necessary, it is performed last.

- Final fixation of the talonavicular joint is performed first by the authors. The subtalar joint is fixed second where it is important to make sure that it has been rotated back underneath the talus, and the calcaneal osteotomy is fixed last to properly align the calcaneus under the ankle.
- Fixation of the osteotomy and subtalar joint can be simultaneously gained with the posterior screws.
- Correction of excessive valgus is important to avoid stress on the deltoid that could fail postoperatively.
- Fixation of the fusion construct is often performed with compression screws or compression staples.
- Fixation of each joint is important, but nonunion is most common in the talonavicular joint.
- Particular care should be taken to ensure good debridement of these curved surfaces while achieving good compression and fixation of this joint.
- For the subtalar joint, one screw can be sufficient fixation when the talonavicular joint is also being fused. The talonavicular joint is often fixed with two screws or one screw and a compression staple. It is very important to compress across the talonavicular joint. For the calcaneocuboid joint, one or two screws, or two staples can be sufficient. Plates utilizing locking screws that also provide compression are a viable alternative.
- The goals of anatomic, plantigrade position and good apposition of the joints in compression should be achieved.

Postoperative Management
These patients are kept non–weight bearing for 6 to 8 weeks. If X-rays show good apposition and early evidence of fusion, then weight bearing is gradually progressed during the next 4 to 6 weeks and the cast removed at 12 weeks. With earlier healing, a removable boot may be used instead of a cast. The boot is often used for 1 month after the cast is removed while the patient transitions to regular shoewear.

Results and Outcome
Triple arthrodesis can give patients considerable pain relief and significant improvement in walking ability. Some patients can be quite active but may have limitations in walking for exercise, and it would be unusual to be able to perform sports that involve running.

Complications
Complications of hindfoot fusions include nonunion and malunion. Proper operative technique can minimize these complications. In particular, position of the foot should be carefully assessed by visually checking the alignment of the heel and forefoot and checking joint position with intraoperative fluoroscopy or X-ray. In situ fusions with significant residual deformity should not be accepted. Although the patient may have good preoperative alignment of the talus in the ankle mortise, on occasion, valgus alignment of the talus can develop in the ankle mortise from an attenuated deltoid ligament, particularly if deformity is not adequately corrected in the foot. Particular care is taken to make sure the first ray is not elevated at the end of the procedure and the heel valgus is well corrected.

Stage IV

Surgical Indications and Contraindications
Surgical options of stage IV disease are limited. A small series of stage IV patients treated operatively has shown correction of the talar tilt within the ankle mortise. If possible, these patients are treated with an ankle brace or AFO. Performing a triple arthrodesis in patients with significant valgus tilt in the ankle mortise has a significant risk of progressive deformity at the level of the ankle. With progressive deformity, arthritis most often occurs. The most reliable method to treat the arthritis and correct the alignment in the ankle is to perform an ankle fusion, thereby giving the patient a pantalar fusion with the considerable activity limitations after that procedure. This procedure should be done only for patients who are unable to do even minimal activities preoperatively. In the patient who has a flexible deformity but considerable valgus tilt in the ankle joint, consideration can be given to correcting the flexible deformity without a triple arthrodesis. However, progressive deformity within the ankle mortise can still occur. Techniques to reconstruct the deltoid have been tried, and there is evidence, with short-term follow-up from the senior author (J.T.D.), that such a technique may be successful as long as the foot deformity is corrected as well.

For patients who are unable to walk and cannot be treated with a brace to allow walking, surgery can be considered. Pantalar fusion is a demanding procedure in which proper positioning is particularly critical because many joints are fused.

Surgical Technique
- The foot is placed back in proper alignment first, which can be done with fixation as described earlier.
- The ankle is then fused, most often with a compression screw technique, through a lateral transfibular approach.
- In patients with remaining valgus or when there is a significant chance of failure of fixation, a lateral plate or retrograde nail is considered.

Postoperative Management
In patients with a pantalar fusion, there is a large lever arm, which can make healing difficult. Therefore, patients should be non–weight bearing until there is good evidence of bony union. This process can take more than 8 weeks. Once union has occurred, a removable boot is used. Because of this stiffness, patients often prefer sneakers or shoes with a rocker bottom and cushioned sole.

Results and Outcome
The results of a pantalar fusion are limited. Even though patients are able to walk, they note significant stiffness and extensive walking is uncomfortable. Functionally, the results are usually no better or worse than in patients with a well-functioning below-the-knee amputation. Some patients may have sufficient deltoid remaining for a total ankle replacement, but with a weak deltoid, there is the risk of deltoid failure and the foot must be well aligned under the ankle.

Algorithm 8.5 considers treatment of PTTD by stage.

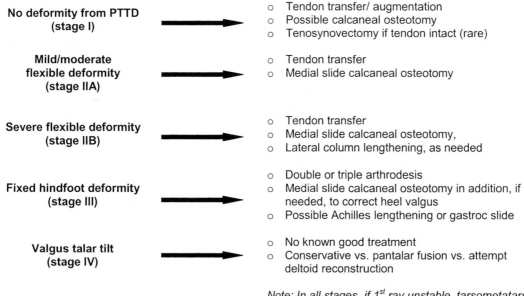

No deformity from PTTD (stage I) →
- Tendon transfer/ augmentation
- Possible calcaneal osteotomy
- Tenosynovectomy if tendon intact (rare)

Mild/moderate flexible deformity (stage IIA) →
- Tendon transfer
- Medial slide calcaneal osteotomy

Severe flexible deformity (stage IIB) →
- Tendon transfer
- Medial slide calcaneal osteotomy,
- Lateral column lengthening, as needed

Fixed hindfoot deformity (stage III) →
- Double or triple arthrodesis
- Medial slide calcaneal osteotomy in addition, if needed, to correct heel valgus
- Possible Achilles lengthening or gastroc slide

Valgus talar tilt (stage IV) →
- No known good treatment
- Conservative vs. pantalar fusion vs. attempt deltoid reconstruction

Note: In all stages, if 1st ray unstable, tarsometatarsal fusion (most common in stages IIB-IV)

Algorithm 8.5　Treatment of PTTD by stage. PTTD, posterior tibial tendon dysfunction.

SUGGESTED READING

Abraham E, Pankovich AM. Neglected rupture of the Achilles tendon. Treatment by V–Y tendinous flap. J Bone Joint Surg Am 1975;57:253–255.

Cetti R, Christensen SE, Ejsted R, et al. Operative versus nonoperative treatment of Achilles tendon rupture. A prospective randomized study and review of the literature. Am J Sports Med 1993;21:791–799.

Deland JT. Posterior tibial tendon dysfunction in clinical orthopedics. Philadelphia: Lippincott Williams & Wilkins, 1999:883–890.

Eckert WR, Davis EA. Acute rupture of the peroneal retinaculum. J Bone Joint Surg Am 1976;58:670–672.

Ellis SJ, Williams BR, Wagshul AD, et al. Deltoid ligament reconstruction with peroneus longus autograft in flatfoot deformity. Foot Ankle Int 2010;31(9):781–789.

Escalas F, Figueras JM, Merino JA. Dislocation of the peroneal tendons. Long-term results of surgical treatment. J Bone Joint Surg Am 1980;62:451–453.

Griend RV. Lateral column lengthening using a "Z" osteotomy of the calcaneus. Tech Foot Ankle Surg 2008;7(4):257–263.

Haddad SL, Mann RA. Flatfoot Deformity in Adults. In: Surgery of the Foot and Ankle. St. Louis: Mosby, 2007:1007–1085.

Hamilton WG, Geppert MJ, Thompson FM. Pain in the posterior aspect of the ankle in dancers. J Bone Joint Surg Am 1996;78:1491–1499.

Heckman DS, Reddy S, Pedowitz D, et al. Operative treatment for peroneal tendon disorders. J Bone Joint Surg Am 2008;90:404–418.

Jacobs D, Martens M, Van Audekercke R, et al. Comparison of conservative and operative treatment of Achilles tendon rupture. Am J Sports Med 1978;6:107–111.

Johnston E, Scranton P Jr, Pfeffer GB. Chronic disorders of the Achilles tendon: results of conservative and surgical treatments. Foot Ankle Int 1997;18(9):570–574.

Kolettis GH, Micheli LJ, Klein JD. Release of the flexor hallucis longus tendon in ballet dancers. J Bone Joint Surg Am 1996;78:1386–1390.

Larsen E, Flink-Olsen M, Seerup K. Surgery for recurrent dislocation of the peroneal tendons. Acta Orthop Scand 1984;55:554–555.

Mandelbaum BR, Myerson MS, Forster R. Achilles tendon ruptures. A new method of repair, early range of motion, and functional rehabilitation. Am J Sports Med 1995;23:392–395.

McLennan JG. Treatment of acute and chronic luxations of the peroneal tendons. Am J Sports Med 1980;8:432–436.

Myerson MS. Adult acquired flatfoot deformity. J Bone Joint Surg Am 1996;78:780.

Ouzonian TJ, Anderson R. Anterior tibial tendon rupture. Foot Ankle Int 1995;16(7):406–410.

Patten A, Pun WK. Spontaneous rupture of the tibialis anterior tendon: a case report and literature review. Foot Ankle Int 2000;21:697–700.

Pomeroy GP, Manoli A. A new operative approach for flatfoot secondary to tibialis posterior tendon insufficiency: a preliminary report. Foot Ankle Int 1997;18:206.

Pomeroy GP, Pike R III, Beals TC, et al. Acquired flatfoot in adults due to dysfunction of the posterior tibial tendon. J Bone Joint Surg Am 1999;81:1173–1182.

Puddu G, Ippolito E, Postacchini F. A classification of Achilles tendon disease. Am J Sports Med 1976;4:145–150.

Schepsis AA, Wagner C, Leach RE. Surgical management of Achilles tendon overuse injuries. A long-term follow-up study. Am J Sports Med 1994;22:611–619.

Scholten PE, Sierevelt IN, van Dijk CN. Hindfoot endoscopy for posterior ankle impingement. J Bone Joint Surg Am 2008;90:2665–2672.

Sobel M, Geppert MJ, Olson EJ, et al. The dynamics of peroneus brevis tendon splits: a proposed mechanism, technique of diagnosis, and classification of injury. Foot Ankle 1992;13:413–422.

Sobel M, Pavlov H, Geppert MJ, et al. Painful os peroneum syndrome: a spectrum of conditions responsible for plantar lateral foot pain. Foot Ankle Int 1994;15:112–124.

Van Dijk CN, de Leeuw PA, Scholten PE. Hindfoot endoscopy for posterior ankle impingement. Surgical technique. J Bone Joint Surg Am 2009;91(suppl 2):287–298.

Wapner KL, Pavlock GS, Hecht PJ, et al. Repair of chronic Achilles tendon rupture with flexor hallucis longus tendon transfer. Foot Ankle 1993;14:443–449.

Zielaskowski LA, Pontious J. Extensor hallicis longus tendon rupture repair using a fascia lata allograft. J Am Podiatr Med Assoc. 2002 Sep;92(8):467–470.

HEEL AND SUBCALCANEAL PAIN

KEITH L. WAPNER

9

INTRODUCTION

Pain about the heel is a common problem presenting to the orthopedic surgeon. Successful treatment depends on a proper identification of the cause of the pain with a careful history and physical examination, so that an appropriate treatment regimen can be initiated. Patients should be informed of the challenge inherent in treating the problem while allowing ambulation. The duration for the resolution of symptoms can be a great source of frustration to the patient and physician. Most authors recommend that conservative modalities should be employed for 6 to 12 months prior to consideration for surgical intervention. Heel pain can be divided into two primary entities: subcalcaneal pain and posterior heel pain syndromes. It has been suggested that although these heel pain syndromes are familiar to all orthopedic surgeons, probably they are not completely understood as yet.

POSTERIOR HEEL PAIN

INTRODUCTION

Pain located in the posterior portion of the calcaneus can be produced by multiple causes and should be distinguished from subcalcaneal heel pain by history and physical examination. Pain in the posterior, superior portion of the calcaneus may arise as a result of the following:

- Retrocalcaneal bursitis
- Enlargement of the superior bursal prominence of the calcaneus known as Haglund deformity (Fig. 9.1)
- Insertional Achilles tendinosis
- Inflammation of an adventitious bursa between the Achilles tendon and the skin (Fig. 9.1).

Each of these entities may exist as an isolated condition or may be part of a symptom complex. Careful analysis of the patient's subjective complaints and objective findings is required for correct diagnosis.

PATHOGENESIS

Etiology

Enlargement of the posterior, superior aspect of the calcaneus (Haglund deformity) can lead to impingement on the insertional fibers of the Achilles tendon, producing irritation over the bony prominence and the tendon fibers. Haglund syndrome is a combination of the enlarged bony prominence creating insertional tendinosis, retrocalcaneal bursitis, and adventitial bursitis. When Achilles tendinosis occurs with Haglund syndrome, it is generally located in the area of the Achilles tendon just at or above the insertion of the Achilles at the posterior portion of the os calcis but not more proximally. Ossification within the Achilles tendon in this area represents ossification in a degenerative area of the tendon. Achilles tendon pathology can be divided into insertional and noninsertional dysfunctions. Insertional tendinosis occurs within and around the Achilles tendon at its insertion and may be associated with Haglund deformity or spur formation within the tendon itself. Insertional Achilles tendinosis represents a biologic disorder of tendon degeneration from constant intrinsic loading, whereas retrocalcaneal bursitis is a manifestation of impingement of the bursa between the Achilles tendon and the calcaneal process. Inflammation of the adventitious bursa, between the Achilles tendon and the overlying skin, is usually caused by pressure of the counter of the shoe against the prominent area. It is more common in women and less common in athletes.

Epidemiology

Retrocalcaneal bursitis tends to manifest in younger populations (30s), whereas insertional Achilles tendinosis with a calcific spur is present in an older population.

Anatomy

The Achilles tendon inserts into the middle of the posterior part of the posterior surface of the calcaneus. A retrocalcaneal bursa located between the Achilles tendon and the superior tuberosity of the calcaneus is a constant finding.

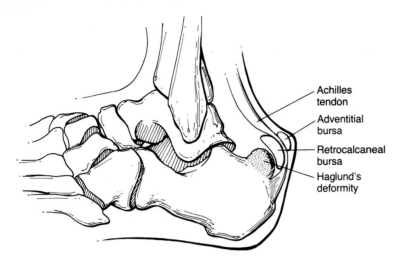

Figure 9.1 Illustration of Haglund deformity with a retrocalcaneal bursa between the Achilles tendon and the superior bursal prominence and an adventitious bursa between the Achilles tendon and the skin. (From Wapner KL, Bordelon RL. Foot and ankle: heel pain. In: DeLee JC, Drez D Jr, Miller MD, eds. DeLee and Drez's orthopaedic sports medicine: principles and practice, 2nd ed, vol 2. Philadelphia: Elsevier, 2003:2447.)

Dorsiflexion of the foot and ankle produces increased pressure in the retrocalcaneal bursa; plantarflexion decreases the pressure in the retrocalcaneal bursa. Anatomically, the retrocalcaneal bursa has an anterior bursal wall comprising fibrocartilage laid over the calcaneus, whereas the posterior wall is indistinguishable from the thin epitenon of the Achilles tendon. It is a disc-shaped structure lying over the posterior superior aspect of the calcaneus, fitting like a cap over the calcaneus and having a concave aspect anteriorly. The retrocalcaneal bursa maintains the relatively constant distance between the axis of the ankle joint and the insertion of the Achilles tendon. If the posterior prominence were not present, there will be shortening of the distance between the ankle joint axis and the insertion of the Achilles tendon during dorsiflexion. As this lever arm shortens, the ability of the gastrocnemius–soleus muscle to function is affected. Thus this projection works as a cam, allowing the tension of the gastrocnemius–soleus muscle group through the Achilles tendon to remain constant with dorsiflexion and plantarflexion.

The superior tuberosity of the os calcis may be hyperconvex, normal, or hypoconvex. The radiographic anatomy of the os calcis has been described in terms of the following anatomic landmarks on the lateral projection.

- The superior aspect of the talar articulation marks the most proximal portion of the posterior facet.
- The bursal projection is the area of the superior tuberosity of the os calcis.
- The tuberosity of the posterior surface marks the site of the Achilles insertion.
- The medial tubercle is the site of insertion of the central portion of the plantar aponeurosis.

Pathophysiology

Retrocalcaneal pain syndrome is commonly associated with a high-arched cavus foot with a varus heel. The combination of these factors tends to produce a foot that does not dorsiflex as readily as a normal foot. There is prominence of the heel, which is more susceptible to increased pressure from the tendons and the counter of the shoe.

Retrocalcaneal bursitis generally occurs in the circumstances of compensated rearfoot varus, compensated forefoot valgus, and a plantar-flexed first ray because of the abnormal motion of the subtalar joint and the frontal and sagittal plane relationships. Varus hindfoot tends to accentuate the posterior superior prominence by making the heel more vertical.

Ruptures of the Achilles tendon occur most commonly in the segment between 2 and 6 cm proximal to its insertion in the os calcis, an area of decreased vascularity and nutrition. This is an important finding relative to the retrocalcaneal bursal syndrome because this classic type of Achilles tendinosis is proximal to the area usually associated with the retrocalcaneal bursal syndrome. This may suggest that insertional tendinosis is brought on by impingement on the tendon because of the morphology of the foot or the prominence of the calcaneus rather than decreased circulation.

DIAGNOSIS

Physical Examination and History

The history in general comprises the following:

- Slow onset of dull ache in the retrocalcaneal area aggravated by activity and certain shoe wear.
- Start up pain after sitting or when arising out of bed in the morning.
- Gradual swelling at the area of the Achilles insertion.

Clinical Features

- Careful palpation of the Achilles tendon down to the area of insertion will allow identification of insertional tendinosis.
- The tendon insertion may be warm, swollen, and tender to palpation.
- If the tendon itself is neither swollen nor tender, palpating the anterior border of the tendon both medially and laterally allows identification of retrocalcaneal bursitis.

- In some instances, ballottement of the bursa is appreciated.
- In the case of retrocalcaneal bursitis, dorsiflexion of the foot increases the pain as it compresses the bursa between the tendon and the calcaneus.
- This condition may coexist with insertional tendinosis with thickening and swelling of the Achilles tendon.
- An adventitial bursa may be located between the skin and the posterior portion of the Achilles tendon rather than deep into the tendon.
- The posterior heel prominence may be warm and the overlying skin may be thickened and inflamed.
- The presence of a Haglund deformity can be palpated through the skin in the area of the superior portion of the heel and may be associated with overlying callus formation.
- There may be an area of periostitis, which is a discrete localized area of tenderness of the calcaneus, usually on the lateral side of the posterior portion and produced by pressure from the shoe counter.
- Passive dorsiflexion of the ankle should be assessed to determine whether there is an Achilles tendon contracture increasing the tension at the insertion of the Achilles tendon.
- This test should be performed with the knee in extension as well as flexion and with the forefoot in both abducted and adducted positions to assess for isolated gastrocnemius tightness.

Radiologic Features

A lateral view of the foot is taken with the patient standing. This allows biomechanical evaluation of the foot as well as evaluation of the specific pointed areas of the calcaneus. The points of the calcaneus are identified as follows:

- The posterior margin of the posterior facet at the superior bursal projection.
- The tuberosity indicating the site of the Achilles tendon insertion.
- The medial tubercle and the anterior tubercle.
- The shape and appearance of the superior bursal prominence are noted.

Radiographic evaluation of the lateral X-ray can include measuring the posterior calcaneal angle that is considered prominent if the angle is greater than 75°. Patients with symptomatic Haglund disease often demonstrate the combination of the posterior calcaneal angle greater than 75° and the angle of calcaneal inclination greater than 90° (Fig. 9.2). Parallel pitch line is measured by placing a line along the medial tuberosity and the anterior tubercle, and a second parallel line is drawn from the posterior lip of the talar articular facet. The bursal prominence is considered abnormal if it extends above this line. Radiographically, the syndrome is characterized by the following:

- Retrocalcaneal bursitis (loss of the lucent retrocalcaneal recess between the Achilles tendon and the bursal projection).
- Achilles tendinitis (an Achilles tendon measuring more than 9 mm located 2 cm above the bursal projection).
- Superficial tendo-Achilles bursitis (a convexity of the soft tissues posterior to the Achilles tendon insertion).
- The cortex is intact, but there is a prominent bursal projection with a positive parallel pitch line.

Some experts do not think X-ray measurements are helpful and rely more on physical examination and the patients history in clinical decision making.

Magnetic resonance imaging (MRI) allows visualization of the Achilles tendon, the bursa, and demonstrates any bony abnormalities in the posterior superior calcaneus (Fig. 9.3). In patients refractory to nonoperative treatment, a preoperative MRI will define the anatomic structures that need to be addressed. The degree of tendinosis present in the Achilles tendon is easily visualized and distinguished from isolated bursitis with MRI.

Laboratory Studies

Retrocalcaneal bursitis may occasionally be a manifestation of systemic arthritis or gout. Specific laboratory studies can be obtained to rule out these disorders. Painful heel syndrome with plantar fasciitis or Achilles tendinosis has been found in patients suffering from a seronegative spondyloarthropathy, but is rare in patients with rheumatoid arthritis.

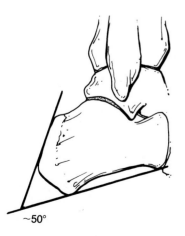 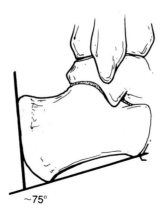

Figure 9.2 Measurement of the posterior calcaneal angle. The normal angle is shown on the left and abnormal on the right. Upper level of normal is considered to be 69°. (From Wapner KL, Bordelon RL. Foot and ankle: heel pain. In: DeLee JC, Drez D Jr, Miller MD, eds. DeLee and Drez's orthopaedic sports medicine: principles and practice, 2nd ed, vol 2. Philadelphia: Elsevier, 2003:2449.)

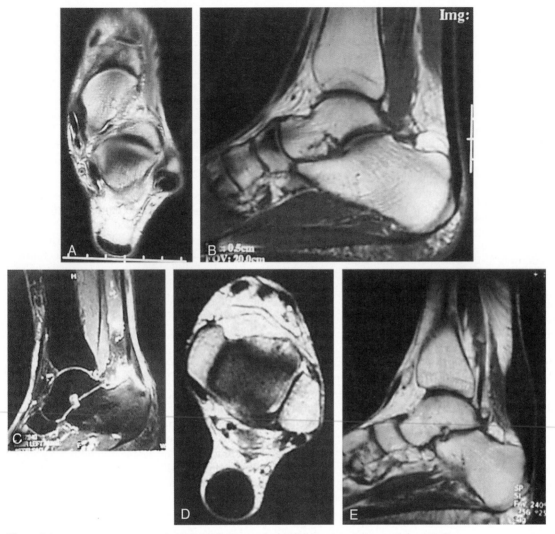

Figure 9.3   (A) Axial MRI scan of normal Achilles tendon showing normal shape of the Achilles. (B) Sagittal MRI scan of normal Achilles tendon showing normal shape of the Achilles. (C) Sagittal MRI scan showing increased signal in the insertion of the Achilles tendon consistent with tendinosis. There is increased fluid demonstrating an inflamed bursa surrounding the Haglund deformity. (D,E) Axial and sagittal MRI scans demonstrating chronic tendinosis of the Achilles with marked fusiform swelling of the tendon. (From Wapner KL, Bordelon RL. Foot and ankle: heel pain. In: DeLee JC, Drez D Jr, Miller MD, eds. DeLee and Drez's orthopaedic sports medicine: principles and practice, 2nd ed, vol 2. Philadelphia: Elsevier, 2003:2451.)

TREATMENT

Nonsurgical Treatment

Conservative management of posterior heel pain includes the following:

- Modification of activity to decrease the load on the tendon.
  - Cross-training with elliptical or stationary bike.
- Stretching activities for the gastrocsoleus complex.
- Modification of shoewear to avoid direct pressure from the counter of the shoe onto the posterior aspect of the heel.
  - Padding of the area will often assist in relieving the pressure.
  - Adjustment of shoe counter material and height.
  - A small heel lift that decreases the pitch angle, allowing the prominent bony projection to slip forward away from the shoe counter.
- Nonsteroidal anti-inflammatory drugs.
- Injection of steroid in this area, if at all, should be done with great care, as this may precipitate tendon rupture.
- The use of night splints to decrease morning pain and assist in improving the flexibility of the Achilles tendon.

Athletes, particularly runners, who presented with acute or chronic posterior heel pain, were successfully managed nonoperatively by activity modification using a combination of the following:

- Decrease in or cessation of the usual weekly mileage.
- Temporary termination of interval training and workouts on hills.
- Change from a harder bank surface to a softer surface.
- Stretching and strengthening the gastrocnemius–soleus complex.

In cases where there is severe pain, significant tendinosis, or failure to respond to conservative modalities, cast immobilization can be employed. Patients can be placed into a short leg walking cast for a period of 4 to 8 weeks until the area becomes nontender to palpation. In instances where there is existing tendinosis, prolonged immobilization with the use of a molded ankle foot orthosis may allow healing over a 6- to 9-month period.

In the pediatric athlete, heel pain may result from osteochondrosis of the apophysis of the calcaneus (Sever disease) or Achilles tendinitis—characterized by pain on palpation of the tendon just above its insertion. In severe cases, there may be crepitation of the tendon. Treatment includes rest and anti-inflammatory agents. In differentiating these two entities it may be helpful to note that the pain due to osteochondrosis occurs on the inferior portion of the os calcis; in Achilles tendinitis, it is proximal to the insertion of the Achilles tendon.

Surgical Treatment

Surgical treatment is recommended in cases refractory to conservative modalities where systemic diseases have been ruled out, or in the case of disruption of the tendon. Surgery should address the specific etiologies producing symptoms in each patient and may include some combination of debridement of the Achilles tendon, retrocalcaneal bursa, superficial Achilles bursa, bursal projection of the os calcis, and tendon transfer as guided by clinical examination and radiologic studies.

To decrease impingement on the bursa and insertion of the tendon, a dorsally based closing wedge osteotomy of the calcaneus has been proposed to unload the soft tissue in dorsiflexion. However, there is no adequate follow-up in patients treated such to justify this procedure.

- For a patient with Haglund exostosis and retrocalcaneal bursa, surgery is done under a tourniquet, with the patient prone.
- Most commonly, a posterolateral or a combination of posteromedial and posterolateral incision is used with care to avoid the sural nerve. The insertion is elevated carefully, so that the insertion of the tendon is not disrupted.
- The retrocalcaneal bursa is excised, and any spur is revealed.
- The posterior, superior tuberosity is resected in a manner that preserves the subtalar joint and the insertion of the Achilles tendon (Fig. 9.4).
- The edges may be smoothed with a rasp, and the tendon may need to be repaired to the bony surface with an anchor.
- Chronically degenerated tissue of Achilles tendinosis is histologically different from the tissue in an acute simple tear.

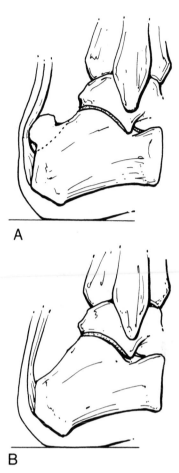

Figure 9.4 (**A**) Diagram of Haglund deformity with prominence of the posterior superior portion of the calcaneus. (**B**) Appearance of the calcaneus after surgical resection of posterior superior prominence for symptomatic Haglund deformity. (From Wapner KL, Bordelon RL. Foot and ankle: heel pain. In: DeLee JC, Drez D Jr, Miller MD, eds. DeLee and Drez's orthopaedic sports medicine: principles and practice, 2nd ed, vol 2. Philadelphia: Elsevier, 2003:2454.)

- In the presence of associated tendinosis and calcification, transfer of the flexor hallucis longus may be necessary to enhance the blood supply and reinforce the Achilles tendon (Fig. 9.5).

Postoperative Management

Immobilization in equinus non–weight bearing for 3 to 4 weeks followed by neutral position partial weight bearing for 3 to 4 weeks, with gradual transition to full weight bearing with physical therapy, is usually successful in most patients. In high-performance athletes, this protocol can be accelerated if the patient is carefully monitored. Casting is used for 2 to 3 weeks with weight bearing permitted after 1 week. In case of pathology within the tendon requiring excision and repair, immobilization is continued for another week or two. Range of motion exercises are emphasized. A graduated program of swimming and stationary bicycling combined with isometric, isotonic, and isokinetic strengthening of the calf muscles is utilized. Jogging is permitted after 8 to 12 weeks. Full return to a competitive level of sports activity usually

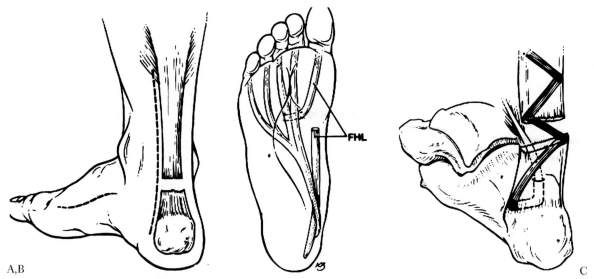

Figure 9.5 (**A, B**) Diagrams of flexor hallucis longus and flexor digitorum longus tenodesis. (**C**) Diagram after weaving the flexor hallucis longus through the Achilles demonstrating the orientation of the tunnel through the posterior calcaneus. (From Wapner KL, Bordelon RL. Foot and ankle: heel pain. In: DeLee JC, Drez D Jr, Miller MD, eds. DeLee and Drez's Orthopaedic sports medicine: principles and practice, 2nd ed, vol 2. Philadelphia: Elsevier, 2003:2455.)

requires 5 to 6 months. Athletes with tendonitis or tenosynovitis usually show a better and faster recovery than those with components of retrocalcaneal bursitis.

Maximum postoperative improvement varies from approximately 6 months for patients with isolated retrocalcaneal bursitis to 1 year for patients with insertional tendinosis and spurs. Satisfaction rates range from 75% to 95%. Complications include the following:

- Avulsion of the tendon
- Recurrent tendinitis
- Sural neuritis and
- Persistent hyperesthesia.

Pearls

- Retrocalcaneal pain is a condition characterized by inflammation of the retrocalcaneal bursa, the Achilles tendon just above its insertion, the bone at the posterior superior aspect of the calcaneus, and at times the bursa between the Achilles and the skin.
- It is generally managed by conservative measures consisting of anti-inflammatory medication, decreased activity, padding to prevent direct pressure on the affected area, orthoses or heel lifts, and most important, stretching and strengthening exercises.
- If it does not respond to these modalities, surgical intervention may be considered.
- Surgery generally comprises excision of the exostosis and the retrocalcaneal bursa and at times the adventious bursa, if present, and repair of the Achilles tendon pathology with an flexor hallucis longus tendon transfer if necessary.
- Although most series do report good results after surgery, in athletes, this condition may prevent continued full activity even after surgical intervention.

SUBCALCANEAL PAIN SYNDROME

PATHOGENESIS

Etiology and Epidemiology

Most patients are 40 to 60 years of age and a large percentage are overweight. Plantar fasciitis usually arises at the medial tuberosity as a traction periostitis with degeneration and microtears of the plantar fascia. Secondary involvement of the adjacent structures such as the medial calcaneal nerve and the nerve to the abductor digiti quinti may coexist. Occasionally, primary entrapment of the nerve to the abductor digiti quinti and the sensory branch of the medial calcaneal nerve may occur. The relationship of the calcaneal heel spur to subcalcaneal pain has not been definitively established. The spur is located in the origin of the flexor digirotum brevis muscle, not in the plantar fascia. A review of 1,000 patients at random with radiographs of the foot noted a 13.2% incidence of heel spurs. Only 39% of those with heel spurs reported any history of subcalcaneal heel pain, indicating only a weak correlation between the spur and the pain. In children, calcaneal apophysitis (Sever disease) is the most common cause of heel pain.

Anatomy

The plantar aponeurosis arises from the calcaneus and comprises three segments. The lateral portion of the planar aponeurosis arises from the lateral process of the tuberosity of the calcaneus and inserts into the base of the fifth metatarsal. The medial portion is thin and covers the undersurface of the abductor hallucis. Clinically, the

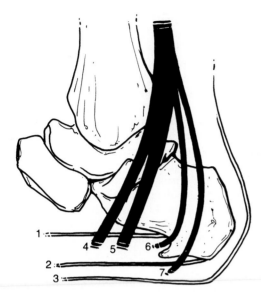

Figure 9.6 Relationship of structures commonly associated with heel pain: (1) long plantar ligament; (2) plantar fascia; (3) skin; (4) medial plantar nerve; (5) lateral plantar nerve; (6) nerve to abductor digiti quinti; and (7) medial calcaneal nerve. Note that the medial calcaneal nerve supplying sensation to the heel passes superficial to the plantar fascia. The nerve to the abductor digiti quinti passes deep to the plantar fascia and beneath the spur. (From Wapner KL, Bordelon RL. Foot and ankle: heel pain. In: DeLee JC, Drez D Jr, Miller MD, eds. DeLee and Drez's orthopaedic sports medicine: principles and practice, 2nd ed, vol 2. Philadelphia: Elsevier, 2003:2460.)

plantar aponeurosis generally refers to the central portion, which extends from the medial tuberosity of the calcaneus and passes to the proximal phalanges of the lesser toes through the longitudinal septa, to the big toe through the sesamoids, and into the skin of the ball of the foot through vertical fibers. Hyperextension of the toes and the metatarsophalangeal joints places tension on the plantar aponeurosis, raises the longitudinal arch of the foot, inverts the

hindfoot, and externally rotates the leg. This mechanism is passive and depends entirely on bony and ligamentous stability and has been termed the *windlass mechanism* by Hicks.

The plantar fat pad below the heel is a complex structure comprising adipose tissue divided by multiple fibrous septae that extend from the calcaneus to the thickened keratinized skin. These U-shaped septae stabilize the adipose tissue and allow forces of direct compression and torsion to be absorbed, thereby, protecting the underlying bone and soft-tissue structures.

The posterior tibial nerve is located on the medial side of the foot behind the medial malleolus and beneath the flexor retinaculum (Fig. 9.6). The medial calcaneal nerve, which may consist of one or two branches, arises at the level of the medial malleolus or below and passes superficially to innervate the skin of the heel. It passes in the subcutaneous tissue between the plantar fascia and the skin. The nerve to the abductor digiti quinti branches off the lateral plantar nerve and, passes deeper, beneath the plantar ligament and underneath the spur, if present, to innervate the abductor digiti quinti and nearby periosteum. Entrapment of the nerve to the abductor digiti quinti occurs between the abductor hallucis and the medial margin of the medial head of the quadratus plantae muscle. Sensory fibers innervate the periosteum and motor fibers branch to the flexor digitorum brevis and abductor digiti quinti muscles. It is important to differentiate the medial calcaneal nerve from the nerve to the abductor digiti quinti during decompression for plantar fasciitis.

The medial and lateral plantar nerves continue to the foot and pass through respective foramina of the abductor muscles. When considering entrapment of the posterior tibial nerve, it is important to note that these nerves may be entrapped either beneath the flexor retinaculum at the level of the medial malleolus or at the point where the medial and lateral plantar nerves exit through separate foramina in the abductor muscles (Fig. 9.7).

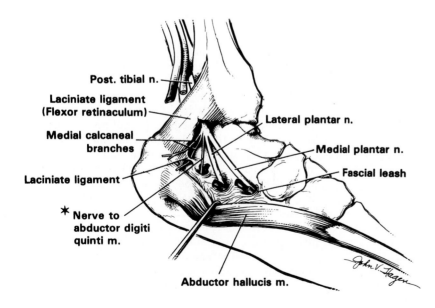

Figure 9.7 Site of entrapment of the posterior tibial nerve and its branches, demonstrating possible entrapment beneath the laciniate ligament and at the point where the nerve passes through the fascia of the abductor hallucis muscle. (From Wapner KL, Bordelon RL. Foot and ankle: heel pain. In: DeLee JC, Drez D Jr, Miller MD, eds. DeLee and Drez's orthopaedic sports medicine: principles and practice, 2nd ed, vol 2. Philadelphia: Elsevier, 2003:2461; redrawn from Baxter DE, Thigpen CM. Heel pain: operative results. Foot Ankle 1984;5:16–25. Copyright American Orthopaedic Foot and Ankle Society.)

Pathophysiology

Cavus and planus feet both have biomechanical implications in plantar fasciitis. A supple foot with a tendency toward a flatfoot deformity will place tension on the origin of the plantar fascia at the calcaneus because the windlass mechanism will be under increased strain in maintaining a stable arch during the propulsive phase of gait. Thus, an orthotic device or strapping with tape to hold the forefoot in adduction and the heel in varus may relieve the pressure on the origin of the plantar aponeurosis during propulsion. When a cavus foot is present, there may be excessive strain on the heel area because the hindfoot lacks the ability to evert to absorb the shock of heel strike.

Many patients with plantar fasciitis are found to have some restricted dorsiflexion with a contracture of both the plantar fascia and the Achilles tendon. Decreased dorsiflexion from a tight Achilles tendon will lead to increased pronation and thus increased load on the plantar fascia resulting in symptoms of overuse with normal activity levels. Once the plantar structures are inflamed, they will tighten at night while the patient sleeps and the foot and ankle assume an equinus position. When the patient arises from bed and begins to ambulate with the foot and ankle in a neutral and dorsiflexed position, this contracted tissue is placed under stretch and may produce pain. Although there is no agreement on the exact cause of plantar fasciitis, restriction of motion and the shape of the foot are factors that are definitely contributory.

DIAGNOSIS

The differential diagnosis of subcalcaneal pain syndrome includes the following (sometimes more than one):

- Plantar fasciitis: most common.
- Lumbar stenosis with atypical radicular symptoms.
- Chronic heel fat pad atrophy.
- Fibromatosis: usually occurs in the arch and can be treated with pressure relief; surgical excision associated with recurrence in approximately 50% of cases.
- Cavus or planus foot deformity.
- Contracture of the Achilles tendon.
- Plantar directed spur (vey uncommon).
- Calcaneal stress fracture.
- Inflammatory arthropathy with associated enthesopathy.
- Plantar fascia rupture.
- Nerve entrapment.

Physical Examination and History

Plantar fasciitis is more common in the middle-aged population and is not restricted to athletic individuals. It is generally unilateral, but may be bilateral in up to 15% to 25% of patients. Patients generally relate a history of a gradual, insidious onset of pain without an acute episode of trauma. The pain is generally described as being along the plantar medial aspect of the heel without distal radiation or paresthesias. A history of proximal or distal radiation, numbness, or paresthesias is suggestive of nerve entrapment or lumbar stenosis. The pain is severe upon arising out of bed in the morning, but as the patient begins to walk and stretch out the plantar structures, the pain will often abate. It will typically be made worse with increasing activity throughout the course of the day. Patients also describe start-up pain after sitting for any extended period. In severe cases, patients can develop an antalgic gait and may describe pain with every step. Acute rupture of the plantar fasciitis may be seen following trauma or following multiple injections of corticosteroids. The patient will generally present with an acute onset or exacerbation of pain, swelling, and tenderness following a painful popping or snapping on the plantar aspect of the foot. Compression of the nerve to the abductor digiti quinti has been identified as a source of pain in patients who generally identify tenderness as being on the medial aspect of the heel, distal to the abductor origin rather than the plantar aspect of the heel.

Clinical Features.
- The patient should be examined standing and while ambulating.
- Patients with a hypermobile supple flat foot may hyperpronate leading to increased pressure through the windlass mechanism leading to strain along the plantar fascia. Patients with a stiff cavus foot may have the inability to dissipate the forces of impact secondary to the rigidity of their foot. Identification of these foot morphologies will be important in devising an appropriate treatment plan.
- Specific examination of the foot reveals acute tenderness along the medial tuberosity of the calcaneus. This tenderness may be at the origin of the central slip of the plantar fascia, or it may be deep with involvement of the nerve to the abductor digiti quinti.
- The medial calcaneal nerve is palpated and tapped to search for paresthesias in the subcutaneous tissues indicative of entrapment.
- Compression over the first branch of the lateral plantar nerve just distal to the origin of the abductor muscle, where the nerve passes deep to the muscle and the fascia, can reveal tenderness also indicating possible nerve entrapment. This pain is distinct from that at the medial tuberosity.
- The plantar fascia is palpated to determine whether it is tender just at its origin or throughout its course. It is also palpated for nodules, the presence of which suggests plantar fibromatosis.
- Palpation is carried out with the toes flexed, so that the plantar fascia is supple as well as with the toes extended, which places tension on the plantar fascia.
- Atrophy of the plantar heel fat pad may reveal tenderness directly over the inferior aspect of the calcaneus.
- Inflammation of the heel pad may also be present and evident with palpation and manipulation of the fat pad.
- In chronic cases, medial and lateral compression over the posterior inferior body of the calcaneus may produce significant pain suggestive of periostitis or stress fracture of the calcaneus.
- The tarsal tunnel is percussed to elicit any tenderness, inflammation, or a Tinel sign of the posterior tibial, medial or lateral plantar, or medial calcaneal nerves.
- Sensation of the foot is evaluated by light touch and pinprick to ascertain the status of the sensory nerves.

If the patient describes proximal or distal radiation of pain, straight leg raise test should be performed to rule out any component of sciatica.

- The range of motion of the hindfoot should be assessed to determine the degree of dorsiflexion with the foot both adducted and abducted.
- Ankle dorsiflexion should be tested with the knee both extended and flexed to distinguish between tightness of the gastrocnemius and soleus muscles.
- Adduction of the forefoot reproduces the position of the foot in the gait cycle at the end of stance phase when the heel initially lifts off the ground. At this point in the gait cycle, pressure is transferred to the plantar fascia and its origin by the windlass mechanism.
- Examination of the muscles that cross the area, such as the posterior tibial, anterior tibial, peroneus longus and brevis, and toe flexors and extensors, is done to determine their motor power and also to see whether any pain is produced with active motor function.
- Neurologic examination of the remainder of the lower extremities and back is performed as indicated.

Radiologic Features

Standing, full-weight-bearing radiographs of the heel will provide information about the osseous structures of the foot as well as specific details of the calcaneus. Standing radiographs will also provide information about the biomechanical status of the foot during the stance phase of gait. Axial non–weight-bearing views of the calcaneus may be taken to provide information in a second plane. A subcalcaneal heel spur may be noted unless a fracture of this heel spur is noted. In children, radiographic irregularity of the calcaneal apophysis is the rule rather than the exception. There is no evidence that treatment alters this radiographic picture.

A technetium-99m bone scan may be performed to provide objective evidence of an inflammatory abnormality in the insertion of the plantar fascia and of the inferior portion of the calcaneus. Significant uptake may be indicative of severe periostitis or insufficiency fracture, which correlates with severe pain on medial and lateral compressions of the calcaneus. Increased activity at the site of insertion of the plantar fascia into the calcaneus in patients with clinical signs of plantar fasciitis may occur in the absence of any radiologic change. In confusing clinical situations, bone scans can be useful in differentiating plantar fasciitis from other etiologies of the painful heel syndrome such as nerve entrapment. An MRI may prove useful in correlating distinct anatomic abnormalities with the findings on physical examination and patient history; however, the cost-effectiveness of these studies has yet to be determined.

Diagnostic Studies

Laboratory studies in most patients with subcalcaneal pain syndrome are normal. With persistent, bilateral, or severe symptoms, consideration should be given to the diagnosis of a systemic disorder such as a seronegative arthropathy. With the subcalcaneal pain syndrome, there may be an incidence as high as 16% of subsequent development of a systemic inflammatory disorder. Surgical treatment is not appropriate in such patients.

Patients with positive HLA-B27 seronegative, pauciarticular arthritis have a higher incidence of low back and buttock pain, Achilles tendinitis, and dactylitis of the toes. This test should be considered part of the systemic work-up for a patient with chronic, recurrent, and/or incapacitating heel pain. Surgery generally yields poor results in patients with a positive HLA-B27 and should be avoided.

Neurologic causes of heel pain should also be considered. Nerve entrapment of the nerves supplying the abductor digiti quinti muscle, calcaneal branches of the tibial nerve, and medial plantar nerve have all been implicated in subcalcaneal pain syndrome. Precise localization of the area of pathology is accomplished by means of differential blocks using a long-acting anesthetic such as bupivacaine in complicated situations. Electromyography is not helpful in the diagnosis of compression neuropathies of the nerve to the abductor digiti minimi. Tarsal tunnel syndrome may be present with referred pain to the heel and sole of the foot. A positive Tinel sign may suggest this diagnosis. Electromyographic and nerve conduction studies should be utilized to assess for this condition. Heel pain may also be referred from the lumbar spine or may be a manifestation of neuropathy from diabetes or alcoholism.

TREATMENT

Nonsurgical Treatment

Management of subcalcaneal heel pain should initially begin with nonoperative treatment for 6 months to 1 year (Algorithm 9.1). Stepwise treatment includes the following:

- Achilles and plantar fascia stretching—two to three times a day especially before running
- Minimize overuse—cross train athletes, weight loss programs
- Night splints to maintain the ankle in dorsiflexion
- Well-padded shoewear such as running shoes or shoes with soft rubber sole
- Nonsteroidal anti-inflammatories
- Soft heel pads or cups, arch support or orthotics
- Physical therapy—supervised stretching, strengthening, modalities (phonophoresis or iontophoresis), low dye taping
- Cast immobilization in refractory patients with a positive bone scan
- Corticosteroid injections should be minimized and should avoid the fat pad, as they increase risk of plantar fascia rupture and fat pad atrophy

The natural history of plantar fasciitis has been shown to be self-limited with good results from nonsurgical therapy in most patients. It is important for the patient to understand that in up to 95% of cases, prolonged utilization of nonsurgical modalities for up to a year will produce complete resolution of their symptoms. Children with the diagnosis of calcaneal apophysitis are treated with soft plastazote orthotics or heel cups in combination with proper athletic footwear.

High-energy extracorporeal shock wave therapy (OssaTron [Health Tronics Surgical Services Inc., Atlanta, GA]) has been shown to be a safe and effective method of

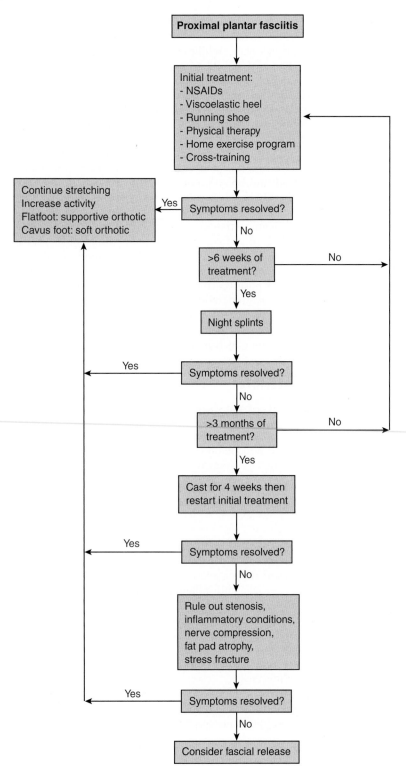

Algorithm 9.1 Algorithm for the treatment of subcalcaneal heel pain.

treating heel pain syndrome that has been unresponsive to nonoperative management in a randomized, 1:1 allocated, placebo-controlled, prospective, double blind clinical study with only minor, transient adverse effects. This treatment theoretically stimulates a healing response at the origin of the plantar fascia on the calcaneus, and it is now FDA approved for this indication.

Surgical Treatment

Surgical management of chronic plantar fasciitis remains controversial. The cause of failure of conservative modalities must be identified prior to consideration for surgery. If a compliant patient has failed an appropriate physical therapy program, has pain resistant to modalities of casting and night splinting, and has undergone workup of seronegative arthropathies, stress fractures, lumbar stenosis, and nerve entrapment, he or she may be a candidate for surgical intervention. The American Orthopaedic Foot and Ankle Society (AOFAS) has issued a position statement on the timing of surgical intervention (Box 9.1).

Surgical Procedures

Surgical alternatives have included fasciotomy (abductor digiti quinti), nerve decompression, drilling of the calcaneus, excision of the calcaneal spur, endoscopic fasciotomy, and some combinations of the above.

There are studies that promote fasciotomy as part of the surgical treatment and that have good and excellent results ranging from 75% to 100% with improvement noted for 6 to 8 months postsurgery. In studies advocating plantar fascial release in athletes, return to running occurred in

---

BOX 9.1 AOFAS POSITION STATEMENT: ENDOSCOPIC AND OPEN HEEL SURGERY

1. Nonsurgical treatment is recommended for a minimum of 6 months and preferably 12 months
2. More than 90% of patients respond to nonsurgical treatment within 6 to 10 months
3. When surgery is considered, a medical evaluation should be considered before surgery
4. Patients should be advised of complications and risks when an endoscopic or open procedure is recommended
5. If nerve compression is coexistent with fascial or bone pain, an endoscopic procedure should not be attempted
6. The AOFAS does not recommend surgical procedures preceding nonoperative methods
7. The AOFAS supports responsible, carefully planned surgical intervention when nonsurgical treatment fails and the workup is complete
8. The AOFAS supports cost constraints in the treatment of heel pain when the outcome is not altered
9. The AOFAS recommends heel padding, medications, and stretching before prescribing custom orthoses and extended physical therapy
10. This position statement is intended as a guide to the orthopaedist and is not intended to dictate a treatment plan

---

88% to 100% of patients from as early as 6 weeks to as late as 4.5 months postsurgery. Others advocate caution citing that in long-term follow-up only 53% of patients had no limitations in activities, only 47% had no pain, and only 49% were totally satisfied.

Surgical Technique

- A medial oblique incision along the heel is made (Fig. 9.8).
- The sensory branch of the medial calcaneal nerve is located, inspected, and protected. Loupe magnification may be utilized.
- If there is entrapment of the medial calcaneal nerve as it comes through the fascia, this is explored and released.
- The medial one-third to one-half of the plantar fascia is released at its origin.
- The spur may be removed using a small rongeur after stripping the muscles.
- The deep fascia of the abductor hallucis and the medial fascia of the quadratus plantae are divided to release the nerve to the abductor digiti quinti as it passes laterally.
- The patient is placed in a short leg cast and kept non–weight bearing for 3 weeks. Weight bearing in a cast or an over-the-counter brace is maintained for 3 more weeks. Activity following this is allowed as tolerated.
- If the patient has a biomechanical foot abnormality, an orthotic device is used postoperatively.

In the patient who has symptoms referred to the posterior tibial nerve as well as pathology of the medial tuberosity, or if he or she has had recurrent or failed surgery, a more extensive procedure is considered. The operation for complex, resistant, or recurrent pain along the medial side of the heel comprises exploration of the posterior tibial nerve from the medial side of the ankle to the point where it exits through the foramina of the abductor muscles and exploration and release of the medial calcaneal nerve and the nerve to the abductor digiti quinti along with release of the central portion of the plantar fascia and excision of the heel spur, if present. The patient is kept non–weight bearing for 3 weeks and then can bear weight in a short leg cast for another 3 weeks; increased activity is started at 12 weeks. This operation is used only for patients with recalcitrant conditions. It carries with it the expectation that the patient will probably, but not certainly, be able to return to his or her preinjury status.

Endoscopic plantar fascia release is being performed also with the potential benefit of less morbidity. The potential risk of overreleasing or underreleasing the central slip and the inability to release any neural structures has received significant attention. Dry needling and platelet-rich plasma injection have also been reported, but to date, there are not adequate data to support the efficacy of these procedures.

Complications

Complications from endoscopic plantar fascial release include stress fractures, pseudoaneurysm formation, numbness and neuroma formation, and recurrence of pain. Because of the high incidence of lateral foot pain,

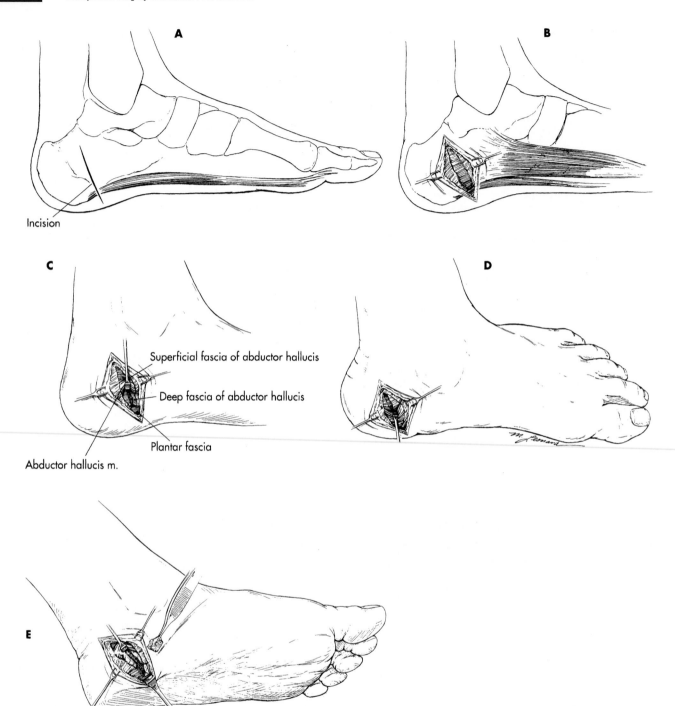

Figure 9.8 Plantar fascia and nerve release. (**A**) Incision. (**B**) Release of the abductor hallucis. (**C**) Abductor hallucis muscle is reflected proximally. (**D**) Abductor hallucis is retracted distally. (**E**) Resection of small medial portion of the plantar fascia. (From Coughlin MJ, Mann RA. Surgery of the foot and ankle, 7th ed. St. Louis: Mosby, 1999:871.)

it is currently recommended that only the medial half to two-thirds of the plantar fascia be released. Complications from open procedures include fracture of the calcaneus following surgical procedures for excision of the calcaneal spur, persistent or recurrent acute plantar fasciitis including rupture, pathology related to arch instability, and structural failure from overload including metatarsal stress fractures, heel numbness, neuroma formation, wound healing problems, and infections. Fasciotomy affects arch stability and should not be performed in patients with evidence of concomitant pes planus deformity because deformity progression may occur.

SUGGESTED READING

Alvarez R. Preliminary results on the safety and efficacy of the OssaTron for treatment of plantar fasciitis. Foot Ankle Int 2002;23:197–203.

Baxter DE, Pfeffer GB. Treatment of chronic heel pain by surgical release of the first branch of the lateral planar nerve. Clin Orthop Relat Res 1992;(279):229–236.

Bordelon RL. Subcalcaneal pain: present status, evaluation, and management. Instr Course Lect 1984;33:283–287.

Davies MS, Weiss GA, Saxby TS. Plantar fasciitis: how successful is surgical intervention? Foot Ankle Int 1999;20:803–807.

Fox JM, Blazina ME, Jobe FW, et al. Degeneration and rupture of the Achilles tendon. Clin Orthop Relat Res 1975;(107):221–224.

Gill LH. Plantar fasciitis: diagnosis and conservative management. J Am Acad Orthop Surg 1997;5:109–117.

Hicks JH. The mechanics of the foot; II: the plantar aponeurosis and the arch. J Anat 1954; 88:25–30

Neufeld SK, Cerrato R. Plantar fasciitis: evaluation and treatment. J Am Acad Orthop Surg 2008;16(6):338–346.

Puddu G, Ippolito E, Postacchini F. A classification of Achilles tendon disease. Am J Sports Med 1976;4:145–150.

Stephens MM. Haglund's deformity and retrocalcaneal bursitis. Orthop Clin North Am 1994;25:41–46.

Wapner KL, Pavlock GS, Hecht PJ, et al. Repair of chronic Achilles tendon rupture with flexor hallucis longus tendon transfer. Foot Ankle 1993;14:443–449.

Watson AD, Anderson RB, Davis WH. Comparison of results of retrocalcaneal decompression for retrocalcaneal bursitis and insertional Achilles tendinosis with calcific spur. Foot Ankle Int 1993;21:638–642.

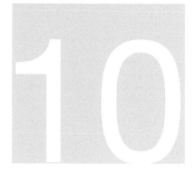

10

DEGENERATIVE JOINT DISEASE OF THE ANKLE AND HINDFOOT

TODD A. KILE
CHRISTOPHER Y. KWEON

Degenerative joint diseases include various clinical entities that are all linked by their common pathologic finding: the destruction of the joint interface. The ankle and the different hindfoot joints can be affected separately or in combination depending on the etiology (Fig. 10.1). Review of the degenerative joint diseases that affect the ankle and hindfoot is made easier by separating these entities using biomechanical and anatomic criteria.

This chapter highlights the important concepts needed to understand ankle degenerative joint disease. The second section discusses the hindfoot. Finally, this chapter presents some of the unique principles regarding combined lesions of the hindfoot and ankle joints.

ANKLE DEGENERATIVE JOINT DISEASE

The ankle joint combines the functions of a weight-bearing surface and allows motion that permits a normal gait cycle. The tibiotalar portion of the ankle joint transmits approximately 80% of the forces crossing the ankle. Shear forces coupled with compression forces are transmitted through this articulation. Compressive forces reach up to five times the body weight at heel rise. Shear forces reach up to 70% of body weight during flatfoot phase. As a result, the cartilage surfaces play a central role in the function of the joint. These surfaces are protected by two primary stabilizing mechanisms: the bony architecture surrounding the talus, shaped in a mortise, and the ligamentous support linking the distal tibia and fibula to the hindfoot. The destruction of either of these mechanisms by a degenerative process of the ankle joint creates unique clinical and radiologic findings, which, when recognized and understood, may help direct both nonsurgical and surgical treatments for patients affected by this disease.

PATHOGENESIS

The commonest cause of degenerative joint disease in the ankle is trauma. Ankle fracture, tibial plafond fracture, talus fracture, chondral trauma, and residual instability represent various pathways that can lead to degenerative arthrosis of the ankle joint. In these cases, the initial trauma is followed by a cascade of events, with all the biochemical and biomechanical changes that occur, leading ultimately to destruction of the joint cartilage.

Systemic diseases can result in ankle degeneration (Box 10.1), but they are less common. Among the inflammatory etiologies, rheumatoid arthritis is the most prevalent with its classic inflamed lymphoid follicles creating the pannus responsible for cartilage and subchondral bone destruction. Psoriatic arthritis can also affect the ankle joint as well as the surrounding skin and soft-tissues.

Metabolic crystalline arthropathies, such as gout or pseudogout, can cause acute and recurrent arthritis of the hindfoot and ankle. These flares, left untreated, can lead to eventual joint destruction. The inflammatory mediators, together with the hypertrophic synovium, cause irreversible injuries to the articular surface. The same kind of destructive pattern can occur in septic arthritis and osteomyelitis, which can cause degenerative joint disease in any joint affected by this condition. Proteolytic enzymes combined with increased intra-articular pressure and lack of nutrition ultimately lead to destruction of the cartilage.

Neuroarthropathy represents a characteristic condition, often confused with infection, which can result in destruction and deformity of the joints. Although the exact pathophysiology is not well understood, it is believed that the loss of protective sensation combined with unrecognized trauma (often subclinical or microtrauma) generates damage that is not adequately protected. This begins a cascade of clinical events—which can be seen radiographically—that can progress to dramatic bone and joint destruction. Diabetes mellitus, nerve and spinal cord

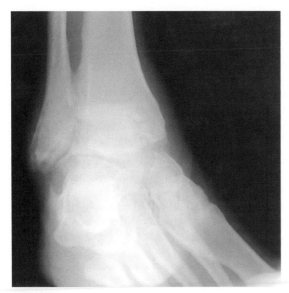

Figure 10.1 Oblique ankle X-ray of a 51-year-old man who shows posttraumatic ankle and subtalar degenerative joint disease.

dysfunction (paralytic injury or trauma), and myelodysplasia represent additional causes of neuroarthropathy at the foot and ankle levels. Interestingly, congenital insensitivity to pain can create similar problems, but remains an unusual clinical entity and seldom leads to destruction of joints.

Hemorrhagic effusions secondary to hemophilia or chronic warfarin therapy can also cause progressive articular destruction. In hemophilia, recurrent hemarthroses create a chronic inflammatory state of the synovium that can eventually affect the integrity of the joint itself by an enzymatic digestion process. Degeneration from septic arthritis and a similar inflammatory and degradative process is also well described.

Other causes of joint degeneration include bone or soft-tissue tumors of the ankle area, iatrogenic trauma, or primary idiopathic degenerative joint disease of the ankle—a diagnosis made by exclusion.

DIAGNOSIS

Physical Examination and History

Despite significant technologic advances in imaging, a complete history remains the most important diagnostic tool when evaluating patients with joint pain. Details regarding any of the possible etiologies previously discussed can be determined and may influence treatment options. Previous trauma should be explored thoroughly because it is the most

BOX 10.1 ETIOLOGY OF DEGENERATIVE JOINT DISEASE OF THE ANKLE

- Trauma
- Inflammatory
- Metabolic
- Neuroarthropathy
- Infectious
- Tumor
- Blood dyscrasia
- Iatrogenic
- Congenital
- Idiopathic

frequent cause of degenerative joint disease of the ankle. The patient's age, occupation, level of activity and autonomy, and past medical and surgical history as well as other joint involvement are important. When surgery is considered, the patient's discontinuation of tobacco use may help to reduce wound or bone healing problems, particularly because decreased fusion rates have been identified in smokers.

- Ankle osteoarthritis usually presents with pain and mechanical symptoms at the anterior aspect of the ankle joint.
  - Pain, which is increased with weight bearing and decreased with unloading, is the most common presenting complaint.
  - Morning pain and stiffness on arising or start-up pain is common.
- Previous treatments such as shoe modifications, orthotics, braces, medications, and changes in activity and their results should be reviewed.
- Neuroarthropathy represents a unique situation in which the patient may notice the appearance of swelling, deformity, and instability associated with relatively little pain at the level of the ankle.

Clinical Findings

- The ankle joint examination is similar to that for other major weight-bearing joints.
  - A complete examination includes gait analysis, inspection, palpation, neurovascular evaluation, active and passive ranges of motion of the ankle and the adjacent joints, strength testing, and ligament stability evaluation.
  - This examination should be compared with the contralateral lower limb findings.
- Gait analysis in the presence of ankle degeneration reveals a decreased velocity and stride length. An antalgic gait pattern is frequently observed.
- Weight-bearing evaluation reveals the clinical magnitude of any deformity.
- Ankle degenerative joint disease commonly presents with decreased range of motion at the ankle joint and usually reproduces the patient's pain.
  - Normal sagittal motion ranges from 25° of dorsiflexion to approximately 30° of plantarflexion rotating about an axis crossing the tip of the medial and the lateral malleoli.
  - Because this approximated axis of rotation is relatively oblique compared with the longitudinal axis of the leg, ankle dorsiflexion is associated with external rotation and plantarflexion with internal rotation of the foot.
- Tendon function and muscle strength are assessed to provide a more complete understanding of the patient's limitations.
- Ligament stability on both the medial and the lateral aspects of the ankle is assessed functionally on examination as well as radiographically, if necessary.

Radiographic Findings

- Degenerative joint disease of the ankle is best visualized using standardized weight-bearing plain X-rays.

- □ The degree of joint degeneration can be underestimated when the X-ray is performed non–weight bearing.
- □ Most institutions use weight-bearing X-rays to ensure a more accurate measurement of the extent of cartilage involvement and to provide a more dynamic picture of the status of the ankle and hindfoot joints (Fig. 10.2).
- Three views—the anteroposterior (AP), lateral, and mortise—of the ankle joint are usually sufficient to reveal the majority of pathologies related to degenerative joint disease of the ankle.
- Positive findings should be correlated with clinical findings.
- The radiographic signs most commonly associated with osteoarthritis include the following:
  - □ Joint space narrowing
  - □ Subchondral sclerosis
  - □ Cysts
  - □ Osteophytes
- Other radiographic findings may depend on the etiology that led to the degenerative joint disease, such as gout or rheumatoid arthritis.
  - □ In patients with inflammatory arthropathies, such as rheumatoid arthritis, symmetric joint involvement with periarticular osteopenia and marginal erosion is common. In addition, the ankle joint and hindfoot frequently demonstrate a severe valgus deformity.
  - □ In the crystalline arthropathies, early involvement of the ankle joint presents as an effusion with soft-tissue swelling.
  - □ Gout is progressive, eventually creating punched-out erosions beneath the joint surfaces.
  - □ Pseudogout or calcium pyrophosphate deposition disease eventually leads to chondrocalcinosis within the joint.
- Other imaging modalities include MRI, which is used to evaluate soft tissues, tendons, cartilage lesions or talus viability in cases of avascular necrosis, and CT

scanning, which provides improved three-dimensional visualization of the bony architecture through the hindfoot.

- Technetium bone scans are a high-sensitivity and low-specificity assessment of changes in bone metabolism and may be helpful when evaluating for occult fractures or acute and subacute chondral injuries. However, the utility of bone scans with respect to degenerative joint disease of the ankle is somewhat limited.

Diagnostic Injections

When doubts persist about the origin of the patient's pain, diagnostic injections of the ankle joint remain an excellent tool to clarify the clinical situation. A typical injection of approximately 5 mL of 1% or 2% Xylocaine with no epinephrine into the ankle joint is performed through the anterolateral (lateral to peroneus tertius) or anteromedial approach (medial to tibialis anterior). The injection may be done under fluoroscopic control, with or without contrast, to ensure intra-articular positioning that can be helpful with severe joint space collapse. Following the injection, the patient evaluates the level of pain and how long this change lasts.

TREATMENT

Nonoperative Treatment

Many nonsurgical options exist for patients with ankle arthritis. Often, the patient is unaware of these options or has not been willing to try them. However, when presented with the surgical risks and a lengthy postoperative recovery process, the patient may opt for a less aggressive approach. General recommendations for treatment of symptomatic degenerative joint disease is similar for all weight-bearing joints of the body and include anti-inflammatory medications, ambulatory aids, and bracing. Although nonsurgical treatment does not cure the degenerative changes, many patients can experience significant pain relief and may be

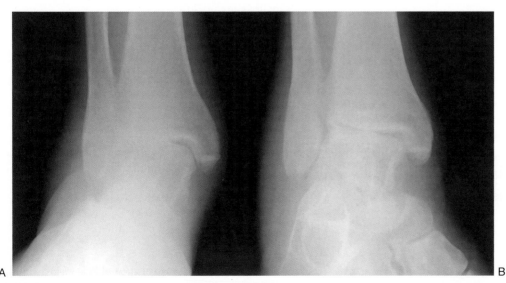

Figure 10.2 Weight-bearing ankle X-ray (**A**) compared with non–weight-bearing view (**B**), demonstrating the value of weight-bearing X-rays to better evaluate the status of the joint.

able to postpone definitive surgical reconstruction until it is more convenient or their symptoms progress.

- Symptomatic pain relief can be obtained by using local and systemic medications.
  - ☐ The local injection of intra-articular steroids two to three times per year may provide substantial relief of the symptoms, especially for inflammatory arthropathy.
  - ☐ Systemic medications may include acetaminophen on a regular basis, nonsteroidal anti-inflammatories, or nutritional supplements such as glucosamine and chondroitin sulfate, but narcotics should be avoided.
- Activity modifications, use of ambulatory aids such as a cane or walker, and orthotic appliances can also be helpful.
  - ☐ It is important to adapt the treatment to the patient's needs and lifestyle.
  - ☐ The University of California Biomechanics Laboratory (UCBL) insert is a low-profile orthosis designed for active patients (Fig. 10.3A). It allows correction of flexible malalignment, but does not immobilize the ankle joint, and it may not work well for end-stage disease.
  - ☐ A flexible brace, such as a lace-up brace, decreases motion and provides some support.
  - ☐ A custom-molded rigid ankle–foot orthosis (AFO) controls ankle motion and remains the gold standard for bracing in ankle degenerative joint disease (see Fig. 10.3C).
  - ☐ Each of these orthotic appliances can be combined with a rocker bottom shoe modification to encourage a more normal gait pattern.

Surgical Treatment

When nonsurgical treatment fails to adequately control the patient's symptoms, surgical intervention may become necessary.

Synovectomy, Loose Body Removal, and Ankle Joint Cheilectomy

The management of early or mild cases of ankle degenerative joint disease is selected according to the underlying etiology.

Chronic inflammatory synovitis, as seen in rheumatoid arthritis or chronic synovitis attributed to recurrent hemarthrosis in hemophilia—which has been symptomatic for greater than 6 months with no satisfactory response to nonsurgical treatment—may be addressed with open or arthroscopic synovectomy. It is important to discuss the goals of the procedure with the patient, which is merely to alleviate the pain. With regrowth of the synovium, the patient usually experiences recurrence of symptoms.

Symptomatic loose bodies in the ankle joint can be excised to control mechanical symptoms and to limit the progression of further cartilaginous lesions. Traumatic lesions with damaging loose bodies, impinging synovial chondromatosis, and displaced intra-articular orthopaedic implants are some other examples that may respond well to excision, either arthroscopic or through open arthrotomy.

Some selected mild and moderate cases of ankle osteoarthrosis with a preserved joint space may benefit from removal of osteophytes (cheilectomy). Osteophytes can be visualized on the anterior distal part of the tibia and the dorsal aspect of the talus (Fig. 10.4), but in one cadaveric study, they were found to rarely be in close contact on forced dorsiflexion. Even so, many patients report symptoms related to anterior impingement with painful limited dorsiflexion of the ankle, which respond well to surgical debridement. In more advanced cases, the patient generally does not feel relief because of the underlying joint disease. When planning incisions, it is important to keep in mind the high likelihood for further surgery in this area, including possible ankle fusion or arthroplasty.

Ankle Arthrodesis

Ankle arthrodesis remains the gold standard for surgical treatment of patients with advanced degenerative joint disease of the ankle that has failed conservative management.

Current surgical techniques designed to obtain bony union continue to rely on basic orthopaedic principles: a large surface area of healthy bleeding cancellous bone apposition combined with compression at the level of the intended fusion site and rigid fixation. In general, patients with rheumatoid arthritis have a higher union rate, possibly because of their relative lack of dense, hypertrophic

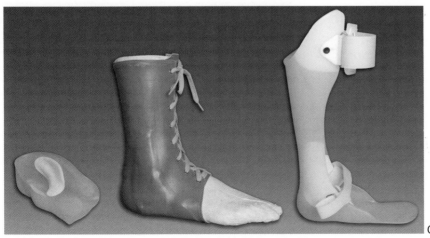

A,B   C

Figure 10.3 Nonsurgical treatment devices: (**A**) example of the UCBL, (**B**) the Arizona Brace, and (**C**) custom-molded rigid AFO.

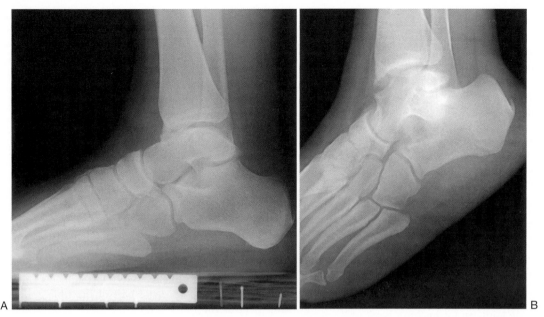

Figure 10.4 Lateral weight-bearing (**A**) and oblique (**B**) foot X-rays of a 33-year-old man with posttraumatic degenerative joint disease. Patient presented with anterior impingement pain when dorsiflexing his ankle joint.

cortical bone. Patients with a higher risk for delayed union or nonunion include smokers or those who are noncompliant and patients with spasticity, significant bone defects, poorly vascularized lower limbs, and infected or neuroarthropathic cases. These conditions may have a significant impact when choosing a particular operative technique or the postoperative management.

Biomechanical Principles. A successful ankle arthrodesis not only provides predictable results with regard to pain relief, but also requires the adjacent joints and low back to compensate for motion loss by absorbing increased stresses. This may lead to early degenerative changes in those areas and should be discussed with the patient before surgery. Ankle fusion eliminates the motion contribution from that joint, which in turn limits sagittal plantarflexion and dorsiflexion by approximately 70%.

The position in which the tibiotalar joint is fused remains paramount to minimizing postfusion-related problems. Obtaining a solid union in neutral dorsiflexion and approximately 5° of hindfoot valgus is optimal. The arthrodesis should also be positioned at about 10° of external rotation, or symmetric to the contralateral ankle (if uninvolved). Slight posterior translation of the talus relative to the distal tibia may provide some biomechanical advantage to assist the fusion while minimizing the tendency to vault over the foot during gait.

Technical Options. Over the years, many different techniques have been described for ankle arthrodesis. Although no one technique has proved clearly superior to the others, several principles have emerged to enhance the chances of a successful outcome. When evaluating each case, several factors may influence the choice of technique, including the patient's biologic makeup (soft tissues, body habitus, expected union rate, quality of bone, etc.), the patient's psychological makeup, the surgeon's experience, and possibly

the patient's preference. No single technique is appropriate for every case.

The spectrum of surgical options ranges from arthroscopic joint preparation with limited internal or external fixation devices to open fusion with more substantial internal fixation using only screws or plates and screws (Box 10.2). Each surgical technique possesses its inherent advantages and disadvantages.

The preparation of the fusion interface can be accomplished arthroscopically in cases that do not require significant correction of deformity or position. This procedure is a less invasive approach, minimizing soft-tissue trauma and postoperative pain, but it carries a significant learning curve for the surgeon (Fig. 10.5A). Alternatively, open debridement permits more extensive visualization of the articular surfaces while allowing the surgeon to correct malalignment more easily. The more recent development

---

BOX 10.2 SURGICAL OPTIONS FOR ISOLATED ANKLE ARTHRODESIS

Articular Surface Debridement
- Arthroscopic
- Mini-open
- Open

Fixation Techniques
External Fixation
- Uniplanar (Charnley)
- Triangular (Calandruccio)
- Circular (Ilizarov)

Internal Fixation
- Steinman pins
- Cannulated compression screws
- Plates and screws
- Blade plate

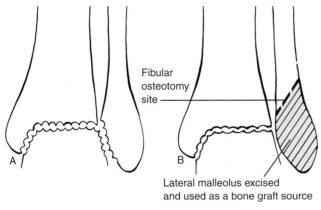

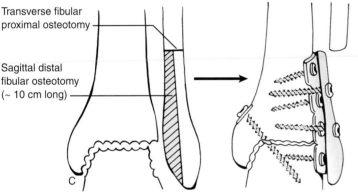

Figure 10.5 Various ankle articular surface debridement options. **A:** The mini-open technique is an option in cases with no significant deformity. **B:** A distal fibular osteotomy 10 cm from the most distal portion provides an excellent source of autologous bone graft. Resection of the medial aspect of the lateral malleolus and fixation using the anterolateral "tension-band technique" is useful in ankles with moderate-to-severe deformity. The remaining lateral cortical strut augments the fixation as shown on the right.

of mini-open approaches, which use extended arthroscopic portal incisions, combines some of the advantages of both open and arthroscopic debridements.

Surgical Technique

- Open ankle arthrodesis remains the standard procedure.
- In the supine position, draping is performed, taking care to allow complete access to the tibia and the knee.
- A thigh tourniquet is routinely used by most surgeons.
- Several approaches can be considered, taking into account the quality of soft tissues, previous incisions, and surgeon's experience.
  - □ A single longitudinal midline anterior approach between the extensor hallus longus and the tibialis anterior tendon has been described, but the disadvantages of this approach include poor access to the medial and lateral gutters and possible neurovascular injury.
  - □ The most common approach uses bilateral longitudinal medial and lateral incisions with a lateral malleolus osteotomy. A skin bridge of at least 7 cm is maintained to protect the vascular supply to the skin. Distal fibular osteotomy allows excellent visualization and constitutes a good autologous source of bone graft (see Fig. 10.5B).
  - □ The posterior approach may be considered in cases with significant soft-tissue scarring anteriorly or multiple prior incisions elsewhere. The Achilles tendon is split longitudinally, and the flexor hallus longus muscle belly is progressively detached from the posterior aspect of the fibula and retracted medially,

protecting the tibial nerve and posterior tibial vessels (Fig. 10.6).
- The joint surfaces are debrided to healthy cancellous bone, preserving as much bone stock as possible. Osteotomes and rongeurs theoretically avoid thermal trauma created by saws and burrs, which may diminish the rate of fusion.
- Bone surface apposition should be maximized while preparing the fusion; feathering or shingling the surfaces to ensure that the sclerotic subchondral bone has been adequately debrided can be helpful.

Fixation has evolved over the years, ranging from external to internal fixation, with most surgeons presently using internal fixation. External fixation devices remain an important tool in the surgeon's armamentarium, especially in cases with infection or occasionally compromised soft tissues. Sir John Charnley developed a uniplanar external fixation device that has evolved into multiplanar external transfixing devices to apply compression more evenly across the ankle fusion site. Ilizarov's principles using circular wire fixators have also been applied, which progressively add compression across the joint.

- Internal fixation can be accomplished with various devices.
  - □ When bone quality permits, screws allow the use of lag technique to create compression across the fusion site.
    - □ Parallel screws, in theory, generate continued compression along the axis of the screws.
    - □ In practice, crossed screws provide even greater purchase with an increased load to failure (Fig. 10.7).

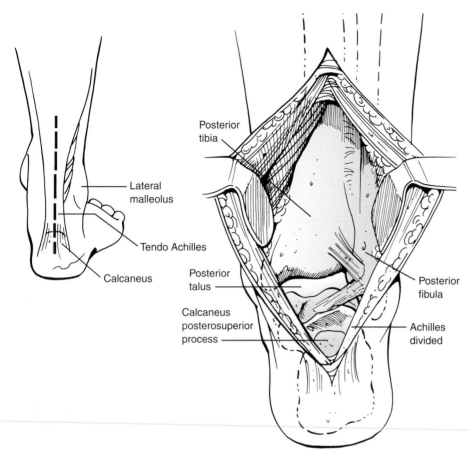

Posterior tibia

Lateral malleolus

Tendo Achilles

Calcaneus

Posterior talus

Calcaneus posterosuperior process

Posterior fibula

Achilles divided

Figure 10.6   Posterior approach to the ankle and subtalar joint. The Achilles tendon can be split longitudinally or coronally and reflected to gain access to the posterior aspect of the ankle as well as the subtalar joint. The flexor hallucis longus muscle belly is released from the posterior fibula and retracted medially, protecting the medial neurovascular structures.

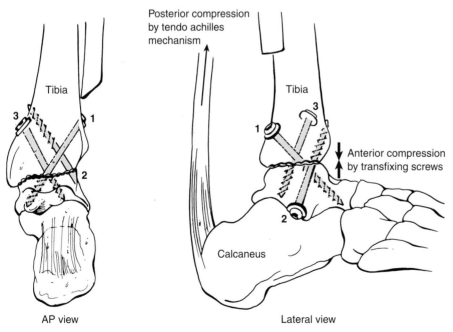

Posterior compression by tendo achilles mechanism

Tibia

Tibia

Anterior compression by transfixing screws

Calcaneus

AP view

Lateral view

Figure 10.7   Ankle fusion technique utilizing anterior compression screws, with the tendo-Achilles posteriorly theoretically providing compression across the fusion site.

☐ In patients with poor bone quality, such as those on chronic steroid therapy or rheumatoid arthritis, Steinman pins may be the only fixation possible.

☐ Alternatively, an "anterolateral tension-band plate technique" creating compression through a reconstruction plate represents one of the most rigid fixation techniques, especially in cases with preoperative moderate to severe deformity (see Figs. 10.8 and 10.5C).

☐ Finally, blade plates provide yet another option to the surgeon for more rigid fixation and have been used with success, particularly in osteoporotic patients or when large bone defects are present.

Bone Grafting. Routine use of bone grafting in primary ankle arthrodesis remains common, but may be unnecessary. Some ankle fusions may be complicated by a significant bone defect or by insufficient bone-to-bone apposition and thus require grafting. Attempting to fuse any unhealthy bone end to another is a risk that can be avoided by adequate debridement, taking into consideration the resulting defect. The use of bone graft should not be considered a replacement for proper preparation of bone surfaces. Although the use of graft material to help in those circumstances is a well-established practice, there is paucity of evidence-based literature to rely on when it comes to choosing one type of graft over another. A great deal of interest has prompted an increase in research regarding bone grafts and bone graft substitutes, and their results need to be closely scrutinized for variables and appropriate controls.

▪ Depending on the size of the defect, a structural or morcellized graft can be used.

▪ Large defects can be best filled with a tricortical iliac crest graft to fill the space and maintain the length of the lower limb.

▪ Autologous graft, allograft products, and synthetic substitutes represent a variety of bone graft options, with their respective advantages and disadvantages.

Postoperative Management

▪ Following the procedure, a compressive dressing and splint are applied to control swelling and maintain appropriate alignment.

▪ The use of a popliteal block for postoperative pain relief can significantly reduce the need for narcotics, both during and after surgery.

☐ Most patients are highly satisfied with their postoperative pain control following a popliteal block. The use of narcotics and hospital stay are also decreased with the use of this block, which lasts on average of 12 to 26 hours.

☐ The technique uses a nerve stimulator or ultrasound and can be safely performed after the patient is under general anesthesia with bupivacaine or ropivicaine (Fig. 10.9).

▪ When swelling allows, a non–weight-bearing short leg fiberglass cast is applied to help maintain neutral alignment.

▪ The expected duration to fusion can vary depending on several factors, and the immobilization is adjusted for each case on the basis of on regular clinical and radiologic assessments.

☐ In general, the patient is kept non–weight bearing for 6 weeks and then put in a walking cast for an additional 4 to 6 weeks. A walking cast boot can be used thereafter until satisfactory bony and clinical union is achieved.

☐ In some cases, such as neuroarthropathy, the period of non–weight bearing and total length of cast immobilization may need to be adjusted, sometimes doubling or tripling the usual recovery process.

Results. Successful ankle arthrodesis occurs in approximately 85% to 90% of cases, but rates have varied widely over the years, from 50% to more than 90%. Long-term follow-up studies, at more than 25 years, reveal the results to be durable and the patients to be satisfied, despite additional degenerative changes seen in the adjacent joints. Some patients may benefit from rocker bottom shoe modifications following ankle fusion, which can improve their gait, particularly if the hindfoot joints have some ankylosis.

Complications. Nonunion remains the most frequent significant complication associated with ankle arthrodesis. Causes vary widely and include biologic and mechanical factors. The initial treatment for symptomatic nonunion includes bracing, activity modification, and other nonsurgical modalities. However, when these fail to control the symptoms, a revision arthrodesis may be considered. In those cases, it is important to identify risk factors for pseudoarthrosis, such as smoking, poor vascularization, patient noncompliance with weight-bearing restrictions, infection, technical errors, or hardware failure. Despite improved techniques, implants, and graft materials, revision ankle arthrodesis continues to yield a disappointing 20% nonunion rate in nonneurologic conditions. Neuroarthropathic patients have a much higher nonunion rate (50% or more).

Malunion of an ankle arthrodesis constitutes another complication. Malposition during surgery or progressive adjacent joint deformity can lead to clinical symptoms. Mild or moderate varus or valgus deformity may be compensated with shoe modifications or orthotic appliances. Relative plantarflexion creates a vaulting type of gait pattern and leads to symptomatic knee pain resulting from a hyperextension or back knee component during the midstance phase of gait. Excessive external or especially internal rotation is difficult to compensate for and can lead to significant gait disturbances. Major malposition may require correction with an osteotomy.

Persistent pain despite solid fusion can often be attributed to underlying subtalar pathology that might have been present preoperatively or might have developed subsequent to the ankle arthrodesis. Diagnostic injection may help to confirm this. Other long-term complications include biomechanical effects due to increased stress and motion in adjacent joints. Overuse of these joints at a supraphysiologic level can lead to progressive degeneration in these articulations as well.

Ankle Arthrodesis Following Tibial Pilon Fracture. Tibial pilon fractures have a high rate of subsequent ankle degenerative joint disease. The more severe

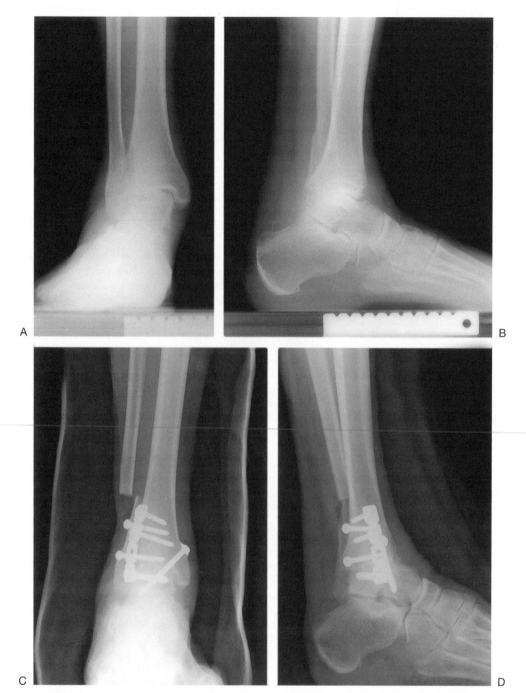

Figure 10.8   Standing AP (**A**) and lateral (**B**) X-rays showing ankle degenerative joint disease. (**C, D**) Ankle fusion was accomplished by using a 4.5-mm pelvic reconstruction plate to apply compression anterolaterally. The Achilles tendon provides posterior compression to counterbalance the plate. The remaining lateral half of the lateral malleolus was used to augment the fusion site.

the articular surface involvement, the greater the likelihood that a patient will require more definitive management.

Ankle arthrodesis can be performed as a primary, a late primary, or a secondary procedure. Choosing between those options remains a matter of judgment and experience. Primary arthrodesis following an acute, highly comminuted pilon fracture allows the definitive treatment to be accomplished in one intervention, but it sacrifices the joint and is a technically demanding surgery. Currently, the trend is to attempt an acute or subacute anatomic reduction with

articular fixation and potentially allow the joint to recover. One goal in treating these fractures acutely includes preservation of bone stock for later reconstruction. If post-traumatic degenerative joint disease develops, a secondary ankle arthrodesis is a reasonable salvage option.

Total Ankle Arthroplasty
Although ankle arthrodesis has traditionally been considered the time-tested standard for end-stage degenerative joint disease unresponsive to nonsurgical treatment, total

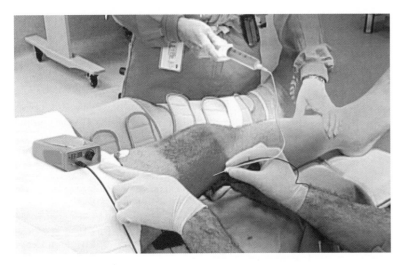

Figure 10.9 Trans-biceps femoris popliteal block performed using a nerve stimulator to provide postoperative pain control. Superficial anatomy landmarks are located, a modification of the lateral technique of McLeod and colleagues, through the biceps femoris to identify the common tibial peroneal nerve sheath. (From Kile TA. Tibiotalocalcaneal arthrodesis. In: Kitaoka HB, ed. Master techniques in orthopaedic surgery: the foot and ankle, 2nd ed. Philadelphia: Lippincott Williams & Wilkins, 2002:553.)

ankle arthroplasty (TAA) has evolved as another viable option in selected patients. TAAs were first performed in the 1970s. The early results revealed high success and satisfaction rates. Enthusiasm diminished as the longer-term results revealed rapid deterioration, such that by the mid-1980s, total ankle replacements were almost completely abandoned.

Despite these poor early results, interest in total joint arthroplasties has persisted and multiple designs of implants in various populations have been performed. Although the popularity of this reconstructive option has waxed and waned, it continues to evolve and greatly improve with new technology development. Recent advances have included the development of highly cross-linked polyethylene, biologic ingrowth fixation to bone, and improved surgical techniques. The decision to perform TAA has become more of a decision to accept the potential complications linked with TAA in an effort to preserve motion at the ankle joint.

Multiple implant designs have been attempted over the years. They have varied in their amount of constraint, interfaces, axes of rotation, and fixation type, among other technical aspects. Most modern TAA systems comprise three components: a flat baseplate on the undersurface of the tibia or stemmed tibial component, a domed component for the resurfaced talus, and a polyethylene spacer between the two metallic (or ceramic) components. In two-piece or fixed-bearing systems, the spacer is attached to the tibial baseplate. In three-piece or mobile-bearing systems, the polyethylene spacer is free to articulate with the talar and tibial components independently.

Proponents of mobile-bearing designs argue that less sheer and torsional forces occur between the polyethylene and the metallic components. Concerns regarding mobile-bearing designs in comparison with fixed-bearing systems include increased backside wear of the polyethylene against the tibial baseplate that could theoretically lead to smaller debris particles that may potentially induce more osteolysis, edge-loading of the polyethylene, and increased risk of dislocation of the mobile spacer. Retrospective case reviews have demonstrated similar clinical outcomes of TAA performed with fixed or mobile-bearing designs.

Indications and Contraindication Although controversy remains regarding the appropriate indications for TAA, some general guidelines are emerging from results obtained in early to midterm follow-up studies. Most authors agree that the ideal candidate is a low-demand, lower body mass index patient older than 60 years of age with minimal deformity. However, there is no clinical evidence to support these guidelines or recommendations, and considerable debate still exists today regarding the selection of patients for TAA.

Similarly, no consensus exists regarding relative contraindications to TAA, but generally they include age less than 45 to 50 years, history of infection, severe malalignment, avascular necrosis of the talus, poor soft-tissue envelope, tobacco use, neuroarthropathy, severe osteoporosis, and morbid obesity. Current active infection and an absent distal fibula are absolute contraindications to TAA.

Surgical Technique

- An anterior approach is routinely used between the anterior tibialis tendon and the extensor hallucis longus.
- A second longitudinal incision may be needed over the lateral aspect of the ankle to gain access to the lateral malleolus and the anterior syndesmosis.
- An external fixator can be used intraoperatively aiding in visualization and correction of deformity, but adds to operating room time, expense, and may have increased risks.
- The goals for preparation of the bone surfaces aim to preserve as much bone as possible, given the prosthetic design, to make bone cuts in a reproducible way to provide for a mechanically neutral final implant position, and to avoid any remaining impingement in the lateral and medial gutters.
- Of particular importance, regardless of the implant selected, is the need to establish adequate soft-tissue balancing.
- Reconstruction of the collateral ligaments may be necessary when there is instability or insufficiency, and it needs to be assessed throughout the procedure.
- Tibial and talar components are then applied using biologic fixation or cement, based on fitting of components and the expected capacity to obtain bone ingrowth between the adjacent bone and the implant (Fig. 10.10).

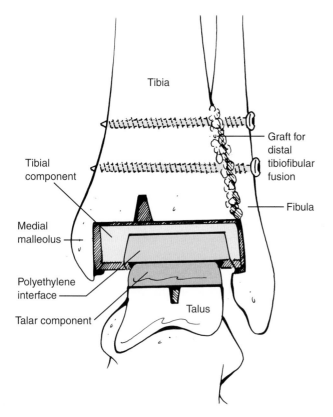

Figure 10.10 TAA with the agility implant. A fusion of the distal syndesmosis provides a more stable platform for the components and prevents subsidence.

■ Intraoperative use of radiographs and fluoroscopy provides critical information regarding the position of the components. In one design system, a distal tibiofibular fusion is created by decortication, bone grafting, and fixing with syndesmosis screws to provide a more stable platform for the tibial component.

■ Finally, before the meticulous multilayer closing is finished, the range of motion and stability of the components are examined during the final check (Fig. 10.11).

Postoperative Management

■ The patient is given a bulky compressive dressing for the immediate postoperative period.

■ A trans-biceps femoris knee block or other regional block preoperatively can be used for improved pain control postoperatively.

■ Prophylactic intravenous antibiotics are routinely given for 24 hours from the anesthetic induction.

■ Rehabilitation programs vary, but generally include progressive range of motion as tolerated once the first dressing is removed and the incisions are healed, with no weight bearing until the distal tibiofibular arthrodesis has healed or early bone ingrowth has occurred—usually around 6 to 8 weeks.

■ A removable cast boot may be used to protect the surgical wound during this time.

Results. The results of TAA have varied widely over the years. With the first generation of cemented implants,

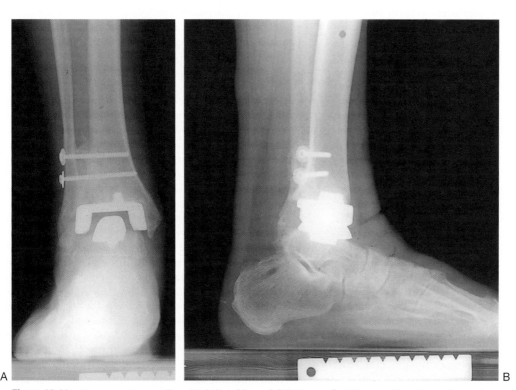

Figure 10.11 Postoperative standing AP (**A**) and lateral (**B**) X-rays of a 69-year-old patient who underwent TAA 10 months ago for symptomatic posttraumatic ankle degenerative joint disease. (Courtesy of R.J. Claridge, MD, Mayo Clinic, Scottsdale, Arizona.)

survival rate of implant ranged from 60% to 100% at follow-up of 1 to 3 years. However, when these patients were evaluated at 5 to 15 years, the implant survival rate was only 10% to 61% leading most surgeons to abandon the procedure altogether. The more modern designs with improved surgical techniques have better early to midterm results with many studies currently being published reporting longer-term follow-up ranging from 8 to 16 years. These recent reports demonstrate implant survival rates ranging from 80% to 93% with patient reports of satisfactory pain relief in about 80% of cases.

When compared with ankle arthrodesis, TAA provides a unique set of complications, uncertainty about long-term survival of the implants, and varying reports of persistent ankle pain. Several recent level III studies have consistently demonstrated similar pain relief between TAA and arthrodesis with increased risk of reoperation with TAA and increased risk of adjacent joint degeneration with arthrodesis. In addition, clinical gait analysis studies comparing TAA and arthrodesis indicate that patients with ankle arthrodesis may have a faster but more asymmetric gait pattern. This seems to be the compromise to retain motion at the ankle joint with arthroplasties (Table 10.1). Postoperative range of motion is generally unchanged from preoperative measurements with the current generation of implants.

Complications. The limited survival of TAA is the most common significant complication (Fig. 10.12). Loosening of implants, talar subsidence, subluxation of components, and malleolar fractures represent different mechanisms of failure. Wound-healing problems are also frequently reported and in the past were found in up to half of the primary total ankle procedures. Deep wound infections are a potentially catastrophic complication, occurring at a rate of 3% to 5%.

Because component failure represents a relatively universal complication of this technique, it becomes essential to have some ideas regarding salvage procedures. If revision to a larger implant or different manufacturer is not an option, implant removal and some form of arthrodesis will be necessary. Depending on the size of the bone defect, quality of the soft-tissue envelope, location of previous skin incisions, and history of an infection, a variety of treatment options

are available. Medial and lateral incisions may afford easy access to the ankle, but may make retrieval of the implants difficult. Anterior or posterior approaches constitute acceptable ways to perform a salvage ankle fusion, each with its wound healing issues.

Structural iliac crest autograft or allograft in the residual defect with external or internal fixation to maintain position and generate compression can be used to obtain a functional ankle fusion. Internal fixation for these challenging revisions can be achieved in various ways using any of the technical options discussed earlier in this chapter. External fixation has been reported by several authors to provide satisfactory results for salvage arthrodeses in failed TAA. Some patients may be better served with a below-knee amputation, particularly in cases of deep sepsis with poor soft tissues.

HINDFOOT DEGENERATIVE JOINT DISEASE

The hindfoot comprises four bones: the talus, the calcaneus, the navicular, and the cuboid. They form three joints:

- Subtalar joint: the link between the talus and the calcaneus
- Talonavicular joint: a mobile joint linking the hindfoot to the medial three rays of the foot
- Calcaneocuboid joint: the link between the hindfoot and the lateral two rays (the lateral column)

These three joints contribute to hindfoot motion. The talonavicular and calcaneocuboid joints form the transverse tarsal or Chopart joint. In early stance phase, the axes of these two joints become parallel or "unlocked," permitting an increased range of motion and flexible hindfoot. In late stance phase, the hindfoot inverts and the axes of the joints are divergent, locking the motion and creating a rigid lever for the foot to provide push off more efficiently.

Any isolated fusion within this complex influences range of motion in the adjacent joints. Specifically, isolated sub-

TABLE 10.1 COMPARISON OF PROPOSED ADVANTAGES AND DISADVANTAGES OF TOTAL ANKLE ARTHROPLASTY VERSUS ANKLE ARTHRODESIS

	Total Ankle Arthroplasty	Ankle Arthrodesis
Pain relief	Excellent	Excellent
Retained ankle joint motion	More	None
Wound healing complications	More	Some
Risk of infection	Higher	Lower
Risk of reoperation	Higher	Lower
Risk of adjacent joint degeneration	Lower	Higher
Postoperative gait speed	Slower	Faster
Postoperative limp	Less	More

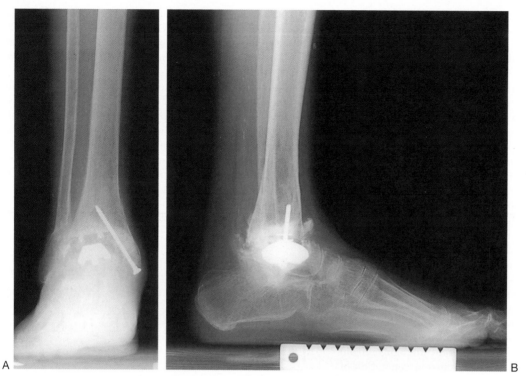

Figure 10.12 Standing AP (**A**) and lateral (**B**) X-rays of a 76-year-old patient who underwent TAA 24 years earlier for posttraumatic degenerative ankle joint disease. The patient sustained a previous medial malleolus fracture that required internal fixation. Note the subsidence of the talar component in this patient whose case was successfully managed with an Arizona brace and a rocker bottom shoe.

talar fusion decreases talonavicular joint motion by about 25% and calcaneocuboid joint motion by approximately 50%. Calcaneocuboid fusion decreases hindfoot motion overall by about one-third. Talonavicular fusion essentially locks hindfoot motion.

PATHOGENESIS

Hindfoot degenerative joint disease may arise from various etiologies; the differential diagnosis is similar to that for the pathogenesis of ankle osteoarthritis. Despite the similarities at that level, some particularities regarding the hindfoot are worth mentioning.

Hindfoot degenerative joint disease remains largely related to posttraumatic changes and inflammatory processes such as rheumatoid arthritis. Of note, deformities caused by neuromuscular disease or classic posterior tibial tendon dysfunction constitute additional specific etiologies to keep in mind. In the adult acquired flatfoot, the progressive loss of the longitudinal medial arch causes subluxation of joints with abnormal biomechanical stresses and inflammation, which can lead to degenerative changes. Neuroarthropathic joint disease is of particular interest with the increasing number of patients affected by diabetes. Although the hindfoot does not represent the most frequent site of Charcot arthropathy, the index of suspicion remains high with the occurrence of severe bone and joint destruction.

DIAGNOSIS

Physical Examination and History

A thorough history constitutes an essential tool in the assessment of the patient with hindfoot disease. Specifically, questions regarding the nature of the symptoms, their location and their progression; aggravating factors; previous attempted treatments; and results are helpful in determining the cause of the patient's symptoms and guide further treatment.

- Subtalar degenerative joint disease typically causes pain over the sinus tarsi area, swelling, stiffness, and difficulty with walking on uneven surfaces. In cases following a calcaneus fracture, a palpable bony bulge and tenderness may be present beneath the tip of the fibula where the lateral wall of the calcaneus may be impinging on the peroneal tendons.
- Some patients note a progressive deformity of the hindfoot area.
- The use of medications, orthotics, or braces and the results obtained also bring valuable clues to the diagnosis and eventually the treatment.

Clinical Features

A systematic approach is necessary to arrive at an accurate diagnosis. Specifically for the hindfoot physical examination, the other joints, bones, and soft tissues need careful assessment to avoid confusion about the primary pathology or pain generator.

- Subtalar degenerative joint disease classically has tenderness directly over the sinus tarsi and may be accompanied by restricted subtalar motion that reproduces the patient's symptoms.
  - ☐ The subtalar joint contributes to movement in the coronal plane. Generally, the patients have approximately 20° of inversion and 5° of eversion.
  - ☐ In practice, it becomes important to understand the hindfoot joints' work as a whole, each contributing varying amounts of motion in the axial plane (internal and external rotations) and in the sagittal plane (plantarflexion and dorsiflexion).
- Talonavicular disease is usually symptomatic on the dorsomedial aspect of the hindfoot and is often confused with anterior ankle joint pain.
  - ☐ Careful palpation over the two sites is usually all that is needed to determine joint that is the true source of the symptoms.
  - ☐ Painful impingement with limited dorsiflexion is usually accompanied by palpable dorsal osteophytes over this joint.
- Deformities involving the hindfoot require both dynamic and static standing evaluation.
- The fixed and flexible portions of hindfoot malalignment need to be identified and addressed because such findings may influence the choice of treatment.
- A complete hindfoot physical examination also includes an evaluation of the Achilles tendon and gastrocnemius–soleus complex to evaluate for tightness with the hindfoot in neutral alignment and the knee in flexion and in extension (Silfverskiold test).
- Many patients with obvious hindfoot deformities have equinus contractures, which may need to be addressed simultaneously with the hindfoot reconstructive surgical procedure.

Radiographic Findings

- Routine roentgenographic evaluation of hindfoot osteoarthritis is performed with weight-bearing foot X-rays, frequently including a weight-bearing AP view of both ankles to evaluate for concomitant ankle joint disease.
- A weight-bearing hindfoot alignment view is occasionally used to document the severity of hindfoot deformity by visualizing the actual dynamic deformity of the hindfoot in the coronal plane as compared with the longitudinal axis of the tibia (Fig. 10.13).
- Other views specific of the subtalar joint include the classic Broden and Canale views.
  - ☐ The medial oblique view described by Broden—the most widely used view—is obtained with the leg internally rotated 45°, varying the cephalad tilt from 10° to 40°. It provides visualization of the posterior facet of the subtalar joint.
  - ☐ The Canale view represents another method to visualize pathology within the sinus tarsi area. It is obtained in the AP plane with 75° of cephalad tilt and 15° of eversion.
- CT scanning has largely replaced these specialized X-rays for additional imaging of the hindfoot. Because of its superior ability to provide three plane reconstructions

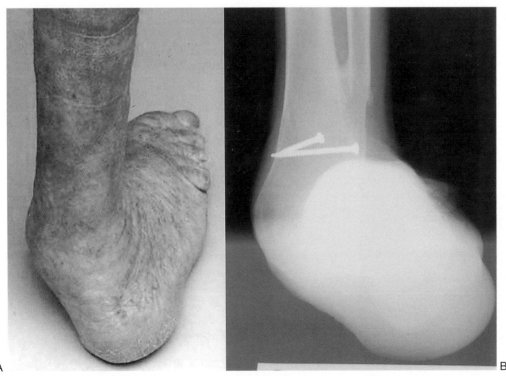

A   B

Figure 10.13 Clinical photo (**A**) and corresponding hindfoot alignment X-ray (**B**) in a 72-year-old patient with rheumatoid arthritis who had previously undergone ankle fusion elsewhere. This X-ray allows measurement of the degree of deformity, both angular and translational in the hindfoot, compared with the mechanical axis of the leg.

(sagittal, tranverse, and coronal), the CT is limited only in that its images are generated in a non–weight-bearing manner.

- MRI is gaining increased popularity in evaluating for hindfoot arthrosis, including subtle articular versus soft-tissue pathology.

Diagnostic Injections

Diagnostic injections constitute a valuable tool in confirming suspected hindfoot joint pathology and formulating a treatment plan (Fig. 10.14). Fluoroscopic guidance is frequently used to confirm the location of the needle tip, and it is used in severe posttraumatic degenerative joint disease with nearly obliterated joint surfaces. Subtalar joint injections can be performed through an anterolateral or a posterior approach. The magnitude of the relief and its duration, or lack thereof, may provide valuable information for diagnosis and offer a potential therapeutic benefit as well when corticosteroids are added to the injection.

TREATMENT

Nonoperative Treatment

The nonsurgical management of degenerative joint disease of the hindfoot is similar to that described for ankle degenerative joint disease, using nonsteroidal anti-inflammatory drugs, bracing, shoe modifications, and activity restriction. In particular, an ankle gauntlet brace (Arizona brace) is well suited for control of hindfoot motion and deformity.

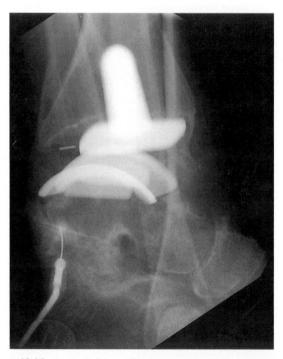

Figure 10.14 Lateral oblique fluoroscopy of a diagnostic injection that was used in this 80-year-old patient with a failed TAA to evaluate the contribution of the subtalar joint as an associated source of pain. Treatment plan was initiated based on the results, as seen in Figure 10.25.

When used in conjunction with intermittent corticosteroid injections, the brace may allow patients to be relatively pain free and avoid surgery indefinitely.

Surgical Treatment

Isolated Subtalar Arthrodesis

When nonsurgical treatment fails to provide adequate control of symptoms, surgical reconstruction may be an option. Isolated subtalar joint arthrodesis permits the correction of deformity and the relief of pain, with good-to-excellent long-term results. Performing a limited fusion of the subtalar joint, compared with performing a triple arthrodesis, allows the patient to maintain a mobile transverse tarsal joint and a relatively high level of function.

The fundamental principles of bone-to-bone fusion are discussed in the section on Ankle Arthrodesis.

Biomechanical Principles. The primary biomechanical consideration when planning an isolated subtalar arthrodesis is the position of the foot. As previously mentioned, slight hindfoot valgus prevents the "locking effect" on the transverse tarsal joint of Chopart (talonavicular and calcaneocuboid joints), by allowing them to remain relatively parallel to one another. This allows for a more flexible foot than would be obtained with slight varus or inversion of the foot.

The ideal position is 5° of hindfoot valgus, but this can be adjusted slightly to maintain the transverse forefoot plane perpendicular to the longitudinal axis of the leg and parallel to the floor. In cases of significant flatfoot deformity, it may be possible to bring the talus back up onto the calcaneus by lengthening the Achilles tendon and thereby avoiding the necessity of a triple arthrodesis.

Technical Options. Subtalar fusions have been performed using many different techniques, but most current practices use some type of large cannulated screws following the debridement of the joint and bone grafting of any dead space within the fusion site. Extra-articular subtalar fusion constitutes an alternative technique that includes the use of structural bone graft to fuse the subtalar joint at the level of the sinus tarsi, but it is generally confined to the pediatric population. In cases with significant loss of height following a calcaneus fracture, subtalar distraction arthrodesis has been successful. This procedure restores the talar angle of declination (an angle that measures the relative longitudinal axis of the talus as compared with the longitudinal axis of the calcaneus in the sagittal plane, on a weight-bearing lateral foot X-ray) using a structural tricortical bone autograft to maintain distraction at the fusion site (Fig. 10.15).

Surgical Technique

- An oblique lateral incision is made directly over the sinus tarsi, starting about 1 cm distal to the tip of the lateral malleolus and curving dorsally (Fig. 10.16).
- The fat pad of the sinus tarsi is dissected and reflected dorsally.

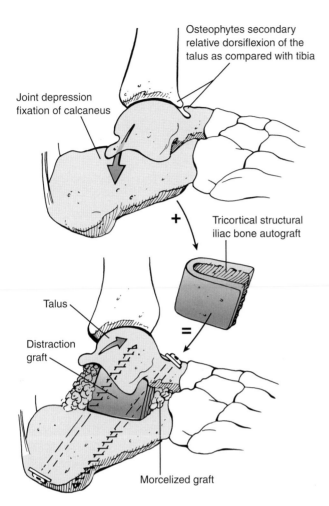

Figure 10.15 Subtalar distraction bone-block arthrodesis. The structural bone graft allows restoration of height through the hindfoot and the normal talar tilt on the calcaneus. A tricortical iliac crest autograft is positioned perpendicularly, taking advantage of the optimal strength of the graft.

- The extensor digitorum brevis muscle is detached inferiorly and reflected distally.
- The posterior margin of the approach is limited by the peroneus brevis and deeply by the calcaneofibular ligament.
- The superior margin includes the anterior talofibular ligament.
- The use of a lamina spreader, small curettes, and curved osteotomes helps to completely remove any remaining articular cartilage and the dense subchondral bone while maintaining the anatomic contour and exposing the underlying cancellous bone.
- A systematic preparation of the three subtalar articular facets begins anteriorly and works posteriorly, focusing on the posterior facet only after the others are completed (Fig. 10.16).
- The flexor hallucis longus tendon is usually visualized in the far posteromedial corner, indicating the limit of the posterior facet.
- The foot is grasped and the talus is reduced, relative to the calcaneus, providing for 5° of hindfoot valgus.
- Bone grafting is performed based on apposition of the surfaces and the patient's biologic makeup.

- The gold standard remains autograft, but donor site morbidity has prompted the development of a wide array of bone graft substitutes, each with its unique set of risks, benefits, and cost issues.

A special case occurs when the patient has arthritis following a malunited calcaneus fracture. They may have significant shortening of the calcaneal height leading to anterior ankle impingement and peroneal tendinitis between the tip of the fibula and the lateral wall of the calcaneus. They require a lateral wall exostectomy to decompress the peroneal tendons and either an osteotomy or a distraction arthrodesis (placement of structural graft into the arthrodesis site) of the calcaneus to restore its height.
- Rigid internal fixation with compression from partially threaded cancellous screws is presently the most common fixation technique used.
  - Screws are placed from the dorsomedial aspect of the talus down into the tuberosity of the calcaneus or vice versa (Figs. 10.17 and 10.18).
- Intraoperative fluoroscopic evaluation facilitates proper positioning of the implants and overall alignment of the hindfoot.
- Once satisfactory fixation is obtained, the closure is completed in a multilayer fashion, with care taken to maintain a meticulous respect for skin fragility.

Postoperative Management

- Perioperative prophylactic antibiotics are frequently used during the initial 24 hours.
- A compression dressing is applied in the operating room and left in place for 1 to 3 days.
- When the postoperative swelling and incisions allow, a short leg fiberglass non–weight-bearing cast is applied for the first 2 weeks, followed by another non–weight-bearing cast for an additional 4 weeks.
- As a general rule, after subtalar fusion, a non–weight-bearing cast is maintained for a total of 6 weeks, followed by 4 to 6 weeks in a weight-bearing below-knee cast or removable cast boot.
- When pain and swelling have subsided, the patient is allowed to wean from the removable cast boot as tolerated.
- Each case remains unique and may require adjustments based on the patient's pain level and the radiographic appearance during the postoperative course.

Results. The long-term satisfaction rate of subtalar fusion in patients with painful end-stage degenerative joint disease of the subtalar joint remains high and is reported in most publications at around 90%.

Generally, a patient with a well-positioned subtalar arthrodesis reaches a higher level of activity compared with a patient who undergoes a triple arthrodesis. Having some difficulty walking on uneven ground is expected, but most patients are able to continue to participate in recreational activities.

Complications Malunion and nonunion are the most common complications associated with subtalar arthrodesis. Union rates range from 70% to 100%. When nonunion

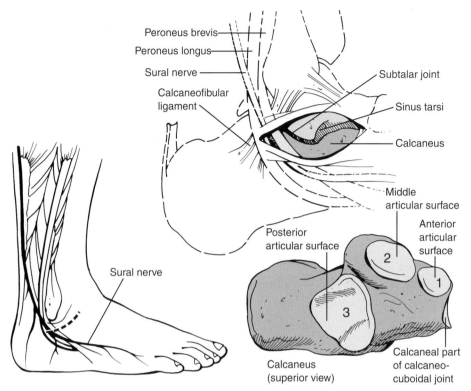

Figure 10.16 Lateral subtalar approach to gain access to the three articular facets (anterior, middle, and posterior) of the talocalcaneal joint. Fat pads over sinus tarsi and extensor digitorum brevis are detached and reflected distally.

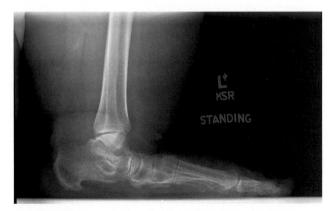

Figure 10.17 Preoperative lateral weight-bearing radiograph of foot with subtalar joint degeneration and significant flatfoot deformity.

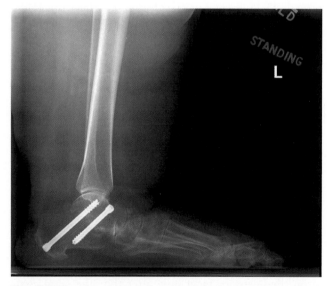

Figure 10.18   Postoperative lateral weight-bearing radiograph of foot after correction of hindfoot deformity and subtalar arthrodesis using two 6.5-mm cannulated screws for fixation.

does occur, revision arthrodesis with autologous bone graft and rigid fixation may be necessary but with an overall lower success rate.

Malalignment of the fusion constitutes another potential complication. Excessive varus locks the transverse tarsal joint and can affect the gait pattern, whereas too much valgus can create lateral impingement pain. Long-term consequences may include adjacent joint stress transfer, particularly through the ankle joint, which can lead to degenerative changes (Fig. 10.19).

Isolated Talonavicular Arthrodesis

The talonavicular joint remains one of the key joints for hindfoot motion. As a result, fusing it essentially eliminates subtalar and calcaneocuboid motion also. Adjacent

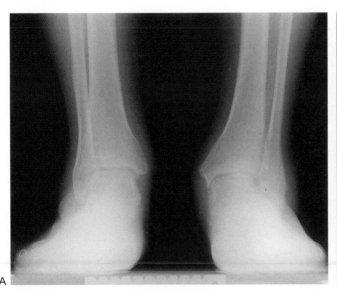
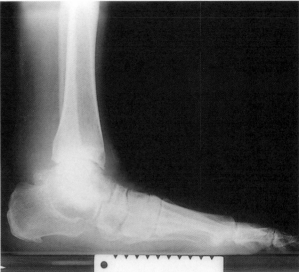

A   B

Figure 10.19   Standing AP (**A**) and lateral (**B**) X-rays 10 years after the subtalar fusion shown in
Figure 10.18. The subtalar fusion healed in valgus and eventually symptomatic ankle joint
degenerative arthritis with valgus collapse of the ankle developed.

joints are subjected to more stress to compensate for
the fused joint and, by necessity, have a higher risk for
development of degenerative joint disease. Thus, more
satisfactory results are possible in sedentary patients
such as in rheumatoid arthritis cases. Some authors have
suggested that patients with higher levels of activity may
benefit from a combined calcaneocuboid arthrodesis
("double arthrodesis"), giving increased stability to the
arthrodesis.

Surgical Technique

- A dorsal longitudinal incision is usually utilized over the
talonavicular joint along the line of the first ray.
- The dorsomedial approach is made between the extensor hallucis longus tendon and the anterior tibialis tendon (Fig. 10.20).
- The capsule is incised, and the joint surfaces are
exposed and resected, paying particular attention to the
dense subchondral bone of the navicular.
- The lateral joint may require additional dissection for
visualization because of the significant convex/concave
nature of the joint.
- Bone graft may be used depending on the presence of a
bone defect or to lengthen the medial column if significant shortening is present at the fusion site.
- The joint is then fixed with compression screws, staples,
or Steinman pins as bone quality dictates (Fig. 10.21).
- The arthrodesis is fixed with the hindfoot in approximately 5° of valgus.
- Cannulated screws may be inserted percutaneously or
through the surgical incision, usually retrograde from
the navicular bone into the talar neck and body, using
intraoperative fluoroscopy to prevent penetration into
the subtalar joint.
- Once satisfactory fixation is obtained, the wound is
closed and the healing of the fusion is protected follow-

ing a protocol similar to the postoperative management
of subtalar joint arthrodesis.

Isolated Calcaneocuboid Arthrodesis
Isolated calcaneocuboid fusion can be considered for
patients with localized degenerative joint disease or with

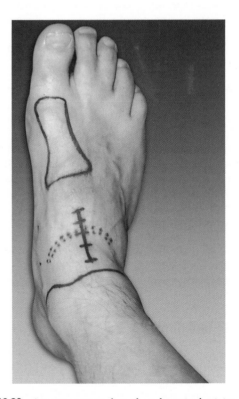

Figure 10.20   Anterior approach to the talonavicular joint
between the extensor hallucis longus and the anterior tibialis
tendon. The medial malleolus and ankle articular line are shown,
as is the base of the first metatarsal. The skin dorsal projection of
the talonavicular joint is illustrated with dotted lines.

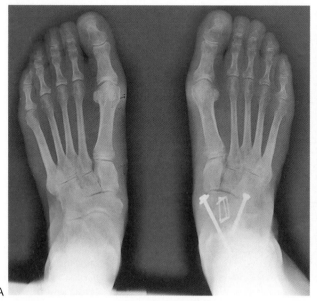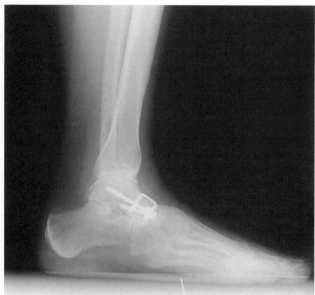

A
B

Figure 10.21   Standing AP (**A**) and lateral (**B**) foot X-rays showing an isolated talonavicular fusion using screws and staples.

rigid adult-acquired flatfoot deformity when choosing to lengthen the lateral column. Theoretically, fusing this joint can decrease the talonavicular motion up to 67% but has little effect on subtalar motion. A longitudinal lateral approach centered over the joint is used to gain access for the fusion procedure. The extensor digitorum brevis is detached from its origin and reflected distally or retracted dorsally. The remainder of the surgical technique shares similar basic principles previously discussed for talonavicular and subtalar fusions.

Double Arthrodesis

The double arthrodesis comprises a fusion of the talonavicular joint and the calcaneocuboid joint. This arthrodesis of the "transverse tarsal joint" (Chopart joint) eliminates subtalar motion, thus functioning as a triple arthrodesis. The hindfoot is placed in approximately 5° of valgus with a neutral abduction/adduction and plantarflexion/dorsiflexion. This type of fusion allows for correction of an abduction/adduction deformity when present.

Double arthrodesis can also be used in younger active patients with isolated talonavicular degenerative joint disease to increase the quality of fixation and provide long-term stability. In some patients, the decision to perform a triple arthrodesis may be needed, depending on the expectations and activity level.

Surgical Technique

- The operative technique and postoperative management combine the previously described details of a talonavicular and a calcaneocuboid joint fusion.
- The talonavicular joint is temporarily fixed first, followed by the calcaneocuboid joint, usually using guide pins from the cannulated screw sets or Steinman pins.
- Clinical alignment in a simulated weight-bearing stance is assessed and then adjusted as necessary.

- Permanent fixation may use screws, staples, or both, depending on bone quality and access.

Triple Arthrodesis

Fusion of all three hindfoot joints (subtalar, talonavicular, and calcaneocuboid) is generally considered only when the patient's arthritis or deformity is untreatable by a more limited fusion, particularly in younger active patients, in whom the increased biomechanical stresses have a more profound effect on the adjacent ankle and midfoot joints.

Many variations of this type of surgery have been published over the years. In the past, triple arthrodesis was frequently used to correct severe neurologic or paralytic deformities, owing in large part to the ability to perform corrections in all three planes (coronal, sagittal, and axial) simultaneously. This powerful tool has been used in a wide variety of hindfoot problems but requires careful attention to detail to avoid malalignment.

Indications and Contraindications.   Indications include the following:

- Subtalar osteoarthritis with either talonavicular or calcaneocuboid degenerative joint disease
- Charcot–Marie–Tooth disease with a fixed deformity
- Polio residuals
- Peripheral nerve injuries with fixed deformities
- Cerebrovascular accident
- Posterior tibialis tendon dysfunction with a fixed deformity
- Painful flexible or fixed rheumatoid hindfoot deformities
- Symptomatic posttraumatic malalignment with hindfoot joint instability
- Nonresectable calcaneonavicular or talocalcaneal coalition.

Relative contraindications include any clinical situation that could be treated with a more limited fusion of an isolated joint. Peripheral vascular disease, diabetes mellitus, neuroar-thropathy, and systemic healing issues need to be considered.

Surgical Technique

- A longitudinal curved incision is made from around 1 cm distal to the tip of fibula toward the base of the fourth metatarsal (Fig. 10.22).
- The extensor digitorum brevis is detached from its origin and retracted dorsally and distally.
- This approach combines the subtalar and calcaneocuboid joints, a technique that has already been described.
- The articular surfaces are then adequately prepared in those two joints and in the lateral aspect of the talonavicular joint.
- A second incision is made dorsomedially over the talonavicular joint, as detailed in the isolated talonavicular fusion portion of this chapter.
- The preparation of the fusion surfaces is completed.
- Once all bone surfaces have been adequately prepared, the hindfoot is positioned into 5° of valgus, neutral abduction/adduction, and neutral dorsiflexion/plantarflexion.
  - Adjustment in the three planes can be done to reach the most ideal position. Correction of varus or valgus of the subtalar joint/hindfoot involves properly rotating the head of the talus over the anterior calcaneus.
- Bone apposition needs to be evaluated and bone grafting can be completed accordingly.
- Satisfactory rigid fixation is achieved by using partially threaded cannulated cancellous screws for the subtalar joint (6.5 mm diameter or greater), 4.0 mm or larger screws for the talonavicular joint, and screws or staples for the calcaneocuboid joint.
  - This order of joint fixation allows for the appropriate foot position to be maintained and verified several times throughout the procedure.

In patients with equinus deformities, which are found frequently with hindfoot pathology, a simultaneous tendo-Achilles lengthening or gastrocnemius recession is necessary. Most experts prefer either a percutaneous triple hemi-section sliding technique or an open gastrocnemius release, each with its advantages and disadvantages (Fig. 10.23).

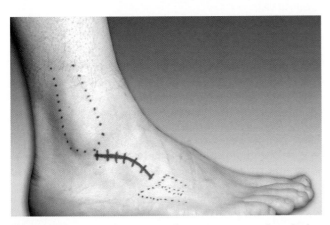

Figure 10.22   Lateral incision used to gain access to the subtalar, talonavicular, and calcaneocuboid joints. Beginning about 1 cm distal to the lateral malleolus, the curved incision is directed toward the base of the fourth metatarsal.

Postoperative Management

- An initial compressive dressing is applied.
- Trans-biceps femoris popliteal block or ankle block can provide assistance for controlling immediate postoperative pain.
- If the patient's ankle is not significantly swollen at the first postoperative visit, a non–weight-bearing below-the-knee fiberglass cast is applied, taking care to maintain neutral alignment.
- Principles of healing and progression to weight bearing and weaning from orthopaedic protective devices are the same as for subtalar joint fusion.

Results.   Triple arthrodesis is a powerful tool that allows correction of significant deformities. Long-term results (average follow-up of 44 years) revealed that 95% of patients were satisfied with the operation despite progressive symptoms and radiographic evidence of degeneration of the joints of the ankle and midfoot.

Triple arthrodesis controls pain and malalignment effectively at the expense of hindfoot motion, which also includes some loss of dorsiflexion, plantarflexion, and tibiopedal motion. Most series show significant improvement of the patients' functional scores postoperatively but reveal persistent serious complications in some, causing many authors to recommend an isolated fusion procedure, when possible.

Complications.   Complications seen most frequently with triple arthrodesis include nonunions and malunions. The nonunion rates vary from less than 5% to 15%. The talonavicular joint is still the most frequent site of pseudoarthrosis. Multiple factors may contribute to a nonunion and are discussed previously.

Malalignment may occur intraoperatively or during the postoperative period. A malaligned triple arthrodesis is closely linked with unsatisfactory results and may eventually necessitate further surgery such as calcaneal osteotomy to correct excessive varus or valgus.

Skin healing problems, sensory nerve damage (sural and superficial peroneal nerve), and long-term degenerative joint disease of the ankle and midfoot constitute other possible complications related to triple arthrodesis.

COMBINED ANKLE AND HINDFOOT DEGENERATIVE JOINT DISEASE

The amount of pain from each joint needs to be evaluated because ideal management is based on more than radiologic findings. Some cases of severe joint space narrowing on weight-bearing X-rays cause no clinical symptoms. The treatment may be dictated by the patient's symptoms and limitations in an effort to obtain the best possible results and to optimize patient satisfaction.

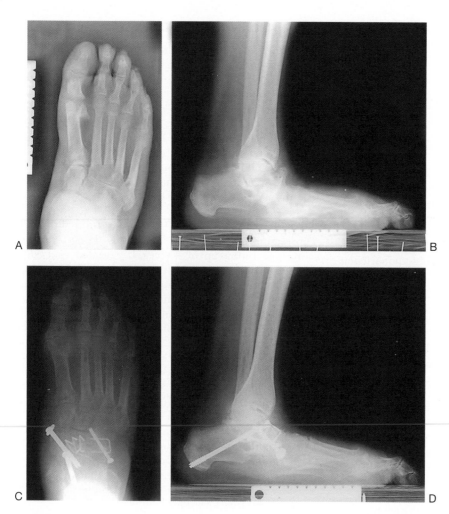

Figure 10.23 Standing AP (**A**) and lateral (**B**) foot X-rays of a 78-year-old patient with preoperative severe hindfoot degenerative joint disease secondary to hemochromatosis arthropathy. This patient was treated with a triple arthrodesis, percutaneous tendo-Achilles lengthening, and an anterior ankle cheilectomy. Postoperative standing AP (**C**) and lateral (**D**) X-rays reveal a satisfactory result.

DIAGNOSIS

A thorough understanding of these challenging cases begins with a complete history and physical examination as well as radiographic evaluations, which are described in the first two sections of this chapter.

Diagnostic injections can be quite helpful, particularly when doubts persist concerning if the symptoms are caused by both joints. Intra-articular injection of local anesthetic, with or without a steroid, using fluoroscopic control if needed, can help evaluate the role of each joint in the ankle and hindfoot complex (Fig. 10.24). Interpreting the results of these injections can be difficult if the location of the needle tip is not well documented. Also, some joints intercommunicate (i.e., ankle and posterior subtalar joint) and some extra-articular leaking could generate false conclusions.

TREATMENT

Nonoperative Treatment

Combined ankle and hindfoot degenerative joint disease can be managed using the same principles discussed earlier for isolated joints of this area. Local injection of steroids, systemic medications such as acetaminophen or nonsteroidal anti-inflammatories, activity modification, cane, walker, shoe modifications (rocker bottoms), and braces such as a custom rigid AFO (Fig. 10.3C) or the Arizona brace (Fig. 10.3B) represent some of the many treatment options available, particularly in patients with multiple medical problems who represent a significant surgical risk.

Surgical Treatment

Ankle and Subtalar Degenerative Joint Disease

Symptomatic involvement of the ankle and subtalar joints, which have failed to obtain satisfactory results with nonsurgical treatment, may benefit from either tibiotalocalcaneal or tibiocalcaneal arthrodesis. These two procedures have been used with success in certain salvage situations. MRI may be useful in cases of avascular necrosis of the talus to determine the extent of involvement. In rare cases, such as a completely extruded talus, the entire talus is involved and a partial or complete talectomy is required to provide for a successful arthrodesis.

Recently, procedures combining hindfoot fusion techniques with TAA for the treatment of combined ankle and subtalar degenerative joint disease have been described. These procedures can be performed simultaneously or in

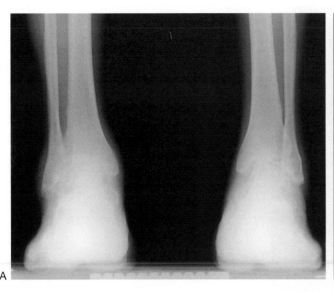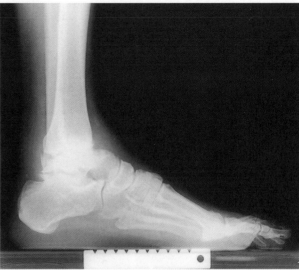

Figure 10.24 Standing AP (**A**) and lateral (**B**) ankle X-rays of a 51-year-old patient with bilateral ankle pain. Note the associated subtalar involvement on the lateral view. A diagnostic injection was used to confirm the clinical symptoms were emanating from the ankle.

a staged fashion. Early reports have demonstrated satisfactory outcomes, but no long-term studies are available.

All the usual considerations related to any foot and ankle arthrodesis or arthroplasty exist when treating cases of combined ankle and subtalar degenerative joint disease. In some cases, the best reconstructive option is a below-knee amputation.

Indications and Contraindications. Tibiotalocalcaneal and tibiocalcaneal arthrodesis represent satisfactory treatment options in clinically symptomatic cases of advanced degenerative arthritis of the ankle and subtalar joints that have failed nonsurgical management. Clinical scenarios include posttraumatic arthritis, posttraumatic avascular necrosis of the talus, failed TAA (Fig. 10.25), and rheumatoid arthritis with involvement of both joints. Severe deformities and chronic pain may not be salvageable and many of these patients should be offered below-knee amputation.

Contraindications are the same as are discussed in the sections on ankle and subtalar arthrodeses individually. As a general rule, when the risks of surgery and the lengthy recovery process become greater than the potential benefit to the patient's quality of life, alternative therapeutic options are recommended.

Technical Options. The planning for tibiotalocalcaneal arthrodesis poses a few important choices that alter the technique to be performed. The approach, using either a posterior approach or a combined medial/lateral approach, determines the position of the patient on the operating table. The posterior approach with the patient prone (described in the section on Ankle Arthrodesis) may represent a more reasonable choice when there is significant anterior soft-tissue damage.

Several fixation devices exist. Each method has been reported to provide satisfactory fixation in selected patients and each device has advantages and disadvantages. Current options include external fixators, used primarily for infected cases, cannulated screws, plate and screws, posterior blade plate, and intramedullary retrograde nails to maintain position and generate compression across the fusion site.

Surgical Technique

- Patients are positioned prone when a posterior approach is chosen, lateral on a beanbag for a lateral, transfibular approach, and supine with a sandbag under the ipsilateral hip when a combined medial/lateral approach is preferred.
- Antibiotics are given prophylactically—preoperatively and for 24 hours after surgery, and a tourniquet is inflated about the thigh of the limb.
- Skin prep and draping are done routinely and the toes are covered with adhesive dressing to minimize the risk of contamination.
- Skin incision and posterior approach are performed through the Achilles tendon as described previously in the section on Ankle Arthrodesis (Fig. 10.6).
- The dissection is extended distally to visualize better the posterior aspect of the talocalcaneal joint.
- When combined incisions are preferred, the lateral incision is made longitudinally, starting 5 to 10 cm proximal to the tip of the lateral malleolus and continuing toward the base of the fourth metatarsal.
- A 7-cm skin bridge between the longitudinal medial and the lateral incision should be maintained.
- Distal fibular osteotomy provides an excellent source of autologous bone graft (Fig. 10.5).
- Both ankle and subtalar joints must be well visualized and prepared as discussed in previous sections.
- The foot is positioned appropriately with neutral dorsiflexion, slight hindfoot valgus, and slight external rotation.
- Bone apposition is assessed and additional bone graft is added as deemed necessary.
  - □ When autograft is not used, bone graft substitutes that contain both osteoconductive and

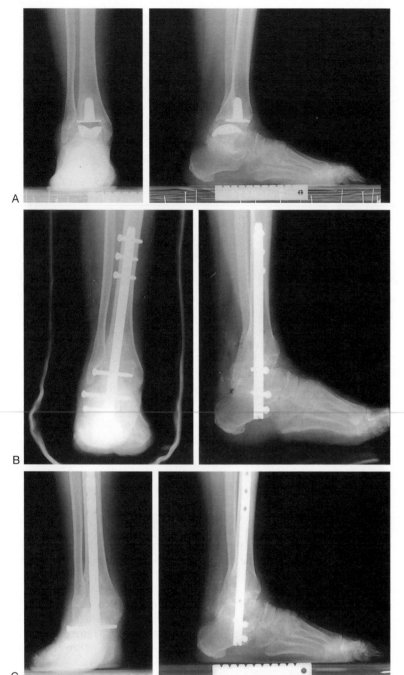

Figure 10.25 (**A**) Standing AP (**left**) and lateral (**right**) ankle X-rays of a failed TAA in an 80-year-old patient who failed nonsurgical management. (**B**) A salvage procedure with a locked retrograde intramedullary nail was performed. (**C**) A delayed union was treated with dynamization of the nail, as visualized on the AP X-ray (**left**) and the nail settled into the tibia proximally allowing the fusion to occur.

osteoinductive agents, such as demineralized bone matrix mixed with fresh autologous bone marrow, may be used.

■ In cases of avascular necrosis, the central portion of the talus can be excised, then replaced with a massive intra-articular and extra-articular bone graft to provide for a solid fusion mass. The next steps depend on the fixation device chosen by the surgeon.

■ When a blade plate is used, a posterior approach may be preferred.

☐ The 95° blade plate is contoured to the posterior aspect of the calcaneus and tibia, then inserted into

the calcaneus and fixed to the posterior aspect of distal tibia and talus.

☐ An allograft fibula, inserted retrograde through the calcaneus and into the tibia, can substantially augment fixation in cases of severe osteoporosis (Fig. 10.26).

■ A locked, retrograde intramedullary nail, designed for the tibiotalocalcaneal region represents an additional option for fixation.

☐ The nail is inserted through a plantar incision, taking care to use anatomic landmarks (heel fat pad and malleoli) to minimize the risk of injury to the lateral plantar artery and nerve.

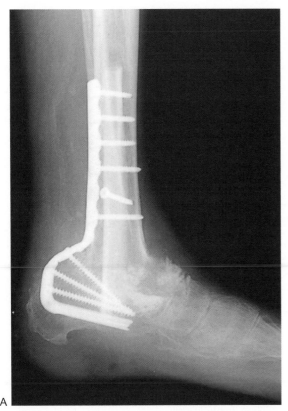

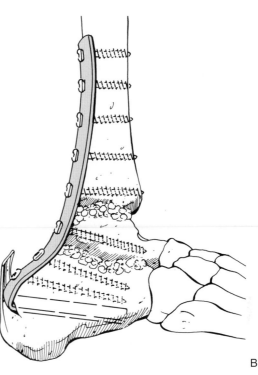

A

B

Figure 10.26 A posteriorly applied and contoured 95° blade plate was used for the tibiocalcaneal fusion in this patient who had undergone prior talectomy with severe residual deformity. **(A)** A posterior approach was used to provide a wide exposure and an allograft fibula was inserted to augment the internal fixation in this severely osteoporotic patient. **(B)** Drawing presenting a typical technique used to achieve a tibiotalocalcaneal fusion.

☐ Reaming is performed, after the foot is confirmed to be appropriately aligned, up to 1 mm less than the planned nail diameter, which improves fixation in the calcaneus.

☐ The nail is inserted while taking care to maintain good clinical and fluoroscopic positioning.

☐ Locking screws are then introduced percutaneously, using fluoroscopy as needed (Fig. 10.27).

▨ Bone grafting is completed as necessary.

▨ A multilayer wound closure is completed after satisfactory clinical and radiologic positions are confirmed.

Postoperative Management

▨ A compressive dressing is used to control swelling and to immobilize the ankle and hindfoot in a neutral position during the immediate postoperative period.

▨ Trans–biceps femoris popliteal block can be used to provide initial pain management as previously discussed.

▨ A non–weight-bearing below-knee fiberglass cast is then applied for a total of 6 weeks after surgery.

▨ At 6 weeks postoperatively, X-rays are obtained and a decision regarding initiation of weight bearing is made.

▨ In general, a fiberglass walking cast is worn for an additional 4 to 6 weeks with progressive weight bearing as symptoms allow.

▨ Serial radiographs are obtained throughout the healing period and compared with prior examinations to corroborate with the clinical evolution of the fusion.

Results. These salvage options have been reported to achieve satisfaction rates approaching 80% when appropriate indications are respected. Success rates in cases involving neuropathic joints are generally lower.

This salvage procedure provides predictable pain relief for symptomatic ankle and subtalar arthritis refractory to nonsurgical treatment but limits the tibiopedal motion and alters the gait pattern. However, it represents a valuable salvage option for these complex cases. Cushioned heel and rocker bottom shoe modifications (Fig. 10.28) may be used to improve the gait pattern.

Complications. Complications associated with tibiotalocalcaneal and tibiocalcaneal fusion are more frequent than with their isolated respective fusions and are related to poor wound healing and inadequate fixation. Most of these patients have multiple prior incisions with compromised soft-tissue and bone vascularity. The nonunion rates are reported to be greater than 10% to 15%. Malunion, skin healing problems, infections, sensory nerve injuries, and long-term degenerative joint disease of Chopart and midfoot joints are additional potential complications to discuss with the patient during the preoperative consultation.

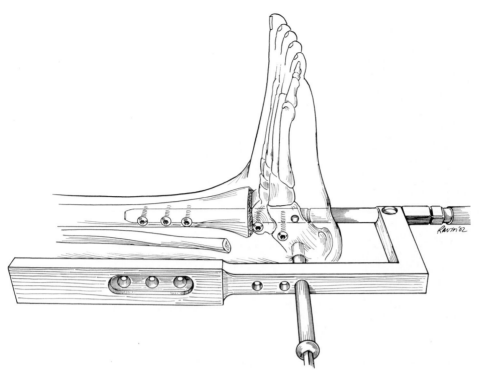

Figure 10.27 Diagram of distal locking of the retrograde intramedullary tibiotalocalcaneal nail. Fluoroscopy is used as needed to verify the proper position of the percutaneous locking screws. (From Kile TA. Tibiotalocalcaneal arthrodesis. In: Kitaoka HB, ed. Master techniques in orthopaedic surgery: the foot and ankle, 2nd ed. Philadelphia: Lippincott Williams & Wilkins, 2002:563.)

The use of a rigid intramedullary retrograde nail has been linked with some specific complications. Tibial cortical hypertrophy and stress fracture near the proximal tip of the nail have generally responded well to nonsurgical management with casting and progressive weight bearing as tolerated. Inadequate distal fixation has also been reported

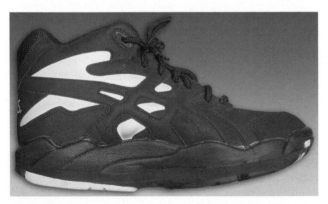

Figure 10.28 Example of a rocker bottom shoe modification. Note the curved black layer buried in the sole of the basketball shoe. Cushioned heel and rocker bottom shoe modification may be used to improve gait pattern in those patients with little or no ankle and hindfoot motion.

but is less common with newer nails allowing posterior to anterior screw insertion in the calcaneus. In cases of hardware sepsis and failure, most have required extensive debridement with hardware removal and culture-directed intravenous antibiotics, and some have resulted in below-knee amputation.

Ankle, Subtalar, and Chopart Degenerative Joint Disease

Symptomatic cases of progressive pantalar arthrosis with multiple joint destruction remains a relatively rare clinical situation that may benefit from pantalar arthrodesis. Patients with severe rheumatoid arthritis or with long-term degenerative joint disease in the ankle following a triple arthrodesis or in the hindfoot following ankle arthrodesis represent the most common presentations for this disabling clinical entity.

Pantalar arthrodesis is a definitive fusion procedure in the ankle and hindfoot area that combines a triple arthrodesis with an ankle fusion. The final position remains vital, and gait pattern changes invariably occur and are significantly more problematic than any of the other fusions described in this chapter. This surgery constitutes a salvage option that may be proposed in rare complex cases but generally does not function as well as a below-knee amputation (Fig. 10.29).

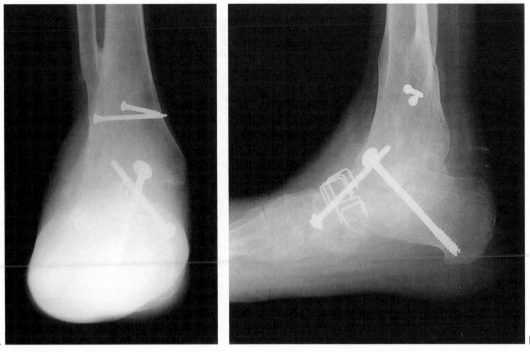

Figure 10.29 (A,B) Salvage pantalar fusion achieved in the rheumatoid arthritis patient mentioned in Figure 10.13. He had a hindfoot valgus collapse, severe pain, and a history of ankle fusion that significantly limited his activities, despite attempts at bracing and shoe wear modifications.

SUGGESTED READINGS

Astion DJ, Deland JT, Otis JC, et al. Motion of the hindfoot after simulated arthrodesis. J Bone Joint Surg Am 1997;79:241–246.

Bednarz PA, Monroe MT, Manoli A II. Triple arthrodesis in adults using rigid internal fixation: an assessment of outcome. Foot Ankle Int 1999;20:356–363.

Chou LB, Mann RA, Yaszay B, et al. Tibiotalocalcaneal arthrodesis. Foot Ankle Int 2000;21:804–808.

Easley ME, Trnka HJ, Schon LC, et al. Isolated subtalar arthrodesis. J Bone Joint Surg Am 2000;82:613–624.

Guyer AJ, Richardson G. Current concepts review: total ankle arthroplasty. Foot Ankle Int 2008;29(2):256–264.

Haddad SL, Coetzee JC, Estok R, et al. Intermediate and long-term outcomes of total ankle arthroplasty and ankle arthrodesis. A systematic review of the literature. J Bone Joint Surg Am 2007;89:1899–1905.

Kile TA. Tibiotalocalcaneal arthrodesis. In: Kitaoka HB, ed. Master techniques in orthopaedic surgery: the foot and ankle, 2nd ed. Philadelphia: Lippincott Williams & Wilkins, 2002:551–568.

Kitaoka HB, Alexander IJ, Adelaar RS, et al. Clinical rating systems for the ankle–hindfoot, midfoot, hallux, and lesser toes. Foot Ankle Int 1994;15:349–353.

Kitaoka HB, Johnson KA. Ankle replacement arthroplasty. In: Morrey BF, ed. Reconstructive surgery of the joints, 2nd ed. Rochester, MN: Mayo Foundation, 1996:1757–1769.

McLeod DH, Wong DH, Claridge RJ, et al. Lateral popliteal sciatic nerve block compared with subcutaneous infiltration for analgesia following foot surgery. Can J Anaesth 1994;41:673–676.

Pell RF IV, Myerson MS, Schon LC. Clinical outcome after primary triple arthrodesis. J Bone Joint Surg Am 2000;82:47–57.

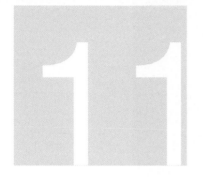

11 DEGENERATIVE JOINT DISEASE OF THE MIDFOOT AND FOREFOOT

CHAD B. CARLSON
MICHAEL E. BRAGE

11.1 MIDFOOT ARTHRITIS

A variety of forms of arthritis affect people of all ages and have significant impact on employment, activities of daily living, and quality of life. It is estimated by the Centers for Disease Control and Prevention that arthritis is the most common cause of disability in the United States and affects nearly 21 million people. The commonest form of arthritis encountered is osteoarthritis (OA), but there are more than 100 other rheumatologic conditions that can cause arthritis-related disability in every age group, ethnicity, and sex.

As physicians, we must be prepared to not only manage the chronic disabilities that fail conservative care but also recognize systemic disease that presents as an isolated foot problem such as the swollen forefoot that on careful examination reveals peripheral symmetric joint involvement as in rheumatoid arthritis (RA).

This chapter encompasses the midfoot and forefoot arthritides, such as primary OA and secondary posttraumatic arthrosis as well as the related topics of hallux rigidus, forefoot RA, crystal-induced arthropathy, and turf toe. The general format will focus stepwise on epidemiology, etiology, pathophysiology, and classification. We then turn to diagnosis clinically and radiographically, giving algorithms when needed. Finally, treatment will be discussed by pinpointing surgical versus nonsurgical modalities, the indications, outcomes, and follow-up of each.

INTRODUCTION

Arthritic disease of the midfoot includes primary degenerative arthritis (OA), secondary posttraumatic arthritis, inflammatory arthritidies (such as RA), seronegative spondyloarthropathies, and crystal-associated arthritis, which includes gout and pseudogout (chondrocalcinosis). The most common forms, primary degenerative arthritis and posttraumatic arthritis of the midfoot, will be the emphasis of this section.

The ability to understand, diagnose, and appropriately treat the midfoot is greatly facilitated by understanding the articular divisions, or columns, of the midfoot, including the following:

Medial—the first metatarsocuneiform joint
Central (middle)—the second and third metatarsocuneiform joints and the intercuneiform joints
Lateral—the cubometatarsal joints.[1]

Some authors combine the medial and middle columns into the medial column as the three tarsometatarsal (TMT) joints are relatively immobile. These columns are enveloped in a stout soft-tissue complex of various ligaments, and the bony architecture of the three cuneiforms and the cuboid forms the transverse arch of the midfoot (Fig. 11.1.1). The significance of the columnar division of the midfoot relates to the amount of motion occurring at each of these articular surfaces. Studies have shown that about 10° of midfoot motion occurs in the sagittal and rotational planes at the lateral column and much less motion in the medial and middle columns. In one cadaver study, it was shown that with increased loads, the medial and middle columns showed significant increases in articular contact forces, whereas the lateral column did not show increased contact forces despite loading up to twice the body weight.[2] Thus, the increased motion and decreased injury incidence occurring in the lateral

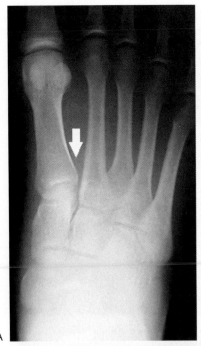

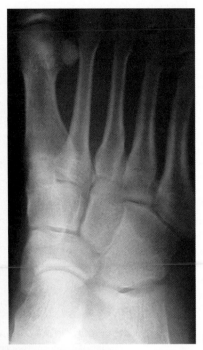

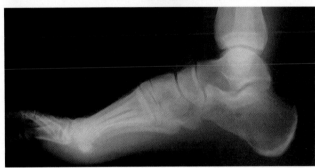

A

B

C

Figure 11.1.1 Radiographs (AP (**A**), oblique (**B**), and lateral (**C**) views) demonstrating the normal columnar division of the midfoot. Medial—the first metatarsocuneiform joint, central (**middle**)—the second and third metatarsocuneiform joints and the intercuneiform joints, and lateral—the cubometatarsal joints. Some authors combine medial and middle into medial column in a two-column model. The transverse arch of the midfoot is formed by the bony architecture of the three cuneiforms and the cuboid (**lateral view**). The primary stabilization of the midfoot is provided by the Lisfranc joint, the transverse tarsometatarsal joint between the base of the second metatarsal and the medial cuneiform (*white arrow*).

column are two important reasons why it is much less involved in arthritis than the other two columns. For this reason and owing to the importance of lateral column motion to foot biomechanics, preservation of lateral motion during midfoot fusions is beneficial and much less debilitating.

Stabilization of the midfoot is based on the ligamentous and bony integrity of the second TMT joint. Lisfranc ligament, the interosseous ligament that runs obliquely from the second metatarsal base to the medial cuneiform, is the largest midfoot ligament and along with the second plantar ligament (intermetatarsus ligament between the second and the third metatarsals) is the strongest ligament in the midfoot.[3] The Lisfranc joint (transverse TMT joint) provides the primary stabilization to the midfoot and is the keystone in creating a "Roman arch-like" effect that resists midfoot collapse (Fig. 11.1.1). As a consequence, small disruptions (displacement and/or alignment changes) to this joint can result in considerable loss of articular contact surface area. Indeed, even subtle injuries with small amounts of displacement or ligamentous disruption to this region can affect midfoot stability and biomechanics, thus predisposing to posttraumatic degenerative changes.

PATHOGENESIS

Epidemiology

OA is a slowly developing degenerative disease affecting many joints of the body. As the most common musculoskeletal disorder worldwide, it exacts a tremendous toll socially and economically in developed countries, establishing itself as the major cause of morbidity in these nations. OA prevalence increases significantly with age and correlates with obesity and high levels of activity or impact loading on the foot. However, secondary arthritis of the midfoot, often the result of previous trauma, is more common than primary OA and can be induced by various injuries. The most common posttraumatic injury leading to midfoot arthritis is injury to the Lisfranc joint, but others include navicular and/or cuboid fracture dislocations as well as metatarsal fractures and ligamentous injuries to the TMT complex.

Etiology and Pathophysiology

In the midfoot TMT complex, arthritis is typically either a primary arthrosis of the TMT complex or a secondary degenerative arthrosis most commonly because of previous trauma or osteochondritis dessicans. Primary degenerative arthrosis (i.e., OA) of the midfoot, regardless of the specific joints affected, generally occurs in older patients and, owing to the gradual nature of disease progression, is typically more advanced and produces greater deformity than that of posttraumatic arthrosis (unless severe). This is especially true when multiple joints are involved, but OA can be present with little deformity when a single joint is involved. A thorough evaluation of associated conditions should always be done including an evaluation to determine whether a gastrocnemius and/or soleus contracture is present.

Posttraumatic midfoot arthrosis is the most common etiology of arthrosis in the midfoot. Both subtle and severe traumatic injuries can result in significant degenerative midfoot arthrosis. Three predisposing factors that will lead to joint degeneration include (a) articular cartilage injury, (b) joint displacement with medial longitudinal arch collapse, and/or (c) persistent joint malalignment. Usually there is a history of high-energy traumatic injury, but even low-energy trauma with Lisfranc complex compromise, which may have been missed or overlooked, can result in significant posttraumatic arthrosis. Along with Lisfranc injuries, other injuries predisposing to midfoot arthrosis are multiple metatarsal fractures, posterior tibial tendon injuries resulting in medial longitudinal arch collapse, and intercuneiform instabilities. Lateral column arthrosis can result from cuboid compression or "nutcracker" fractures. Understanding of the complex anatomy of this region and how it is stabilized is vital to both diagnosis and treatment of primary and secondary arthroses of the midfoot.

DIAGNOSIS

Clinical Features

As with arthritis in general, the commonest complaint of midfoot arthritis is pain. Patients may also complain of shoe wear problems owing to bony prominences or deformity. Physical examination should reveal tenderness and often limited motion at these painful areas. A standing and sitting examination of both feet should be included to determine whether deformity, motion limitations, neurovascular compromise, or focal tenderness is present and to what extent. A weight-bearing examination is essential to determine the degree and extent of deformity. In both primary and posttraumatic midfoot arthroses, deformity and swelling may be present and the characteristic flatfoot appearance of pronation, dorsiflexion, and abduction seen (Fig. 11.1.2). In general, midfoot pain is due to articular surface injury/wear/inflammation with normal joint movement and no obvious instability or abnormal movement at a joint—with or without articular surface changes. Ligamentous injuries at the Lisfranc joint often result in the latter (abnormal movement), whereas, at least initially, primary arthrosis typically results from the former (articular surface changes). When it is difficult to assess exact origins of pain, localized injections have been advocated. These may be difficult to interpret owing to the different compartments of the foot, the diffusion into or from the joint where the anesthetic is injected, and the plane in which it enters. However, when

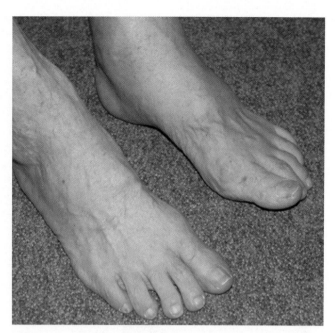

Figure 11.1.2 Clinical appearance of the characteristic flatfoot deformity seen with midfoot arthritis (comparison of arthritic left foot with uninvolved right foot).

anesthetic injections are assisted by radiography and result in prolonged pain relief, they can be extremely valuable in determining the joint that is the source of pain.[4,5]

Radiologic Features

Standing images of both feet in the anteroposterior (AP), lateral, and 30° oblique planes are most helpful. In assessing the degree of deformity, comparison with non–weight-bearing views and with the other foot is useful, as is evaluating for loss of talar head coverage by the navicular. Joint space narrowing and subchondral bone sclerosis may be seen (Fig. 11.1.3). Although significant bony displacement or arthrosis of the midfoot articulations may be easily seen, subtle injuries or single joint involvement may be difficult to appreciate on plain radiographs. Furthermore, physical examination findings and plain radiographic appearance may not be easily correlated with the significant painful symptoms of arthritic disease. Therefore, some advocate CT or bone scan for further determination of the specific location and extent of arthrosis in the midfoot, especially in cases of preoperative planning. This, however, remains controversial, and CT results should be evaluated for consistency with plain radiographs, examination, and intra-operative findings.

In the presence of posttraumatic arthrosis, it is still important to decipher whether the Lisfranc midfoot injury exists. Careful evaluation of weight-bearing X-rays should include colinearity of the medial aspect of the middle cuneiform with the second metatarsal on an AP view; the medial border of the cuboid should be colinear with the medial aspect of the fourth metatarsal on the oblique view; and any dorsal displacement of the metatarsal complex on the lateral view is indicative of a ligamentous injury. Further evaluation can include abduction/pronation and adduction/supination stress radiographs of the foot, contralateral films for comparison, and perhaps CT scan, bone scan, or MRI

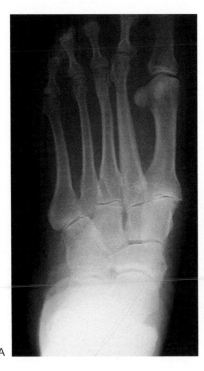

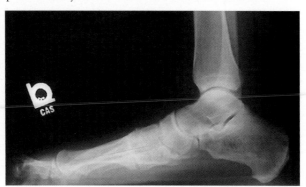

Figure 11.1.3 AP (**A**) and lateral (**B**) radiographs demonstrating primary degenerative arthrosis of the midfoot with predominantly medial and middle column involvement.

A

B

of the affected foot. Chronic Lisfranc injuries, possibly missed after a previous injury, often present only with painful gait and minor tenderness and might be identified only by stress radiographs that reveal widening between the first and the second metatarsals. Both weight-bearing and stress radiographs may be more representative and better tolerated by using an ankle block anesthetic. These further studies can be helpful in the posttraumatic setting to evaluate the extent of medial, middle, and lateral column arthroses, especially when operative intervention is being considered.

TREATMENT

The options for the treatment of primary or secondary degenerative arthrosis in the midfoot depend on the patient's pain and activity levels (Algorithm 11.1.1). Nonoperative treatment may alleviate enough pain to allow for increased levels of activity and function for a variable time while not being overly restrictive. Decisions to operatively intervene should come after nonoperative measures have been tried and pain/loss of function remains unacceptable.

Nonoperative Treatment

Nonsurgical management should be focused on relieving pain and providing midfoot stability and support. This is especially valuable to the osteopenic patient and should begin early in the course when arthrosis of the midfoot or forefoot is suspected. Nonsteroidal anti-inflammatory drugs (NSAIDs) often help, as do weight loss and activity modifications, especially in conjunction with supportive shoe wear. Bony osteophytes often protrude around the joint and into soft tissues, needing pressure relief by padding or stretching of the overlying shoe. Orthotic devices

can provide padding, with added support for the longitudinal arch and relief of some pain at the metatarsal head. However, when significant deformity is present, arch support is often not well tolerated. An ankle–foot orthosis (AFO) with a stiffened foot plate may also provide some relief. In general, orthotics that decrease motion of painful degenerative joints will contribute significantly to pain control. Dorsal osteophytes may be especially troublesome, but padding and modifying shoe wear can decrease pressure in that region to relieve some pain.

Surgical Considerations

Surgical indications for patients with primary and secondary midfoot arthroses include instability and/or continued pain that affects activities of daily living, despite attempts at nonoperative management. Although debridement and resection of osteophytes—especially when skin irritation or nerve impingement is occurring—are useful and can bring symptomatic relief, the main surgical options for degenerative arthrosis generally involve arthrodesis, excisional arthroplasty, and sometimes osteotomy of the involved joints. In general, medial and middle column midfoot arthrodesis is the preferred surgical modality for arthrosis in these regions, whether the cause is primary degenerative disease, posttraumatic arthrosis, or inflammatory arthritis in particular (Fig. 11.1.4). The operative management of lateral column midfoot arthrosis is discussed later.

In Situ Fusion

When deformity is not present, in situ fusion is indicated and should include rigid internal fixation of every involved joint. Surgical approaches vary, but in general the first TMT joint can be approached dorsally or dorsomedially. When approaching the second and third TMT joints or the

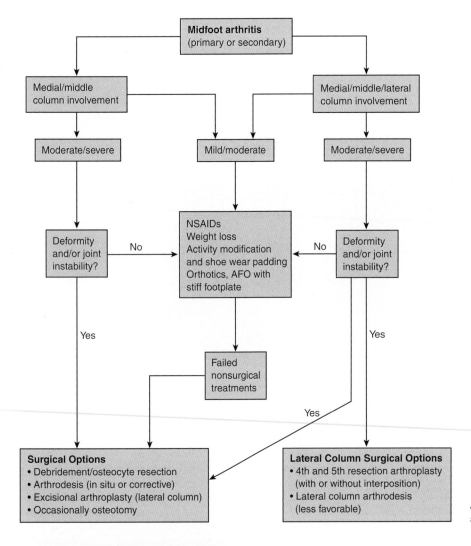

Midfoot arthritis
(primary or secondary)

Medial/middle
column involvement

Medial/middle/lateral
column involvement

Moderate/severe

Mild/moderate

Moderate/severe

Deformity
and/or joint
instability? ——No——→

NSAIDs
Weight loss
Activity modification
and shoe wear padding
Orthotics, AFO with
stiff footplate

←——No—— Deformity
and/or joint
instability?

Yes

Yes

Failed
nonsurgical
treatments

Yes

Surgical Options
• Debridement/osteocyte resection
• Arthrodesis (in situ or corrective)
• Excisional arthroplasty (lateral column)
• Occasionally osteotomy

Lateral Column Surgical Options
• 4th and 5th resection arthroplasty
  (with or without interposition)
• Lateral column arthrodesis
  (less favorable)

Algorithm 11.1.1. Treatment algorithm for midfoot arthritis.

Figure 11.1.4 Six-month postoperative AP (**A**) and lateral (**B**) radiographs demonstrating midfoot arthrodesis with interfragmentary screw fixation for primary degenerative arthritis. The lateral column was asymptomatic and was left unfused even though mild degenerative changes are present.

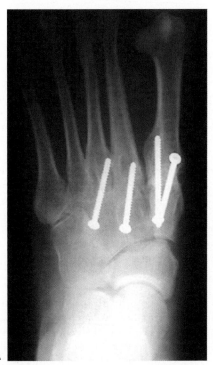

A

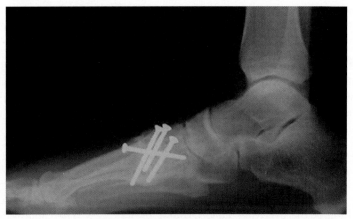

B

fourth and fifth TMT joints, longitudinal incisions between the second and the third metatarsals or the fourth and the fifth metatarsals, respectively, can be used. Following the approach, the joint should be exposed and all articular cartilage removed. Underlying subchondral bone should be perforated using an osteotome or multiple drill holes. For fixation and compression, standard lag screw techniques can be utilized using 3.5-mm fully threaded screws in a number of screw configurations crossing the joint involved. Some surgeons also use dorsal plates—locked or unlocked (Fig. 11.1.4). Fixation of intercuneiform or intermetatarsal joints can be achieved often in a medial to lateral fashion. Supplemental bone grafting is usually not necessary but can be used either with local bone graft or from drillings. Lateral midfoot motion should be preserved if not affected by painful arthrosis, and in general the cubometatarsal joints infrequently require arthrodesis. Naviculocuneiform joint fixation can be accomplished in medial to lateral fashion as well and may be facilitated by joint release. Fixation at each level should consider the anatomic positions and weight-bearing function of each TMT (and even metatarsophalangeal [MTP]) joint. For example, first metatarsocuneiform joint arthrodesis accomplished by fixation and shortening of the medial column may require first metatarsal plantarflexion to distribute forces evenly for weight-bearing.

Corrective Fusion

When deformity is present, corrective fusion using bone graft and soft-tissue lengthening or shortening is indicated. The extent of deformity required for correction will vary, but in general, any deformity with greater than 2 mm or 15° of displacement should be corrected. For midfoot medial column deformity, bony resection is often necessary and fixation can be achieved by interfragmentary screw fixation after meticulous joint preparation. Plating the medial column may be helpful as well, especially in osteoporotic bone, or if screw purchase is poor. More important, the lateral column may require lateral soft-tissue lengthening (especially the peroneus brevis tendon) to achieve appropriate medial column deformity correction. Kirschner wires (K-wires), laminar spreader, or external fixator on the lateral column can assist in achieving adequate reduction/correction as well.

Lateral Column Arthrosis

The most common long-term complication of midfoot arthrodesis is the development of symptomatic arthritis in adjacent motion segments, albeit the midfoot has a lower incidence of this than other areas of the foot and ankle.[6] Other causes of lateral column midfoot arthrosis include Lisfranc complex injuries as well as degenerative and inflammatory arthritidies, isolated lateral midfoot trauma (cuboid "nutcracker" type fracture) and base of fifth metatarsal fracture sequelae.[7] TMT joint arthrodesis for post-traumatic arthrosis is well reported where the incidence of lateral column symptoms is fairly small (from 6% to 25%).[1,8,9] In the study by Komenda et al.,[1] 2 of 32 patients were symptomatic enough to require lateral column fusion. This study, as well as those by Mann et al.[8] and Sangeorzan et al.,[9] did not reveal complications specific

to lateral column fusions but suggested that an alternative was "welcomed" and that appropriate diagnosis of lateral column arthrosis as the true source of pain was imperative. Indeed, the majority of midfoot motion is through the cuboid-fourth/fifth metatarsal articulation, and fusion of this region can be disabling, leaving the patient with a very stiff foot.

An alternative to lateral column arthrodesis is tendon arthroplasty for basal fourth and fifth metatarsal arthritis, as proposed by Berlet and Anderson.[7] In this study, 12 patients who failed nonoperative treatment for lateral column arthrosis underwent resection arthroplasty of the base of the fifth or fourth and fifth metatarsals with tendon interposition. Average follow-up was 25 months, and patients were evaluated with the American Orthopaedic Foot and Ankle Society (AOFAS) clinical midfoot scale—a visual analogue scale for pain and disability perception and a satisfaction index. The AOFAS score was 64.5, and pain scores improved an average of 35%, whereas disability scores improved by 10%. Overall, the operation was deemed satisfactory in 75% of patients. All patients had lateral column motion preservation, although the amount of motion was not used as an assessment tool as the authors felt there was too much inaccuracy in its measurement and was difficult to reproduce in the clinical setting. The authors believe that lateral column TMT resection arthroplasty "is an effective salvage operation when lateral column midfoot arthritis is confirmed by differential injection and nonoperative measures have provided inadequate relief."[7] This procedure gives the surgeon a motion-sparing alternative for lateral column arthritis and stresses the importance of truly identifying the lateral column as the source of a patient's arthritic complaints by differential injection. Indeed, patients with higher postoperative AOFAS scores were statistically more likely to have had a positive differential anesthetic injection preoperatively.[7] This is important because lateral column arthritic changes identified on radiographs do not always lead to lateral midfoot pain or functional impairment.[1,10]

Technique. Following local (ankle block), regional or general anesthesia, limb exsanguination and tourniquet placement, a dorsolateral incision is made paralleling the long axis of the foot. Center the incision on the fourth metatarsocuboid joint, taking care to avoid sural nerve injury. Expose the fourth toe long extensor tendon as well as the peroneus tertius tendon—the latter should be released proximally and retracted out of the wound. The long extensor tendon of the fourth toe can be used when this tendon is absent. Open the fourth and fifth metatarsocuboid joint capsule dorsally and debride the joints. Debridement should be carried down to subchondral bone distally to create an approximately 1-cm space (proximal-distal) while maintaining the plantar and medial ligamentous supports as well as the lateral capsule. Insert the rolled up peroneus tertius tendon graft into the joint(s).[7] Joint alignment in approximately neutral can be maintained by 0.062-in K-wire insertion from distal-lateral to proximal-medial and through the tendon graft. If inadequate tendon is available, an allograft or synthetic ball can be used for interposition.

Postoperative care comprises rigid splint placement in the operating room and non-weight bearing for 6 to 8 weeks, at which time the K-wire is removed. Weight bearing as tolerated commences at 6 to 8 weeks, and the patient is kept in a walker boot or short leg cast for four additional weeks. A shoe is then used after this time. Concomitant procedures may modify this regimen.

RESULTS AND OUTCOMES

Patients undergoing nonoperative treatment have a variable course, depending on the location, extent, and duration of arthrosis of the midfoot. A significant proportion will go on to require midfoot arthrodesis and/or osteophyte resection. Studies indicate that the outcome of midfoot arthrodesis for primary and posttraumatic degenerative arthrosis is good, with one study showing a 93% satisfaction rate and 98% union rate (176 of 179 joints) in 40 patients followed for an average of 6 years.[8] Deformity correction was approximately 8° in this study. Another study by Komenda et al.[1] in 32 patients requiring midfoot arthrodesis for posttraumatic arthrosis demonstrated only one asymptomatic nonunion and substantial improvement in the clinical foot score. Extent or location of the arthrodesis, patient age, or need for revision surgery did not have a significant effect on outcome in this study. Malunion occurred in 7 of the 32 patients. The malunions involved second metatarsal plantarflexion in all seven patients and in addition, third or first metatarsal plantarflexion in four patients. Surgical correction for these malunions was required only in two patients and involved dorsal closing-wedge osteotomies.

11.2 FOREFOOT ARTHRITIS

INTRODUCTION

Arthritis typically affecting the forefoot includes OA, RA, the seronegative spondyloarthropathies, and the crystal-induced arthritidies. Some of these arthritic conditions have a predilection for the forefoot (e.g., RA, gout). The focus of this section will be on hallux rigidus, RA of the forefoot, gout, pseudogout, and turf toe injuries, a predisposing factor for first MTP joint arthrosis.

HALLUX RIGIDUS

PATHOGENESIS

Epidemiology

Hallux rigidus is a painful arthritic condition of the first MTP joint characterized by restricted dorsiflexion and dorsal osteophytes. Normal range of motion is approximately 30° of plantarflexion and nearly 100° of dorsiflexion with approximately 60° of dorsiflexion required for normal gait and activities of daily living. It is generally seen in a younger population of patients than with other conditions of arthritis, and the incidence is estimated to be 1 in 45 of the adult population aged 60 years or older. However, this disorder occurs in two age groups. The much less common subset of patients affected are adolescents, with an incidence of 1 in 4,500. The adolescent form is characterized by localized osteochondral lesions rather than the more generalized diffuse arthrosis seen in the adult form.

Etiology

The precise etiology of hallux rigidus is still unknown; however, many authors have noted predisposing factors that have been proposed to cause increased stress across the hallux MTP joint. These include flat metatarsal head, a long first metatarsal, a dorsiflexed first metatarsal, improper shoe wear, a long slender foot, congenital deformities, gastrocnemius contracture, pes planus, and a pronated foot. Besides these factors, the degenerative process can be caused by trauma, accumulated microtrauma secondary to eccentric loading, systemic diseases, osteochondritis dissecans, turf toe injuries, or infection. Even with this list of predisposing conditions and anatomic factors, many cases have an unknown cause.

Pathophysiology

In understanding first MTP joint pathology, it is important to recall that the first MTP joint is cam shaped with a convex metatarsal head and concave proximal phalangeal base. Stability comes mainly through strong medial and lateral collateral ligaments, a thick plantar plate, and metatarsosesamoid suspensory ligaments. Motion at the first MTP joint is mainly dorsiflexion (with less plantarflexion) and functions by a sliding action along the metatarsal head.

The pathology of hallux rigidus, whatever the cause, is the result of an imperfect ball and socket joint and altered joint kinematics leading to early compressive forces during dorsiflexion and subsequent arthrosis.[11] The degenerative process begins with synovitis and associated articular degeneration of the dorsal metatarsal head. Impingement of the base of the proximal phalanx on the dorsal metatarsal head occurs with forced dorsiflexion leading to chondral or osteochondral injuries of the articular cartilage. Cartilage erosions and dorsal and lateral osteophyte formations follow. The osteophytes become larger and more prominent thus restricting range of motion. The mechanical impingement dorsally causes jamming instead of gliding of the proximal phalanx on the metatarsal head. The pain associated with this destructive joint process is secondary to synovitis, motion of the arthritic joint, and dorsal impingement of the osteophytes with dorsiflexion. Stretching in plantarflexion of the synovium, digital nerves and capsule over the osteophytes also causes irritation and produces pain.

DIAGNOSIS

Clinical Features

Hallux rigidus usually presents with an insidious onset of a painful, stiff, and swollen first MTP joint without any history of trauma. Most often the pain is activity related and progresses to a point that makes shoe wear difficult, especially those with elevated heels. Occasionally patients with acute osteochondral lesions may remark about a clicking or catching sensation with range of motion. It is important to elicit from the history not only the hallmarks of this condition, pain, loss of dorsiflexion, and increased bulk of the first MTP joint but also the limitations of the patient's activity level. This will help guide treatment recommendations.

Physical examination findings can vary with the severity of the disease but the characteristic finding is restricted active and passive dorsiflexion, which reproduces the patient's pain. This dorsal impingement syndrome is caused by marginal osteophytes—typically present dorsally and, less commonly, laterally. The first MTP joint is usually tender to palpation about the dorsal prominence and the dorsolateral ridge. There may also be dorsal skin changes over a prominent osteophyte (Fig. 11.2.1A). The first MTP joint can demonstrate varying degrees of swelling, which can be both seen and palpated. Neuritic signs, pain, and paresthesias with percussion along the dorsal medial and lateral digital nerves to the great toe can also be a finding on physical examination. Gait abnormalities, such as supination of the forefoot and walking on the lateral border of the foot to avoid pushing off through the first MTP joint, occur as a late finding because normal walking requires only 15° of dorsiflexion.

Patients with osteochondral injuries do not have bony proliferative changes until late. Early physical examination findings with osteochondral lesions can include clicking and pain with passive range of motion and compression across the first MTP joint. This may be relieved with joint distraction during range of motion.

Radiologic Features

Radiographic evaluation should comprise weight-bearing AP, lateral, and oblique views of the foot. These views are used to evaluate the degree of joint space narrowing. The AP view is also useful for evaluating the presence of medial or lateral osteophytes and is the best view to assess osteochondral lesions. The lateral view demonstrates the presence of dorsal osteophytes and the degree of impingement as well as the presence of any loose bodies (Fig. 11.2.1B). The oblique projection can show flattening of the metatarsal head and can also be useful for assessing the amount of joint space remaining if the joint space is obscured by dorsal osteophytes on the AP view. Other radiographic modalities are seldom indicated, but occasionally a bone scan or MRI will detect early degenerative changes or an osteochondral defect before any plain radiographic evidence can be seen.

Classification

Classification schemes based on plain radiographic findings have been developed. However, radiographic images can range from totally normal to severe joint destruction, and the degree of radiographic involvement of the first MTP joint does not necessarily correlate with the degree of symptoms. One such classification system comprises three grades: grade I—minimal to no joint space narrowing with dorsal osteophytes, grade II—more extensive narrowing with only the plantar joint space preserved, and grade III—complete joint space narrowing and severe arthrosis.[12] The utility of this classification system in developing treatment algorithms is debatable owing to poor correlation between radiographic involvement and symptom level. Another system includes a grade IV, where in addition to complete loss of joint space, the patient has pain throughout the MTP joint range of motion.

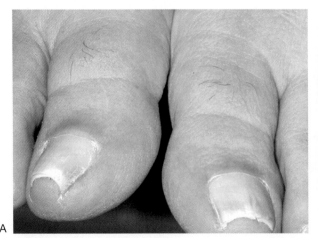
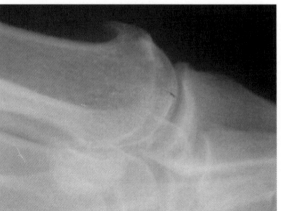

A   B

Figure 11.2.1   **A:** Clinical appearance of hallux rigidus with characteristic swelling and dorsal prominence of the first MTP joint (uninvolved left great toe shown for comparison). **B:** Lateral radiograph showing large dorsal osteophyte and joint space narrowing.

TREATMENT

Treatment for hallux rigidus is based on the patients' complaints, age, and degree of interference with their activity requirements. Conservative care comprises mainly orthotic devices directed at preventing and relieving symptoms by relieving stress across the first MTP joint. Shoe modifications must provide a wide/deep toe box to accommodate the increased bulk of the arthritic joint and provide a rigid rocker sole to diminish joint motion. For work shoes, a stiff-soled shoe can be used, and for athletics, a rocker-sole insert across the MTP joint can be used with a sneaker. Occasionally a rocker bottom sole, metatarsal bar, or steel-shanked shoe can be tried, but the cumbersome nature of these orthotic devices has a low degree of patient acceptance. Although orthotics can be used to stiffen the sole and decrease motion, they also occupy space within the toe box. This diminished room in the toe box can aggravate symptoms, and therefore, if these devices are used, the shoe must be large enough to house the enlarged MTP joint as well as the orthotic. Nonsteroidal anti-inflammatory medication, both oral and transdermal, can also be used to relieve symptoms, and intra-articular steroid injections can provide temporary relief in acute flare-ups.

If conservative management has failed to provide relief, the pain becomes disabling in everyday activities, and significant symptoms persist—surgical intervention should be considered. The goal of surgery is to alleviate pain, maintain motion when possible, correct deformity, and preserve length.

Many surgical options exist, but generally they fall into two categories:

Joint preserving (debridement, cheilectomy, and dorsiflexion osteotomy of the proximal phalanx) for milder cases.

Joint sacrificing (resection arthroplasty, interposition arthroplasty, prosthetic replacement, rarely if ever, and arthrodesis) for more advanced disease (Table 11.2.1).

The optimal surgery is occasionally based on what is found at the time of surgery after the articular cartilage of the metatarsal head is evaluated. However, all these procedures have a high likelihood of satisfactory results with the best procedure for the patient depending on the extent of pathology present and the goals and expectations of that patient.

Cheilectomy

For patients who present with clicking or catching complaints, have few or no radiographic findings, and their examination correlates with a loose body or osteochondral lesion, an open or arthroscopic debridement may be indicated. However, most patients will present with early degenerative joint changes on radiographs, a dorsal spur, and pain with dorsiflexion. In these patients, a cheilectomy, a procedure that removes the impinging osteophytes, should be the primary procedure of choice. This operation is relatively simple, has a short recovery period, and does not interfere with future operations that might be required. The indication for cheilectomy is early hallux rigidus with dorsal impingement,

TABLE 11.2.1 SURGICAL OPTIONS FOR TREATING HALLUX RIGIDUS

Procedure	Indications	Goals	Technique	Pitfalls
Cheilectomy	Dorsal osteophytes Mild to moderate arthrosis	Pain relief Improved motion	Remove up to one-third dorsal MT head	Insufficient bony resection Severe arthrosis
Dorsiflexion osteotomy (Moberg procedure)	Young, active patients Preserved plantar flexion, loss of dorsiflexion	Increased dorsiflexion Pain relief	Dorsal closing wedge osteotomy of proximal phalanx	Inadequate fixation (nonunion)
Interposition arthroplasty	Advanced arthrosis Desire to maintain motion Instead of Keller procedure in older, sedentary patients	Pain relief Maintained motion	Resection base of proximal phalanx Varied interposition techniques	Shortened hallux Transfer metatarsalgia Push off weakness
Prosthetic arthroplasty	Advanced arthrosis Generally not recommended	Functional joint motion Preserved length	prosthetic replacement	Implant failure Synovitis Joint instability Young, active patient
Arthrodesis	End-stage arthrosis	Pain relief Stability Durability	Rigid fixation MTP Position: 15°–20° valgus 25°–30° DF to MT shaft 10°–15° DF to ball of foot	Nonunion Malunion (dorsiflexion, loss of hallux weight bearing)

but there is debate in the literature as to whether cheilectomy is indicated in patients with significant joint space narrowing. There are no absolute contraindications for this procedure, however, and patients with severe arthrosis must be prepared for some postoperative arthritic pain symptoms if this procedure is attempted in advanced cases.

Many authors have demonstrated consistently good results in regard to relief of pain and improvement in range of motion with cheilectomy. Mann et al.[13] demonstrated excellent results in 22 of 25 patients and noted an average of 20° improvement in range of motion with average follow-up of 56 months. Feltham et al.[14] looked at age-based outcomes of cheilectomy for hallux rigidus and found 91% of patients to be better than before surgery. Patients aged 60 years and older demonstrated higher mean scores on outcome measures than any other age group, and they concluded that cheilectomy was the procedure of choice for predominantly extra-articular symptoms in patients older than 60 years. Most poor results are related to insufficient removal of bone from the dorsal metatarsal head and failure to achieve intraoperative dorsiflexion of 70° to 90° at the time of surgery.

Technique

Cheilectomy is performed through a dorsal or medial approach exposing the dorsal osteophytes of the first metatarsal. A capsulotomy with a complete synovectomy is carried out, along with excision of the proliferative osteophytes dorsally as well as laterally. The amount of bone removed depends on the degree of cartilage destruction, but most authors recommend removal of the dorsal 25% to 35% of the metatarsal head with achievement of intraoperative dorsiflexion at the MTP joint of 70° to 90° without bony impingement. The resection of the metatarsal head is accomplished with the use of a sagittal saw or osteotomes. If there is significant articular damage and osteophytes of the proximal phalanx, the dorsal one-quarter of the base can be removed. It is important to explore the lateral joint and remove these osteophytes as well. The majority of poor results are related to insufficient bone resection or severe arthrosis with unrealistic patient expectations.

Postoperative management with a hard-soled shoe and dressing is used until the wound heals. Early range-of-motion exercises are begun after a few days. Eventual range of motion will usually be less than that achieved at the time of surgery, but most patients can expect an increase of about 25° of dorsiflexion. This increase varies considerably and is related to compliance with the postoperative range-of-motion exercises.

Moberg (Proximal Phalanx Osteotomy) Procedure

The Moberg procedure comprises a dorsal closing wedge osteotomy of the proximal phalanx.[11] This procedure can be combined with a cheilectomy if large dorsal osteophytes are present. This procedure is mainly indicated in younger active patients with preserved cartilage and who require more dorsiflexion for activities such as running. These patients tend to have preserved plantarflexion but loss of dorsiflexion related to impingement and plantar

soft-tissue contracture. The patient must demonstrate adequate plantarflexion for this procedure to be successful. The procedure changes the arc of motion to provide greater dorsiflexion but does not change the absolute range of motion. Pitfalls associated with this procedure are inadequate fixation of the osteotomy or insufficient extension of the proximal phalanx with the closing wedge osteotomy. A recent review comparing dorsal closing wedge osteotomy with arthrodesis for the treatment of hallux rigidus noted fewer complications with the Moberg procedure and less callus formation postoperatively.[15] This procedure is recommended to preserve motion and prevent callus formation in younger patients with hallux rigidus and arthrodesis is recommended as a salvage procedure for failures.

Technique

A medial or dorsal approach to the first MTP joint is used with exposure of the shaft of the proximal phalanx. An osteotomy is created removing a dorsal wedge of bone approximately 5-mm wide to place the proximal phalanx in about 25° to 30° of extension relative to the metatarsal shaft. We prefer two crossed K-wires for fixation but staples or screws can also be used. They can be removed at 4 to 6 weeks, when the osteotomy is healed. If this is performed in conjunction with a cheilectomy, range-of-motion exercises need to be delayed until bone healing occurs at the osteotomy site.

Resection and Interposition Arthroplasty

Resection arthroplasty with removal of one-third to one-half of the proximal phalanx to decompress the MTP joint was first described by Keller in 1904. Problems have been encountered with long-term follow-up of patients who underwent this procedure. These problems result from resection of the base of the proximal phalanx with inherent detachment of the plantar plate and flexor hallucis brevis muscles. Cock-up deformity of the first toe, difficulty with push off, shortening of the hallux, instability with subsequent valgus drift of the hallux, and transverse metatarsalgia are problems related to the Keller procedure. To address these problems, modifications to the Keller procedure have centered on interpositional arthroplasty with removal of less of the base of the proximal phalanx and interposing capsular tissue, extensor hallucis brevis (EHB) tendon, rolled up plantaris tendon, or with a regenerative tissue matrix.[16–21] Indications for the Keller procedure as originally described consist of older sedentary patients with severe first MTP arthrosis and a desire to retain some motion of the first MTP joint. In a younger patient with advanced hallux rigidus (too advanced for a cheilectomy), with a desire to retain MTP joint motion and avoid an arthrodesis, interposition arthroplasty is a good choice. Many authors feel that interpositional arthroplasty relieves pain, corrects the deformity, provides good range of motion, avoids hallux shortening, and maintains joint stability. A contraindication to these procedures is a short first metatarsal because of the potential for transfer metatarsalgia.

Results of Keller arthroplasty and interpositional arthroplasty have been mixed. In elderly individuals, O'Doherty et al.,[22] in a prospective study comparing arthrodesis with the Keller arthroplasty, showed similar patient satisfaction and symptomatic pain relief with either operation. However, in younger patients, this procedure has fallen out of favor due to problems mentioned earlier of cock-up deformity, shortening of the hallux and weakness with push off at long term follow-up. In these patients, interpositional arthroplasty has become a more favored procedure. Berlet et al. described an interpositional arthroplasty technique using human acellular regenerative tissue matrix as a spacer to resurface both the MTP and sesamoid articulations with promising early results. Hamilton et al.[18] also described their modification to the Keller arthroplasty with interposition of the capsule and EHB. However, Lau et al.[21] noticed weakness of the great toe and less satisfaction with interpositional arthroplasty for moderate/severe hallux rigidus even though pain relief and range of motion were comparable with those seen after cheilectomy. They stated that interpositional arthroplasty has less predictable results than arthrodesis for severe hallux rigidus.

Technique

Berlet et al. described this technique for interpositional arthroplasty using human acellular regenerative tissue matrix as a spacer to resurface both the MTP and sesamoid articulations. A dorsal approach was utilized and a cheilectomy was performed with a release of the adhesions surrounding the sesamoid articulation using a McGlamery elevator. A modified Keller osteotomy was performed. The metatarsal head was then contoured, and the regenerative tissue matrix was sized and prepped. Two drill holes were then made at the metatarsal neck and a suture passer was utilized to pass the regenerative matrix to fix the graft to the metatarsal. The wound was then copiously irrigated and closed in a standard fashion. Postoperatively the patient was kept heel weight bearing in a postop shoe until the incision healed. After the skin healed, range of motion was instituted, and by 4 weeks the patient was placed into a lace-up shoe along with formal physical therapy if necessary.

Implant Arthroplasty

Prosthetic replacement for the treatment of hallux rigidus first gained popularity with the use of a single-stem hemiarthroplasty of the proximal phalanx. However, the success of this procedure has been met with mixed results. The advantages of implant arthroplasty include preservation of some functional joint motion and the length of the first ray. Even though short-term results are generally good, longer-term follow-up has revealed many problems with reports of implant failure (loosening, fragmentation), synovitis, soft-tissue foreign body reaction, joint stiffness, joint instability, osteolysis, and silicone wear. A risk factor for poor survival of first MTP joint implant arthroplasty is the young active patient. Most patients with unsatisfactory results showed fragmentation of the implant and bone/soft-tissue reaction about the prosthesis. Newer designs of implant arthroplasty include the use of titanium grommet liners and a double stemmed prosthesis. The use of titanium grommets has been shown to improve the long-term durability of implant arthroplasty secondary to fewer problems with

implant fracture and particulate reactivity, especially in the rheumatoid population.[23] Long-term follow-up for these newer designs is still forthcoming; therefore, widespread use of implant arthroplasty is still not recommended.

First MTP Joint Arthrodesis

For severe arthrosis of the first MTP joint, arthrodesis provides predictable pain relief and is currently the most widely used procedure for end-stage hallux rigidus. The advantages of arthrodesis are that it provides predictable pain relief, stability, and durability. However, these are accomplished at the expense of motion. After first MTP arthrodesis, patients can walk fast, ride a bike, and play golf, although they will have difficulty running and will have limitations on shoe wear, especially with respect to heel height of more than 1 in. A successful arthrodesis depends on bony union and acceptable position of the first toe. The toe should be fused in 10° to 15° of valgus, 25° to 30° of dorsiflexion with respect to the metatarsal shaft, or 10° to 15° of dorsiflexion with respect to the ball of the foot with neutral rotation (Fig. 11.2.2).

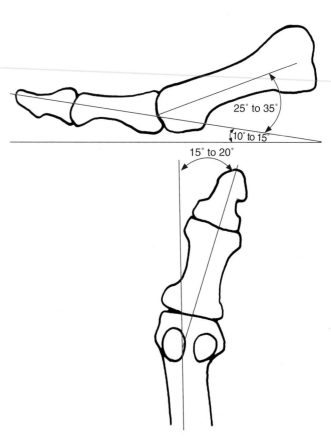

Figure 11.2.2 Diagram demonstrating optimal position for first MTP joint arthrodesis: 25° to 35° of dorsiflexion with respect to the metatarsal shaft, 10° to 15° of dorsiflexion with respect to the sole of the foot, and 15° to 20° of valgus with respect to the first metatarsal. (Adapted from Katcherian DA. Pathology of the first ray. In: Mizel MS, Miller RA, Scioli MW, eds. Orthopaedic knowledge update, foot and ankle, 2nd ed. Rosemont: American Academy of Orthopaedic Surgeons, 1998:154.)

Many techniques for internal fixation have been described and include longitudinal Steinmann pins, crossed or oblique compression screws, Herbert screws with tension band wiring, and dorsal plates. Bone grafting has not been found to be necessary. A disadvantage to the use of dorsal plating is the bulk of the implant and the potential for irritation with a need for a second procedure for hardware removal. Recent modifications to the dorsal plate have included low profile designs, alterations in plate design (no screw holes over the fusion site), and changes in manufacturing material (vitallium instead of stainless steel), which have increased the strength of the plate. Theoretical disadvantages to compression screws or Steinmann pins include the potential stress riser at the site of insertion with the potential for stress fracture. Biomechanical studies have been performed to determine the optimal method of internal fixation for first MTP arthrodesis.[24,25] One recent study comparing the use of dorsal plates, Steinmann pins, oblique compression screws, and Herbert screws found that dorsal plating required the greatest force to failure, provided the largest initial stiffness, and concluded that the dorsal plate was significantly stronger than other internal fixation methods.[24]

First MTP arthrodesis provides long-term predictable pain relief for end-stage hallux rigidus with an average union rate greater than 90% regardless of what type of internal fixation is used.[15,26–29] Complications from first MTP arthrodesis include nonunion, malunion, and interphalangeal (IP) arthritis. The incidence of degenerative changes of the IP joint of the great toe is variable (30% to 40%); however, the majority of patients are asymptomatic, and its presence is of little clinical significance. Adequate valgus positioning will help minimize this complication. The most common positioning error is too much dorsiflexion, and this leads to problems with shoe impingement and loss of hallux weight bearing (Fig. 11.2.3).

Technique

The dorsal plating technique is performed through a dorsal approach, exposing the cartilage surfaces of the proximal phalanx and first metatarsal. The articular cartilage surfaces can be prepared with the use of conical reamers producing a convex metatarsal head and a concave proximal phalanx or by freehand using a burr and oscillating saw to remove the articular cartilage. The exposed subchondral bone is then perforated with multiple small drill holes to allow apposition of two bleeding cancellous bony surfaces across which the fusion will occur. The joint is reduced into the position of fusion (15° of dorsiflexion with respect to the plantar surface of the foot and 10° to 15° of valgus) and provisionally fixed in this position with K-wires. The position of arthrodesis is checked by simulating weight bearing of the foot on a flat tray[30] (Fig. 11.2.4A and B). One should be able to slide a fingertip under the toe tip to verify good position. The dorsal plate is then applied in compression across the MTP joint (Fig. 11.2.4C and D). The postoperative regimen includes immediate weight bearing in a postoperative hard-soled shoe.

RA OF THE FOREFOOT

EPIDEMIOLOGY, ETIOLOGY, AND PATHOGENESIS

RA is a progressive systemic inflammatory disorder primarily affecting the synovial tissues and is the commonest inflammatory disorder to affect the foot. Approximately 1% of the population in the United States has RA and, as in OA, the incidence increases with age, peaking between 40 and 60 years. RA is three times more common in women and affects all ethnic groups.[31] Foot involvement in RA is extremely common, with the hindfoot and forefoot being more affected than the midfoot. It is reported that nearly 50% of patients with RA have active foot and ankle symptoms with forefoot involvement present in 100% after 10 years of active RA disease.[32,33] The forefoot is generally involved early in RA with up to 15% of patients presenting with forefoot pain as the first symptoms of having the disease. This pain is caused by the inflammatory synovitis seen with this disorder. Joint involvement is typically symmetric, but RA can also affect the extra-articular tissues, contributing to the observed pain and deformity of this disorder. The forefoot deformities seen with RA can vary and may include hallux valgus/varus, hammer or claw toes, and variable levels of intermetatarsal deviations and/or widening.

The pathogenesis of RA is driven by the immune system through an autoimmune phenomenon. A predilection for developing RA may exist in those who are HLA-DR4 positive. Although controversial, some studies support an infectious etiology to RA. Immunologically, up to 80% of adults with RA are seropositive for rheumatoid factor (RF) and reactive antinuclear antibody (ANA). In fact, higher levels of RF are associated with more severe disease, whereas both RF and ANA seronegativity have a lower incidence of extra-articular disease and a better prognosis. Other markers of disease activity, mostly indicating immune system reactivity, are C-reactive protein (CRP), erythrocyte sedimentation rate (ESR), circulating immune complexes, and platelet count.[34]

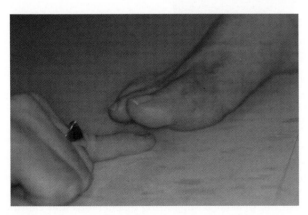

Figure 11.2.3 Complications after first MTP arthrodesis. Shown here is the most common positioning problem; too much dorsiflexion can lead to problems with shoe impingement and loss of hallux weight bearing.

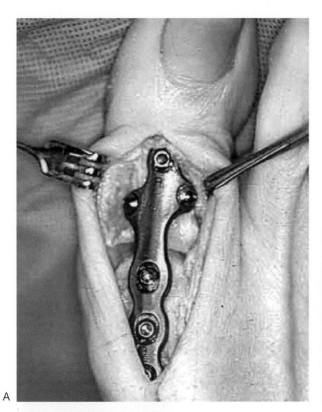

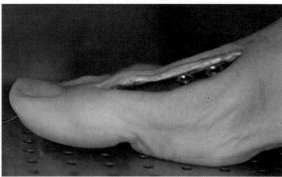

A

B

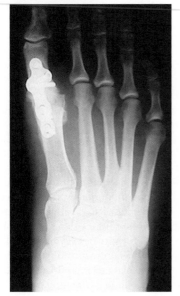

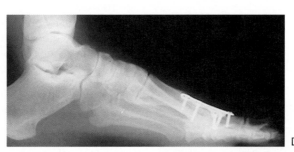

C

D

Figure 11.2.4   Intraoperative clinical AP (**A**) and lateral (**B**) views of a first MTP joint arthrodesis. The metal tray allows the surgeon to check adequate dorsiflexion positioning of the great toe by simulating weight bearing (**C and D**). Postoperative AP and lateral radiographs of first MTP joint arthrodesis. Notice the low-profile dorsal plate design and the absence of screw holes over the fusion site, which decreases the incidence of hardware failure.

Immune system reactivity leads to an inflammatory synovitis that invades and destroys the capsular tissue, cartilage, bone, and ligamentous structures. This migrating, destructive inflammatory pannus leads to joint instability and destroys the smooth articular surface. Pathologically, synovial hypertrophy and ligamentous laxity appear to develop first, followed by an inflammation-mediated destruction of the cartilage and surrounding tissue. The resulting deformities then occur as mechanical stresses traverse the weakened supporting ligamentous and capsular tissues of the joint. As with OA, the extent of deformity in RA depends on the time active disease has been present. An important distinction of RA is that of juxta-articular joint destruction owing to the invasive inflammatory synovitis.

In the foot and ankle, tenosynovitis is a common finding, most commonly involving the peroneal and posterior tibial tendons. Vasculitis may also occur, where involvement of the subdermal vessels in connective tissue may predispose to the development of rheumatoid nodules.

DIAGNOSIS

Clinical Features

The diagnosis of RA is a clinical one, supported by several laboratory findings, a detailed examination, and characteristic roentgenographic findings (Table 11.2.2). In the midfoot, chronic synovitis generally leads to joint space loss and pain, but manifestations otherwise are not specific. In the forefoot, metatarsalgia is most commonly the presenting complaint. Nearly every toe deformity has been described in forefoot RA, including the commonest one—severe hallux valgus often with metatarsus primus varus (Fig. 11.2.5A). The toes may eventually sublux dorsally and may even dislocate as the synovitis progresses to plantar plate destruction, and the MTP joints become gradually incompetent. The plantar fat pad of the forefoot is pulled distally by this dorsal subluxation and becomes more of an anterior structure. When this occurs, the lesser toes become even more dorsally displaced. These deformities lead to gait changes, increased pressure "metatarsalgia," and a thick plantar callus (Fig. 11.2.5B). The findings seen in the lesser toes are variable and include claw toe, curly toe, and hammer toe deformities as well as cock-up (dorsal subluxation) deformity of the fifth toe. These may be fixed or flexible deformities. Claw toe deformity is the result of severe MTP joint dorsiflexion/hyperextension combined with flexion deformity at the IP joints. Hammer toe is a flexion deformity at the IP joint with extension at the MTP and distal IP joints. Rheumatoid nodules may be present at a variety of forefoot areas leading to location-specific symptoms. If intermetatarsal, nodules can lead to spreading of adjacent toes and can potentially be misdiagnosed as an interdigital neuroma. The IP joints are often in hyperextension in patients with forefoot RA, leading to pain in this region. MTP dislocation causes severe pain and bursitis at the metatarsal heads. Extensive nodules in these plantar regions may ulcerate, with the potential for the development of osteomyelitis. The anterior drawer test can evaluate the stability of the MTP joint. By applying dorsally directed pressure at the base of the proximal phalanx while holding the metatarsal head, joint displacement may be appreciated, which may reproduce the patients' symptoms.

Radiologic Features

The duration and activity of the disease process are the most important factors associated with finding radiographic changes in RA.[35] The clinical progression of RA disease occurs ahead of radiographic findings. AP, lateral, and oblique views of the feet should be obtained. Initial forefoot changes often occur at the MTP joints, especially at the first, fourth, and fifth MTP joints (Fig. 11.2.5C). Radiographic features are typically symmetric, most commonly showing osteoporosis starting at the subchondral bone. Another classic early change in RA is periarticular marginal erosions, with secondary OA occurring later. Osseous ankylosis of the midfoot may occur late, but spontaneous MTP joint fusion is uncommon. Lateral foot radiographs often reveal the extent of proximal phalanx hyperextension at the MTP joint. The AP or oblique foot view will show dislocations of the lesser MTP joints. On AP radiographs, one may see the "gun barrel" sign as the dislocated second proximal phalanx is viewed end on.

TREATMENT

Clinical Management

Clinically, the treatment of early foot RA comprises physical therapy and medical management. These treatments are aimed primarily at limiting the synovitis of RA. Physical therapy is designed to prevent deformity and loss of range of motion. Regimens should comprise muscle and ligament stretching and strengthening exercises. Shoe wear modifications can be used, especially for fixed deformities of

---

TABLE 11.2.2 CLINICAL, RADIOGRAPHIC, AND LABORATORY FINDINGS OF RA OF THE FOOT

Clinical Features	Radiographic Features	Laboratory Features
Forefoot pain; inflammatory synovitis; metatarsalgia	Osteoporosis starting at the subchondral bone	HLA-DR4±
±Tenosynovitis (peroneal and posterior tibialis tendons most common)	Periarticular marginal erosions	RF±
Ligamentous laxity, dorsal subluxation/dislocation at the MTP joints	Joint malalignment/subluxation/dislocations	ANA±
Plantar fat pad migration/callus formation	Osseous ankylosis—late finding	*Increased* CRP, ESR, and platelet counts
Rheumatoid nodules	"Gun barrel sign"—AP view of second proximal phalanx on end	Circulating immune complexes
Toe deformities (hammer toe, claw toe, curly toe)		

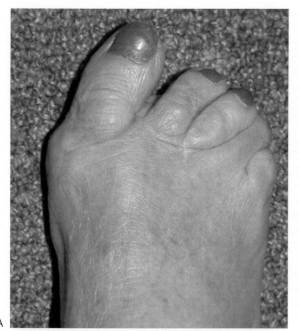

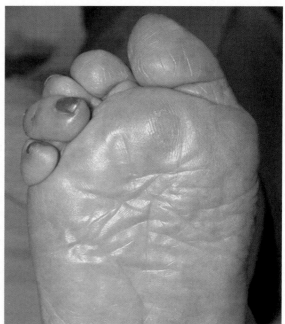

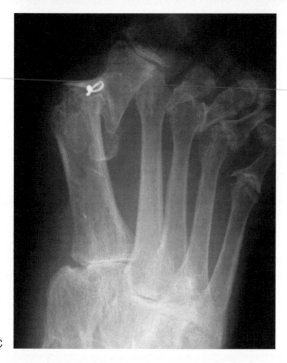

Figure 11.2.5 The forefoot in RA. **A:** Clinical appearance demonstrating characteristic hallux valgus and lesser toe deformities. **B:** Plantar view demonstrating distal displacement of the plantar fat pad and thick callus formation. **C:** Radiographic features of osteopenia, periarticular erosions, hallux valgus, and subluxation/dislocation of the great toe and lesser toe MTP joints.

the forefoot. Soft orthotic devices, widened, extra-depth accommodative shoe wear, and padding all may help. These modalities are designed to unload the forefoot and metatarsal heads while relieving lesser toe discomfort. (AFOs or University of California–Berkley Laboratories (UCBLs) bracing may be effective as well. For rheumatoid nodules, regardless of location, shoe wear modification is generally employed and, if unsuccessful, surgical excision may relieve local symptoms.

First-line medical therapies focus on limiting inflammation-related pain and swelling but do not impact disease progression.[36] Oral salicylates, high-dose nonsteroidal anti-inflammatory medications, or low-dose prednisone (5 mg per day) predominate in this situation. The

"disease-modifying" medications are second-line therapy for RA and are used when there is persistent synovitis despite first-line therapies, or when radiographic erosions or clinical deformity is present, or when there is extra-articular disease.[36] These agents include the gold salts, antimalarials, methotrexate, azathioprine, D-penicillamine, cyclosporine A, sulfasalazine, and combination therapies. Intramuscular weekly gold injections or oral gold salt twice a day can be useful. Gold toxicity leading to bone marrow suppression, dermatitis, or possibly membranous nephropathy must be monitored. Methotrexate at doses from 2.5 to 15 mg per week is a first-line remitting agent as well, but the development of stomatitis and bone marrow suppression are concerns that should be monitored.

Dihydrochloroquine at a dose of 400 mg per day (retinal screening should be performed) or 1 to 2 mg per day of azulfidine (must not have sulfa allergy) can be very effective as remittive RA therapies as well. The use of intra-articular steroid injections may help alleviate mild synovitic symptoms in RA and can be repeated if relief occurs.

Surgical Considerations

Patients with RA may require multiple procedures, possibly symmetric or combined, owing to the nature of the disease. However, limiting postoperative motion and restricting weight bearing are important but in patients with active disease, this may further promote debility and possible deformity. Management of the patient's medical therapies with the involvement of the rheumatologist in the perioperative period should be aimed at optimizing bone and soft-tissue healing while minimizing disease activity.

Operative indications depend on the severity of active disease, the patient's level of function and debility, and the extent of deformity. Ideally, the optimal candidate is a patient with an isolated deformity and low levels of active inflammatory markers, whereas high inflammatory indicators combined with continually worsening disease in multiple areas is less preferable. Numerous surgical procedures have been reported to be successful, ranging from synovectomy to arthrodesis, or even forefoot amputation. In this regard, it is important to remember that patients with advancing stages of RA have a progressive decrease in overall functioning. Historically, "soft tissue only" techniques have generally done poorly and have higher recurrence rates in these patients. Bone resection and arthrodesis have been used in RA to lessen the chances of recurrent deformity. With further advancements in the medical management of RA joint preservation procedures have become more common. Hallux valgus deformities in RA patients can be treated with arthrodesis, or rarely with Keller-type interpositional arthroplasty or implant arthroplasty. Surgical procedures to correct nonrheumatic hallux valgus other than these have high recurrence rates and are not recommended. Hallux rigidus is discussed in detail in the previous section and is treated as mentioned, by cheilectomy, interpositional arthroplasty, implant arthroplasty, or arthrodesis. IP joint arthrosis can be treated with stiffened shoes to prevent motion and decrease pain or with arthrodesis of the joint. In general, first MP joint deformities should be corrected prior to lesser toe deformities.

Surgical Forefoot Reconstruction

Historically, the most accepted surgical correction of forefoot RA is first metatarsalphalangeal joint arthrodesis and resection of the lesser metatarsal heads. Resection or implant arthroplasty of the hallux is problematic and can lead to higher recurrence of deformity. Operative reconstruction of the forefoot aims to give medial post stabilization with first MTP joint arthrodesis. Thordarson et al. have shown that joint preservation surgery without first MTP fusion has a high failure rate. First MTP fusion combined with reducing the plantar fat pad to its appropriate position by resection arthroplasty of the lesser MP joints decompresses the forefoot and improves metatarsalgia. With improvement of medical management of RA, joint preservation has been a proposed treatment option with first ray correction along with lesser toe reconstruction using proximal interphalangeal (PIP) arthroplasty or arthrodesis with shorter-term results. Other techniques reported include decompression by extensor tenotomy or proximal phalanx removal. In RA it is important to remember that even if one or two lesser MTP joints do not have "obvious" involvement, all the lesser toe MTP joints should be included in the forefoot arthroplasty especially to avoid transfer metatarsalgia. Other surgical considerations include wound and bone healing along with recession of the gastrocnemius to potentially decrease forefoot load.

Technique. Longitudinal incisions should be dorsal to the first MTP joint, dorsally between metatarsals 2 and 3, and again between metatarsals 4 and 5. The second through the fifth metatarsal heads should be resected stepwise from medial to lateral, with dorsal-distal to plantar-proximal beveling parallel to the floor. K-wires should be used for MTP region fixation with long extensor tendon interposition.

Surgical Correction of Lesser Toe Deformity

Operative correction of the lesser toes is indicated when conservative measures fail to alleviate symptoms, the patient cannot tolerate the pain, and/or if activities of daily living are being affected. Early in RA, synovectomy to remove inflamed tissue helps decompress the joint and lessen pain. When used in combination with first MTP joint arthrodesis, results are improved. However, the progressive nature of RA in the forefoot will usually require further surgical correction of the progressive deformity of the lesser MTP joints and toes.

Hammer and Claw Toe Deformity Correction. Hammer toe and claw toe deformities are treated surgically by the same principles, by correcting each level of deformity and in most cases correcting any MTP deformity before correcting PIP deformity. Surgical treatment is aimed at bringing the MTP and PIP joints into a neutral position, ultimately to allow pain-free ambulation. Although approaches vary, a dorsal approach is preferred, which prioritizes a scarless plantar surface and protects plantar neurovascular structures. Although dorsal longitudinal incisions are generally preferred for isolated joint reconstructions, a single transverse incision to access the metatarsal heads for their resection can be beneficial. While obtaining good alignment, care must be taken to excise enough of the metatarsal heads and part of the neck to limit the potential for bone-on-bone irritation postoperatively. Following resection, callosities on the plantar surface may resolve as the plantar fat pad relocates, decreasing stresses on the skin in this region. For flexible claw or hammer toe deformities, flexor tendon transfer can be utilized often with MTP joint capsule release and extensor tenotomies. Fixed deformities can be corrected by MTP joint release as well, or by Du Vries resection arthroplasty, where the distal portion of the articular surface of the metatarsal head is resected with an osteotome. Surgical correction may also require collateral ligament release. Lesser toe deformities can be corrected simultaneously with first MTP arthrodesis and metatarsal head resection. Stabilization of the lesser toes postoperatively can be accomplished by K-wires or a supportive soft dressing changed weekly. This protects the toes during scar tissue formation and may decrease the risk of recurrence. Correction of skin contractures should not be overlooked and should be alleviated when possible.

Joint Preservation Surgery

Joint preservation surgery is an evolving concept in the management of the RA forefoot. First ray stabilization at the TMT joint with correction of hallux valgus deformity through a modified Lapidus procedure or first metatarsal osteotomy has been advocated in the RA forefoot. Correction of lesser toe deformity can then be done using traditional soft-tissue releases combined with shortening metatarsal osteotomies if necessary and PIP arthroplasty, arthrodesis, or closed manipulation, which has been advocated most frequently in the literature. Metatarsal head preservation can make salvage operations easier and can preserve forefoot biomechanics with more normal forefoot motion. Preservation of bone and forefoot motion can restore the balance of forefoot load in stance and toe off. Potential difficulties include recurrence of metatarsalgia and need for revision surgery along with the potential for disease advancement and later salvage procedures.

There are no specific absolute contraindications to surgical intervention in RA other than those requiring medical risk stratification prior to surgery.

RESULTS AND OUTCOMES

Although shoe modifications, physical therapy, and medical therapies may limit disease progress, outcomes vary depending on the duration of active disease and degrees of deformity corrected.

In general, outcomes are good. In a study of 20 patients undergoing hallux arthrodesis, 19 achieved fusion and were satisfied with the procedure. Only 10% of these patients had postoperative painful callosities.[37] Patients have been noted to do better with forefoot reconstruction when the hallux is managed by arthrodesis than by other means. Currently, it appears that less aggressive or more joint-sparing procedures have higher recurrence rates of deformity. Despite 83% of patients at 6 years reporting satisfactory results following a modified procedure, namely metatarsals 2-to-5 shortening oblique osteotomy and MTP joint synovectomy, with hallux valgus reconstruction using an implant arthroplasty or osteotomy, there were a 12% plantar callosity recurrence rate and 30% lesser ray deformity recurrence rate.[38] This emphasizes the importance of reserving joint-sparing procedures for those younger, active patients who may require repeat procedures.

CRYSTAL-INDUCED ARTHROPATHY OF THE FOREFOOT

PATHOGENESIS

Gout and pseudogout are crystalline deposition disorders that may present with foot involvement (Table 11.2.3). Gout is characterized by the presence of intra-articular monosodium urate crystals, which are needle shaped and demonstrate the classic negative birefringence under polarizing light microscopy. Pseudogout, which is also known as CPPD crystal deposition disease, is characterized by the presence of CPPD crystals of variable shapes in joint or periarticular

TABLE 11.2.3 COMPARISON OF TWO CRYSTAL-INDUCED ARTHROPATHIES AFFECTING THE FOREFOOT

	Gout	Pseudogout
Clinical	Stiffness Swelling Severe pain Hallux most common location	Less severe clinical picture Variable location, less common in foot, most common in knee
Radiographic	Late stages: periarticular erosions	Chondrocalcinosis (usually linear)
Crystal Analysis	Monosodium urate crystals, needle-shaped, Negative birefringence under polarized light Elevated serum uric acid	Calcium pyrophosphate dihydrate (CPPD) crystals, variable shape Weak positive birefringence under polarized light
Treatment	Rest NSAIDS/indomethacin Colchicine Suppressive therapy	Rest NSAIDS/indomethacin Colchicine

tissues and have weak positive birefringence under the polarizing microscope. Both disorders produce an acute inflammatory synovitis most commonly involving the first MTP joint.

Gout results from a disorder of purine metabolism resulting in increased uric acid synthesis. Renal disorders can also cause increased uric acid levels secondary to poor renal clearance of urate. The plasma becomes saturated with uric acid, and this saturation allows precipitation of monosodium urate crystals in the relatively avascular tissues of distal peripheral joints. The presence of these crystals causes an acute inflammatory synovitis that can be monarticular or polyarticular in nature. In most cases of gout, the reason for increased uric acid synthesis is unknown, but it can be associated with certain diseases (lymphoma, leukemia, or psoriasis), certain medications (cyclosporine for organ transplants), or certain foods with high purine content (alcoholic beverages). Serum uric acid levels are often normal. Gout is more frequent in men than in women, and the hallux is the most commonly affected region, accounting for 50% to 70% of initial attacks. The first MTP joint will be affected in 90% of patients with gout at some point during their lifetime. Other regions of the foot that can be involved include the dorsum of the foot, the instep, the heel, and the ankle. Besides joint involvement, urate crystals can precipitate into subcutaneous nodules known as tophi (Fig. 11.2.6).

The etiology of CPPD deposition disease is unknown. However, frequent associations include previous trauma, gout, and hyperparathyroidism. Symptomatic disease usually appears in patients older than 60 years of age and both sexes are affected equally. Most commonly this disorder is encountered in the knee, hip, ankle, wrist, and shoulder, but it can also affect the first MTP joint by causing an acute synovitis owing to calcium pyrophosphate deposition. The inflammatory response is usually less severe than that seen in gout, but it is unclear why a more intense reaction occurs with urate crystals than with calcium pyrophosphate crystals.

DIAGNOSIS

The onset of an acute gouty attack is manifested by severe pain, swelling, erythema, stiffness, warmth about the involved joint, and a sudden onset of symptoms. The attack usually lasts from several days to a week. It usually occurs without provocation; however, it may be preceded by mild trauma or the consumption of purine-rich foods. Gouty attacks are frequently seen after an operation in the acute postoperative period. Diagnosis is confirmed by joint aspiration and crystal analysis of the synovial fluid. However, usually the diagnosis can be inferred clinically with the history of symptoms, the characteristic location of the first MTP joint, and the frequent polyarticular nature in the presence of an elevated serum urate level. Septic arthritis can have a similar appearing clinical picture. If uncertainty exists or the presentation is of monoarticular involvement of the knee, ankle, or wrist, aspiration is mandatory to rule out infection. Crystal analysis shows the classic negatively birefringent needle-shaped crystals. Occasionally, gout can present in a chronic fashion with enlarging prominences about the first MTP joint caused by hypertrophic bone and tophaceous deposits. Some patients debilitated by other medical problems such as neuropathy, diabetes, or vascular disease will present with chronic ulcerations over these prominent tophaceous deposits. With an initial gouty attack, radiographic features of the bone and joint surfaces are unremarkable; however, with more advanced disease periarticular erosions classically described as rat bite lesions can be seen on both sides of the joint. The articular surface is often spared, but in chronic cases joint destruction may be severe.

An acute pseudogout attack usually presents with a less severe clinical picture than that seen with gout. Most commonly, pseudogout is seen in the knee, hip, ankle, wrist, or shoulder, but it can present with first MTP joint involvement. Again physical examination findings of erythema, swelling, stiffness are present, but the intensity of pain is usually less severe than seen with gout. Diagnosis can be confirmed only by joint aspiration and the presence of CPPD crystals as no blood tests are diagnostic. These crystals are weakly positively birefringent and variably shaped. Radiographic features of pseudogout include the presence of chondrocalcinosis, fine linear calcifications in articulate cartilage, or fibrocartilage; however, joint destruction is uncommon.

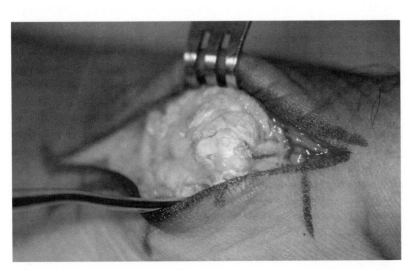

Figure 11.2.6 Intraoperative view demonstrating characteristic appearance of tophaceous gout affecting the first MTP joint.

TREATMENT

Treatment for acute gout and pseudogout attacks is identical. Rest, elevation, and the use of a wooden sole, open toe postoperative shoe should be used for symptomatic relief. Medical management comprises either high-dose nonsteroidal anti-inflammatory medication or colchicine. If there are no medical contraindications such as gastrointestinal bleeding, coagulopathies, or renal insufficiency, 50 mg of indomethacin three times a day for 3 to 5 days is usually an effective regimen. Colchicine is also an effective therapy for acute attacks if initiated within the first 24 to 48 hours of onset. The response is usually dramatic and the dose is 1 mg by mouth every 2 hours until a response is obtained or until diarrhea occurs. No more than 7 mg should be given in 48 hours. Severe electrolyte imbalances can be seen with colchicine-induced diarrhea and therefore, the medication should be discontinued upon onset, and electrolytes should be monitored. Colchicine is also used chronically to lessen the frequency of attacks by daily administration of tablets between 0.5 and 1.5 mg dose.

Surgical treatment is seldom indicated in the treatment of gout or pseudogout. In chronic tophaceous gout, debridement of symptomatic or draining deposits can be attempted (Fig. 11.10). If severe joint destruction has occurred with either gout or pseudogout, the treatment is similar to that of degenerative arthrosis of the first MTP joint or hallux rigidus. Joint debridement, interpositional arthroplasty, or arthrodesis are all reasonable surgical options in the presence of moderate-to-severe joint involvement and destruction.

TURF TOE

PATHOGENESIS

Bowers and Martin[39] coined the term "turf toe" in 1976 after correlating an increased incidence of great toe soft-tissue injuries in football players wearing a more flexible soccer style shoe on artificial turf playing fields. Since that time, the term has been expanded to include all first MTP sprains, whether or not they occur on artificial turf. Turf toe results from severe hyperextension of the first MTP joint and its occurrence and recognition have increased since the advent of artificial turf. However, these injuries can occur in many ways including automobile accidents, equestrian stirrup injuries, chronic overuse problems in ballet dancers, and athletic competition injuries. Turf toe can be significantly disabling in both the acute period and with long-term follow-up. Some studies have shown that turf toe injuries account for more missed practice and playing time than ankle sprains, even though they occur less often.[40] These injuries also have the potential to lead to chronic problems (hallux rigidus, hallux valgus, or hallux varus) because most players and coaches perceive this injury as trivial and return to athletic competition without sufficient recovery time. In a review of 20 athletes with prior turf toe injuries and greater than 5 years of follow-up, 50% of the patients had persistent symptoms, and specific problems included early onset hallux rigidus and hallux valgus.[40] These late sequelae of turf toe injuries can lead to chronic disability and early retirement from professional athletics.

Many different factors have been implicated in the increased incidence of turf toe injuries. Most authors agree that the increased hardness of artificial turf over time and the increased flexibility of turf type shoes result in increased stress faced by the MTP joint. These issues combined with patient factors such as weight, age, sport, player position, pes planus, restricted first MTP motion, flat metatarsal head, increased ankle dorsiflexion, and prior injury all have been postulated to contribute to turf toe. Although these injuries have been implicated in all sporting events, they are most common in football players.

The mechanism of injury relates to forced dorsiflexion of the first MTP joint. This occurs when an external force drives the first MTP joint of a firmly planted foot on the ground into further dorsiflexion. The proximal phalanx is compressed in extension against the dorsal articular surface of the metatarsal head as the taut plantar capsule attempts to restrict dorsiflexion beyond its normal limit. When this occurs the plantar soft-tissue restraints are either stretched or torn. The normal dorsiflexion range of motion of the first MTP joint ranges from 30° to 100°; therefore, for athletes with baseline decreased motion of the MTP joint, less dorsiflexion is tolerated before stressing the plantar capsular restraints. A soft-soled shoe with increased flexibility contributes to the mechanism of turf toe injury by failing to restrict first MTP joint dorsiflexion. Varus or valgus stresses at the first MTP joint may also be associated with this forced dorsiflexion causing collateral capsular ligament strain, ligament rupture, or avulsion fracture from the base of the proximal phalanx.

DIAGNOSIS

Clinical findings can vary according to the severity of injury. The history can reveal either a single acute event or multiple episodes of jamming the great toe. Some patients may recall a single injury in the past with relatively uneventful recovery, but gradually after several mild recurrent injuries the symptoms of pain, swelling, and stiffness have persisted. Turf toe can include mild sprains, tears of the capsuloligamentous structures, bruising of the articular cartilage, osteochondral fracture, sesamoid fractures, subluxation, dislocation, and fracture dislocation of the first MTP joint. Physical examination findings include a dorsally tender, swollen first MTP joint. This is usually accompanied by varying degrees of ecchymosis. Range of motion is painful and limited. Tenderness can be mild and localized to very intense and diffuse. Weight bearing is usually tolerated with some pain, but in more severe injuries weight bearing may be accompanied by a limp or not tolerated at all. During athletic competition, patients with mild injuries usually report being able to resume play with some pain but in severe cases of turf toe, the athlete is usually not able to return to practice or the game.

Radiographic evaluation can be used to further delineate the extent of injury. Some authors feel radiographs should be obtained for all turf toe injuries, whereas others feel that clinical findings of a more severe injury will dictate the need for radiographs. They can be used to evaluate for fractures, articular joint incongruity, and pre-existing arthritic conditions. Serial radiographs can be obtained to follow fracture healing, monitor for sesamoid migration or widening, and evaluate for subchondral bone resorption seen in chondral injuries. Recently MRI has been used to evaluate turf toe injuries and define the extent of the soft-tissue capsuloligamentous pathology.[41] The widespread utility of MRI is still in question.

Classification of these injuries has been proposed by some authors to direct treatment and determine short-term prognosis[40,42] (Table 11.2.4).

- Grade I sprains are a stretch injury to the capsuloligamentous structures of the first joint with only minor tearing of the soft-tissue restraints. Tenderness is usually localized and range of motion is only slightly decreased. Weight bearing is tolerated with minor pain, and with mild symptoms, the patient can usually participate in athletics.
- Grade II injuries are partial tears of the soft-tissue restraints and tenderness and ecchymosis are more intense and diffuse. Range of motion is moderately limited. Usually weight bearing is tolerated with a limp, and usually the patient cannot perform normally in athletic competition.
- Grade III injuries represent complete tears of the capsuloligamentous structures with or without bony avulsion fractures. Significant pain, swelling, and ecchymosis are seen with marked limitation in motion. Weight bearing

---

TABLE 11.2.4 CLASSIFICATION AND ACTIVITY GUIDELINES FOR TURF TOE INJURIES[40]

Classification

Grade I
Capsuloligamentous stretch injury to first MTP joint
Minor tears of soft-tissue restraints
Able to continue activity as tolerated
Return to athletics as symptoms allow

Grade II
Partial tears of capsuloligamentous structures
Tenderness, ecchymosis, ROM limitations
Weight bearing with limp, limited activity
Return to athletic activities as tolerated after approximately
  2 wk rest/adjuvant therapies

Grade III
Complete tears of capsuloligamentous structures with or
  without bony avulsion fractures
Pain, swelling, ecchymosis, marked ROM limitation
Weight bearing not tolerated, unable to perform athletic
  activities
Crutch use, ± taping/shoe wear modification
Usually no athletic competition 2–6 wk, return to athletics with
  resumption of pain-free motion

ROM, range of motion.

is not tolerated, and the patient is unable to perform athletic activities.[40]

TREATMENT

Most turf toe injuries are treated nonsurgically. An initial assessment to rule out fractures or dislocations is made, and then treatment is directed at protecting the soft tissues and allowing for functional rehabilitation. The standard rest, ice, compression, and elevation/R.I.C.E. protocol is indicated with rest and restriction of motion, ice during the first 48 hours after injury, application of a compressive dressing and elevation. Nonsteroidal anti-inflammatory medication can be used as an adjuvant therapy. To minimize the loss of motion, early active range-of-motion exercises should be instituted as soon as symptoms allow. Adjuvant therapy to increase range of motion includes whirlpool and ultrasound with cold compression, which helps improve motion by actively reducing edema and mobilizing scar. Taping of the hallux to splint the first MTP joint and protect the injured soft tissues can provide symptomatic relief by restricting hyperextension at the first MTP joint. This is accomplished by using a 0.5-in tape crosslooped over the top of the proximal phalanx. Successive overlapping loops are placed over the toe and again cross over themselves on the plantar surface of the foot. These are anchored in place with another band of tape around the forefoot.

Surgical treatment is rarely necessary; however, indications for acute surgical intervention include displaced intra-articular fractures, irreducible dislocations, and unstable ligamentous avulsion injuries with displacement. If the avulsion fragment is too small, then excision with ligament repair is indicated. Delayed surgical intervention after a trial of nonoperative treatment is indicated for symptomatic loose bodies, osteochondral lesions, or sesamoid nonunions. Chronic long-term sequelae of turf toe include acquired hallux rigidus, hallux valgus, and hallux varus, and these may require late surgical intervention.

Return to athletic competition is relative to the severity and grade of injury. Rest, which is vital to limiting prolonged disability, is difficult to control because of the perception that this injury is trivial. Returning to competition too early can lead to chronic problems, and the importance of physicians, trainers, coaches, and players recognizing the severity of injury cannot be overstated. A general guideline for resumption of athletic competition depending on the grade of turf toe injury has been recommended.

- Grade I sprains—return to athletic competition as symptoms allow, that is, when swelling has decreased and painless passive extension of the first MTP joint to 90° has returned.
- Grade II sprains usually require up to 2 weeks of rest and then return to activity when swelling and range of motion allow.
- Grade III sprains usually require crutch usage and gradual return to weight bearing over the first week. Players are usually out of athletic competition from 2 to 6 weeks, and again resumption of range of motion will dictate when play can be resumed.

Players with turf toe injuries may benefit from taping to restrict excessive dorsiflexion of the first MTP joint and the use of a stiff-soled shoe design or insert to reduce stress and limit motion of the first MTP joint. Shoe modifications can include a steel forefoot plate that resists torque and bending to help prevent recurrent injury. It is also important for proper shoe fit after injury, and adjustments may need to be made in width to accommodate the injured hallux.

SUGGESTED READINGS

Midfoot Arthritis

Myerson MS, Fisher RT, Burgess AR, et al. Fracture dislocations of the tarsometatarsal joints: end results correlated with pathology and treatment. Foot Ankle 1986;6(5):225–242.

Turf Toe

Watson TS, Anderson RB, Davis WH. Periarticular injuries to the hallux metatarsophalangeal joint in athletes. Foot Ankle Clin 2000;5(3):687–713.

REFERENCES

1. Komenda GA, Myerson MS, Biddinger KR. Results of arthrodesis of the tarsometatarsal joints after traumatic injury. J Bone Joint Surg Am 1996;78(11):1665–1676.
2. Lakin RC, DeGnore LT, Pienkowski D. Contact mechanics of normal tarsometatarsal joints. J Bone Joint Surg Am 2001;83-A(4):520–528.
3. de Palma L, Santucci A, Sabetta SP, et al. Anatomy of the LisFranc joint complex. Foot Ankle Int 1997;18(6):356–364.
4. Khoury NJ, el-Khoury, GY, Saltzman CL, et al. Intraarticular foot and ankle injections to identify source of pain before arthrodesis. AJR Am J Roentgenol 1996;167(3):669–673.
5. Lucas PE, Hurwitz SR, Kaplan PA, et al. Fluoroscopically guided injections into the foot and ankle: localization of the source of pain as a guide to treatment—prospective study. Radiology 1997;204(2):411–415.
6. Bibbo C, Anderson RB, Davis WH. Complications of midfoot and hindfoot arthrodesis. Clin Orthop Relat Res 2001;(391):45–58.
7. Berlet GC, Hodges Davis W, Anderson RB. Tendon arthroplasty for basal fourth and fifth metatarsal arthritis. Foot Ankle Int 2002;23(5):440–446.
8. Mann RA, Prieskorn D, Sobel M. Mid-tarsal and tarsometatarsal arthrodesis for primary degenerative osteoarthrosis or osteoarthrosis after trauma. J Bone Joint Surg Am 1996;78(9):1376–1385.
9. Sangeorzan BJ, Veith RG, Hansen ST Jr. Salvage of Lisfranc's tarsometatarsal joint by arthrodesis. Foot Ankle 1990;10(4):193–200.
10. Brunet JA, Wiley JJ. The late results of tarsometatarsal joint injuries. J Bone Joint Surg Br 1987;69(3):437–440.
11. Moberg E. A simple operation for hallux rigidus. Clin Orthop Relat Res 1979;(142):55–56.
12. Love TR, Whynot AS, Farine I, et al. Keller arthroplasty: a prospective review. Foot Ankle 1987;8(1):46–54.
13. Mann RA, Clanton TO. Hallux rigidus: treatment by cheilectomy. J Bone Joint Surg Am 1988;70(3):400–406.
14. Feltham GT, Hanks SE, Marcus RE. Age-based outcomes of cheilectomy for the treatment of hallux rigidus. Foot Ankle Int 2001;22(3):192–197.
15. Southgate JJ, Urry SR. Hallux rigidus: the long-term results of dorsal wedge osteotomy and arthrodesis in adults. J Foot Ankle Surg 1997;36(2):136–140, discussion 161.

16. Barca F. Tendon arthroplasty of the first metatarsophalangeal joint in hallux rigidus: preliminary communication. Foot Ankle Int 1997;18(4):222–228.
17. Cosentino GL. The Cosentino modification for tendon interpositional arthroplasty. J Foot Ankle Surg 1995;34(5):501–508.
18. Hamilton WG, O'Malley MJ, Thompson FM, et al. Roger Mann Award 1995. Capsular interposition arthroplasty for severe hallux rigidus. Foot Ankle Int 1997;18(2):68–70.
19. Hamilton WG, Hubbard CE. Hallux rigidus. Excisional arthroplasty. Foot Ankle Clin 2000;5(3):663–671.
20. Harper MC. A modified Keller resection arthroplasty. Foot Ankle Int 1995;16(4):236–237.
21. Lau JT, Daniels TR. Outcomes following cheilectomy and interpositional arthroplasty in hallux rigidus. Foot Ankle Int 2001;22(6):462–470.
22. O'Doherty DP, Lowrie IG, Magnussen PA, et al. The management of the painful first metatarsophalangeal joint in the older patient. Arthrodesis or Keller's arthroplasty? J Bone Joint Surg Br 1990;72(5):839–842.
23. Sebold EJ, Cracchiolo A III. Use of titanium grommets in silicone implant arthroplasty of the hallux metatarsophalangeal joint. Foot Ankle Int 1996;17(3):145–151.
24. Rongstad KM, Miller GJ, Vander Griend RA, et al. A biomechanical comparison of four fixation methods of first metatarsophalangeal joint arthrodesis. Foot Ankle Int 1994;15(8):415–419.
25. Curtis MJ, Myerson M, Jinnah RH, et al. Arthrodesis of the first metatarsophalangeal joint: a biomechanical study of internal fixation techniques. Foot Ankle 1993;14(7):395–399.
26. Mann RA, Oates JC. Arthrodesis of the first metatarsophalangeal joint. Foot Ankle 1980;1(3):159–166.
27. Lombardi CM, Silhanek AD, Connolly FG, et al. First metatarsophalangeal arthrodesis for treatment of hallux rigidus: a retrospective study. J Foot Ankle Surg 2001;40(3):137–143.
28. Fitzgerald JA, Wilkinson JM. Arthrodesis of the metatarsophalangeal joint of the great toe. Clin Orthop Relat Res 1981;(157):70–77.
29. Coughlin MJ, Mann RA. Arthrodesis of the first metatarsophalangeal joint as salvage for the failed Keller procedure. J Bone Joint Surg Am 1987;69(1):68–75.
30. Harper MC. Positioning of the hallux for first metatarsophalangeal joint arthrodesis. Foot Ankle Int 1997;18(12):827.
31. Smith CA, Arnett FC. Epidemiologic aspects of rheumatoid arthritis. Current immunogenetic approach. Clin Orthop Relat Res 1991;(265):23–35.
32. Michelson J, Easley M, Wigley FM, et al. Foot and ankle problems in rheumatoid arthritis. Foot Ankle Int 1994;15(11):608–613.
33. Vainio K. The rheumatoid foot. A clinical study with pathological and roentgenological comments. 1956. Clin Orthop Relat Res 1991;(265):4–8.
34. Persselin JE. Diagnosis of rheumatoid arthritis. Medical and laboratory aspects. Clin Orthop Relat Res 1991;(265):73–82.
35. Caruso I, Santandrea S, Sarzi Puttini P, et al. Clinical, laboratory and radiographic features in early rheumatoid arthritis. J Rheumatol 1990;17(10):1263–1267.
36. Kerr LD. Arthritis of the forefoot. A review from a rheumatologic and medical perspective. Clin Orthop Relat Res 1998;(349):20–27.
37. Mann RA, Schakel ME II. Surgical correction of rheumatoid forefoot deformities. Foot Ankle Int 1995;16(1):1–6.
38. Hanyu T, Yamazaki H, Murasawa A, et al. Arthroplasty for rheumatoid forefoot deformities by a shortening oblique osteotomy. Clin Orthop Relat Res 1997;(338):131–138.
39. Bowers KD Jr, Martin RB. Turf-toe: a shoe-surface related football injury. Med Sci Sports 1976;8(2):81–83.
40. Clanton TO, Ford JJ. Turf toe injury. Clin Sports Med 1994;13(4):731–741.
41. Tewes DP, Fischer DA, Fritts HM, et al. MRI findings of acute turf toe. A case report and review of anatomy. Clin Orthop Relat Res 1994;(304):200–203.
42. Bowman MW. Athletic injuries of the great to metatarsophalangeal joint. In: Adelaar RS, ed. Disorders of the great toe. Rosemont: American Academy of Orthopaedic Surgeons, 1997:1–22.

ACUTE ANKLE SPRAIN, CHRONIC ANKLE INSTABILITY, AND SUBTALAR LAXITY

GREGORY C. BERLET
G. ALEXANDER SIMPSON

ACUTE ANKLE SPRAINS AND CHRONIC ANKLE INSTABILITY

PATHOGENESIS

Ankle sprains are the most common sports-associated injury, accounting for as much as 40% of all athletic injuries. It has been estimated that ankle sprains account for up to 10% of all visits to the emergency department and have an incidence of up to one inversion injury of the ankle per 30,000 people each day and 2 million per year.

Epidemiology

Sprains of the ankle occur in many sports. The incidence of ankle injuries appears to be equal among males and females when compared within specific sporting activities. The peak ages of injury range between 10 and 19 years. They account for 45% of all basketball injuries and 31% of soccer injuries. In football, 10% to 15% of all time lost to injuries is attributable to ankle injuries. One-third of all military recruits sustain an inversion ankle injury that requires medical care during a 4-year tenure.

Long-term sequelae from lateral ankle sprains have been estimated to occur in up to 60% of patients. The grade of acute ankle sprains does not correlate well with chronic symptoms. Interestingly, the factor most predictive of residual symptoms, 6 months following an ankle injury, was a syndesmosis sprain and not mechanical instability. The most common complaints in patients with chronic ankle instability are swelling, giving way, frank instability, and pain.

Anatomy

The lateral ankle is supported by both static and dynamic restraints. The static restraints are provided by the bony configuration of the ankle and the ligaments. The dynamic restraints are the peroneal tendons—longus and brevis. The shape of the joint contributes about 30% of the resistance to rotational forces about the ankle, whereas the soft tissues provide the other 70%.

The configuration of the talus, with its flared anterior half, provides a bony restraint to lateral motion when the talus is engaged in the mortise in dorsiflexion. In plantarflexion, the narrowest surface of the talus is in the mortise, rendering less bony stability and an increased risk to inversion injury.

The lateral collateral ligaments of the ankle include (Fig. 12.1) the following:

■ Anterior talofibular ligament (ATFL) from the anterior border of the lateral malleolus to the lateral talar body
■ Calcaneofibular ligament (CFL) from the anterior tip of the lateral malleolus to the lateral posterior calcaneus
■ Posterior talofibular ligament (PTFL)

In neutral position, the ATFL runs parallel to the axis of the foot, whereas in plantarflexion, it is vertical and functions as a collateral ligament. The CFL is taut in dorsiflexion. The CFL works in concert with the ATFL and is rarely injured alone. The ATFL is the primary restraint to inversion throughout ankle plantarflexion and dorsiflexion.

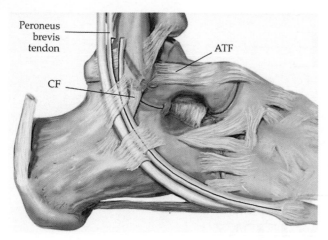

Figure 12.1 Lateral aspect of the ankle. The anterior half of the peroneus brevis tendon is harvested. The superior peroneal retinaculum is preserved.

BOX 12.1 TYPES OF ANKLE INSTABILITY

Functional Instability
- Subjective giving way
- Motion beyond voluntary control but not necessarily exceeding the physiologic range of motion
- Peroneal muscle weakness
- Decreased peroneal reaction time
- Subtalar instability
- Proprioceptive defects
- Poor balance
- Physical therapy is mainstay of treatment

Mechanical Instability
- Motion beyond the normal physiologic limits
- Excessive anterolateral laxity
- Physical therapy program tried
- Persistent mechanical lateral ankle instability is an indication for surgical stabilization of the ankle

---

At the lateral malleolus, the peroneal tendons run through a fibro-osseous tunnel under the superior peroneal retinaculum, and distally they pass deep to the inferior peroneal retinaculum. The superior peroneal retinaculum and CFL run parallel. Anteriorly, the peroneal tendons are stabilized by the posterior surface of the distal fibula in the retromalleolar sulcus. The peroneus brevis inserts on the base of the fifth metatarsal, and the peroneus longus courses under the cuboid to insert on the base of the first metatarsal and medial cuneiform. The peroneals act primarily as evertors, with the peroneus brevis being the stronger of the two. The peroneal muscles work dynamically to stabilize both the ankle and the subtalar joint.

Classification

A classification scheme for ankle sprains is given in Table 12.1. Chronic ankle instability has been estimated to occur in up to 40% of patients with acute ankle sprains with two types of instability: mechanical and functional (Box 12.1).

TABLE 12.1 CLASSIFICATION SCHEME FOR ANKLE SPRAINS

Grade	Description
I	Mild ligamentous stretch, minimal swelling and tenderness, no instability, little functional loss
II	Partial tears, increased swelling and tenderness, mild to moderate instability
III	Complete rupture of the ATFL with variable injury of CFL with severe swelling and tenderness, loss of function, significant instability

ATFL, anterior talofibular ligament.

DIAGNOSIS

History and Physical Examination

- The physical examination is used to confirm the working diagnosis and to rule out associated injuries.
- Patients with chronic ankle instability typically present with pain, instability, or a combination of pain and instability.
- Patients will typically provide a history of severe inversion injury or a history of multiple ankle sprains.
- A key feature of the history is whether pain is present in the intervals between ankle sprains.
  - If pain is present in the intervals between sprains, a secondary diagnosis, in addition to ligamentous instability, should be entertained (Table 12.2).

Clinical Features

- A complete physical examination of the ankle includes the following:
  - Examination of the joint above (knee) and below (subtalar)
  - Assessment of lower extremity alignment
  - Ankle range of motion
  - Eliciting the point of maximal tenderness
  - Anterior drawer and varus stress test
  - Assessing for peroneal pathology
  - Assessment of ankle proprioception
- The assessment of point tenderness includes a systematic examination of the bony and soft-tissue anatomy of the foot and ankle with palpation of the following:
  - ATFL
  - PTFL
  - CFL
  - Syndesmosis
  - Calcaneocuboid joint
  - Posterior tibial and peroneal tendons
  - The base and shaft of the fifth metatarsal
  - Medial and lateral malleoli

TABLE 12.2 LESIONS TO CONSIDER IN PATIENTS WITH CHRONIC SYMPTOMS FOLLOWING ANKLE INSTABILITY

Type	Characteristics
Bone	Anterior process of the calcaneus fracture
	Lateral and posterior talar process fracture
	Malleoli fracture
	Base of fifth metatarsal fracture
	Tibiotalar bony impingement
	Osseous and fibrous tarsal coalition
Cartilage	Osteochondral lesions (i.e., OCD) of the talus and tibia
Ligamentous	Functional lateral ligamentous instability
	Mechanical lateral ligamentous instability
	Subtalar instability
	Syndesmosis injury
Neural	Neurapraxia of the superficial peroneal nerve
	Neurapraxia of the sural nerve
Tendinous	Os peroneum syndrome
	Tear of the peroneus longus at the peroneal tubercle
	Peroneal brevis tear
	Peroneal instability at the superior peroneal retinaculum
Soft tissue	Sinus tarsi syndrome
	Anterolateral ankle soft-tissue impingement

- Lower extremity alignment should be assessed with the patient both weight bearing and seated.
- Varus hindfoot alignment should be assessed, as it predisposes the ankle to inversion injury.
- Tarsal coalitions may present as recurrent sprained ankles.
  - A patient with a tarsal coalition will most commonly have hindfoot valgus with a variable but decreased amount of subtalar motion.
  - Hindfoot malalignment needs to be assessed for flexibility.
  - The hindfoot malalignment may need to be corrected at the time of ligamentous reconstruction.
  - The functional range of motion is 10° of dorsiflexion to 25° of plantarflexion.
- Subtalar motion is rotation around an oblique axis running from the medial side of the talar neck to the posterolateral aspect of the calcaneus.
  - Total subtalar motion is around 20°, but is difficult to accurately measure clinically.
  - Subtalar motion is often referred to as a percentage of the contralateral limb.
- The anterior drawer test is designed to test the competency of the ATFL.
  - The test is performed with the patient sitting and the knee flexed at 90°.

- The tibia is stabilized and an attempt is made to draw the talus forward.
- With intact medial structures and incompetent lateral ligaments, the displacement is rotatory.
- More anterior displacement of the talus relative to the tibia on the injured side compared with the contralateral side or excessive displacement signifies a positive test.
- A positive anterior drawer test has been described to be translation of 5 mm more than on the contralateral side or an absolute value of 9 to 10 mm.
- A firm end point on stressing is less likely to indicate instability of the ATFL.
- A positive test is significant only when it correlates with symptoms because only one-half of patients with a positive anterior drawer test have symptomatic instability.
- Peroneal tendon assessment includes strength of eversion, stability of the tendons behind the fibula, and tenderness along the course of the tendons.
  - Patients with chronic tendon subluxation may describe snapping and discomfort with repeated episodes of giving way in the ankle.
  - The best provocative test for subluxation or dislocation of the tendons is active eversion of the foot with ankle dorsiflexion against resistance.
  - Peroneal eversion strength is considered adequate if the examiner is unable to overcome the peroneals with a maximal eversion effort.
  - Weakness should mandate a search for peroneal pathology before a diagnosis of deconditioned peroneal muscles is made.
- Proprioceptive defects may present as giving way.
  - The mechanism of nerve injury is traction with damage occurring after as little as 6% nerve elongation.
  - Severe (grade III) ankle sprains have been associated with more than 80% injury rate to the tibial and peroneal nerves.
  - Proprioception can be assessed with a modified Romberg test by having the patient stand first on the uninjured limb and then on the injured limb with eyes open and then closed.
  - Stabilometry is an objective means to measure postural equilibrium and has been shown to correlate with functional instability.

Radiologic Features

- Three plain radiographic views of the ankle (AP, lateral, and mortise) help rule out associated bony lesions and degenerative arthritis.
- If a tarsal coalition is suspected, oblique and axial hindfoot views are helpful. Magnetic resonance imaging is useful to evaluate ligamentous injury, peroneal tendon pathology, and suspected osteochondral injuries.
- Use of stress radiography is controversial.
  - The use of a standardized testing apparatus such as a Telos device using the contralateral ankle as a control to measure talar tilt and anterior talar translation may help improve consistency, but the high degree of interobserver variability of ligamentous laxity prevents any strict recommendations for surgery based on stress radiography.

Associated Conditions

Anterior ankle impingement exostoses (footballer's ankle) may create a loss in ankle dorsiflexion, anterior ankle pain, and a compromise in ankle proprioception. They are most common in athletes, particularly dancers. Spurs may coincide with degenerative joint disease, although there is no conclusive evidence that chronic ankle instability leads to degenerative joint disease. Recurrent capsular strains may lead to these exostoses.

Subtalar disorders are recognized as a cause of chronic lateral hindfoot pain following an inversion injury. Patients with lateral instability of the ankle have 10% to 25% incidence of subtalar instability with the most common pathology being a tear of the interosseous talocalcaneal ligament.

Pain over the peroneal tendons may represent tendonitis or a tear. Peroneal tendonitis and traumatic rupture may be related to severe ankle sprains. Patients with tendonitis present with pain, swelling, and warmth over the peroneal tendons. Pain may be reproduced by plantarflexion–inversion or dorsiflexion–eversion. A thickening of the tendon may be detected. Partial and complete tears are commonly associated with tenosynovitis. Tendon degeneration and complete rupture usually occur in areas of stenosis, such as the retromalleolar sulcus, the peroneal tubercle, and the cuboid groove.

Osteochondritis dissecans (OCDs) of the talus presents with pain and sometimes catching with walking or active ankle motion. Talar OCD lesions are typically either posteromedial or anterolateral. The etiology of these OCD lesions is controversial, but it appears that most anterolateral talar lesions are transchondral fractures. Anterolateral OCD lesions have been produced in cadavers by impaction of the talus on the fibula with ankle inversion and dorsiflexion. Posteromedial OCD lesions are frequently asymptomatic and often lack a history of trauma. A posteromedial OCD lesion may be secondary to repetitive microtrauma. The most common OCD lesion location is on the central medial talus.

TREATMENT

Acute Ankle Sprains

Grades I and II sprains are best treated with a three-phase program called *functional treatment* (Table 12.3). Functional treatment rehabilitation has led to faster return to sport in high-level athletes. Some controversy exists regarding grade III sprains. The current recommendations remain nonoperative treatment of grade III sprains as outlined in Table 12.3. Some experts have argued that primary repair of the torn ligaments can lead to better results, but numerous studies comparing surgical versus conservative care typically have shown no improvement in results with surgical treatment. However, surgical intervention is believed to decrease prevalence of ligament reinjury.

Chronic Ankle Instability

Indications and Contraindications

The indication for lateral ligamentous reconstruction of the ankle is persistent, symptomatic, and mechanical instability, despite appropriate conservative management. The

TABLE 12.3 FUNCTIONAL TREATMENT OF GRADES I AND II ACUTE ANKLE SPRAINS

Phase	Therapy
I	Rest, ice, compression, and elevation
II	Short period of relative immobilization and protection (bracing, taping, or bandaging)
III	Active range of motion exercises, weight bearing, proprioceptive training on a tilt board, peroneal strengthening

contraindications for surgery include pain with no instability, peripheral vascular disease, peripheral neuropathy, and inability to be compliant with postoperative management.

Nonoperative Treatment

- [ ] Physical therapy is indicated in the treatment of functional ankle instability and in the treatment of mechanical instability when the peroneal muscles are weak.
- [ ] Stretching, proprioception, and peroneal strengthening are most important.
- [ ] The optimal duration of physical therapy varies according to initial strength deficiencies and intensity of the rehabilitation program.
- [ ] Strength (i.e., Cybex) testing before and after strength training provides a quantitative measure of progress and can aid in patient motivation.
- Orthotic devices or shoe wear modifications may be used for foot and ankle malalignment and instability.
  - [ ] Lateral ankle instability, particularly in running athletes with dynamic supination, is benefited by an external lateral heel wedge.
  - [ ] If the patient has a flexible valgus forefoot with compensatory varus hindfoot, a lateral forefoot post on the orthotic may be beneficial.
  - [ ] A heel lift can help open the anterior tibiotalar joint and aid anterior impingement symptoms.
- External stabilization of the ankle joint by taping and wrap dressings can be used, but recently reusable braces have gained popularity.
- Taping provides effective stabilization of the tibiotalar joint, but the support from taping deteriorates with a reduction of initial support of 50% after 10 minutes of exercise and minimal support after 1 hour of exercise.
- Various braces significantly reduce the talar tilt in patients with unstable ankle joints, and their effectiveness is not diminished with exercise.
- Prophylactic bracing in volleyball athletes does not alter the incidence of ankle sprains.
  - [ ] Volleyball players without previous ankle injury were shown to have a decreased incidence of ankle sprain.
  - [ ] Rigid ankle supports offered better protection than nonrigid supports.
  - [ ] The higher cost and skin irritation by tape has led us to recommend reusable ankle orthoses instead of prophylactic taping.

Surgical Treatment

More than 80 surgical operations have been described for the treatment of chronic lateral ligamentous instability of the ankle. These procedures may be divided into nonanatomic reconstruction techniques (i.e., peroneus brevis augmentation) and anatomic repair methods (i.e., Broström repair). Our choice for lateral ankle ligament reconstruction is influenced by the patient's body habitus and activity pattern:

- Anatomic repair (modified Broström) is indicated for the majority of patients. Patients must not have general ligamentous laxity. It is only rarely indicated for revision ankle stabilization.
- Modified Broström–Evans (hybrid) procedure for all patients who do not fit the above criteria.
- Chrisman–Snook (split peroneus brevis) reconstruction for obese patients, athletes at high risk for reinjury (e.g., football lineman), connective tissue disease (e.g., Ehlers–Danlos), or following failed ankle instability surgery. Some surgeons advocate allograft reconstruction to avoid donor site morbidity but this includes the risk of disease transmission.

Arthroscopy is indicated for the treatment of osteochondral lesions of the talus and anterolateral and anterior soft-tissue impingement lesions. In these situations, arthroscopy is done as the primary procedure followed by the ligamentous reconstruction. If anterior impingement caused by exostoses is suspected and confirmed with radiographic studies, an arthroscopic or open anterior ankle decompression is done in combination with the ligamentous reconstruction.

Modified Broström Anatomic Lateral Ligament Reconstruction. The Broström anatomic ligament repair includes a direct late repair of the lateral ligaments of the ankle. The ligaments of the ATFL and CFL are disrupted but present. In the modified Broström technique, the lateral aspect of the extensor retinaculum is advanced to the fibula over the Broström repair, which reinforces the repair, limits inversion, and helps correct the subtalar component of the instability. Direct late repair has the advantage of preserving normal anatomy and avoiding morbidity associated with autologous tendon grafts. The disadvantage of this technique is that it relies on good quality tissue for a strong repair.

Surgical Technique.
- The patient is placed supine with a bump under the ipsilateral hip.
- A thigh tourniquet is used.
- Two incisions have been described:
  - An anterior incision is used when the surgeon is confident that there is no peroneal pathology.
  - A posterior curvilinear incision is used when exposure of the peroneal tendons and anterolateral ankle is desired.
- The posterior curvilinear incision extends from 4 to 5 cm proximal to the tip of the lateral malleolus following the course of the peroneal tendons to 2 cm proximal to the base of the fifth metatarsal, avoiding branches of the superficial peroneal and sural nerves.

- The skin flaps are elevated to expose the anterior ankle capsule, the anterior fibula, and the peroneal tendons.
- The lateral extent of the extensor retinaculum is identified and mobilized for later reconstruction.
- The peroneal sheath is opened proximally and distally, preserving the superior peroneal retinaculum.
- The anterior incision is curvilinear made along the anterior and distal border of the fibula.
  - The incision begins at the level of the ankle joint and stops at the peroneal tendons.
  - The dissection is carried down to the joint capsule along the anterior border of the lateral malleolus.
- The extensor retinaculum is identified and mobilized for later reconstruction.
- An arthrotomy at the anterolateral ankle joint is made, dividing the ATFL in its midsubstance.
- This ligament is often attenuated and cannot be identified until the divided capsule is inspected for ligamentous fibers.
- The CFL is identified under the peroneal tendons, its course paralleling the superior peroneal retinaculum.
  - An intraoperative stress test can be performed to determine the integrity of the CFL.
  - If the ligament is attenuated, an imbrication is warranted.
  - The CFL is divided in its midsubstance.
- A segmental resection of scar tissue is performed to allow coaptation of ligament to ligament.
- Up to 5 mm of redundant tissue is excised from both the ATFL and the CFL.
- Two 2-0 nonabsorbable sutures are placed in a pants-over-vest fashion into the CFL.
- Two or three 0 nonabsorbable sutures are placed into the ATFL in a pants-over-vest fashion. Another option is to anchor the cut ligament to the fibula directly with suture anchors.
- The sutures in the CFL are secured with the ankle in slight plantarflexion and eversion.
- The ATFL sutures are tied with the posterior heel suspended, avoiding anterior subluxation of the talus.
- If insufficient length of ligament is available, a periosteal sleeve from the fibula can be advanced in a turn-down fashion to augment the ligament repair
- The ankle is taken through a full range of motion, making sure that the sutures hold.
- The anterolateral ankle capsule is then repaired with absorbable sutures in a fashion that tightens the local soft tissue.
- The extensor retinaculum and local tissues are then advanced and secured with absorbable sutures to the periosteum of the distal fibula, thereby covering the ligament and capsular repair. Absorbable sutures for this part of the repair decrease the incidence of irritable suture knots in this subcutaneous location
- The skin is closed and the patient is placed in a splint in neutral plantarflexion and slight eversion.

Postoperative Management.
- The patient remains non–weight bearing for 2 weeks and then wears a weight-bearing cast for 3 weeks in the neutral position, followed by a bootwalker for 3 weeks.

- A circumferential ankle brace, with rotation control, is then worn in the shoe until physical therapy is completed and also during at-risk activities for 1 year.
- Physical therapy is begun at 8 weeks.
- Physical therapy protocol scores patients on commencement of PT and prior to physician appointment at 4 months.
- Return to sport is estimated to occur at 4 months post-surgery.

Results. Good and excellent results have been reported in approximately 90% of patients in most series. Factors thought to be associated with a poorer outcome were greater than 10 years of instability, generalized ligamentous laxity, and osteoarthritis of the ankle.

Modified Broström–Evans Procedure

The Evans procedure, a tenodesis of the whole peroneus brevis, involves rerouting it through the fibula and reattaching to its proximal stump. Another option is to augment the Broström reconstruction with the anterior one-third of the peroneus brevis. This modified Broström–Evans procedure has been shown to add static restraint without a significant sacrifice of dynamic peroneal restraint and is indicated in the heavier, more demanding, nonathletic population (Fig. 12.2).

Surgical Technique.
- A posterior curvilinear incision is made from 4 to 5 cm proximal to the tip of the lateral malleolus following the course of the peroneal tendons to 2 cm proximal to the base of the fifth metatarsal, avoiding branches of the superficial peroneal and sural nerves.
- The peroneus brevis tendon is exposed while preserving the superior peroneal retinaculum.
- The anterior third of the tendon is isolated distally and split from this distal position to the musculotendinous junction proximally.
- It is transected proximally, but it remains attached on the base of the fifth metatarsal.
- A modified Broström procedure is performed as described previously.

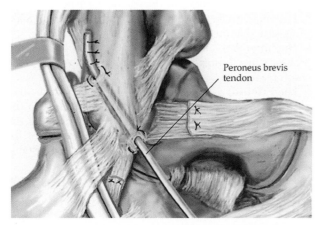

Figure 12.2 End-to-end repair of the CFL and ATFL is achieved with nonabsorbable suture. The anterior half of the split peroneus brevis tendon is routed through a drill hole in the fibula and secured at the entrance and exit with nonabsorbable suture.

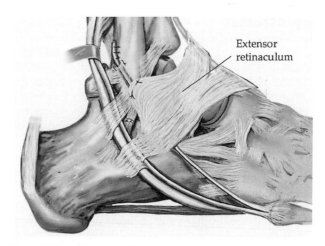

Figure 12.3 Gould and colleagues' modification completes the lateral repair in the modified Broström and modified Broström–Evans reconstructions. The extensor retinaculum is advanced to the distal fibula.

- After the sutures are placed, but not tied, a hole is drilled from anterior to posterior, exiting 2.5 cm proximal to the tip of the fibula.
- The split portion of the peroneus brevis tendon is passed through the drilled hole in a distal to proximal direction.
- The sutures in the CFL and the ATFL are tied in slight plantarflexion and eversion.
- The static peroneal tendon transfer is tensioned with the foot in mild plantarflexion and eversion and sutured to the periosteum at both the entrance and the exit sites on the fibula.
- The residual tendon is excised so as not to interfere with easy peroneal passage behind the fibula.
- The ankle is taken through a full range of motion, making sure that the sutures hold.
- The remaining capsular closure and extensor retinaculum are repaired as described earlier (Fig. 12.3).
- Postoperative management is the same as for the Broström procedure.

Chrisman–Snook Reconstruction

Chrisman and Snook modified the Elmslie procedure, a nonanatomic ligament reconstruction with fascia lata, by using a split portion of the peroneus brevis instead of a strip of fascia lata. They believed that the success of the Elmslie technique was because the vectors of both ATFL and CFL were reconstructed. We prefer allograft hamstring tendon with an average length of the graft necessary being 12 to 19 cm.

Surgical Technique.
- A posterior curvilinear incision extending from 4 to 5 cm proximal to the tip of the lateral malleolus following the course of the peroneal tendons to 2 cm proximal to the base of the fifth metatarsal is made.
- The course of the peroneus brevis graft is designed to recreate the vectors of the ATFL and CFL.
- Two fibular bone tunnels are used to recreate the fibular insertions of the ATFL and CFL.
- The first tunnel begins at the ATFL insertion of the fibula angling superiorly at 30° and exiting the posterior fibula

approximately 2.5 cm proximal to the tip of the fibula and superior to the superior peroneal retinaculum.

■ The second bone tunnel angles from the CFL footprint on the fibula anterior and superior to intersect the ATFL tunnel. This tunnel is unicortical and stops once it intersects the first tunnel that was created.

■ The calcaneal insertion of the CFL is identified by dissection distal and posterior to the fibula revealing the lateral wall of the calcaneus. A unicortical drill hole, appropriate for the diameter of the allograft tendon, is made in preparation to anchor the graft with an interference screw into the calcaneus.

■ The talar neck insertion of the ATFL is located and an appropriate diameter hole is made bicortical paralleling the superior surface of the talus. Intraoperative imaging can be helpful to guide this tunnel parallel to the joint.

■ The tendon allograft is passed through the fibular tunnel using a suture passing instrument that engages the grasping sutures on the ends of the graft. It is often accomplished most easily by passing the graft from anterior to posterior and then redirecting out the inferior tunnel of the fibula.

■ Posterior to the fibula, the tendon graft is positioned deep to the peroneus longus and remaining peroneus brevis in the retromalleolar sulcus.

■ The graft is pulled into the calcaneal drill hole delivering only the sutures medially. The interference screw is advanced into the calcaneus.

■ The graft is then delivered through the talar tunnel from lateral to medial. A small incision is necessary to free the medial tendon from the soft tissues as the graft is pulled taut

■ The ankle is held in neutral dorsiflexion and in slight eversion, as the interference screws is placed in the talar neck from lateral to medial.

■ Additional interference screws may be placed in the fibular bone tunnels, at the surgeon's discretion.

■ Nonabsorbable sutures can be used to secure the tendon graft to periosteum at the entrance and exit of all bone tunnels.

■ Postoperative management is the same as for the other ligament repairs.

Results. At 10-year follow-up, more than 90% of patients have a good or excellent result in most series. Generally, patients with fair or poor results had a reinjury. Some loss

of inversion is an expected and desirable outcome of this procedure.

Future Consideration

One direction of current research has explored arthroscopic repair of the lateral ankle ligaments for ankle instability using concepts popularized in the shoulder. There are only small case series (level IV evidence), but the concept deserves further consideration. Better bracing and focused rehabilitation efforts to speed the return of proprioception are ongoing. Finally, isolating objective measures of fitness for return to sport will also help guide future rehabilitation efforts.

SUBTALAR INSTABILITY

PATHOGENESIS

It is not unusual for the subtalar joint to be injured after an inversion injury to the ankle joint. However, instability of this joint is difficult to diagnose and treat. Approximately 25% of patients with chronic ankle instability are estimated to have associated subtalar instability. Injuries to the subtalar joint can be described by four types (Table 12.4). The motion about this joint has been defined as primarily inversion and eversion. The lateral ligaments of the subtalar joint may be described in three layers:

■ Superficial layer includes the lateral limb of the inferior extensor retinaculum.

■ Intermediate layer includes the intermediate root of the inferior extensor retinaculum and the cervical ligament.

■ Deep layer comprises the medial root of the extensor retinaculum, lateral talocalcaneal ligament, and the interosseous ligament.

DIAGNOSIS

History and Physical Examination

Clinical Features
■ On physical examination, the anterior drawer may elicit a click and be positive in isolated subtalar instability, but it is not as obvious as in ankle instability.

TABLE 12.4 CLASSIFICATION SCHEME FOR INJURIES TO THE SUBTALAR JOINT

Type	Description
I	Occurs with forced supination of the hindfoot; ATFL can be injured if the foot is plantarflexed; cervical ligament is torn first followed by the CFL
II	Includes the above plus disruption of the interosseous ligament
III	Occurs with the ankle in dorsiflexion and involves the CFL and interosseous ligaments
IV	Severe soft-tissue disruption with involvement of all the ligaments

ATFL, anterior talofibular ligament; CFL, calcaneofibular ligament.

- The commonest finding in subtalar instability is pain in the sinus tarsi.
- Patients may have increased internal rotation of the calcaneus relative to the noninvolved side.
- They may also exhibit increased anterior/distal translation of the calcaneus.

Radiologic Features

- Several methods of diagnosis have been described, including stress views, stress Broden's views, and arthrograms. No accepted standard has gained clinical acceptance.
- Subtalar arthroscopy has gained some popularity for diagnosing instability.
- Increased motion and opening of the posterior facet with varus stress is thought to be indicative of subtalar instability.
- MRI will often show sinus tarsi inflammation and intact lateral ankle ligaments. When combined with a clinical examination of instability this guides the differential diagnosis toward subtalar instability.

TREATMENT

Nonoperative Treatment

- Treatment of subtalar instability is similar to the rehabilitation of the ankle as described previously.
- Nonsurgical management should include Achilles stretching, peroneal strengthening, and proprioception training. These are the same protocols as utilized with ankle instability.
- Bracing can be effective if the heel can be captured and subtalar motion limited.

Surgical Treatment

Surgical management should include ankle ligament repairs that cross the subtalar joint as the instability almost always involves the ankle also. The modified Broström–Evans and the Chrisman–Snook procedures, as described earlier, can be used to successfully treat subtalar instability. Other procedures—one using half of the peroneal brevis tendon placed through drill holes in the fibula and then secured to the posterior aspect of the calcaneus, and another being a triligament reconstruction using a plantaris tendon in a weave from the calcaneus, through the talus and fibula, and back onto the posterior aspect of the calcaneus—have been described.

SUGGESTED READING

Broström L. Sprained ankles. VI. Surgical treatment of "chronic" ligament ruptures. Acta Chir Scand 1966;132:551–565.

Clanton TO. Instability of the subtalar joint. Orthop Clin North Am 1989;20:583–592.

DiGiovanni CW, Brodsky A. Current concepts: lateral ankle instability. Foot Ankle Int 2006;27:854–866.

Frey C, Feder KS, Sleight J. Prophylactic ankle brace use in high school volleyball players: a prospective study. Foot Ankle Int 2010;31(4):296–300.

Harrington KD. Degenerative arthritis of the ankle secondary to long-standing lateral ligament instability. J Bone Joint Surg Am 1979;61:354–361.

Maffulli N, Ferran NA. Management of acute and chronic ankle instability. J Am Acad Orthop Surg 2008;16(10):608–615.

Malliaropoulos N, Ntessalen M, Papacostas E, et al. Reinjury after acute lateral ankle sprains in elite track and field athletes. Am J Sports Med 2009;37(9):1755–1761.

Pihlajamäki H, Hietaniemi K, Paavola M, et al. Surgical versus functional treatment for acute ruptures of the lateral ligament complex of the ankle in young men: a randomized controlled trial. J Bone Joint Surg Am 2010;92:2367–2374.

Snook GA, Chrisman OD, Wilson TC. Long-term results of the Chrisman–Snook operation for reconstruction of the lateral ligaments of the ankle. J Bone Joint Surg Am 1985;67:1–7.

ANKLE AND SUBTALAR ARTHROSCOPY

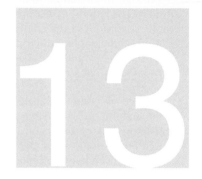

13.1 ANKLE ARTHROSCOPY

JEFFREY D. JACKSON ■ RICHARD D. FERKEL ■ ELLIS K. NAM

The first arthroscopic inspection of a cadaveric knee joint was performed by Takagi in Japan in 1918. In 1939, he reported on an arthroscopic examination of an ankle joint in a human patient. With the advent of fiber-optic light transmission, video cameras, instruments for small joints, and distraction devices, arthroscopy has become an important diagnostic and therapeutic modality for disorders of the ankle. Arthroscopic examination of the ankle joint allows direct visualization and stress testing of intra-articular structures and ligaments about the ankle joint. Various arthroscopic procedures have been developed and proven to be successful and will be discussed in this chapter.

PATIENT SELECTION

Indications

Patients undergoing ankle arthroscopy frequently present with pain, swelling, stiffness, instability, hemarthrosis, locking, or abnormal snapping or popping. Operative indications for ankle arthroscopy include the following:

- Loose body removal
- Chondral or osteochondral injury
- Soft-tissue impingement
- Osteophyte removal
- Biopsy
- Synovectomy
- Arthrodesis
- Ankle fracture intra-articular evaluation and treatment
- Ankle instability
- Hardware removal

Contraindications

Absolute contraindications for ankle arthroscopy include localized soft-tissue or systemic infection and severe, rigid degenerative joint disease. With end-stage degenerative joint disease and joint narrowing, successful distraction may not be possible, precluding visualization of the ankle joint. Relative contraindications for ankle arthroscopy include moderate degenerative joint disease with restricted range of motion (ROM), severe edema, reflex sympathetic dystrophy, and tenuous vascular supply.

Patient Evaluation

- Successful outcome of ankle arthroscopy depends on accurate diagnosis and preoperative planning.
- Patient evaluation includes a thorough history, physical examination, and radiologic evaluation.
- The chief complaint should be carefully sought, with emphasis on the duration, severity, and provocative events.
- A careful inquiry of pain, swelling, stiffness, instability, snapping, popping, or locking should be performed.
- A general medical history should be obtained, with special attention to rheumatologic disorders.
- Physical examination should include inspection and palpation of localized areas of tenderness.
- ROM as well as stability of the ankle joint should be assessed and compared with that of the uninvolved side.
- The subtalar joint should also be tested for instability.
- Often, a local anesthetic agent can be injected into a specific joint to aid in diagnosis.
- Routine blood tests to check for systemic and rheumatologic conditions and infection should be performed.

- Aspiration of the ankle joint and analysis of the joint fluid can be helpful in distinguishing inflammatory from septic conditions of the ankle joint.
- Routine radiographs (anteroposterior [AP], lateral, and mortise view) should be obtained for all patients.
- Stress radiographs can be obtained when instability is suspected.
- Advanced imaging modalities such as CT or MRI are often helpful in evaluating osteochondral lesions or soft-tissue lesions about the ankle.
- Three-phase bone scans can also aid in distinguishing soft tissue from bony pathology.

OPERATING ROOM SETUP

Equipment

Arthroscopes are available in various sizes, ranging from the 1.9-mm to the 4.0-mm diameter scope (Fig. 13.1.1). The 2.7-mm arthroscope is preferred by the authors, particularly in tighter areas such as the medial and lateral gutters and the posterior aspect of the ankle. In the past, the 4.0-mm arthroscope afforded an improved picture quality to that of the smaller arthroscopes; however, with the advent of improved technology, the picture quality is now almost equivalent. As opposed to traditional knee arthroscopes, small joint arthroscopes that are shorter are preferred (67-mm long) to prevent chondral injury and instrument breakage. Another important variable is the inclination of view, defined as the angle of projection at the objective end of the arthroscope. Because of the rotational ability of the arthroscope, a 30° arthroscope increases the field of view compared with a 0° arthroscope. The 30° view, the most practical and the most commonly used, permits excellent visualization within the ankle and subtalar joints. The 70° arthroscope is also valuable in the ankle joint as it allows the surgeon to see around corners (i.e., the medial and lateral gutters). The 70° scope requires more experience because it is less commonly used and a central blind spot is present (Fig. 13.1.2).

Various instruments, specifically designed for the ankle, are needed to perform effective arthroscopy, including probes, dissectors, graspers, basket forceps, knives, curettes, osteotomes, rongeurs, and suction baskets (Fig. 13.1.3). In addition, small-joint motorized shaver and burr systems are available to perform different tasks quickly and efficiently. These instruments are shorter than those used in the knee and shoulder, and smaller in diameter. Various tip designs are available, and run at speeds between 1,500 and 6,000 rpm. In tight spaces, smaller 2.0- and 2.9-mm tips are used; where more space is available, larger 3.5- and 4-mm tips are utilized to lessen clogging and to perform the task more efficiently.

A high inflow and outflow system can be achieved by gravity drainage from a third portal (i.e., posterolaterally). Occasionally, if the posterior portal is difficult to obtain or a high hydrostatic pressure is desired, an arthroscopic pump can be used. However, care must be taken not to extravasate excess fluid into the surrounding soft tissues, leading to increased compartment pressure.

Particularly important in performing ankle arthroscopy is achieving adequate distraction. Inadequate distraction will preclude complete inspection of the central and posterior aspects of the ankle. The ankle can be distracted by noninvasive and invasive techniques. Guhl popularized the use of an invasive distraction device with pins in the distal tibia and calcaneus. This affords a large amount of distraction force. However, the disadvantages are the risk of neurovascular damage, infection, scarring, and fracture. In recent years, noninvasive techniques have replaced invasive devices almost completely. Yet, noninvasive distraction can also result in neurovascular compromise caused by excessive and prolonged pressure; thus periodic relaxation of the distraction strap is recommended to prevent potential complications. The authors use a noninvasive disposable soft-tissue distraction strap that grips around the posterior aspect of the heel and the dorsum of the foot. This attaches to a sterile device that grips the table (Fig. 13.1.4).

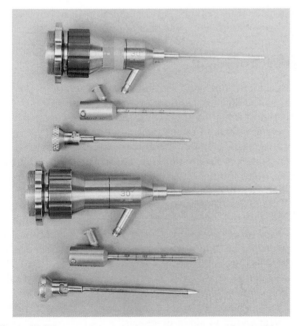

Figure 13.1.1 Small joint arthroscope with interchangeable cannulae is helpful in ankle and foot arthroscopy. A 1.9-mm 30° oblique arthroscope is pictured at top, and a 2.7-mm 30° oblique arthroscope is pictured below. (From Ferkel RD. Instrumentation. In: Arthroscopic surgery: the foot and ankle. Philadelphia: Lippincott-Raven, 1996:51.)

Positioning

Ankle arthroscopy is usually performed either in the lateral decubitus or in the supine position. Newer techniques for prone arthroscopy will be discussed at the end of the chapter. At our institution, we prefer the supine position with a padded thigh support, as it allows "hands-free" positioning of the ankle without having to hold the extremity. In addition, this position allows the surgeon to be more readily oriented with the video monitor as well as affording easy access to the anterior and posterior portals.

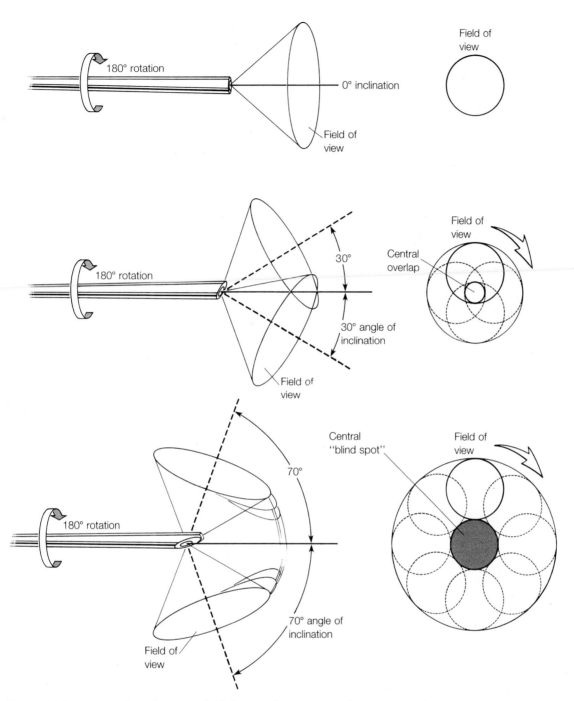

Figure 13.1.2   Rotating the arthroscopic field of view enhances viewing by creating overlapping circular images with a 30° arthroscope (**center**). With a 0° arthroscope (**top**), the field of view is unchanged with rotation. With a 70° arthroscope (**bottom**), rotation occurs around a central blind spot. (From Ferkel RD. Instrumentation. In: Arthroscopic surgery: the foot and ankle. Philadelphia: Lippincott-Raven, 1996:53.)

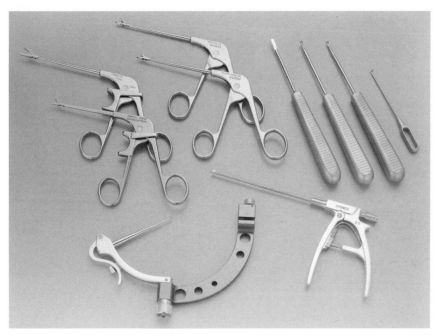

Figure 13.1.3   Small-joint instrumentation, including a drill guide (MicroVector), graspers, basket forceps, suction punch, elevator, curettes, and probe, can facilitate ankle arthroscopy.

- After the tourniquet is secured on the upper thigh, the leg is placed onto a thigh support and positioned with the hip flexed 45° to 50°.
- The thigh support is placed proximal to the popliteal fossa and is well padded to avoid injury to the *sciatic nerve*.
- The patient is then rotated so the knee and ankle point directly to the ceiling.
- The pad is removed from the end of the table to facilitate posterior ankle access.

- The patient is prepped and draped so that good access is available posteriorly.
- The tourniquet is inflated at the surgeon's discretion.
- The noninvasive distraction strap is then placed onto the foot and attached to a sterile holder.
- If subtalar arthroscopy is being performed, the posterior strap should be placed below the tip of the fibula.
- This foot holder is secured to the operating table over the surgical drape by a sterile clamp.

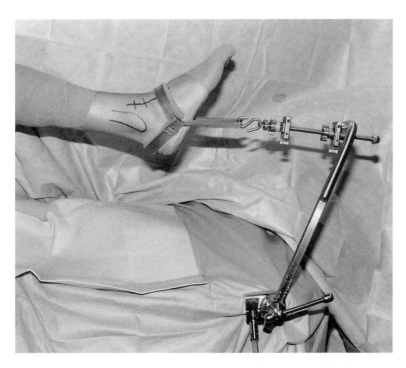

Figure 13.1.4   Patient positioning using a thigh support with a noninvasive strap attached to a distraction device.

SURGICAL TECHNIQUE

Arthroscopic Portals

As in arthroscopy involving other joints, ankle arthroscopy mandates proper portal placement for adequate visualization. Therefore, a thorough knowledge of ankle anatomy is required to avoid potential complications. It is very important to mark out potential structures at risk before performing ankle arthroscopy.

■ Before applying the distraction strap, the *dorsalis pedis artery, deep peroneal nerve, greater saphenous vein, anterior tibial tendon, peroneus tertius tendon,* and *superficial peroneal nerve and its branches (intermediate and medial dorsal cutaneous nerves)* should be identified and outlined on the surface of the ankle using a marking pen.
■ By inverting and plantarflexing the foot, branches of the *superficial peroneal nerve* can be readily visualized.
■ Similarly, the joint line is identified by dorsiflexing and plantarflexing the ankle.

Anterior Portals

The anteromedial and anterolateral portals are the most commonly used anterior portals.

■ The anteromedial portal is placed first just medial to the *anterior tibial tendon* at the joint line.
  □ Proper technique is mandatory in creating the antero-medial portal as the *greater saphenous vein* and *saphenous nerve* traverse the joint line along the anterior edge of the medial malleolus. After incising the skin, the soft tissues and joint capsule are bluntly divided.

■ The anterolateral portal is placed just lateral to the peroneus tertius tendon at or slightly proximal to the joint line.
  □ A branch of the *superficial peroneal nerve* (the most commonly injured nerve in ankle arthroscopy) can be disrupted in creating this portal if care is not taken.
■ The anterocentral portal is established between the tendons of the extensor digitorum communis, but we do not recommend this portal because of the increased risk of damage to the *deep peroneal nerve* and the *dorsalis pedis artery* and *vein,* which traverse between the *extensor hallucis longus* and the medial border of the *extensor digitorum communis* (Fig. 13.1.5).

Accessory Anterior Portals

The accessory anterior portals are used in addition to the usual anteromedial and anterolateral portals when working in the tight confines of the medial and lateral gutters for instrumentation or excision of soft tissue or bony lesions. Two accessory anterior portals are most commonly used, the anterolateral and the anteromedial (Fig. 13.1.5).

■ The accessory anteromedial portal is established 0.5 to 1 cm inferior and 1 cm anterior to the anterior border of the medial malleolus.
  □ It is especially useful in facilitating the evaluation of the medial gutter and deltoid ligament, particularly for the removal of ossicles adherent to the deep portion of the deltoid ligament while visualizing from the anteromedial portal.
■ The accessory anterolateral portal is established 1 cm anterior to and at or just below the tip of the anterior

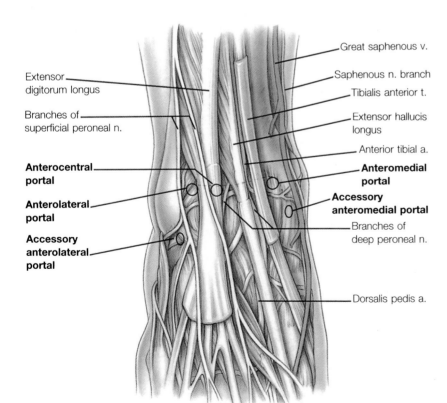

Extensor digitorum longus

Branches of superficial peroneal n.

Anterocentral portal

Anterolateral portal

Accessory anterolateral portal

Great saphenous v.

Saphenous n. branch

Tibialis anterior t.

Extensor hallucis longus

Anterior tibial a.

Anteromedial portal

Accessory anteromedial portal

Branches of deep peroneal n.

Dorsalis pedis a.

Figure 13.1.5 Anterior anatomy. Three anterior and two accessory anterior portals are used in ankle arthroscopy. (From Ferkel RD. Diagnostic arthroscopic examination. In: Arthroscopic surgery: the foot and ankle. Philadelphia: Lippincott-Raven, 1996:104.)

border of the lateral malleolus, in the area of the anterior talofibular ligament.

- ☐ When visualizing ossicles from the anterolateral portal, an instrument can be inserted through the accessory anterolateral portal to facilitate removal as well as probing of the anterior talofibular ligament, the posterior talofibular ligament, and surrounding bony architecture.

Posterior Portals

The three described posterior portals are the posterolateral, trans-Achilles, and the posteromedial portal.

- ▨ The posterolateral portal, the most commonly used and safest portal, is located directly adjacent to the lateral edge of the Achilles tendon, in the soft spot, about 1.2 cm above the tip of the fibula; the exact level depends on the type of distraction used.
  - ☐ This portal is usually at or slightly below the joint line. Branches of the *sural nerve* and the *lesser saphenous vein* must be avoided with this portal which is why it is made adjacent to the Achilles tendon (Fig. 13.1.6).
- ▨ The trans-Achilles portal is established at the same level as the posterolateral but through the center of the Achilles tendon.
  - ☐ In our experience, this portal does not allow easy mobility of the instruments and may lead to increased iatrogenic damage of the Achilles tendon. For these reasons, we do not recommend this portal.
- ▨ The posteromedial portal is created just medial to the Achilles tendon at the joint line. The *posterior tibial artery* and the *tibial nerve* must be avoided, and the tendons of the flexor hallucis longus (FHL) and flexor digitorum longus must also be protected.
  - ☐ The calcaneal nerve and its branches may separate from the tibial nerve proximal to the ankle joint and traverse in an interval between the tibial nerve and the medial border of the Achilles tendon.
  - ☐ It is critical that this portal be made lateral to the FHL to avoid neurovascular injury.
  - ☐ Because of the potential for serious complications, the posteromedial portal is seldom made in the supine position, but it is routinely used with prone positioning.

Accessory Posterior Portal

- ▨ The accessory posterolateral portal is made at the same level as or slightly higher than the posterolateral portal.
  - ☐ It is established posterior to the fibula and lateral to the FHL. This is 1 to 1.5 cm lateral to the posterolateral portal, and extreme caution must be exercised to avoid injury to the sural nerve and small saphenous vein.
  - ☐ This portal is particularly useful for the removal of posterior loose bodies when posterior visualization is necessary, and for the debridement and drilling of extremely posterior osteochondral lesions of the talus (OLT).

Portal Placement Technique

- ▨ The anteromedial portal is created first. While palpating the anterior tibial tendon, a 22G needle is used to find the correct trajectory medial to the tendon. Sterile lactated Ringer's solution is then infused into the ankle joint.
  - ☐ Backflow from the needle confirms entry into the ankle joint.
  - ☐ A "nick-and-spread" technique is used to establish the portal. A no. 11 scalpel is used to cut through the skin just medial to the tibialis anterior tendon in a vertical fashion. This is done with the index

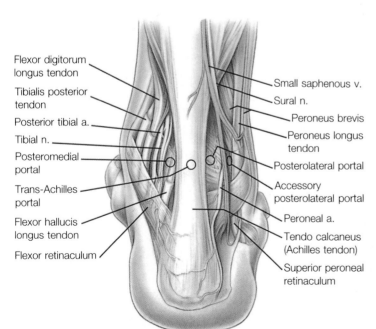

Flexor digitorum longus tendon
Tibialis posterior tendon
Posterior tibial a.
Tibial n.
Posteromedial portal
Trans-Achilles portal
Flexor hallucis longus tendon
Flexor retinaculum

Small saphenous v.
Sural n.
Peroneus brevis
Peroneus longus tendon
Posterolateral portal
Accessory posterolateral portal
Peroneal a.
Tendo calcaneus (Achilles tendon)
Superior peroneal retinaculum

Figure 13.1.6 Posterior anatomy. There are three posterior portals and one accessory posterior portal in the ankle. Usually only the posterolateral portal is used. (From Ferkel RD. Diagnostic arthroscopic examination. In: Arthroscopic surgery: the foot and ankle. Philadelphia: Lippincott-Raven, 1996:106.)

finger on the anterior tibial tendon to avoid injury to it. A mosquito clamp is then used to bluntly dissect through the subcutaneous tissue down to the capsule and puncture through it (Fig. 13.1.7).

- [ ] A blunt trocar with attached arthroscopic cannula is placed into the ankle joint and the trocar is exchanged for the arthroscope.
- [ ] The joint is then examined from the anteromedial portal.
- [ ] Continued joint distension is accomplished by manually injecting fluid through the arthroscopic cannula with a 50-mL syringe.

Using a technique similar to that for the anteromedial portal, the anterolateral portal is established. Under direct arthroscopic vision, a 25G needle is carefully inserted into the ankle joint to locate the position of the anterolateral portal.

- [ ] Location of the anterolateral portal varies depending on the pathology.
- [ ] Sequential examination of intra-articular anatomy can then be performed.

The posterolateral portal is established under direct visualization by taking the arthroscope from the anteromedial portal and maneuvering it through the notch of Harty from anterior to posterior (Fig. 13.1.8).

- [ ] The tip of the fibula is then palpated, and approximately 1.2 cm above it, an 18G spinal needle is inserted directly adjacent to the Achilles tendon, in

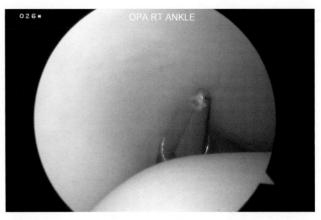

Figure 13.1.8 To establish the posterolateral portal, the arthroscope is placed in the anteromedial portal and brought through the notch of Hardy to visualize the posterior stuctures.

line with the ankle joint and angled 45° toward the medial malleolus (Fig. 13.1.9).

- [ ] Arthroscopically, the needle should be seen medial to the posteroinferior tibiofibular and transverse tibiofibular ligaments.
- [ ] The cannula should be inserted with care to avoid injury to the branches of the sural nerve and the lesser saphenous vein.

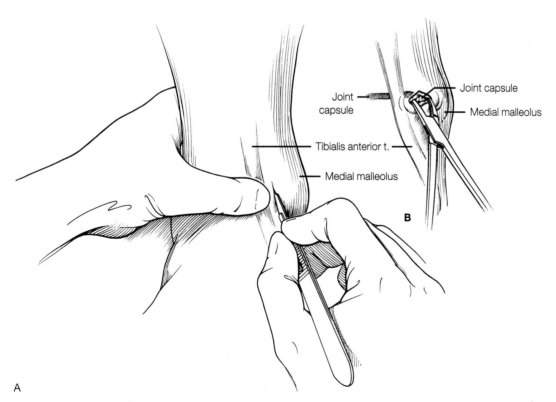

Figure 13.1.7 Establishing the anteromedial portal. (**A**) An incision is made medial to the anterior tibial tendon while the tendon is palpated with the thumb. (**B**) Blunt dissection is performed with a clamp through the skin to the capsule. (From Ferkel RD. Diagnostic arthroscopic examination. In: Arthroscopic surgery: the foot and ankle. Philadelphia: Lippincott-Raven, 1996:108.)

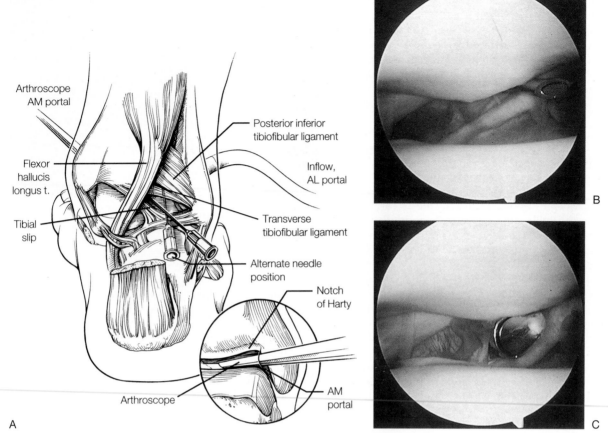

Figure 13.1.9   Establishing the posterolateral portal. (**A**) Posterior view. Inflow is placed through the AL portal and the arthroscope is inserted through the AM portal. Inset: The arthroscope is maneuvered through the notch of Harty to visualize the posterior structures. A spinal needle is then inserted to determine the appropriate direction for the posterolateral portal. (**B**) Arthroscopic view from the anteromedial portal, demonstrating the spinal needle penetrating the joint capsule medial to the transverse tibiofibular ligament. (**C**) After the spinal needle determines the appropriate direction, an interchangeable cannula is inserted through the posterolateral portal under direct vision, medial to the transverse tibiofibular ligament. AL, anterolateral; AM, anteromedial. (From Ferkel RD. Diagnostic arthroscopic examination. In: Arthroscopic surgery: the foot and ankle. Philadelphia: Lippincott-Raven, 1996:109.)

☐ The posterolateral portal is primarily used as an inflow portal, and may also be used for visualization or instrumentation through an interchangeable cannulae system.

Arthroscopic Examination

The normal intra-articular anatomic structures of the ankle have been well described.

▪ A 21-point arthroscopic examination of the ankle is recommended to ensure a systematic evaluation of the ankle.
▪ The eight-point anterior examination includes the deltoid ligament, medial gutter, medial talus, central talus, lateral talus, talofibular articulation, lateral gutter, and anterior gutter (Fig. 13.1.10).
▪ The six-point central examination includes the medial, central, and lateral portions of the tibiotalar articulation. By maneuvering the arthroscope from the anteromedial portal to view the posterior structures, three additional points can be seen, including the posteroinferior tibiofibular ligament, transverse tibiofibular ligament, and capsular reflection of the flexor hallucis tendon (Fig. 13.1.11).
▪ The seven-point posterior examination includes the medial gutter and deltoid ligament, posteromedial talar dome and tibial plafond, central talus, lateral talus,

Figure 13.1.11   Six-point central examination, viewed from the anteromedial portal. It is performed by maneuvering the arthroscope into the center of the ankle and examining the tibiotalar articulation. The arthroscope is then placed more posteriorly to examine the posterior capsular structures. (From Ferkel RD. Diagnostic arthroscopic examination. In: Arthroscopic surgery: the foot and ankle. Philadelphia: Lippincott-Raven, 1996:112.)

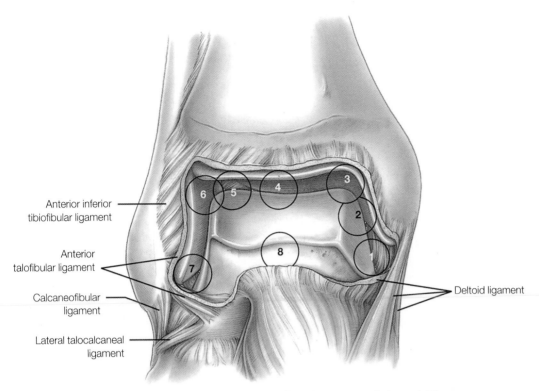

Figure 13.1.10 Eight-point anterior examination viewed from the anteromedial portal. The anterior ankle is examined starting at the tip of the medial malleolus and making a circle within the ankle joint. (From Ferkel RD. Diagnostic arthroscopic examination. In: Arthroscopic surgery: the foot and ankle. Philadelphia: Lippincott-Raven, 1996:110.)

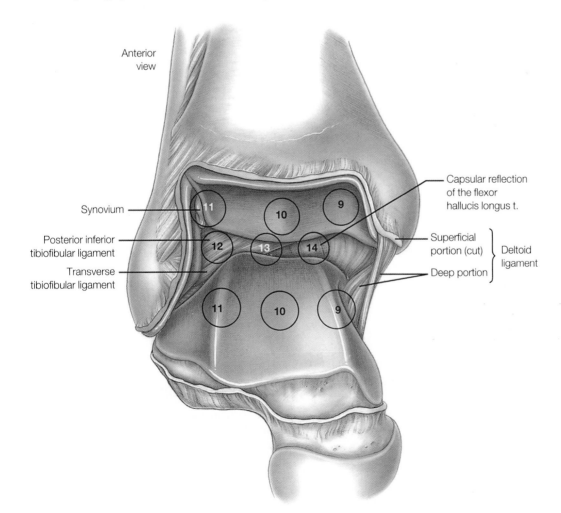

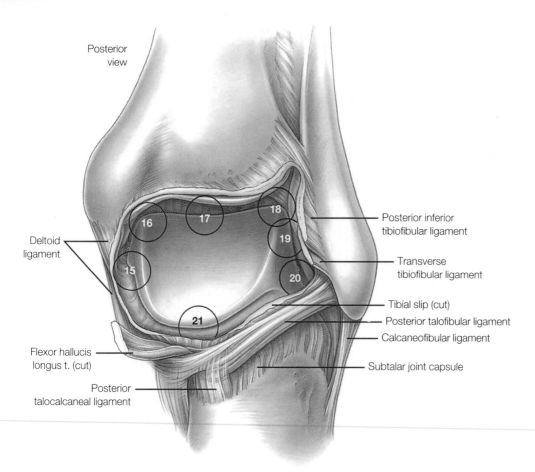

Posterior
view

Deltoid
ligament

Flexor hallucis
longus t. (cut)

Posterior
talocalcaneal ligament

Posterior inferior
tibiofibular ligament

Transverse
tibiofibular ligament

Tibial slip (cut)

Posterior talofibular ligament

Calcaneofibular ligament

Subtalar joint capsule

Figure 13.1.12 Seven-point posterior examination viewed from the posterolateral portal. The examination is initiated along the posteromedial malleolar–talar articulation and is carried clockwise to end in the posterior recess. (From Ferkel RD. Diagnostic arthroscopic examination. In: Arthroscopic surgery: the foot and ankle. Philadelphia: Lippincott-Raven, 1996:114.)

talofibular posterior articulation, lateral gutter, and posterior gutter (Fig. 13.1.12).
- In general, the anteromedial, anterolateral, and posterolateral portals provide excellent visualization of the entire joint.
- With the three-portal system, adequate inflow can be maintained with gravity drainage so that there is no need for an arthroscopic pump.

LOOSE BODIES

The presence of loose bodies is an indicator of an underlying pathologic disorder involving the synovium, cartilage, or underlying bone. Thus, to effectively treat this entity, the underlying pathology must be addressed as well.

PATHOGENESIS

Loose bodies may be either chondral or osteochondral and may arise from defects in the talus or tibia, osteophytes, or degenerative joint disease. They may result from major trauma to the ankle joint or from a relatively innocuous injury such as a lateral ligament sprain. Multiple loose cartilaginous or osteocartilaginous bodies may also form in synovial chondromatosis. This disorder is more common in larger joints, but it may also occur in the ankle. In this disorder, metaplastic mesenchymal cells in the joint capsule develop into chondroblasts, which produce small clusters of cartilage. These nodules of cartilage can protrude into the joint and break off to form small loose bodies. As the cartilage mass grows, the central portion may become necrotic and calcify. The loose bodies then become visible on routine radiographs (Fig. 13.1.13).

DIAGNOSIS

History and Physical Examination

- A small loose body may cause catching symptoms with joint motion along with pain, swelling, and decreased ROM.
- Symptoms of internal derangement may resolve if a small loose body becomes fixed to the synovial lining, ceasing to cause joint irritation.

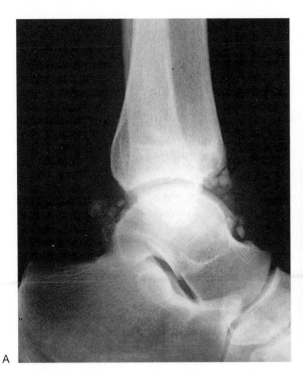

A

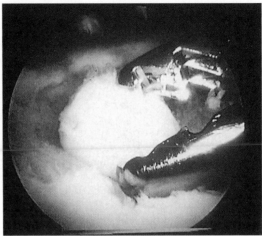

B

Figure 13.1.13 (**A**) Lateral radiograph shows numerous loose bodies in the anterior and posterior recesses of the ankle joint. (**B**) Arthroscopic view shows removal of the loose body with a grasper. (From Ferkel RD. Articular surface defects, loose bodies, and osteophytes. In: Arthroscopic surgery: the foot and ankle. Philadelphia: Lippincott-Raven, 1996:173.)

- A loose body may grow by proliferation of chondro-blasts/osteoblasts, or may shrink owing to the action of chondroclasts/osteoclasts.
- The physical examination may not be very revealing, with vague areas of tenderness, possible limitation of motion, and catching.
- Seldom is a loose body palpable.
- As with all ankle pathology, a careful physical examination must rule out extra-articular entities that can cause symptoms similar to intra-articular lesions.
- Peroneal tendon subluxation, posterior tibial tendon attrition or rupture, tarsal tunnel syndrome, sinus tarsi syndrome, stress fracture, and tendinitis must be carefully excluded by both physical examination and ancillary studies.

Radiologic Features

- Plain radiographs can reveal an osseous loose body unless it is superimposed on other bony structures, but chondral loose bodies are not visible on routine radiographic studies.
- Arthrography, especially a CT arthrogram, usually reveals the loose bodies.
- Bone scans are seldom informative, although MRI holds promise for showing chondral lesions not seen on other types of studies.
- The plain radiographs, arthrogram, CT scan, and/or MRI scan should be scrutinized to discover the origin of the loose body, such as a defect of the talar dome, tibial plafond, or osteophyte.
- Lesions that appear on routine radiographs to be loose bodies may actually be intra-articular, intracapsular, or extra-articular in location, particularly in the posterior ankle joint.

- □ The location of the lesions should be carefully determined preoperatively to avoid performing an arthroscopic examination for loose body removal, only to find the joint free of any abnormality.
- □ An arthrogram, an arthrogram–CT scan, or an MRI study is best suited to make the distinction between an intra-articular and an extra-articular abnormality.

TREATMENT

- Loose bodies localized to the anterior compartment, particularly in patients with ligamentous laxity, can be approached with a routine setup using anteromedial, anterolateral, and posterolateral portals. However, the posterior joint should also be examined for the presence of loose bodies, which can be hidden in the posterior recess of the joint. Joint distraction is helpful to visualize this area. In the case of an ankle with tight ligamentous support, joint distraction may be mandatory.
- □ Loose bodies in the anterior joint can generally be retrieved from anterior portals.
- □ However, if there is instrument crowding, then the arthroscope can be placed in the posterolateral portal and the loose bodies removed using the anteromedial or anterolateral portal.
- □ Retrieval of loose bodies in the posterior aspect of the joint can be more problematic.
- □ Rarely, a carefully placed anterocentral portal may be used to triangulate into the posterior joint.
- □ This portal should be placed directly through the common digitorum extensor longus tendon sheath.

☐ With the arthroscope placed in either of the anterior portals, removal may be best accomplished with a loose body clamp placed in the posterolateral portal.

■ After removal of the loose bodies, a careful evaluation of the joint surfaces should be performed to find the source.

☐ If a chondral or osteochondral defect is found, it should be debrided (see OLT).

☐ If an osteophyte is responsible for the loose body, it should be debrided with an arthroscopic burr, an osteotome, or a pituitary rongeur.

■ The wounds are closed with a 4-0 nylon suture.

Postoperative Management

■ Postoperatively, a bulky compressive dressing with a posterior splint is applied.

■ The sutures and splint are removed 5 to 7 days postoperatively and exercises to regain ROM are begun.

■ The exercise regimen then advances to include strengthening and proprioceptive training.

Results

The clinical results after loose body removal are quite good in patients who do not have associated abnormalities. When degenerative or posttraumatic arthritic changes or significant chondral defects are present, the results are less predictable.

SOFT-TISSUE IMPINGEMENT

PATHOGENESIS

Epidemiology

Ankle sprains are one of the most common injuries in sports. One inversion ankle sprain occurs per 10,000 persons per day. In a study at West Point, 30% of cadets suffered an ankle sprain in their 4 years at the school. Furthermore, it has been estimated that 10% to 50% of patients will have some degree of chronic ankle. The differential diagnosis of chronic pain after an ankle sprain include the following:

■ OLT
■ Calcific ossicles at the medial or lateral malleolus
■ Peroneal tendon tears or subluxation
■ Tarsal coalition
■ Degenerative joint disease
■ Nerve entrapment
■ Occult fractures of the talus or calcaneus
■ Subtalar dysfunction
■ Reflex sympathetic dystrophy/complex regional pain syndrome
■ Soft-tissue impingement

The primary cause of chronic pain after an ankle sprain is soft-tissue impingement. This can occur along the syndesmosis, medial and/or lateral gutters, the syndesmotic interval between the tibia and the fibula, or posteriorly in the syndesmosis and posterior gutter.

Pathophysiology

Soft-tissue impingement is most commonly seen anterolaterally because of the inversion mechanism of most ankle sprains. In 1950, Wolin et al. first described a meniscoid band of hyalinized tissue between the talus and the fibula as a source of ankle pain. They thought that impingement of this meniscal tissue led to pain and that removal would result in symptomatic relief. Waller, in 1982, termed this pathology anterolateral corner compression syndrome and noted pain localized along the anteroinferior border of the fibula and the anterolateral talus. These findings, confirmed arthroscopically by Ferkel and others, are thought to reflect a chronic synovitis and fibrosis. Adjacent talar or fibular chondromalacia may also be associated with this lesion.

Anterolateral soft-tissue impingement (ASTI) usually occurs in the superior portion of the anterior talofibular ligament but can also be localized to the distal portion of the anterior inferior tibiofibular (syndesmotic) ligament (Fig. 13.1.14). A separate or accessory fascicle of the anteroinferior tibiofibular ligament has been reported as a source of soft-tissue impingement. Furthermore, soft-tissue impingement can occur along the entire lateral gutter.

Syndesmotic impingement may involve any or all of the following structures: the anterior inferior tibiofibular

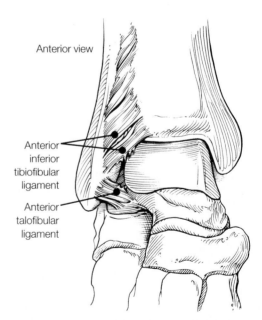

Figure 13.1.14 Anterolateral ankle anatomy: soft-tissue impingement sites. Note the accessory fascicle of the anterior inferior tibiofibular ligament, which can impinge across the lateral talar dome. (From Ferkel RD. Soft-tissue lesions of the ankle. In: Arthroscopic surgery: the foot and ankle. Philadelphia: Lippincott-Raven, 1996:125.)

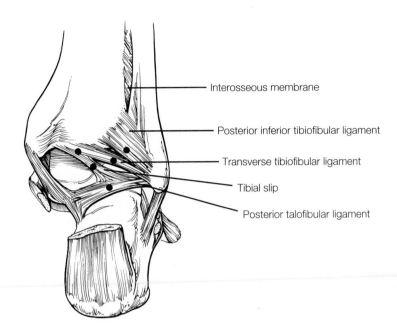

- Interosseous membrane
- Posterior inferior tibiofibular ligament
- Transverse tibiofibular ligament
- Tibial slip
- Posterior talofibular ligament

Figure 13.1.15 Posterior impingement sites. The tibial slip (posterior intermalleolar ligament) can also be an area of soft-tissue impingement. (From Ferkel RD. Soft-tissue lesions of the ankle. In: Arthroscopic surgery: the foot and ankle. Philadelphia: Lippincott-Raven, 1996:134.)

ligament and its fascicle; the posterior inferior tibiofibular ligament, including its distal and deep component, the transverse ligament; and the interosseous membrane (Fig. 13.1.14). Injuries to the syndesmosis are vastly underestimated and often occur with sprains and fractures that go undetected. Syndesmotic sprains have been estimated to occur in 10% of all ankle injuries, and tend to be most common in collision sports such as ice hockey, football, and soccer.

Posterior soft-tissue impingement usually occurs along the posterolateral or posterocentral portion of the ankle and involves the posterior tibiofibular ligament, including the transverse tibiofibular ligament, and occasionally the tibial slip (also known as the posterior intermalleolar ligament, Fig. 13.1.15). This impingement can occur alone or in combination with anterolateral and syndesmosis impingement. However, usually a more generalized posterolateral impingement occurs with fibrosis, capsulitis, and synovial swelling along the posterior portions of the ankle.

Medial soft-tissue impingement has been less frequently described in the literature compared with anterolateral impingement. It has been hypothesized that medial impingement involving the deltoid ligament may occur secondary to either direct trauma, scarring from a twisting injury, prior surgery, or increased anterior to posterior laxity from a tear of the ATFL. Patients with medial impingement can be treated with arthroscopic debridement in a similar fashion to anterolateral impingement.

DIAGNOSIS

History and Physical Examination

- Typically, in ASTI, the patient complains of vague anterior pain, usually along the anterior and anterolateral aspect of the ankle, sometimes involving the syndesmosis and sinus tarsi regions.

- Pain is usually absent at rest and present with most activities, limiting the patient's ability to participate in a given sport.
- Physical examination may reveal tenderness along the syndesmosis, anterior gutter, including the anterior talofibular ligament and the calcaneofibular ligament, and many times also the posterior subtalar joint or sinus tarsi. It is important to differentiate lateral gutter pain from subtalar pain, especially in the sinus tarsi.
- In syndesmotic impingement, the patients have exquisite tenderness along the syndesmosis and more proximally on the interosseous membrane.
- A positive squeeze test can be seen with this injury besides a positive external rotation stress test.
- Because posterior impingement may occur with anterior and syndesmotic impingement, the physical findings may be similar, with the addition of pain located posteriorly between the distal tibia and the fibula.

Radiologic Features

- Radiologic evaluation may reveal calcification or heterotopic bone in the interosseous space, which suggests previous injury to the distal tibiofibular syndesmosis, with ossicles along the tip of the fibula and the lateral talar dome consistent with injuries of the anterior talofibular ligament.
- Ossicles can also be seen medially indicative of a deltoid ligament injury.
- X-rays are often normal, as are bone scans and CT scans.
- In approximately 30% of cases, MRI may indicate pathology in the lateral gutter.
- Stress X-rays in this group are usually negative, ruling out ankle instability.
- Recently, Ferkel et al. reported on the efficacy and reliability of MRI in detecting ASTI of the ankle. The

diagnosis was generally made using the sagittal T1 and Short Tau Inversion Recovery images. Twenty-four patients with an arthroscopically and clinically confirmed diagnosis of anterolateral impingement of the ankle were compared with 16 controls. MRI was found to have an accuracy of 78.9%, a sensitivity of 83.3%, and a specificity of 78.6%. We believe MRI is an excellent modality to evaluate the ankle for possible soft-tissue impingement (Fig. 13.1.16).

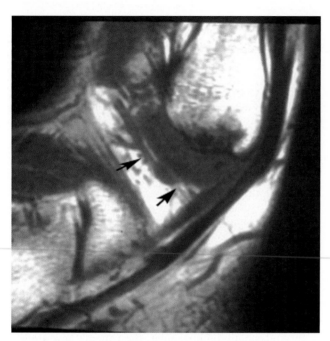

Figure 13.1.16 Sagittal T1 MRI of the ankle showing a low-signal intensity mass in the anterolateral gutter. This is consistent with ASTI of the ankle.

TREATMENT

At arthroscopy, the medial malleolar–talar articulation and the central portion of the ankle and anterior gutter are usually normal. In ASTI, pathology is generally limited to the syndesmosis and the lateral gutter. Synovitis surrounding the anterior inferior tibiofibular ligament, both in front and behind as well as synovitis of the anterior talofibular ligament is usually present. Fibrosis of the lateral gutter and chondromalacia of the talus and fibula may be present in some cases. In addition, a small ossicle or loose body may be hidden in the soft tissues at the tip of the fibula (Fig. 13.1.17). In syndesmotic impingement, inflamed synovitis involves the anterior and posterior aspects of the syndesmotic ligament, and sometimes the ligament is torn and frayed. It is important to note that posterior impingement may be easily missed if careful anterior and posterior viewing is not done. Without some type of distraction device, it can be difficult to see some of the synovial pathology involving the posterolateral corner of the ankle. Using motorized shavers, burrs, graspers, and baskets, the inflamed synovium, thickened adhesive bands, osteophytes, and loose bodies are debrided (Fig. 13.1.18). Care must be taken not to excise the anterior talofibular ligament remnant. Previous cadaver studies indicate that approximately 20% of the anterior inferior tibiofibular ligament is viewed intra-articulary, and no instability has been produced at the syndesmostic joint by resecting this intra-articular portion.

Postoperative Management

◼ After surgery, patients are placed in a posterior splint for 1 week.

◼ They are then put in a controlled active motion (CAM) walker boot for an additional 2 to 3 weeks.

◼ Subsequently, they are given a small ankle brace to wear inside a tennis shoe and begin formal physiotherapy.

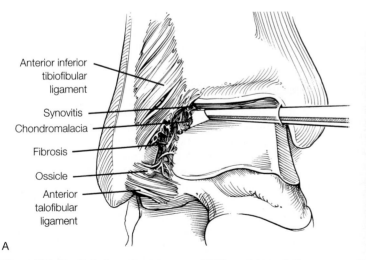

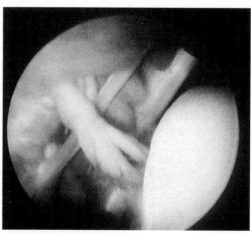

Anterior inferior tibiofibular ligament

Synovitis

Chondromalacia

Fibrosis

Ossicle

Anterior talofibular ligament

A

B

Figure 13.1.17 Soft-tissue impingement. (**A**) Viewed through the anteromedial portal, ASTI with synovitis and fibrosis and chondromalacia in the anterolateral gutter. (**B**) Arthroscopic view of the anterolateral impingement lesion. Note the hemosiderin staining of the lateral gutter and associated scar bands and synovitis. (From Ferkel RD. Soft-tissue lesions of the ankle. In: Arthroscopic surgery: the foot and ankle. Philadelphia: Lippincott-Raven, 1996:127.)

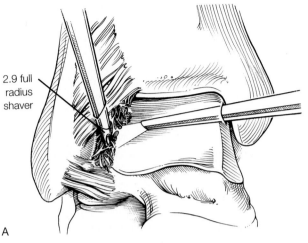

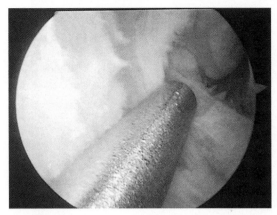

Figure 13.1.18 Debridement of the lateral gutter. (**A**) Debridement is performed with a small-joint shaver and includes removing inflamed synovium, thickened adhesive bands, osteophytes, and loose bodies. (**B**) Arthroscopic view through the anteromedial portal. A full-radius shaver is debriding the lateral gutter while avoiding injury to the anterior talofibular ligament. (From Ferkel RD. Soft-tissue lesions of the ankle. In: Arthroscopic surgery: the foot and ankle. Philadelphia: Lippincott-Raven, 1996:129.)

▪ Patients can return to full activity, including sports, when all the goals of rehabilitation have been achieved.

Results

Arthroscopic treatment of ASTI of the ankle has proven successful, alleviating chronic ankle pain that patients exhibit after an inversion ankle sprain. Between 1983 and 2011, the senior author has treated more than 350 patients arthroscopically for ASTI. Our initial group of 31 patients with more than 2 years of follow-up has been reported, with 26 of 31 (84%) rated as excellent/good, subjectively and objectively; 4 of 31 (13%) fair, and 1 poor. In subsequent cases, the results have remained similar. Numerous other authors have reported a high percentage of the good/excellent results after arthroscopic treatment for anterolateral impingement.

Medial impingement of ankle, a less common entity, has received much less attention in the literature than anterolateral impingement. Egol and Parisien described a case of medial impingement of the ankle following a hypothesized eversion injury to the deep deltoid ligament that was relieved with arthroscopic debridement. Liu and Mirzayan reported a case of chronic posteromedial impingement following an ankle injury that resulted in soft-tissue impingement between the medial talus and the tibial plafond. Open treatment has also been reported as successful in small case series. Arthroscopic debridement seems to be effective as well, but larger case series are needed to evaluate this further.

SYNOVIAL DISORDERS

The arthroscopic surgeon must understand certain points to diagnose and treat these problems correctly. Our discussion will focus on rheumatoid arthritis (RA), pigmented villonodular synovitis (PVNS), synovial chondromatosis, and hemophilia.

PATHOGENESIS

RA is a chronic systemic inflammatory condition characterized by the method in which it affects joints. Although the etiology is unknown and various causes have been postulated, including a cell-mediated immune response (T cell), no consensus exists as to its exact cause.

PVNS is thought by some to be a benign neoplasm involving the synovium. It occurs most commonly in the knee, but it can involve the ankle. Both generalized and localized forms occur. The localized solitary lesion is more common in the ankle than the former type.

Synovial chondromatosis is seldom seen in the ankle and is almost always monoarticular. This entity involves multiple foci of cartilage metaplasia within the synovium. As these masses grow, they form nodules within the synovial tissue and then become excrescences. These nodules can calcify or ossify.

Hemophilia is a bleeding disorder caused by a factor VIII deficiency (hemophilia A) or factor IX deficiency (hemophilia B). This disorder, which commonly affects the ankle, manifests in repeated hemarthroses owing to minor trauma, which in turn leads into eventual cartilage destruction and joint deformity.

DIAGNOSIS

▪ The clinical presentation in RA is highly inconsistent, ranging from pauciarticular illness of brief duration to progressive destruction with polyarthritis and vasculitis.
   ▫ Although RA can affect any diarthrodial joint, it initially involves the small joints of the hands, wrists, knees, and feet.
   ▫ The disease may progress to affect the elbow, shoulder, ankle, talonavicular, and subtalar regions.
   ▫ Radiographs are characteristic for RA, often demonstrating periarticular erosions and osteopenia.

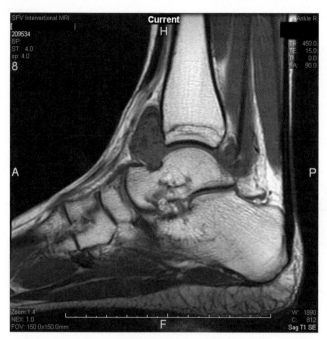

Figure 13.1.19 Sagittal T1-weighted MRI of the ankle showing a nodular soft-tissue mass in the anterior and posterior gutters of ankle. This MRI is consistent with PVNS.

☐ Preoperatively, it is important to aspirate the ankle or subtalar region.

☐ A CT scan or MRI may be useful to look for synovitis, effusion, articular damage, and other unsuspected abnormalities.

■ In PVNS, physical examination reveals a warm, swollen, and tender ankle with decreased ROM.

☐ Aspiration of the joint reveals dark, serosanguinous fluid, and X-rays are occasionally helpful in the diagnosis.

☐ The arthrogram may show nodular masses and MRI can demonstrate swollen synovial tissue and cartilage erosions (Fig. 13.1.19).

■ Diagnosis of synovial chondromatosis is made by noting limited ROM, locking, swelling, and visualization of multiple calcifications on X-rays of the ankle.

☐ Synovial biopsy will often make the diagnosis.

■ Hemophilia should always involve consultation with a hematologist for diagnosis and treatment.

☐ Acutely the joint is swollen, red, and tender, and extensive loss of joint space can occur.

☐ On X-ray, effusion with spurs and sclerosis can be seen.

☐ Infection should always be included in the differential diagnosis.

TREATMENT

Indications and Contraindications

Surgery in RA is based on correct timing, with careful assessment of the region and estimation of the patient's general condition. In the ankle, chondromalacia and synovitis may be seen, depending on the severity of the disease. In some situations, areas of articular cartilage necrosis on the tibial plafond or the talar dome may be the primary pathology. If the conservative treatment fails, ankle arthroscopy should be considered after consultation with a rheumatologist. The main indications for surgery are pain, swelling, and locking/catching sensations. Arthroscopic synovectomy should be reserved for early joint involvement, as extensive degenerative changes will preclude a good result. Synovectomy may be performed using 2.9-, 3.5-, or 4.5-mm full-radius shaver blades. As always, careful attention should be paid to the neurovascular structures adjacent to the capsule, and use of distraction is helpful in performing a complete synovectomy. Although some investigators have questioned the benefit of synovectomy, in general, the results are improved if minimal cartilage involvement is seen. Thus, if on preoperative X-ray films, significant joint disruption has occurred, synovectomy should be avoided. Even under the best circumstances, debridement and synovectomy slow down but do not prevent articular destruction, and they provide only temporary relief (Fig. 13.1.20).

In PVNS, arthroscopy is helpful to confirm the diagnosis when synovitis, papillary formation, and hemosiderin deposits are seen. In addition, brownish-red or yellow components may be visible on the surface of the lesion. As in RA, treatment includes total synovectomy aided by a distractor. With the localized form of PVNS, arthroscopic excision of the lesion is usually curative. However, with the generalized form, synovectomy may not give lasting results, as recurrences are more common (Fig. 13.1.21).

Arthroscopic treatment of synovial chondromatosis involves loose body removal in the earlier stages, and debridement and loose body removal without synovectomy in the late stage. With open surgery, approximately 5% of the problems recur, but no series of arthroscopic treatment has been reported. Even with recurrence, arthroscopy is recommended for repeat surgery.

In chronic repetitive hemarthrosis secondary to hemophilia, arthroscopic synovectomy may be helpful. Along with proper medical supervision for administration of deficient clotting factors, arthroscopic synovectomy may decrease the number and severity of future bleeding episodes.

Postoperative Management

■ Postoperatively, a compression dressing and a posterior splint should be applied for 7 to 14 days to allow swelling and inflammation to subside.

■ Early motion should be initiated as soon as soft-tissue swelling has abated and pain is controlled.

OSTEOCHONDRAL LESIONS OF THE TALUS

OLT include many pathologic entities, such as osteochondritis dissecans, chondral and osteochondral loose bodies, osteophytes, chondral and osteochondral fractures of the tibia and talus, cystic lesions of the talus, fracture defects,

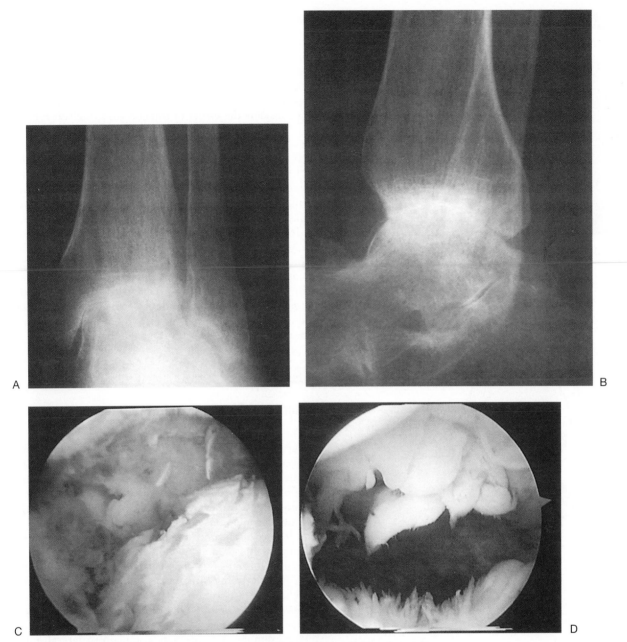

Figure 13.1.20 Rheumatoid arthritis. Preoperative AP (**A**) and lateral (**B**) radiographs of a 53-year-old woman with RA. The loss of joint space is severe. (**C**) Arthroscopic view of the same patient shows loss of articular cartilage and hemorrhagic synovium. (**D**) Synovitis and degeneration of the articular cartilage in a 45-year-old man with RA. (From Ferkel RD. Soft-tissue lesions of the ankle. In: Arthroscopic surgery: the foot and ankle. Philadelphia: Lippincott-Raven, 1996:139.)

and arthritis. Controversy persists regarding the etiology, treatment, and prognosis of osteochondral and chondral lesions of the ankle.

PATHOGENESIS

There is more than one etiology for OLT. Although trauma is believed to play a major role, idiopathic avascular necrosis, may be a potential cause, supported by the fact that most patients with OLT have no history of antecedent trauma.

Medial lesions are more common than lateral lesions; they tend to be more posterior, more cup-shaped, and deeper than lateral lesions. Unlike lateral lesions, medial lesions are generally nondisplaced. Lateral lesions are more commonly induced by acute trauma and are more anterior than medial lesions; they are usually shallow, wafer shaped, and frequently displaced (Fig. 13.1.22).

The type of lesion can give insight into the nature of the initial injury. A superficial lesion generally comprises sheared off flakes of cartilage with an intact subchondral plate. More severe lesions penetrate deeper into the

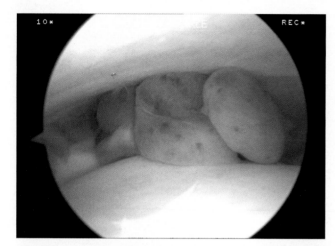

Figure 13.1.21   Arthroscopic view from the anteromedial portal showing extensive hemorrhagic, nodular masses in the posterior ankle, consistent with PVNS.

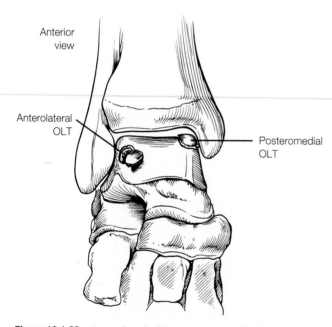

Figure 13.1.22   Osteochondral lesion size varies by location. Lateral lesions tend to be shallower and wafer shaped; medial lesions are deeper and cup shaped. (From Ferkel RD. Articular surface defects, loose bodies, and osteophytes. In: Arthroscopic surgery: the foot and ankle. Philadelphia: Lippincott-Raven, 1996:147.)

subchondral bone creating a bone bruise. The fate of the lesion is dependent on whether the bone bruise extends to the surface of the subchondral bone. If the subchondral bone has a defect, synovial fluid can enter the bone and eventually a cyst can form. This is further exacerbated by weight bearing as positive and negative pressures can drive the fluid in and out of the bone defect with each step. Persistent fluid in the bone prevents healing and results in cyst formation.

Classification

A radiographic staging of OLT was described by Berndt and Harty. Four stages were proposed to describe the amount of destruction and displacement of the fragment. Ferkel and Sgaglione proposed a CT staging system that not only corresponds to the stages described by Berndt and Harty but also considers the extent of osteonecrosis, the subchondral cyst formation, and the separation of fragments that are not seen radiographically (Fig. 13.1.23 and Table 13.1.1). MRI has also been used by Anderson to stage OLT (Table 13.1.2). In 1986, Prtisch and associates developed a staging system based on arthroscopic appearance of the overlying cartilage. They classified OLT into three grades: (1) Intact, firm, and shiny cartilage; (2) intact but soft cartilage; and (3) frayed cartilage. They noted a poor correlation between the X-ray appearance and arthroscopic findings and felt that arthroscopic findings were the most significant determinants of outcome. Ferkel, Cheng, and Applegate correlated CT and MRI with a new arthroscopic staging system, and found the imaging appearance cannot always predict the arthroscopic findings (Table 13.1.3). They also found that arthroscopic appearance correlated best with long-term results.

DIAGNOSIS

History and Physical Examination

- The diagnosis of OLT requires a high index of suspicion because in many cases the clinical symptoms and findings are so mild that routine radiographs are not done.
- The presentation can be acute after injury, but more often it is associated with persistent ankle pain, particularly after a trauma such as an inversion injury of the lateral ligamentous complex.
- A history of chronic lateral ankle pain or chronic ankle sprain pain is commonly noted.
- In addition, a history of associated injuries such as ankle or lower extremity fractures or falls from a height may be elicited.
- Location of pain often does not correlate with the location of the lesion.
- For example, patients may complain of lateral ankle pain with a medial lesion.
- Usually symptoms are intermittent but can include stiffness and pain of a deep aching nature aggravated by weight bearing, swelling, catching, clicking, locking, and less commonly giving way.

Radiologic Features

- After careful clinical examination, three views of the ankle should be done (AP, mortise, and lateral).
- However, plain X-rays do not always demonstrate the lesion.
- Alexander and Barrack reported that mortise and AP views can be taken in various degrees of plantarflexion and dorsiflexion to demonstrate the lesion.
- In a study by Zinman and associates, CT scans have been found to be superior to X-rays for both diagnosis and follow-up of OLT (Fig. 13.1.24).

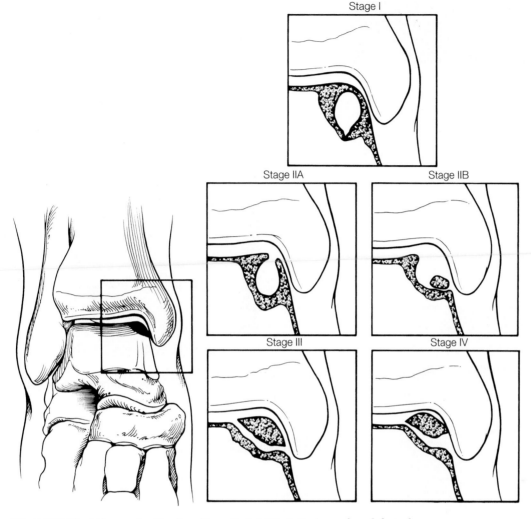

Figure 13.1.23   CT scan classification. (From Ferkel RD. Articular surface defects, loose bodies, and osteophytes. In: Arthroscopic surgery: the foot and ankle. Philadelphia: Lippincott-Raven, 1996:151.)

TABLE 13.1.1 CLASSIFICATION SYSTEM FOR OLT BASED ON CT FINDINGS

Stage	Description
I	Cystic lesion within dome of talus, intact roof on all views
IIA	Cystic lesion with communication to talar dome surface
IIB	Open articular surface lesion with overlying nondisplaced fragment
III	Undisplaced lesion with lucency
IV	Displaced fragment

From Ferkel RD, Sgaglione NA. Arthroscopic treatment of osteochondral lesions of the talus: long term results. Orthop Trans 1993–1994;17:1011.

TABLE 13.1.2 CLASSIFICATION SYSTEM FOR OLT BASED ON MRI FINDINGS

Stage	Description
I	Subchondral trabecular compression Plain radiograph normal, positive bone scan Marrow edema on MRI
IIA	Formation of subchondral cyst
II	Incomplete separation of fragment
III	Unattached, undisplaced fragment with presence of synovial fluid around fragment
IV	Displaced fragment

From Anderson IF, Crichton KJ, Grattan-Smith T, et al. Osteochondral fractures of the dome of the talus. J Bone Joint Surg Am 1989;71:1143.

TABLE 13.1.3 CLASSIFICATION SYSTEM FOR OLT BASED ON ARTHROSCOPIC APPEARANCE \ING CARTILAGE

Grade	Description
A	Smooth, intact, but soft and ballottable
B	Rough surface
C	Fibrillations/fissures
D	Flap present or bone exposed
E	Loose, undisplaced fragment
F	Displaced fragment

From Ferkel RD, Zanotti RM, Komenda GA, et al. Arthroscopic treatment of chronic osteochondral lesions of the talus. Am J Sports Med 2008;36:1750–1762.

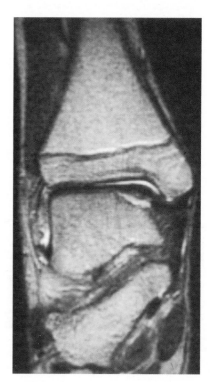

Figure 13.1.25 MRI can be useful in diagnosing OLT as well as soft-tissue pathology. Notice fluid under the OLT indicating the fragment is loose.

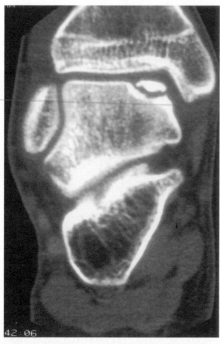

Figure 13.1.24 CT scan clearly demonstrates an osteochondral lesion of the talus affecting the medial talar dome. The lucency under the fragment often is a fibrous membrane that inhibits bone healing.

- MRI has been advocated as being comparable to CT in evaluating OLT lesions.
- Anderson and coworkers compared CT with MRI in 24 cases and found that CT scans failed to detect stage I lesions in four patients, whereas MRI clearly showed these lesions.
- At Southern California Orthopaedic Institute, we reviewed X-rays, CT, MRI, and intraoperative videos in 80 cases, and concluded that CT in the coronal, sagittal, and axial planes is the study of choice if there is a known diagnosis of OLT.
- However, if the X-ray films and clinical examinations are nondiagnostic, MRI may be more valuable because of its ability to image both bone and soft tissue (Fig. 13.1.25).

TREATMENT

Treatment of OLT depends on the severity and duration of symptoms, age of the patient, and the appearance or stage of the lesion. Conservative treatment has been advocated for nondisplaced osteochondral lesions and arthroscopy or arthrotomy for displaced fragments. The authors recommend conservative treatment for both acute and chronic OLT in CT stages I and II. Conservative treatment comprises 6 to 12 weeks of casting with duration dependent on the size of the lesion. Because there is little evidence that non–weight bearing leads to better results, patients are allowed to gradually bear weight in the cast. If the patient remains symptomatic after conservative treatment, arthroscopic evaluation and treatment are recommended. Arthroscopy is advocated for all symptomatic CT stages III and IV lesions. The only exception is for children with grade 3 lesions whose growth plates remain open at the distal tibial and fibular epiphysis. For this patient group, conservative treatment with casting is recommended.

Open treatment for OLT usually requires extensive arthrotomy and/or transmalleolar osteotomy for exposure, excision of loose bodies, drilling, and bone grafting. These approaches are associated with malleolar nonunion, malunion, and joint stiffness. Given the morbidity involved in these approaches, arthroscopic surgery has become the preferred method to address these lesions. Decision making for removal versus repair of the lesion depends on the size and presence of bone on the fragment, and whether it is acute or chronic.

Acute OLT

Most acute, small, loose chondral fragments should be removed followed by addressing the bony bed (microfracture, drilling, etc.). However, if significant bone remains attached to the osteochondral lesion, the fragment should be reattached, if at all possible. This is especially important when the fragment is large and anatomic reduction is feasible. An acute lesion is secured in place by absorbable pins, screws, or K-wires. Lateral lesions that are located anteriorly are more amenable to pinning than medial lesions. Absorbable pins allow for accurate fixation and early motion and maintain hyaline cartilage covering. In our experience, all acute lateral lesions involving the anterolateral talus are inverted. We have termed these "LIFT lesions" (lateral inverted osteochondral fractures of the talus; see Figs. 13.1.26 to 13.1.28).

Chronic OLT

With chronic OLT, it is also critical to identify the lesion and its extent carefully. This can be performed by correlating the imaging results with the arthroscopic findings. Usually these lesions cannot be reattached and will need to be removed. This leaves an exposed bony bed. Different techniques have been advocated to induce cartilage repair of penetrating subchondral bone, including resecting the sclerotic subchondral bone, drilling through the subchondral bone, abrading the articular surface, and creating small-diameter defects with a sharp instrument (microfracture). Penetration of the subchondral bone disrupts subchondral blood vessels with subsequent formation of a clot rich in fibrin. Fibrocartilaginous repair tissue often forms over the surface to protect it from excessive loading. Experimental studies have shown that cells responsible for a new fibrocartilaginous articular surface enter the fibrin clot from the marrow. These cells start as undifferentiated mesenchymal cells and then differentiate into chondroblasts and chondrocytes.

Although the current literature does not indicate the methods that produce the best articular cartilage surface, the authors prefer to drill small to medium lesions and to drill and microfracture large lesions. A comparison of abrasion with

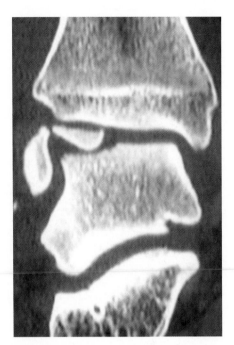

Figure 13.1.27 Coronal CT image of the right ankle demonstrating a stage IV LIFT lesion.

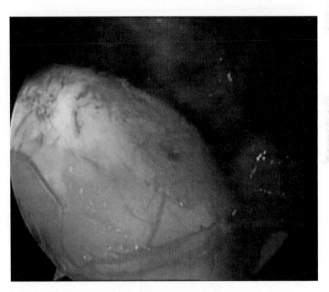

Figure 13.1.28 Picture of a LIFT lesion reduced with three absorbable pins on the lateral talar dome.

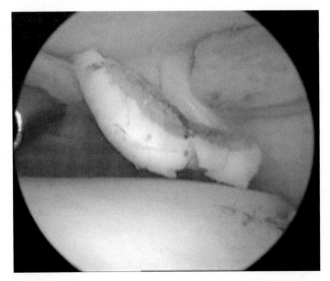

Figure 13.1.26 Arthroscopic picture shows a displaced LIFT lesion.

drilling for treatment of experimental chondral defects in the rabbit demonstrated that long-term results of drilling appear to be better than those of abrasion.

In the chronic situation, OLT that are intact but soft should be drilled by the transmalleolar or transtalar approaches. If the lesion is loose, it should be removed. Debridement of the lesion is performed by using a full-radius resector, high-speed burr, minicurettes, graspers, and banana knife. Drilling is performed through three portals or through transmalleolar or transtalar techniques, using 0.045- or 0.062-in K-wires at 3- to 5-mm intervals to a depth of approximately 10 mm to increase vascular access and formation of new fibrocartilage. A small-joint drill guide (MicroVector) can facilitate accurate drilling (Fig. 13.1.29).

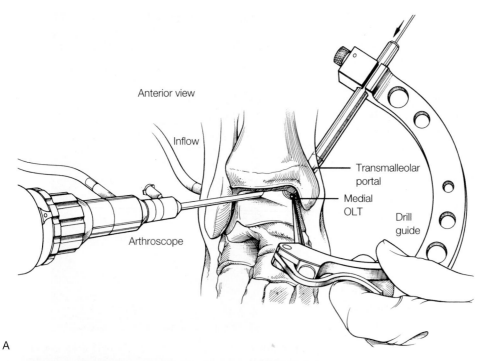

A

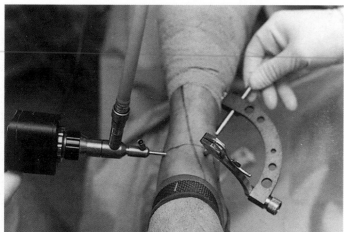

B

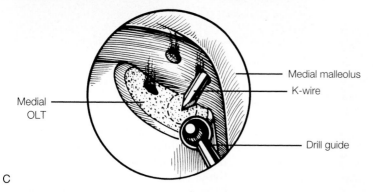

C

Figure 13.1.29 Transmalleolar drilling with the arthroscope in the anterolateral portal. (**A**) If the lesion is anterior enough, it can be visualized through the anterolateral portal and the drilling performed through the anteromedial portal. (**B**) A soft-tissue distraction device in place with the typical setup using small-joint instrumentation. (**C**) Once the K-wire is advanced through the distal tibia, the probe is retracted to allow the K-wire to pass into the talus. (From Ferkel RD. Articular surface defects, loose bodies, and osteophytes. In: Arthroscopic surgery: the foot and ankle. Philadelphia: Lippincott-Raven, 1996:163.)

Microfracture

Microfracture is a popular technique used to address osteochondral lesions because of its limited invasiveness, technical simplicity, and low postoperative morbidity. Microfracture in the ankle is similar to other joints. First, the affected area is delineated and a sharp, perpendicular border is created on the edges. The area is cleaned of any fibrous tissue or remaining cartilage, and the debridement is carried down removing the calcified cartilage layer, preserving the subchondral bone. Microfracture holes are made with an awl penetrating 3 to 4 mm deep and spaced 3 to 4 mm apart. The holes are first placed around the periphery of the defect and spiral in a circular manner into the center of the lesion. At the end of the procedure, the tourniquet is released and blood and marrow elements can be visualized exiting the holes.

Postoperative Management

- Postoperatively, a bulky compressive dressing is applied with a posterior splint in the neutral position.
- ROM exercises are begun at approximately 1 week after the portal sites have healed.
- Weight bearing is restricted for a period of 6 to 8 weeks, depending on the size of the lesion.

Results

The results of arthroscopic management for OLT are comparable to those of open procedures, with lower morbidity and recovery time. Ferkel reported on his results of more than 100 patients treated arthroscopically for OLT. Sixty-six percent involved the medial talar dome, 27% involved the lateral dome of the talus, and 7% were central lesions. Overall results were 83% good to excellent, graded by three different methods. The two poor results had CT stage III lesions that were drilled but not excised; subsequently, one of the patients had excision and further drilling with resolution of his symptoms. The lateral lesions that were acute were either excised and drilled or internally fixated. The medial lesions were either drilled or excision and drilling was performed. The average follow-up was 50 months. Outcome was not significantly affected by a delay in diagnosis.

A recent study by Schimmer et al. examined the results of diagnostic and operative arthroscopy in the treatment of 36 OLT cases. These authors found that despite the use of preoperative MRI, arthroscopy helps in assessing the extent and stability of the OLT and in defining the treatment strategy, including continued conservative care in the case of stage I lesions. Their results support a conservative approach to stages II and III medial lesions as well.

In 2009, Lee et al. reported on 35 ankles with isolated OLT less than 1.5 cm^2 treated with microfracture. Postoperative AOFAS scores were excellent in 46%, good in 43%, and poor in 11% cases. Mean scores improved from 63 to 90 points at final follow-up. They found microfracture to be an effective treatment for OLT.

Recently, clinical management of articular cartilage defects has generated significant research interest in the orthopaedic community. Attempts to stimulate a hyaline cartilage response have included transplantation of various cells including periosteal and perichondral tissues, woven carbon-fiber pads as well as osteochondral auto- or allografts. In addition, chondrocyte transplantation has been studied extensively in Europe and more recently in the United States. With further research, it is hoped that osteochondral defects may be successfully covered by articular cartilage instead of fibrocartilage replacement.

AUTOLOGOUS CHONDROCYTE IMPLANTATION

Indications and Contraindications

Autologous chondrocyte implantation (ACI) has been evolving since 1965 when Smith first isolated and grew chondrocytes in culture. There are currently three generations of ACI (Table 13.1.4). ACI is generally reserved for patients who have failed previous surgery or who present with large lesions with cystic changes. Lesions should be larger than 1 cm^2. Patients with bipolar lesions and patients older than 55 years of age are not good candidates for ACI. Lesions that are uncontained (do not have a circumferential healthy cartilage border) are not ideal lesions for this technique.

TREATMENT

ACI is performed as a two-stage technique. The initial surgery consists of cartilage harvest. This is usually done from the intercondylar notch of the ipsilateral knee but can also be done from the talus. The cartilage biopsy is sent to the laboratory for cell culture. Ankle arthroscopy is done at the first stage to document the lesion size and the status of the surrounding cartilage and to treat associated pathology. The second stage is performed at least 4 weeks after the first surgery. A medial or lateral osteotomy is performed to access the OLT. The lesion is debrided of any fibrinous soft tissue or cartilage, and sharp borders or walls are created with the surrounding healthy articular cartilage. The bone is cleaned, but the subchondral bone is not penetrated. A type I or III collagen membrane is used or an autogenous periosteal graft is harvested. This graft is sewn onto the periphery of the defect and the cultured cells are then injected into the space under the graft (Fig. 13.1.30). Newer techniques are being developed in an attempt to make this a single-stage operation.

TABLE 13.1.4 THE THREE GENERATIONS OF ACI

Generation	Description
I	Cartilage cells suspended under a periosteal flap
II	Cartilage cells inserted under a tissue patch or onto a carrier scaffold
III	Carrier-free, immature cartilage tissue

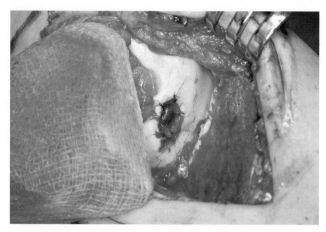

Figure 13.1.30 Medial malleolar osteotomy of the right ankle revealing a type I or III collagen membrane sewn over an osteochondral defect of the talus. The autologous chondrocytes will subsequently be injected under the membrane.

Postoperative Management

▪ The patient is kept non–weight bearing in a cast for 2 weeks.
▪ Then motion is advanced and partial weight bearing is allowed in a CAM walker boot as the osteotomy heals.
▪ Return to low-impact activities is started at 4 to 6 months, repetitive impact activities at 6 to 8 months, and high-level sports at 12 months.

Results

Several surgeons have published their series of results of ACI in the ankle with overall good results in the majority of patients. The short-term results seem to be similar to those reported for drilling, microfracture, and osteochondral autograft transplantation. We recently reported our long-term results using first generation ACI for failed OLT. At an average of 70 months, the results were 9 "excellent," 14 "good," 5 "fair," and 1 "poor." Newer generations of ACI-type transplants may yield better outcomes, but more research is needed.

OSTEOCHONDRAL TRANSPLANTATION

Osteochondral transplantation has demonstrated encouraging results. In this technique, autologous ostechondral grafts are taken from the ipsilateral knee joint (femoral condyle) and inserted into the OLT by an arthrotomy. Scranton et al. reported on 50 patients, with large cystic lesions of the talus treated with arthroscopically harvested, cored osteochondral graft taken from the ipsilateral knee (usually intercondylar notch). They found 45 patients (90%) had a good-to-excellent score, at a mean follow-up of 36 months. This procedure is technically demanding but can yield good results if performed well.

In 2010, Zengerink et al. published a meta-analysis that shared the best treatment options for OLT. They found that osteochondral autograft transplantation system (OATS), bone marrow stimulation (BMS), and ACI scored success

TABLE 13.1.5 GUIDELINES FOR TREATING OSTEOCHONDRAL TALAR LESIONS

Lesion	Treatment
Type 1: asymptomatic lesion	Conservative
Type 2: symptomatic lesion <10 mm	Debridement and drilling/microfracture
Type 3: symptomatic lesion 11 to 14 mm	Consider debridement and drilling/microfracture, fixation, an osteochondral graft, or ACI with sandwich procedure
Type 4: symptomatic lesion >15 mm	Consider fixation, graft, or ACI
Type 5: large talar cystic lesion	Consider retrograde drilling ± bone transplant or ACI with a sandwich procedure or osteochondral transplant
Type 6: secondary lesion	Consider osteochondral transplant

From Zengerink M, Szerb I, Hangody L, et al. Current concepts: treatment of osteochondral ankle defects. Foot Ankle Clin 2006;11:331–359.

rates of 87%, 85%, and 76%, respectively. Retrograde drilling and fixation scored 88% and 89%, respectively. Together with the newer techniques such as OATS and ACI, BMS was identified as an effective treatment strategy for OLT. Because of the relatively high cost of ACI and the knee morbidity seen in OATS, they concluded that BMS is the treatment of choice for primary osteochondral talar lesions. However, owing to great diversity in the articles and variability in treatment results, no definitive conclusions can be drawn. We have found patient symptoms and the size of the lesion useful in determining surgical management (Table 13.1.5).

TIBIOTALAR OSTEOPHYTES

Osteophytes may form as a consequence of degenerative joint disease of the ankle; however, they may be associated with posttraumatic conditions. With the advent of arthroscopic excision of these lesions, patient morbidity and return to function has improved over conventional open approaches.

PATHOGENESIS

Osteophyte formation can occur anterolaterally between the talus and the distal tibia, on the anterior aspect of the medial malleolus, and the posterior aspect of the distal tibia. With anterior spurs, the beak-like prominence of the distal tibia is often associated with a "kissing" lesion of the talar neck. This lesion may be the result of forced dorsiflexion following trauma or capsular avulsion from forced plantarflexion. These spurs are prevalent in dancers and other jumping athletes. Anterior tibiotalar osteophytes are frequently found in soccer players. In 2002, Tol et al. looked at the potential etiology of these osteophytes analyzing foot position during the kicking motion and ball contact areas of soccer players. They found that osteophytes are likely caused by repetitive trauma to the anterior capsule and synovium rather than distraction of the capsule owing to hyperplantarflexion.

Classification

A classification system for anterior spurs was developed by Scranton and McDermott comprising four grades, based on the size of the spur and the extent of the ankle arthritis (Fig. 13.1.31). Scranton and McDermott compared open with arthroscopic resection of anterior impingement spurs and showed that grades 1, 2, and 3 spurs are amenable to arthroscopic resection with half the recovery time compared with an open arthrotomy group. Grade 4 lesions were thought to be inappropriate for arthroscopic

resection; however, with increasing experience, the authors have demonstrated successful resection of grade 4 lesions arthroscopically.

DIAGNOSIS

History and Physical Examination

■ The patient can present with symptoms of pain, decreased ROM, catching, and joint swelling.
■ The patient may describe anterior ankle pain, especially with stair climbing, squatting, or running.
■ On examination, tenderness is elicited anteriorly and exacerbated by passive dorsiflexion.

Radiologic Features

■ Plain radiographs will demonstrate the anterior osteophyte.
■ Normally, the angle between the distal end of the tibia and the talus is greater than 60°.
■ However, with an anterior osteophyte, this angle diminishes to less than 60°.
■ A lateral stress radiograph in dorsiflexion may demonstrate impingement of the osteophytes anteriorly.

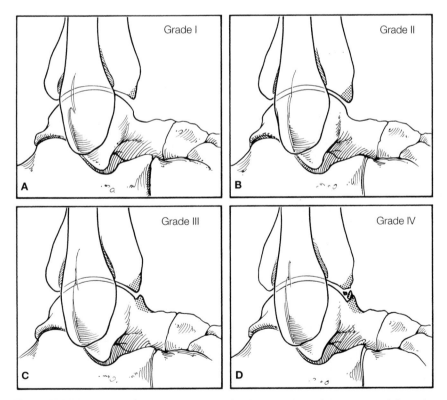

Figure 13.1.31   Grades of ankle spurs as classified by Scranton and McDermott. (**A**) Grade 1: synovial impingement. Radiograph shows inflammatory reaction with spurs as large as 3 mm. (**B**) Grade 2: osteochondral reaction exostosis. Radiograph shows spurs of more than 3 mm. No other talar spur is seen. (**C**) Grade 3: severe exostosis with or without fragmentation. In addition, secondary spur formation is noted on the dorsum of the talus, often with fragmentation of the osteophytes. (**D**) Grade 4: pantalocrural osteoarthritic destruction. Radiograph suggests degenerative osteoarthritic changes medially, laterally, or posteriorly. (From Ferkel RD. Articular surface defects, loose bodies, and osteophytes. In: Arthroscopic surgery: the foot and ankle. Philadelphia: Lippincott-Raven, 1996:179.)

■ Stoller and colleagues have demonstrated that most anterior osteophytes are asymptomatic; therefore, patients with anterior tibiotalar ostephytes need additional diagnostic study.

■ A bone scan, MRI, or CT scan usually shows an abnormal area at the impingement site in symptomatic individuals, and occasionally it will reveal a fracture or nonunion of the osteophyte (Fig. 13.1.32).

TREATMENT

First, conservative treatment should be initiated. This includes rest, nonsteroidal anti-inflammatory drugs, heel lift, or intra-articular injections. If symptoms persist, then operative treatment can be considered. Visualization of the anterior ankle joint and particularly the inferior and superior confines of the osteophyte can be improved with mechanical distraction. However, sometimes distraction puts the anterior capsule under tension over the osteophyte. When this problem occurs, distraction should be decreased to allow the anterior capsule to relax and provide more working room anteriorly. It is critical to identify the anterior and superior borders of the osteophyte, and this often requires careful elevation or peeling of the soft tissues from the osteophyte (Fig. 13.1.33). The neurovascular

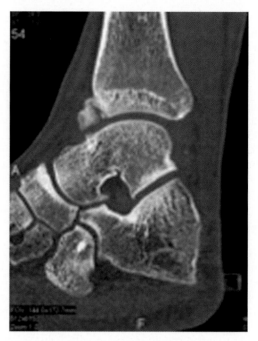

Figure 13.1.32   Sagittal CT scan showing a fractured anterior osteophyte in a professional basketball player.

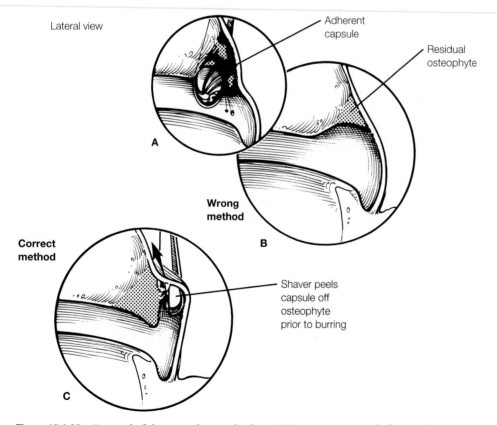

Figure 13.1.33   Removal of the osteophyte with a burr. (**A**) Incorrect removal of osteophyte secondary to the adherent capsule to the distal tibia. (**B**) Residual anterior distal tibial osteophyte is present after burring because the anterior aspect of the spur is not visualized. (**C**) Correct method of removing an osteophyte using a shaver to peel the anterior capsule off the anterior border of the osteophyte. (From Ferkel RD. Articular surface defects, loose bodies, and osteophytes. In: Arthroscopic surgery: the foot and ankle. Philadelphia: Lippincott-Raven, 1996:176.)

structures must not be injured during this process. Once the borders of the osteophyte have been defined, it can be removed with a small burr, pituitary rongeur, or osteotome (Fig. 13.1.34). The surgical instruments should be alternated between the anteromedial and anterolateral portals to obtain a complete resection. Attention should then be directed to the anterior talar neck to ensure that it is smooth. An intraoperative lateral X-ray is recommended before completion of the procedure to confirm that the osteophyte resection is complete and the normal angle between the talar neck and the anterior tibia has been reestablished. Occasionally, visualization through the posterolateral portal is necessary to facilitate removal of large osteophytes and to verify complete removal of anterior osteophyte. As the presence of osteophytes may induce a significant inflammatory synovial reaction, a partial synovectomy may be required in the initial phase of the arthroscopic procedure to gain visualization of the lesion.

Results

In general, patients whose symptoms are caused by impinging osteophytes have significant pain relief after arthroscopic resection and often have increased ankle motion in dorsiflexion. The actual result in a given patient depends on the coexisting ankle pathology. Martin and colleagues suggested that patients with isolated osteophytes were more amenable to arthroscopic resection than patients with generalized joint disease. The former condition may represent a less severe or less advanced stage of the degenerative process. In a report of 58 patients undergoing arthroscopic resection of anterior osteophytes, Branca et al. found good results in the majority of their patients, however, they noted recurrence in four patients with stages III and IV disease. Ogilvie-Harris and associates reported on 18 patients after arthroscopic resection for anterior bony impingement of the ankle. At 39 months, significant improvements were seen in levels of pain, swelling, stiffness, limping, and activity besides an improvement in dorsiflexion.

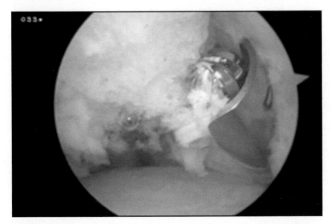

Figure 13.1.34 Intraoperative photograph demonstrating the burr in the anteromedial portal being used to remove the osteophyte. Notice the sheath of the blade is anterior, protecting the capsule and adjacent neurovascular structures.

Postoperative Management

Postoperatively, a splint to eliminate ankle motion reduces pain, allows healing of the arthroscopic portals, and discourages the formation of a synovial sinus. After 5 to 7 days of immobilization, the patient is encouraged to rehabilitate the ankle with active ROM exercises and graduated weight bearing.

DEGENERATIVE ARTHRITIS OF THE ANKLE JOINT

Degenerative arthritis of the ankle can be a debilitating condition greatly affecting the patient's quality of life. Traditionally, end-stage arthritis of the ankle has been treated by an open arthrodesis. However, with improvements in arthroscopic technique and instrumentation of the ankle, it has become possible to apply open arthrodesis techniques using minimal incisions. The advantages of arthroscopic ankle arthrodesis include reduced morbidity and hospitalization, rapid fusion rate, better cosmesis, decreased complications, and optional use of a tourniquet. Disadvantages include a difficult learning curve for the surgeon, the need for expensive arthroscopic equipment, and the inability to correct significant varus, valgus, or rotational problems.

PATHOGENESIS

Although osteoarthritis is the commonest form of arthritis, this entity is not well understood. It may be classified as primary (intrinsic) or secondary (trauma, infection, or congenital pathology). In both forms, progressive deterioration of the hyaline cartilage occurs, with the development of osteophyte formation. Eventually, subchondral cysts form secondary to microfractures and attempted bone repair.

DIAGNOSIS

- The diagnosis of osteoarthritis is generally straightforward, with a patient giving a history of progressive pain, decreased ROM, and a decreased ability to perform daily tasks.
- Radiographs are diagnostic, which demonstrate osteophyte formation, joint space narrowing, and subchondral cyst formation.

TREATMENT

Indications and Contraindications

As always, a conservative approach should be attempted initially. Activity modification, orthotics, canes, and anti-inflammatories should be prescribed to alleviate the stresses placed across the ankle joint. After these methods have been exhausted, surgical treatment may be considered. Indications for arthroscopic ankle arthrodesis include significant and unrelenting pain at the tibiotalar joint that does not respond to conservative measures. Contraindications include varus or valgus malalignment greater than 15°, malrotation of the ankle, significant bone loss, active infection, previous failed fusion, complex regional pain syndrome, a neuropathic destructive process in the tibiotalar joint, and anterior–posterior translation of the tibiotalar joint requiring correction to planar joint surfaces.

Surgical Technique

The principles of arthroscopic arthrodesis are similar to an open procedure, involving debridement of all hyaline cartilage and underlying necrotic bone, appropriate position of fusion (5° of valgus, neutral dorsiflexion) and maintenance of the

joint contour. Fixation of the arthrodesis is accomplished by percutaneously placed cannulated screws through the medial and lateral malleoli or medial malleolus alone.

- The patient is placed in a supine position, and the ankle must be accessible to fluoroscopy.
- Ankle distraction is performed to allow for maximal visualization and access. The entire articular surface of the tibial plafond, talar dome, and the medial and lateral talomalleolar surfaces should be systematically removed with a ring curette, rongeur, osteotome, and motorized shaver and burr.
- All hyaline cartilage and sclerotic bone must be removed to expose the underlying cancellous bone (Fig. 13.1.35).
- Care must be taken to maintain the normal anatomic contour of the talar dome and tibial plafond.
- Mild degrees of existing varus/valgus deformity must be corrected at this time.

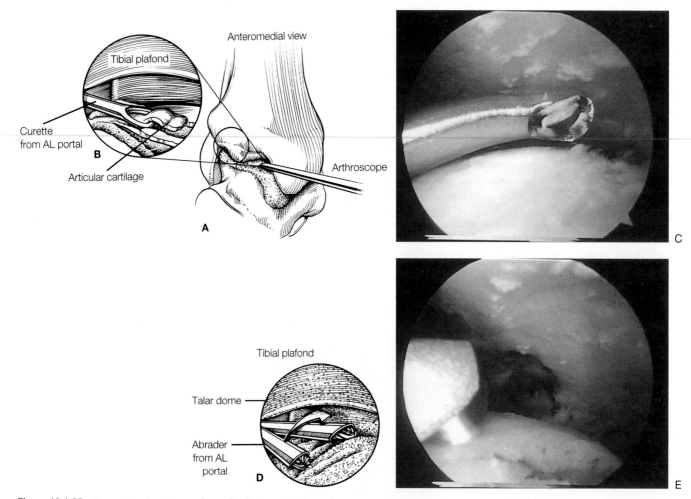

Figure 13.1.35   Preparing the joint surfaces for fusion. (**A**) The arthroscope is inserted anteromedially and instruments are inserted anterolaterally. (**B**) Strong ring curettes are used to remove the diseased articular cartilage. (**C**) Arthroscopic view demonstrating the use of a curved curette on the distal tibia. (**D**) The subchondral plate is denuded to a bleeding surface using a motorized burr. (**E**) Arthroscopic view using a 5.5-mm burr. (From Ferkel RD. Arthroscopic ankle arthrodesis. In: Arthroscopic surgery: the foot and ankle. Philadelphia: Lippincott-Raven, 1996:224.)

■ Avoid resecting too much bone or squaring off the surfaces to prevent varus/valgus deformity.

■ In general, the posterior compartment can be abraded from the anterior portals. If the burr cannot reach the posterior gutter, then a 15° angled curette can be used.

■ The anterolateral and anteromedial portals are used interchangeably to perform most of the debridement. Instruments can also be inserted from the posterolateral portal to abrade the posterior compartment while viewing from the anterior portal.

■ Approximately 1 mm of bone is removed to promote bleeding.

■ After a complete debridement, the burr should be used to make "dimples" or "spot welds" along the talus and tibia to enhance vascularization and promote fusion.

■ Anterior tibiotalar osteophytes should be removed so that they do not block reduction of the talar dome convexity onto the plafond.

■ Once cancellous bone with viable vascularity is established over the entire fusion surface, two or three guide pins from a cannulated 6.5- or 7.3-mm cancellous screw set are placed percutaneously through the medial and lateral malleolus.

■ There are several options for screw placement, including two screws placed through the medial malleolus, and one screw through the medial and lateral malleoli.

■ A third option is to place a screw through the medial malleolus, lateral malleolus, and then through either the posterior aspect of the tibia into the talus, or from the anterior aspect of the tibia into the talus.

■ The authors prefer medial and lateral screws with occasional supplementation with an additional medial malleolar screw or a screw from the anterior distal tibia into the talus to improve fixation.

■ The first pin is drilled from the proximal portion of the medial malleolus just above the joint line, and is angled 30° coronally and 30° sagittally, which allows maximum purchase in the body of the talus.

■ The placement of the guide pin is facilitated by the use of a small joint drill guide. The tip of the guide is placed so that the pin enters at the junction of the tibial plafond and medial malleolus intra-articularly.

■ The lateral pin is inserted through the posterolateral corner of the fibula so it enters the lateral dome of the talus at the intersection between the horizontal and vertical walls, and is also angled 45° to 50° sagittally and 30° coronally.

■ Once the pins are visualized arthroscopically and their position verified, they should be backed out so that their tips are in level with the denuded surfaces of the tibial plafond. Allograft paste can be inserted, particularly if cystic lesions are removed.

■ At this point, distraction and arthroscopic instruments are removed and the fusion surfaces are reduced under image intensification by manual dorsiflexion of the ankle and foot to a neutral position.

■ While holding this position, the medial and then lateral pins are inserted. The ankle is checked fluoroscopically for appropriate position, particularly so that the pins do not enter the subtalar joint.

■ The cannulated screws are then inserted over the guide pins and position again is checked (Figs. 13.1.36 and 13.1.37).

■ A third screw or washers can be used if the bone is soft. Occasionally, it may be difficult to achieve neutral position of the ankle after debridement, and a percutaneous Achilles tendon lengthening should be performed.

Postoperative Management

Postoperatively, the ankle is immobilized in a posterior splint or cast. After 1 week, a short leg non–weight-bearing cast is

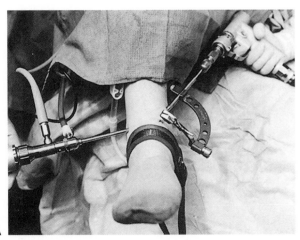
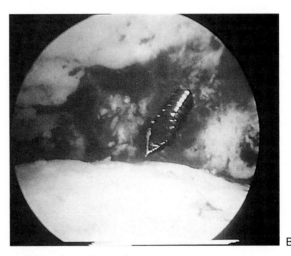

A   B

Figure 13.1.36 Inserting the cannulated screws. (**A**) A small-joint drill guide can be used to assist in the accurate placement of the guide pin in the medial malleolus. (**B**) Visualizing from the anterolateral portal, the guide pin position can be assessed as it enters the medial ankle joint.

(continued)

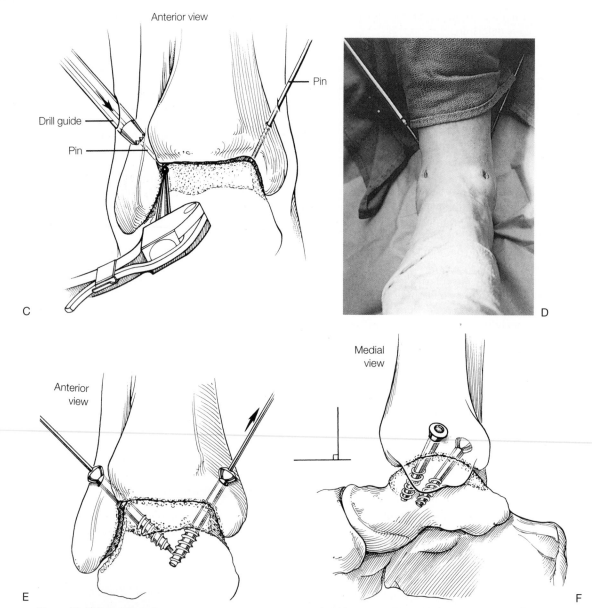

Figure 13.1.36 (continued)   (C) The medial pin is inserted angled 30° coronally and 30° sagittally. The lateral pin is started from the posterior aspect of the fibula and angled 45° to 50° sagittally and 30° coronally. (D) With the ankle stabilized in the neutral position, a 6.5-mm to a 7.3-mm self-drilling, self-tapping screw is inserted. (E) Both screws are inserted so that no threads cross the tibiotalar joint. (F) After the guide pins are removed, the screws are tightened further and the screw tip positions are checked fluoroscopically to verify that the subtalar joint has not been violated. (From Ferkel RD. Arthroscopic ankle arthrodesis. In: Arthroscopic surgery: the foot and ankle. Philadelphia: Lippincott-Raven, 1996:226.)

applied for 2 weeks, followed by a short leg walking cast or removable CAM walker boot for an additional 4 to 6 weeks. The time of immobilization depends on the quality of bone, fixation, and patient compliance. All protection is discontinued when X-rays reveal solid arthrodesis of the ankle.

Results

Several surgeons have reported their results with arthroscopic ankle fusion. Ferkel and Hewitt reported on

35 patients with end-stage ankle arthritis who underwent arthroscopic fusion. The overall fusion rate was 97% with an average fusion time of 11.8 weeks. In this series and others, arthroscopic arthrodesis seems to yield high fusion rates with low complication rates. In a study comparing open versus arthroscopic arthrodesis, fusion and recovery time was found to be much faster in the arthroscopic group. This procedure is especially appealing in elderly patients and those with RA who are unable to tolerate prolonged non–weight bearing postoperatively.

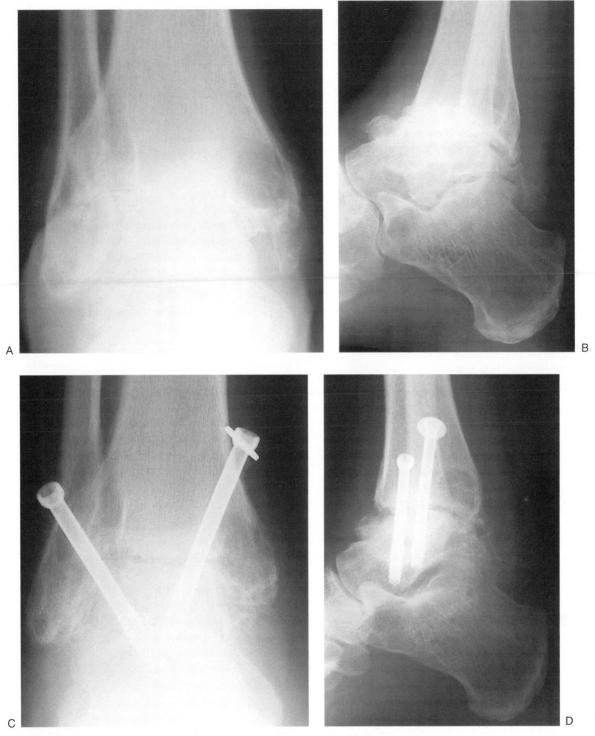

Figure 13.1.37 Tibiotalar arthritis treated with arthroscopic ankle arthrodesis. Preoperatively, AP (**A**) and lateral (**B**) views demonstrate severe ankle arthritis. Postoperatively, AP (**C**) and lateral (**D**) views demonstrate secure fixation with medial and lateral screws.

ANKLE INSTABILITY

Lateral ankle sprains are common injuries. Many of them heal uneventfully; however, recurrent ankle sprains can lead to chronic instability that does not respond to conservative treatment. Historically, open approaches for repair/reconstruction of the ankle ligaments have been successful for patients refractory to conservative treatment (see Chapter 12). Arthroscopic repair is a relatively new approach for the repair of recurrent instability. Often, chronic lateral ankle instability can be associated with intra-articular abnormalities. In one study, 92% of patients had intra-articular pathology, including loose bodies, synovitis, OLT, ossicles, osteophytes, adhesions, and chondromalacia. Failure to recognize these associated lesions can compromise results; therefore, the authors advocate an arthroscopic examination prior to a stabilization procedure. Arthroscopic ligament stabilization has been described by Hawkins for patients with mild instability.

PATHOGENESIS

Strain gauge analysis of normal ankle ligaments and biomechanical testing indicate that the anterior talofibular ligament is the primary restraint to anterior translocation, internal rotation, and inversion of the talus at all angles tested. Cadaver stress tests have shown that the anterior talofibular ligament always fails before the calcaneofibular ligament. Studies by Broström showed that rupture of the calcaneofibular ligament is rare in chronic lateral instability. Thus, the ideal ligament reconstruction would recreate the anterior talofibular ligament in an anatomic fashion without restricting subtalar motion. Procedures that restrict subtalar motion are thought to be less desirable than those that correct the laxity of the anterior talofibular ligament unless there is associated subtalar instability.

DIAGNOSIS

History and Physical Examination

- The major complaint of patients with chronic instability of the ankle is pain and swelling after each episode of injury.
- The second most frequent complaint is giving way or a sense of instability.
- The problem of not being able to predict when the ankle will "give out," adds a sense of insecurity and inability to rely on the ankle.
- Other complaints include weakness, stiffness, tenderness, a sense of looseness, sensitivity to damp or cold weather, and giving way unexpectedly.
- On physical examination, there is a positive anterior drawer test caused by rupture or laxity of the anterior talofibular ligament.
- The examiner may also elicit tenderness over the anterior talofibular ligament and note related swelling and crepitus with motion.

- Another reliable test is the inversion stress test, which elicits pain with plantarflexion and inversion of the ankle.

Radiologic Features

In addition to the three standard views of the ankle, increased "talar tilt" on stress inversion radiographs are seen, ranging from 6° to 17°. It is important to compare this value with the contralateral normal ankle. Some surgeons also perform an anterior drawer stress radiograph but it is more difficult to measure and thus less reliable.

TREATMENT

Patients with chronic lateral ankle instability at arthroscopy demonstrate an attenuated anterior talofibular ligament with scarring of the lateral gutter and syndesmosis (Fig. 13.1.38). Associated pathology, such as osteochondral lesions, loose bodies, and chondromalacia should be evaluated. Arthroscopic lateral ankle stabilization is a technically difficult procedure that requires skill in arthroscopic surgery.

- We prefer, at this time, an open modified Broström procedure as our procedure of choice (see Chapter 12).
- Arthroscopic stabilization has been described with the use of staples and suture anchors.
- In both techniques, the anterior talofibular ligament and associated capsular structures are plicated to a prepared talar bed.
- Using an abrader, the articular surface of the talus approximately 1 cm anterior to the tip of the fibula is denuded down to bleeding bone.
- In the anchor technique, two or three sutures on "O" suture anchors are inserted into the fibula or talus and

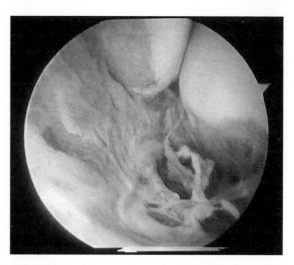

Figure 13.1.38 Arthroscopic view of a right ankle demonstrating the lateral gutter. The fibula is to the left, the talus is to the right, and the anterior talofibular ligament is thinned with scarring at its attachment to the talus. (From Ferkel RD. Arthroscopic approach to lateral ankle instability. In: Arthroscopic surgery: the foot and ankle. Philadelphia: Lippincott-Raven, 1996:205.)

the suture limbs from the adjacent anchors are tied together, thus plicating the ligament.

Postoperative Management

▓ Touch-down weight bearing is allowed at 3 weeks, with full–weight bearing at 4 weeks while in a cast.

▓ At 6 weeks the patient goes into a boot and a graduated rehabilitation program is started, stressing on cycling and swimming.

▓ A lightweight brace with medial and lateral supports is recommended for sports or physical activity after the ankle has been full rehabilitated.

Results

Results with a modified Broström procedure are very good from many authors. In a series of 21 patients, we found that all patients had restored stability, and 96% reported good or excellent results at a mean of 60 months follow-up. Thermal energy has also been utilized to do lateral ankle ligament stabilization. In 2002, Berlet et al. reported on a series 16 patients who underwent thermal capsular shrinkage for pain over the ATFL. Thirteen of the 16 patients had mild laxity. At a mean of 14.5 months, AOFAS scores improved from 60.2 preoperatively to 88.5 postoperatively. Despite this, concerns regarding collagen cross-link destruction related to thermal necrosis of the capsule exist and we currently do not recommend this procedure for mechanical instability.

Arthroscopic treatment of ankle instability still has limited utility today. New, more refined arthroscopic techniques will be developed in the future.

ANKLE FRACTURES

Although the long-term results of ankle fractures treated in either closed or open fashion have significantly improved over the last 50 years, problems still exist with postfracture stiffness, pain, swelling, and discomfort. In the past, the extent of intra-articular injury had not been comprehensively studied because there was no method to look at the entire ankle joint. Recently, excellent results with arthroscopic reduction and stabilization of tibial plateau fractures have stimulated the development of similar techniques in the ankle.

PATHOGENESIS

In 1950, Lauge-Hansen developed a classification system for ankle fractures based on clinical, radiographic, and experimental observations. It is beyond the scope of this chapter to discuss the mechanism of various ankle fractures; however, like all ankle fractures, an important factor is determination of articular involvement. Arthroscopy permits evaluation of injured ligaments and removal of loose debris that may cause eventual articular damage. It is also helpful in facilitating open reduction and internal fixation in certain types of ankle fractures and allows the surgeon to understand and correct the full extent of damage that has occurred.

DIAGNOSIS

History and Physical Examination

▓ The diagnosis of an ankle fractures is usually straightforward, with the patient giving a history of injury to the ankle, with associated pain and inability to bear weight on the affected limb.

▓ As always, a careful neurovascular examination should be performed and the site of tenderness as well.

Radiologic Features

▓ Standard radiographic evaluation will determine the type of fracture, and occasionally, MRI and/or CT scan are useful to determine the extent and degree of involvement of the articular surface.

TREATMENT

Indications and Contraindications

The indications for arthroscopy of the ankle in the acute setting include all intra- and extra-articular ankle fractures with any likelihood of articular damage. In addition, arthroscopically assisted reduction and internal fixation can be accomplished in certain fractures with minimal to mild displacement, easily reducible by manipulation, where minimal-to-mild ankle swelling has occurred and there is no neurovascular injury. Arthroscopy can also be useful to evaluate and treat syndesmosis disruptions, to evaluate posterior malleolar fixation of the tibial plafond, and to assist in the removal of debris and reduction of talus fractures (Fig. 13.1.39). Ankle arthroscopy is contraindicated in an open fracture, with preexisting neurovascular injury, and with moderate-to-severe ankle swelling. Fracture dislocations are not considered a contraindication, and ankle arthroscopy can be used for reduction in selected cases. Arthroscopy should be performed with caution in an acutely fractured ankle, and care must be taken to avoid excessive fluid extravasation, swelling, and potential compartment syndrome.

Surgical Technique

▓ Initially, visualization is difficult because of the amount of fracture debris, hematoma, and cartilage and bony fragments present.

▓ A shaver is inserted to remove the hematoma and debris present.

▓ After the fracture lines are visualized, the fracture fragments are then reduced manually or with reduction forceps. K-wires are then used to skewer the fracture fragments under arthroscopic visualization.

▓ Cannulated screws can then be inserted after anatomic reduction is achieved (Fig. 13.1.40).

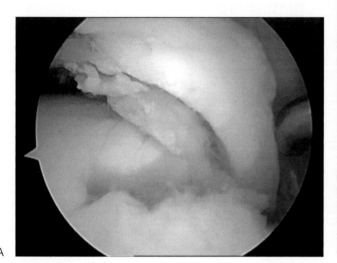

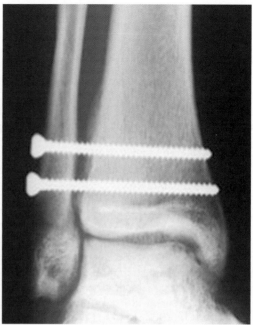

A   B

Figure 13.1.39 Syndesmotic disruption after patient slid into second base. (**A**) Arthroscopic picture, visualizing from the anterolateral portal, an acute OLT of the lateral talar dome. This cartilage injury may not have been visualized without arthroscopy. (**B**) Mortise X-ray of the right ankle after reduction of the syndesmosis with two fully-threaded screws across four cortices.

Postoperative Management

■ Postoperatively, the fracture should be treated in a standard fashion, including a posterior mold/cast with elevation, and non–weight bearing.

■ Gradual weight bearing should be progressed as radiographic demonstration of fracture healing occurs.

Results

In a prospectively randomized study assessing the benefits of ankle arthroscopy in the treatment of ankle fractures, Thordarson et al. found no difference in the clinical outcomes between patients who had plate fixation and ankle arthroscopy versus patients undergoing plate fixation alone. However, eight out of nine patients in the arthroscopy-treated group had articular damage to the talar dome. Furthermore, this was a short-term study. In another recent

study, Ferkel and Loren also found a high incidence (63%) of traumatic articular surface lesions involving both the tibia and the talar articular surface. Most of these lesions were found to be unstable or displaced; therefore, the authors concluded that arthroscopy is a valuable tool in the diagnosis and treatment of concomitant articular injuries associated with ankle fractures. Stufkens et al. reported on 288 ankle fractures with arthroscopic evaluation and/or treatment. They found that patients with an articular lesion at the time of surgery were much more likely to develop subsequent traumatic arthritis (odds ratio (OR) = 3.4) and have a suboptimal clinical outcome (OR = 5.0). Lesions on the anterior and lateral aspects of the talus and on the medial and lateral malleolus correlated with a worse clinical outcome. The added surgical time and morbidity appear minimal; however, a well-powered, randomized, prospective study needs to be carried out to determine whether it is beneficial to use ankle arthroscopy in evaluation and reduction of ankle fractures.

Figure 13.1.40 Medial malleolar fracture. (**A**) Preoperative X-ray shows displaced medial malleolar fracture with malrotation. (**B**) Arthroscopic view of left medial malleolar fracture. There is a fragment missing from the anterior portion of the fracture that had to be removed. (**C**) Intraoperative fluoroscopic view of K-wire insertion used to reduce the fracture. (**D**) After the fracture is reduced, the K-wires are advanced proximally and the fracture reduction is assessed arthroscopically. (**E**) Fracture reduction verified with fluoroscopy. (**F**) Postoperative X-ray at 9 months showing healed medial malleolus. (From Ferkel RD. Arthroscopic treatment of acute ankle fractures and postfracture defects. In: Arthroscopic surgery: the foot and ankle. Philadelphia: Lippincott-Raven, 1996:192.)

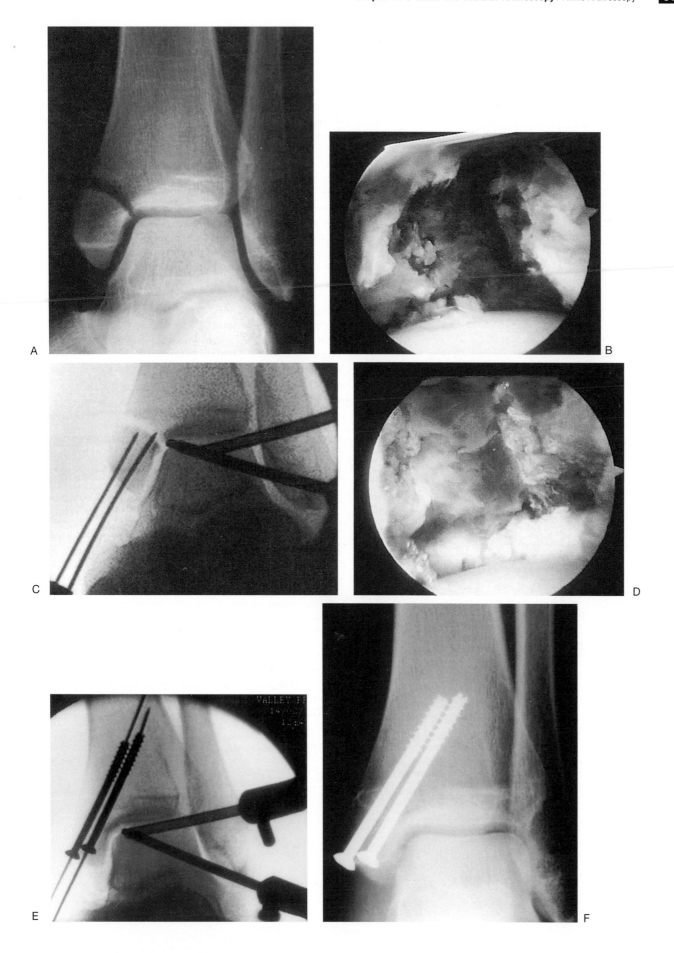

COMPLICATIONS OF ANKLE ARTHROSCOPY

There are many potential complications associated with ankle arthroscopy. Ferkel et al. reported an overall complication rate of 9% in a series of 612 cases. The most common complication was neurologic (49%), primarily involving the superficial branch of the peroneal nerve (15 of 27 or 56%), sural nerve (6 of 27 or 22%), saphenous nerve (5 of 27 or 18%), and the deep peroneal nerve (1 of 27 or 4%). Neurologic damage can be caused by the placement of the distraction pins or operative instruments through the portal sites or by overly aggressive shaving, especially of the anterior capsule. Neurologic and arterial damages have been reported with the use of anterocentral and posteromedial portals.

Other complications included superficial infections, adhesions, fractures, deep infection, instrument failure, ligament injuries, and incisional pain. It is crucial that a surgeon has a "golden retriever" available at all times to help retrieve broken instruments. A golden retriever is a magnetic wand with a suction attached to it (Fig. 13.1.41).

Invasive distraction was used in 317 of 612 cases. Distraction pins were associated with some transient pin tract pain. Two stress fractures of the tibia occurred early in the series because of inappropriate pin placement and too rapid rehabilitation. One stress fracture of the fibula occurred owing to pin placement in the fibula. Statistically, the overall complication rate was not affected by the use of invasive distraction. Superficial wound infections appeared to be related to closeness of portal placement, types of cannulae used, early mobilization, and using tapes (instead of sutures) to close portals. Deep wound infection is associated with a lack of perioperative antibiotic coverage. Increased experience of the arthroscopist is also associated with a lower complication rate. More recently, Young et al. reported on complications using noninvasive distraction. Their complication rate of 6.8% was lower than prior studies that included pin distraction.

Careful preoperative planning, knowledge of surface anatomy, use of appropriate distraction, and instrumentation techniques help avoid complications (Table 13.1.6). In the last 12 years we have used noninvasive distraction exclusively to avoid the problems with pins. The majority of complications reported with ankle arthroscopy are transient and minor, although, serious complications do occur. The surgeon must exhibit exceptional care and attention to detail when performing ankle arthroscopy to minimize potential complications.

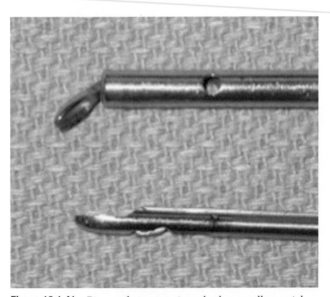

Figure 13.1.41 Picture demonstrating a broken small synovial rongeur. The top image shows a "golden retriever" (a magnetic wand with a suction attached to it) with the broken instrument tip. The bottom image shows the rest of the instrument.

TABLE 13.1.6 AVOIDING COMPLICATIONS IN ANKLE ARTHROSCOPY

- Incise the skin using a scalpel, followed by blunt dissection down to the capsule, which minimizes the risk to neurovascular structures and tendons
- Avoid use of the anterocentral and posteromedial portals because of potential damage to neurovascular structures and tendons
- Use an arthroscopic cannula to minimize soft-tissue trauma around the portals
- Suture the portals to minimize wound problems
- Administer prophylactic antibiotics
- Avoid multiple portals in close proximity
- When necessary, insert invasive distraction pins through one cortex through cannulae with blunt dissection from the skin to the bone surface
- Currently, noninvasive distraction is usually used to avoid pin problems

13.2 SUBTALAR ARTHROSCOPY

Refinements in arthroscopic instrumentation and technique have allowed small joint arthroscopy to become more feasible and popular. Subtalar arthroscopy was first described by Parisien in 1985. There have been only a few isolated reports in the literature on this subject. It is important to note that subtalar arthroscopy generally refers to arthroscopy of the posterior subtalar joint or the posterior talocalcaneal joint. The sinus tarsi, anterior and middle facets are not accessible to arthroscopy without debridement of the tissues to expose them more clearly.

PATIENT SELECTION

Indications

The diagnostic indications for posterior subtalar arthroscopy include persistent subtalar pain, swelling, stiffness, locking, or catching that has been recalcitrant to conservative management. The therapeutic indications for subtalar arthroscopy include the treatment of degenerative joint disease, synovitis, loose bodies, chondromalacia, posttraumatic arthrofibrosis, sinus tarsi syndrome, painful os trigonum, OLT, and fractures. Severe degenerative arthritis may require subtalar arthrodesis and recently Tasto has described his technique of arthroscopic subtalar arthrodesis with excellent fusion rates. Other indications for subtalar arthroscopy will no doubt arise as expertise in this area increases.

Contraindications

Absolute contraindications to subtalar arthroscopy include localized infection and advanced degenerative joint disease with deformity. Relative contraindications include severe edema, poor vascularity, and severe arthrofibrosis that preclude visualization of anatomy.

Patient Evaluation

- Subtalar evaluation begins with a detailed history followed by careful physical examination.
- Weight-bearing radiographs must be performed and should include oblique views to see both the ankle and the subtalar joints.
- Occasionally, special views such as Broden views and stress X-rays are necessary to assess the problem.
- Prior to surgery, all patients are treated conservatively with nonsteroidal anti-inflammatories, ice, bracing, casting, and physical therapy.
- Physical therapy should emphasize on modalities to control inflammation (such as phonophoresis and iontophoresis), stretching, and strengthening of the foot and ankle, and proprioceptive training.
- Shoe modification as well as orthotic inserts should be considered.
- A trial of immobilization using a removable short leg orthosis or cast may be of some benefit in selected cases of chronic subtalar pain and swelling.
- Occasionally, a lidocaine injection, with or without cortisone, may be of both diagnostic and therapeutic benefit in the subtalar joint.
- In patients with persistent symptoms, further diagnostic testing is indicated.
- A CT scan in the coronal, axial and sagittal planes is helpful to detect degenerative joint disease, loose bodies, osteochondral lesions, nonunion of the os trigonum, and other abnormalities.
- A three-phase technetium bone scan can identify and localize occult pathology.
- An MRI scan may be beneficial in evaluating soft-tissue pathology, including the surrounding tendons and ligaments as well as osteochondral lesions and marrow edema.

OPERATING ROOM SETUP

Equipment/Positioning

Subtalar arthroscopy is performed in a similar position and manner to ankle arthroscopy. The operative equipment includes a tourniquet, a thigh holder, and small joint instruments similar to those used in the ankle. Small joint arthroscopes of 2.7- and 1.9-mm as well as small joint shavers, burrs, and other small joint instrumentation are used. Initially, a short 2.7-mm 30° oblique arthroscope is used. A 2.7-mm 70° oblique scope is used to look around corners and to facilitate instrumentation. A small 1.9-mm 30° oblique arthroscope is sometimes required in particularly tight joints. For most cases, a 2.9-mm full radius synovial resector and a 2.9-mm burr are adequate, but a smaller 2.0-mm shaver and burr should be available as needed. Other often-used instruments include probe, baskets, knives, graspers, and curettes. Soft-tissue distraction techniques are similar to those used for the ankle.

SURGICAL TECHNIQUE

Arthroscopic Portals

Primary Portals

- Arthroscopy of the posterior subtalar joint is performed on the lateral side of the hindfoot using three portals (Fig. 13.2.1).
- It is important to outline pertinent bony and soft-tissue anatomy prior to subtalar arthroscopy.

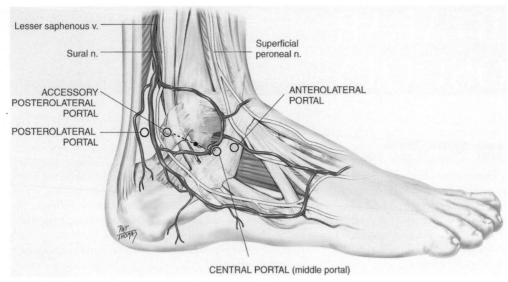

Figure 13.2.1   Location of subtalar arthroscopic portals and related anatomy. (From Ferkel RD, Cheng JC. Ankle and subtalar arthroscopy. In: Kelikian AS, ed. Operative treatment of the foot and ankle. New York: McGraw-Hill, 1998:321–350.)

☐ The *superficial* and *deep peroneal nerve, the dorsalis pedis artery*, the *sural nerve*, and *lesser saphenous vein* should be marked with a pen.

☐ The tip of the fibula and the Achilles tendon serve as the anatomic landmarks for the subtalar portals.

■ The posterolateral portal is made at or slightly above the tip of the fibula, just lateral to the Achilles tendon (Fig. 13.2.2).

☐ The *sural nerve, peroneal tendons*, and *short saphenous nerve* are at risk when this portal is placed.

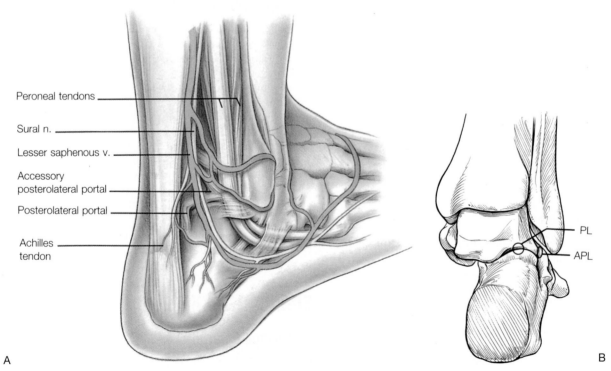

Figure 13.2.2   Posterolateral portals. (**A**) Posterolateral view. The posterolateral portal is established just lateral to the Achilles tendon; the accessory posterolateral portal is made behind the peroneal tendons, with care taken not to injure the neurovascular structures. (**B**) Posterior view showing the relation of the posterolateral portals to the subtalar bony anatomy. (From Ferkel RD. Subtalar arthroscopy. In: Arthroscopic surgery: the foot and ankle. Philadelphia: Lippincott-Raven, 1996:240.)

- The central portal (sometimes called the middle portal) is normally placed slightly anterior and inferior to the tip of the fibula.
- The anterolateral portal is about 2 cm anterior and 1 cm distal to the fibula tip.
  - Adequate separation must be maintained between the central and anterolateral portals to allow for triangulation and prevent instrument crowding.

Accessory Portals

The accessory anterolateral and posterolateral portals are used for additional instrumentation.

- The accessory posterolateral portal is established lateral to the posterolateral portal with extreme care to avoid injury to the *sural nerve, lesser saphenous vein,* and the *peroneal tendons.*
- The accessory anterolateral portal is seldom used unless additional access is needed to the sinus tarsi and anterior facet.

Establishment of Portals

- The joint is first distended by inserting a 19G needle into the posterolateral portal.
  - The correct position of the needle is parallel to the joint surfaces.
  - Once the needle is positioned appropriately, backflow of fluid confirms correct needle placement into the joint.
  - When locating the portal it is important to avoid angulating the portal too proximally or the posterior ankle might be entered inadvertently.
- Next, a 19G needle is placed into the central portal and angled toward the posterolateral subtalar joint.

- Correct placement of the central portal is verified by injecting fluid through the posterior needle and observing good flow out of the central needle.
- Branches of the *superficial peroneal nerve* are particularly at risk with placement of the central portal.
- The central and posterolateral portals are used for subtalar joint assessment and instrumentation.
- Usually, the third portal, anterolateral, is then made so that inflow is through a dedicated cannula.

The accessory portals are utilized as needed to address pathology and facilitate flow. Occasionally, subtalar and ankle arthroscopies are performed in the same patient. In this instance, subtalar arthroscopy should be performed first because after ankle arthroscopy, fluid extravasation can make it difficult to properly locate the subtalar joint. It is important to remember that the posterior subtalar joint is very close to the posterior ankle joint. The authors use the same skin incision for the posterolateral portal but change the level of capsular penetration when doing simultaneous ankle and subtalar arthroscopy.

Arthroscopic Examination

As with diagnostic arthroscopy of other joints, it is important to have a reproducible, systematic method for anatomic review. The authors recommend a 13-point arthroscopic evaluation system starting from anterior to posterior.

- The diagnostic examination begins with the scope in the central portal (Fig. 13.2.3).
  - The interosseous talocalcaneal ligament is initially observed. Both the deep and superficial portions of the interosseous ligament are noted.

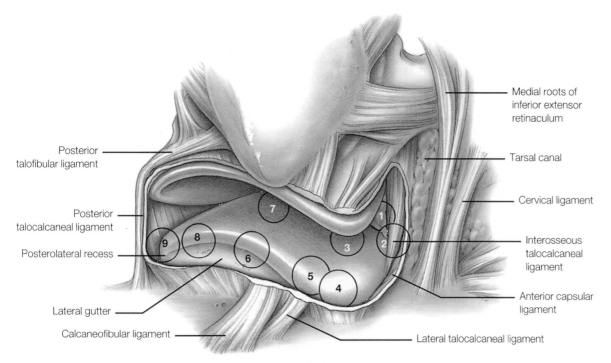

Figure 13.2.3   Lateral view of the six-point examination of the subtalar joint, viewed from the central portal. The posterior subtalar joint is examined starting at the most medial portion of the talocalcaneal joint, progressing laterally and then posteriorly. (From Ferkel RD. Subtalar arthroscopy. In: Arthroscopic surgery: the foot and ankle. Philadelphia: Lippincott-Raven, 1996:247.)

- ☐ As the arthroscope lens is rotated from medial to lateral, the anterior aspect of the saddle-shaped posterior talocalcaneal joint is visualized.
- ☐ Further laterally, the anterolateral corner is examined and the ligamentous reflections of the lateral talocalcaneal ligament and the calcaneofibular ligament are seen.
- ☐ The calcaneofibular ligament is posterior to the lateral talocalcaneal ligament.
- ☐ As the arthroscope lens is rotated medially, the central articulation and the posterior gutter are seen.
- The arthroscope is then switched to the posterolateral portal, and the inflow may be placed in the anterolateral portal or through the arthroscope (Fig. 13.2.4).
  - ☐ The joint is once again examined from anterior to posterior.
  - ☐ Anteriorly, the interosseous ligament may be seen through the bony articulation.
  - ☐ The lateral talocalcaneal ligament and the calcaneofibular ligament reflections are observed from the posterior view.
  - ☐ As the arthroscope is withdrawn posteriorly, the posterolateral recess and posterior gutter are identified.
  - ☐ The arthroscopic lens is then rotated medially to observe the posteromedial recess and the posteromedial corner.
  - ☐ The final structure seen is the posterior aspect of the talocalcaneal articulation.
- The arthroscope is then placed in the anterolateral portal and visualization is repeated.

CHRONIC POSTSPRAIN PAIN AND SINUS TARSI SYNDROME

PATHOGENESIS

Chronic pain in the subtalar joint is often caused by repeated inversion type injuries affecting the ankle and/or subtalar ligamentous structures. Scarring and fibrosis may cause an impingement-like syndrome. Sinus tarsi syndrome was first described by O'Connor in 1958. Approximately 70% of cases involve trauma, usually a significant inversion sprain of the ankle. The exact etiology is not clearly defined, but scarring and degenerative changes to the soft-tissue structures of the sinus tarsi are thought to be the most common causes of pain in this region. The presence of nerve endings in the ligamentous tissue within the sinus and tarsal canals suggest the possibility that injury to these nerves and loss of their proprioceptive function could be a factor in this condition.

DIAGNOSIS

- The exact location of chronic postsprain pain can be difficult to determine because of the close proximity of the

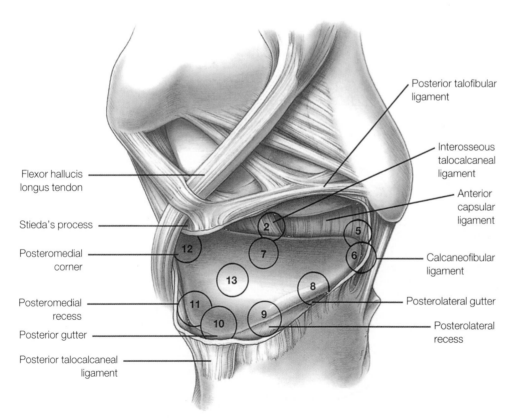

Figure 13.2.4 Seven-point examination of the subtalar joint, viewed from the posterolateral portal. The posterior examination starts by visualization along the lateral gutter, going posterolaterally, then posteriorly and medially, and ending centrally. (From Ferkel RD. Subtalar arthroscopy. In: Arthroscopic surgery: the foot and ankle. Philadelphia: Lippincott-Raven, 1996:248.)

sinus tarsi, subtalar joint, and the inferior aspect of the lateral gutter of the ankle.

- Selective injections may assist in determining the location of the pain and the appropriate treatment.
- Patients with sinus tarsi syndrome will have pain on the lateral side of their foot, in the area of the lateral opening of the sinus tarsi, that is most severe with deep palpation, standing, and walking on uneven ground, and during rotation of the subtalar joint.
- The patient may also have a feeling of instability or giving way of the ankle, particularly on uneven surfaces.
- Routine X-rays and stress examination reveal no evidence of instability of the ankle or subtalar region.
- Selective injections in the subtalar and ankle joints can be helpful for diagnostic and therapeutic purposes.
- If conservative treatment fails, surgery may be necessary.

TREATMENT

In some cases when pain in the ankle and subtalar joint is difficult to differentiate, patients with such complaints usually undergo arthroscopy of both areas concurrently. In patients with chronic sprain pain, the subtalar joint can have fibrosis, synovitis, and scarring, with pathology localized to the lateral gutter of the ankle and subtalar joints.

- If subtalar fibrosis and scarring is found, it is debrided as needed.
- In patients with sinus tarsi syndrome, part of the interosseous ligament, cervical ligament, and fibrofatty tissue is removed in the lateral 1 to 1.5 cm of the sinus to avoid injury to the blood supply of the talus.
- Postoperatively, the wounds are closed with 4-0 nylon stitches and a compression dressing and posterior splint are applied.
- The splint and stitches are removed at 5 to 7 days and ROM exercises are begun.
- A compressive below-the-knee stocking is also used postoperatively while swelling resolves.

OS TRIGONUM

PATHOGENESIS

An os trigonum is an accessory bone located just posterior to the talus, which is present in approximately 2% to 14% of the population. This accessory bone may be a source of posterior heel pain. Although an os trigonum may remain as a separate ossicle, at times it may fuse with the lateral tubercle of the posterior talus, called the Stieda process. From repetitive dorsiflexion/plantarflexion, the os trigonum may eventually fracture from the lateral tubercle. Moreover, the os trigonum may fail to re-unite, causing a painful condition.

DIAGNOSIS

- A painful os trigonum can be diagnosed by pain over the region of the os trigonum, which may be exacerbated in

maximum plantarflexion of the ankle with positive X-ray and bone scan changes.

- A marked increase in activity of the os trigonum, as demonstrated on bone scan, represents a nonunion in this area (Fig. 13.2.5A).
- MRI of the posterior talus may show bone marrow edema, fluid, and soft-tissue swelling in patients with injury of the os trigonum (Fig. 13.2.5B).
- In addition, a CT scan can occasionally be helpful in demonstrating the fibrous nonunion (Fig. 13.2.5C).

TREATMENT

- The 2.7-mm, 30° and 70° arthroscopes are used from the central portal to look around the corner to visualize the os trigonum, and instrumentation can be inserted posterolaterally.
- The os trigonum is evaluated with a probe and also dynamically, by moving the ankle and subtalar joints.
- A nonunion of the os trigonum reveals significant motion at its fibrous attachment to the talus and irregularity and sometimes chondromalacia and fibrosis at its insertion.
- Extreme caution is needed when excising the os trigonum to avoid injuring the FHL and neurovascular bundle, which are just medial to it.
- A banana knife is inserted, and the fibrous capsular and posterior talofibular ligament attachments to the talus are released (Fig. 13.2.5D).
- A shaver and reverse-angle curette are then used to free the os trigonum by further releasing the surrounding ligaments and capsule allowing it to be "shelled out."
- Instruments should be used only under direct visualization.
- Once the fragment is loose, it is removed with a grasper (Fig. 13.2.5E).
- In the series reported by the senior author, 14% of patients treated with operative subtalar arthroscopy underwent an arthroscopic excision of the os trigonum.
- Postoperatively, the patient is immobilized in a below-the-knee cast or removable cast boot for 3 weeks, followed by a rehabilitation program.

DEGENERATIVE ARTHRITIS OF THE SUBTALAR JOINT

Traditionally, subtalar arthrodesis has been performed by an open technique. Recently, an arthroscopic subtalar arthrodesis technique has been developed similar to the ankle with good results.

PATHOGENESIS

Similar to the ankle joint, subtalar joint arthritis can be caused by primary degenerative joint disease or secondary causes, such as trauma or an inflammatory etiology. In

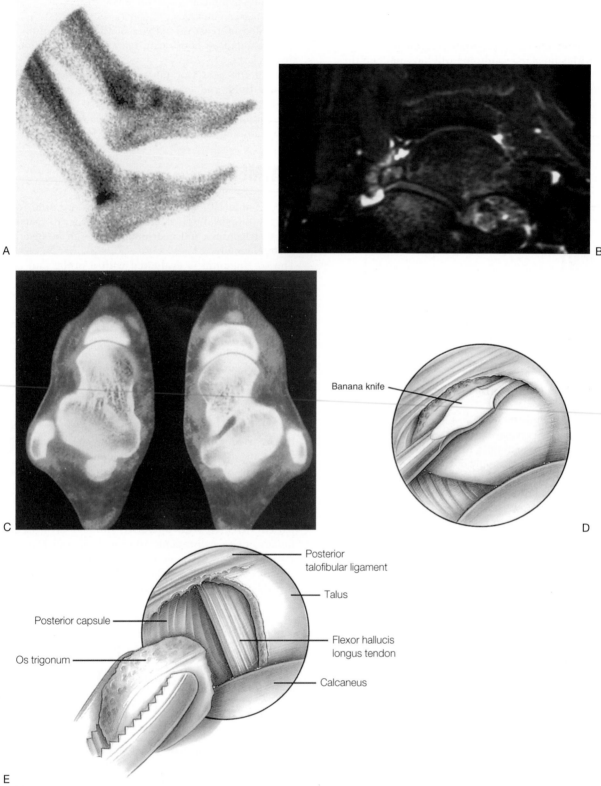

A

B

C

D

E

Banana knife

Posterior
talofibular ligament

Talus

Flexor hallucis
longus tendon

Calcaneus

Posterior capsule

Os trigonum

Figure 13.2.5 Excision of os trigonum. (**A**) Bone scan demonstrates marked increased activity of the os trigonum, representing a nonunion in this area. (**B**) Sagittal T2 MRI showing a bony edema of an os trigonum. (**C**) Axial bilateral hindfoot CT scan showing the os trigonum present on the right ankle but absent on the left. (**D**) A banana knife is used to release the soft-tissue attachments to the os trigonum, with extreme care being taken to avoid injuring the FHL and the neurovascular bundle medially. (**E**) Once the os trigonum is free, it is removed with a grasper. (From Ferkel RD. Subtalar arthroscopy. In: Arthroscopic surgery: the foot and ankle. Philadelphia: Lippincott-Raven, 1996:249–250.)

general, the most common reason for performing subtalar arthrodesis is posttruama.

DIAGNOSIS

- Patients may give a history of a traumatic event. In general, they will complain of daily pain in the hindfoot with weight bearing, usually associated with swelling, often complaining of start-up pain in the morning.
- Ambulating on uneven surfaces will exacerbate their symptoms, secondary to the loss of the normally accommodating subtalar motion.
- Relief of symptoms after a diagnostic injection of local anesthetic can be extremely helpful with the diagnosis.
- Standard radiographs of the foot and ankle as well as Broden views can be helpful in assessing the subtalar joint and additional pathology.
- A CT scan of the subtalar joint will be diagnostic.

TREATMENT

Indications and Contraindications

The indications for subtalar arthrodesis are similar to those for ankle fusion, and patients with persistent unremitting pain that do not respond to conservative methods are candidates for this procedure. Ideally, isolated degenerative changes of the subtalar joint should be present, such as after a calcaneal fracture, with a normal talonavicular and calcaneocuboid joint. Similar to ankle arthrodesis, this procedure is indicated in subtalar joints that do not have significant angular or rotatory deformity, significant bone loss that often precludes this technique after a calcaneus fracture or severe ankylosis.

Technique

- All three portals previously discussed are utilized.
- Portals are alternated to debride the entire articular surfaces of the talocalcaneal joint.
- The soft tissues are debrided and articular surfaces resected using a ring curette and shaver.
- A burr is used to abrade the surface to a good bleeding cancellous surface and to make multiple "dimples" or "spot welds."
- The foot is then put in the appropriate position (5° valgus) and compressed together.
- A small incision is made medial to the tibialis anterior tendon and the anterosuperior aspect of the talar neck is exposed.
- Using an ACL drill guide, a 0.125-in guide wire is then placed superiorly from the talar neck across the subtalar joint, exiting the heel just lateral to the Achilles tendon.
- One or two 6.5- or 7.3-mm cannulated screws are then inserted retrograde from the calcaneus into the talar neck.
- The tip of the screw should be checked so that it does not protrude out of the talar neck and abut against the distal tibia.
- Tasto reported on his results of arthroscopic subtalar fusions and found average time to union is 10 weeks with no nonunions or other complications.

- Postoperatively, the patient is seen at 1 week and the splint and sutures are removed.
- The patient is placed in a short leg cast until radiographic evidence of union is noted.
- Weight bearing is gradually progressed as bony healing occurs.

COMPLICATIONS OF SUBTALAR ARTHROSCOPY

Similar complications can be expected with subtalar arthroscopy as has been reported with ankle arthroscopy. In the senior author's initial series of 50 subtalar arthroscopies, there were no major complications noted and only one minor complication of postoperative ecchymosis, which resolved uneventfully. Neurologic damage during portal placement can occur. The *sural nerve, superficial peroneal nerve,* and *lesser saphenous vein* are particularly vulnerable. The skin should not be incised below the dermis, and the subcutaneous tissues should be bluntly dissected with a small hemostat when placing arthroscopic cannulae. Attention to detail when establishing portals will minimize complications.

Prone Ankle Arthroscopy

Prone ankle arthroscopy has become increasingly used to assess and treat pathology of the posterior ankle joint. Many surgeons find this technique easier, as they do not use a posterolateral portal routinely. With posterior ankle arthroscopy, and particularly the use of the posteromedial portal, one must be familiar with the anatomic structures that are present in this area.

Indications and Contraindications

Prone posterior ankle arthroscopy can be used for the following:

- Painful os trigonum
- Posterior ankle soft-tissue impingement
- Posterior ankle impingement with osteophyte formation
- Loose body removal
- Soft-tissue debridement of the ankle (i.e., PVNS)
- FHL stenosis or tenonsynovitis
- Haglund deformity/retrocalcaneal bursitis and
- Posterior OLT.

Posterior prone ankle arthroscopy with establishment of a posteromedial portal is contraindicated when there is a soft-tissue infection involving the area or the patient does not have a posterior tibial pulse. In dysvascular cases, an MRI can be used to assess the vascular anatomy in this area. Prior surgery involving the posteromedial ankle can distort the anatomy and may endanger important neurovascular structures. Other relative contraindications include severe edema and diabetic vascular disease.

Positioning

- The patient is placed in the prone position on the operating room table (Fig 13.2.6).
- A thigh tourniquet is placed and the knees are padded.

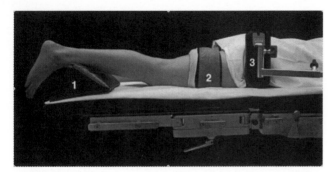

Figure 13.2.6   For prone ankle arthroscopy, the patient is positioned prone with a tourniquet applied to the upper thigh and a small support is placed under the lower leg. A hip rest is placed on the ipsilateral side to allow for tilting of the table when needed. (Reproduced with permission from van Dijk CN, de Leeuw PAJ, Scholten PE. Hindfoot endoscopy for posterior ankle impingement: surgical technique. J Bone Joint Surg Am 2009;91(suppl 2):287–298.)

- A bump is placed anterior to the distal tibia with the ankle allowed to hang over the end of the table.
- This will allow for ankle plantarflexion and dorsiflexion during the case.
- Distraction is not needed.

Portals

- Posteromedial and posterolateral portals are used.
- Both portals are made adjacent to the Achilles tendon (4 to 5 mm) at the level of the tip of the fibula (Fig. 13.2.7).
- The ankle joint is marked out anteriorly on the skin to assist with orientation and penetration of instruments.
- The posterolateral portal is usually made first at the level of, or slightly proximal to, the tip of the lateral malleolus.

- A "nick-and-spread" technique is used, puncturing the skin with a no. 11 blade followed by spreading with a small hemostat.
- The hemostat is aimed toward the first web space (Fig. 13.2.8).
- Before penetrating the fascia, the hemostat is exchanged for the arthroscope sheath with blunt trocar and it is left at this level.
- The posteromedial portal is created at the same level adjacent to the Achilles tendon with the same "nick-and-spread" technique.
- A hemostat is used to spread down to the level of the arthroscope sheath.
- When felt, the scope sheath is withdrawn slightly, and the arthroscope is introduced and the hemostat tip is visualized.
- Space is created by spreading the hemostat, and a 5-mm full radius shaver is used to remove all fat and soft tissue from the posterior ankle joint lateral to the FHL tendon.
  - The crural fascia (Rouviere ligament) overlying the posterior talar process at this level may be thick.
- At this point, the capsular layer can be entered easily with a small hemostat.
- The FHL tendon is the medial boundary for portal placement.
- After the pathology is addressed, the wounds are closed with 4-0 nylon sutures.

Postoperative Management

- Management is dependent on the pathology addressed.
- For most patients except those who had a cartilage procedure, patients are placed in a posterior splint or soft, functional dressing.
- Active ROM is begun on postoperative day 2.
- Touch-down weight bearing is allowed after 2 to 4 days.
- Sutures are removed postoperative 10 to 14 days.

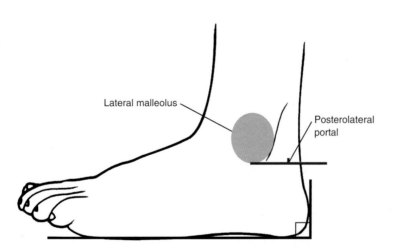
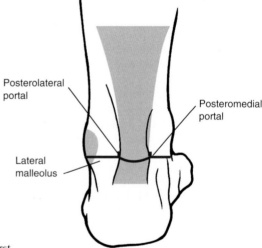

Figure 13.2.7   In prone arthroscopy of the ankle, the posterolateral portal is made first. This portal is made at the level of the tip of the lateral malleolus and 4 to 5 mm off the lateral border of the Achilles tendon. The posteromedial portal is made at the same level and position on the other side of the Achilles tendon. (Adapted from van Dijk CN, de Leeuw PAJ, Scholten PE. Hindfoot endoscopy for posterior ankle impingement: surgical technique. J Bone Joint Surg Am 2009;91(suppl 2):287–298.)

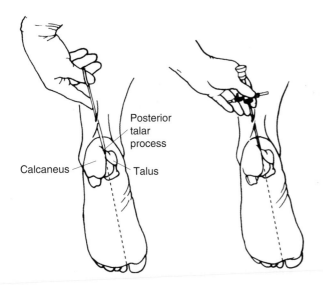

Figure 13.2.8 The posterolateral portal is made with a "nick-and-spread" technique. As the hemostat and the arthroscope are introduced through the skin incision, the instruments are directed toward the first web space. (Adapted from van Dijk CN, de Leeuw PAJ, Scholten PE. Hindfoot endoscopy for posterior ankle impingement: surgical technique. J Bone Joint Surg Am 2009;91(suppl 2):287–298.)

Results

Results reported for posterior ankle arthroscopy have been uniformly positive. In 2008, Scholten et al. reported on their results of prone ankle arthroscopy to treat posterior impingement of the ankle in 56 patients. At a mean of 36 months follow-up, the mean AOFAS score increased from 75 to 90 points. They also noted that results were slightly better in patients with overuse pathology rather than posttraumatic pathology. The complication rate was very low (<3%), with only one patient experiencing a transient deficit of medial heel sensation. This complication rate compares favorably with that of open procedures (10% to 24%).

Prone ankle arthroscopy is an effective method to address pathology present in the posterior ankle. It is critical to understand the anatomy of the posterior ankle, specifically and posteromedial side, but when understood procedures can be performed in a safe and reproducible manner.

SUGGESTED READINGS

Albritton MJ, Ferkel RD. 21 point arthroscopic examination of the ankle. AAOS Video, 2006.

Bazaz R, Ferkel RD. Results of endoscopic plantar fascia release. Foot Ankle Int 2007;28(5):549–556.

Berndt AL, Harty M. Transchondral fractures (osteochondritis dissecans) of the talus. J Bone Joint Surg Am 1959;41:988.

Branca A, Di Palma L, Bucca C, et al. Arthroscopic treatment of anterior ankle impingement. Foot Ankle Int 1997;18(7):418–423.

Corte-Real NM, Moreira RM. Arthroscopic repair of chronic lateral ankle instability. Foot Ankle Int 2009;30(3):213–217.

Egol KA. Parisien JS. Impingement syndrome of the ankle caused by a medial meniscoid lesion. Arthroscopy 1997;13: 522–525.

Ferkel RD. Arthroscopic surgery—the foot and ankle. Philadelphia: Lippincott-Raven, 1996.

Ferkel RD, Chams RN. Chronic lateral instability: arthroscopic findings and long-term results. Foot Ankle Int 2007;28(1):24–31.

Ferkel RD, Heath DD, Guhl JF. Neurologic complications of ankle arthroscopy. Arthroscopy 1996;12:200–208.

Ferkel RD, Hewitt M. Long-term results of arthroscopic ankle arthrodesis. Foot Ankle Int 2005;26(4):275–280.

Ferkel RD, Karzel RP, Del Pizzo W, Friedman MJ, Fischer SP. Arthroscopic treatment of anterolateral impingement of the ankle. *Am J Sports Med* 1991;19: 440–446.

Ferkel RD, Scranton PE Jr. Arthroscopy of the ankle and foot. J Bone Joint Surg Am 1993;75(8):1233–1242.

Ferkel RD, Scranton PE Jr, Stone JW, et al. Surgical treatment of osteochondral lesions of the talus. Instr Course Lect 2010;59:387–404.

Ferkel RD, Tyorkin M, Applegate GR, et al. MRI evaluation of anterolateral soft tissue impingement of the ankle. Foot Ankle Int 2010;31(8):655–661.

Ferkel RD, Zanotti RM, Komenda GA, et al. Arthroscopic treatment of chronic osteochondral lesions of the talus: long-term results. Am J Sports Med 2008;36:1750–1762.

Gregush RV, Ferkel RD. Treatment of the unstable ankle with an osteochondral lesion: results and long-term follow-up. Am J Sports Med 2010;38:782–790.

Hermanson E, Ferkel RD. Bilateral osteochondral lesions of the talus. Foot Ankle Int 2009;30:723–727.

Lauge-Hansen N. Fractures of the ankle. II. Combined experimental-surgical and experimental-roentgenologic investigations. Arch Surg 1950;60:957.

Liu SH, Mirzayan R. Posteromedial ankle impingement. Arthroscopy 1993;9: 709–711.

Loren GJ, Ferkel RD. Arthroscopic assessment of occult intra-articular injury in acute ankle fractures. Arthroscopy 2002;18:412–421.

Nam EK, Ferkel RD, Applegate GR. Autologous chondrocyte implantation of the ankle: A 2- to 5-year follow-up. Am J Sports Med 2009;37(2):274–284.

Nery C, Raduan F, Del Buono A, et al. Arthroscopic-assisted Broström-Gould for chronic ankle instability: a long-term follow-up. Am J Sports Med 2011;39(11):2381–2388.

Schimmer RC, Dick W, Hintermann B. The role of ankle arthroscopy in the treatment strategies of osteochondritis dissecans lesions of the talus. Foot Ankle Int 2001;22(11):895–900.

Scholten PE, Sierevelt IN, van Dijk CN. Hindfoot endoscopy for posterior ankle impingement. J Bone Joint Surg Am 2008;90:2665–2672.

Scranton PE, Frey CC, Feder KS. Outcome of osteochondral autograft transplantation for type-V cystic osteochondral lesions of the talus. J Bone Joint Surg Br 2006;88:614–619.

Sitler DF, Amendola A, Bailey CS, et al. Posterior ankle arthroscopy: an anatomic study. J Bone Joint Surg Am 2002;84:763–769.

Tasto JP. Arthroscopic subtalar arthrodesis. Tech Foot Ankle Surg 2003;2:122–128.

Tol JL, Struijs PA, Bossuyt PM, Verhagen RA, et al. Treatment strategies in osteochondral defects of the talar dome: a systematic review. Foot Ankle Int 2000;21:119–26.

Van Buecken KP, Barrack MD, Alexander AH, Ertl J. Arthroscopic treatment of transchondral talar dome fractures. Am J Sports Med 1989;17:350.

Van Dijk CN, de Leeuw PAJ, Scholten PE. Hindfoot endoscopy for posterior ankle impingement: surgical technique. J Bone Joint Surg Am 2009;91(suppl 2):287–298.

Van Dijk CN, Reilingh ML, Zengerink M, et al. The natural history of osteochondral lesions of the ankle. Instr Course Lect 2010;59:375–386.

Waller JM. Hindfoot and midfoot problems of the runner. Symposium on the foot and leg in running sports. St. Louis: Mosby, 1982.

Williams MM, Ferkel RD. Subtalar arthroscopy: indications, techniques, and results. Arthroscopy 1998;14:373–381.

Wolin I, Glassman F, Sideman S, Levinthal DH. Internal derangement of the talofibular component of the ankle. Surg Gynecol Obstet 1950;91:193–200.

Young BH, Flanigan RM, Digiovanni BF. Complications of ankle arthroscopy utilizing a contemporary noninvasive distraction technique. J Bone Joint Surg Am 2011;93(10):963–968.

Zengerink M, Szerb I, Hangody L, et al. Current concepts: treatment of osteochondral ankle defects. Foot Ankle Clin 2006;11:331–359.

Zinman C, Reis ND. High resolution CT scan in osteochondritis dissecans of the talus. Acta Orthop Scand 1982;53:697–700.

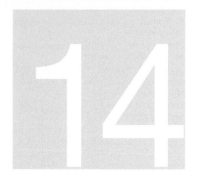

FOOT AND ANKLE TRAUMA

DAVID B. THORDARSON

Although foot and ankle injuries are not life threatening, the long-term disability resulting from them is well established. Two studies have compared multiply injured patients with and without foot injuries and found that those who survive their injuries are far more impaired functionally if they had a foot injury in addition to multisystem trauma. This chapter provides a summary of foot and ankle trauma, including the mechanism of injury, clinical presentation, appropriate radiographic evaluation, and classification and treatment for fractures and dislocations of the foot and ankle region.

ANKLE FRACTURES

PATHOGENESIS

Although technically ankle fractures include any injury to the ankle joint, fractures involving the weight-bearing dome (plafond–pilon fracture) are discussed in a separate section because they have a far worse prognosis and are more difficult to treat. The usual mechanism of injury for most ankle fractures is a rotational injury to the ankle. The position of the ankle at the time of injury and subsequent direction of force generally dictates the fracture pattern. These mechanisms are highlighted in the classification systems (e.g., Lauge–Hansen), which are discussed subsequently. Special cases include severe external rotation injuries to the ankle when in neutral position, which can lead to syndesmotic injuries, associated on occasion with high fibular fractures (Maisonneuve).

DIAGNOSIS

Physical Examination and History

Clinical Features

Patients should present with a mechanism of injury consistent with an ankle fracture. Occasionally, a diabetic patient presents with a history of little or no trauma, which should raise the suspicion of Charcot neuroarthropathy. Other pertinent

historical factors besides the mechanism include medical comorbidities such as diabetes and peripheral vascular disease, which could complicate wound healing, and use of tobacco, which can interfere with wound and fracture healing.

- Physical examination is pertinent for the presence of deformity and the amount of soft-tissue swelling.
- Occasionally, injuries are open; these should clearly be noted and treated on priority.
- Neurovascular status should likewise be noted, especially in the presence of dislocation that increases the likelihood of neurovascular compromise.

Radiologic Features

- A standard radiographic series of the ankle, including an anteroposterior (AP), lateral, and mortise radiograph, is generally sufficient to classify these injuries and plan treatment.
- Occasionally, if a patient has more proximal leg tenderness or medial clear space widening with no obvious fibular fracture, full-length radiographs of the tibia and fibula should be obtained to rule out the presence of a high fibular fracture as in the case of a Maisonneuve injury.

Classification

Two common classification systems are used for rotational ankle fractures. The Dennis–Weber classification system is shown in Table 14.1 (Figs. 14.1 to 14.3). In the Lauge–Hansen system (Table 14.2 and Fig. 14.4), the classification describes the position of the foot at the time of injury and the deforming force with the resultant injury pattern.

TREATMENT

- Initial treatment for all displaced ankle fractures is closed reduction and placement of a splint or cast.
- If anatomic reduction of the joint is achieved the fracture can be treated closed, generally with 6 weeks in a short nonwalking cast followed by a variable period of protected weight bearing in a cast or removable boot.

TABLE 14.1 THE DENNIS–WEBER CLASSIFICATION SYSTEM FOR ROTATIONAL ANKLE FRACTURES

Type	Description
A	Fracture below the syndesmosis. Probable avulsion injuries associated frequently with oblique or vertical medial malleolar fractures (correlates with supination adduction injury; Fig. 14.1)
B	Fracture begins at joint level and extends proximally in an oblique fashion. May be accompanied by transverse, medial malleolus fracture or with deltoid ligament rupture (correlates with supination external rotational injury; Fig. 14.2)
C	Fractures above the joint line, generally with syndesmotic injury. Can be associated with transverse avulsion medial malleolus fracture or deltoid ligament rupture (similar to pronation eversion fracture; Fig. 14.3)

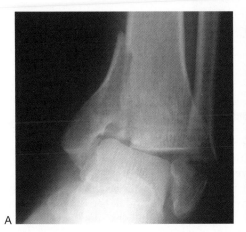
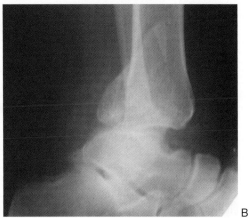

A   B

Figure 14.1   AP (**A**) and lateral (**B**) X-rays demonstrating Weber A fracture of the ankle. Note transverse fracture of fibula below the level of plafond and vertical fracture of the medial malleolus.

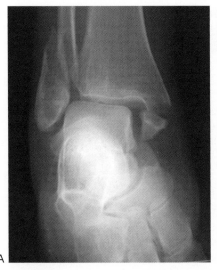
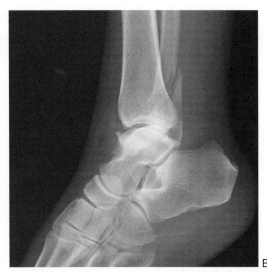

A   B

Figure 14.2   AP (**A**) and lateral (**B**) X-rays demonstrating Weber B fracture of the ankle. Note the bimalleolar pattern with transverse fracture of the medial malleolus and oblique fracture of fibula beginning at the mortise.

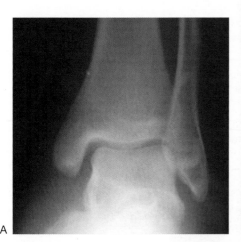
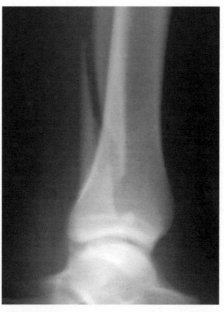

Figure 14.3 AP (**A**) and lateral (**B**) X-rays demonstrating Weber C ankle fracture. Note fibular fracture above the level of the plafond with intact medial malleolus in this case.

- Regular follow-up is necessary to rule out redisplacement of the fracture fragments during fracture healing
- A special case exists with SER type II injuries in which there is no medial ankle injury. These are stable injuries and can be treated with weight bearing as tolerated throughout the course of treatment usually in a cast or boot, but some have advocated using just a stirrup brace for protection.
- Persistent displacement after closed reduction of greater than 1 to 2 mm of the talus should be treated with operative reduction if there is no medical contraindication. Previous studies have demonstrated a significant increase in intra-articular contact stresses with minimal residual displacement of the talus. One study demonstrated that displacement of the fibula in a PER fracture model increases contact stresses most with shortening of the fibula, followed by lateral translation, and external rotation.

In general, bimalleolar fractures are not amenable to closed reduction and casting because there is no stable direction to reduce the ankle (Fig. 14.5). PER fractures have a higher rate of persistent displacement because the ligaments are disrupted to the level of the fibular fracture. In general, the higher the level of the fibula fracture, the greater the amount of instability.

In addition to anatomic reduction of the fracture site, syndesmotic stability must be assessed following operative reduction. Most surgeons advocate intraoperative stability assessment after plating fibular fractures above the level of the ankle where syndesmotic and interosseous membrane

TABLE 14.2 LAUGE–HANSEN CLASSIFICATION SYSTEM FOR ROTATIONAL ANKLE FRACTURES

Type	Description
Supination–external rotation (SER)	Correlates to Weber B Important distinction is SER fracture type II, in which there is no medial injury because these are mechanically stable injuries, do not require surgery, and can begin immediate weight bearing to tolerance
Pronation–external rotation (PER)	Correlates to Weber C Injury including fracture proximal to the plafond with associated syndesmotic and interosseous membrane injury to the level of fracture
Supination–adduction	Correlates to Weber A Transverse fracture of the lateral malleolus inferior to the ankle joint with oblique versus vertical fracture of the medial malleolus
Pronation–abduction	Oblique fracture of fibula above ankle mortise with medial malleolar fracture or deltoid ligament tear (Fig. 14.4)

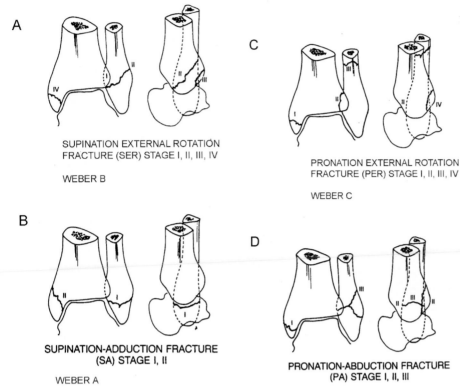

A

SUPINATION EXTERNAL ROTATION
FRACTURE (SER) STAGE I, II, III, IV

WEBER B

B

SUPINATION-ADDUCTION FRACTURE
(SA) STAGE I, II

WEBER A

C

PRONATION EXTERNAL ROTATION
FRACTURE (PER) STAGE I, II, III, IV

WEBER C

D

PRONATION-ABDUCTION FRACTURE
(PA) STAGE I, II, III

Figure 14.4 **A–D**: Lauge–Hansen classification of ankle fractures. Note the subclassifications for each fracture type (from 1 to 4). Supination–adduction pattern correlates with Weber A, SER pattern correlates with Weber B, and PER fracture correlates with Weber C. The position of the foot at the time of injury is either in supination or pronation, and the direction of force causing the fracture is the second part of the name (i.e., external rotation or adduction/abduction). (From Weber ME. Ankle fractures and dislocations. In: Chapman MW, ed. Operative orthopaedics. Philadelphia: JB Lippincott, 1988:471–485.)

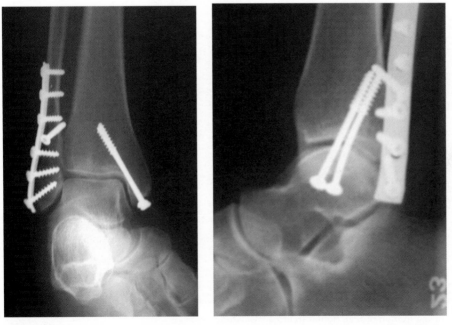

A

B

Figure 14.5 Postoperative AP (**A**) and lateral (**B**) X-rays demonstrating fixation of bimalleolar Weber B SER ankle fracture.

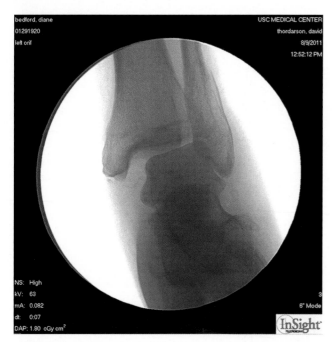

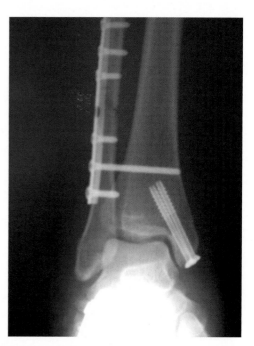

Figure 14.6 Intraoperative external rotation stress view with Weber B–SER IV equivalent fracture. Note marked medial instability indicating ruptured deltoid ligament thus an unstable fracture pattern.

Figure 14.7 AP X-ray of patient who underwent open reduction and internal fixation (ORIF) of Weber C–PER IV ankle fracture with standard medial and lateral plate fixation and stainless steel 3.5-mm cortical screw through three cortices.

injury have occurred (Fig. 14.6). Less stability is present in patients with deltoid ligament rupture rather than a medial malleolus fracture because internal fixation of the medial malleolar fragment does restore some degree of medial stability through the attached deltoid ligament. In cases of deltoid ligament rupture or higher fibular fracture, especially more than 4.5 cm above the joint, a greater degree of syndesmotic instability usually persists after fixation of the fibular fracture.

In those cases, most surgeons place a syndesmotic screw to stabilize the syndesmosis while soft-tissue healing occurs. No consensus exists regarding the method of stabilization with some surgeons using smaller (3.5 mm) versus larger (4.5 mm) screws or three-cortex versus four-cortex fixation following these injuries (Fig. 14.7). In addition, some have begun to use suture button devices as they are flexible and do not

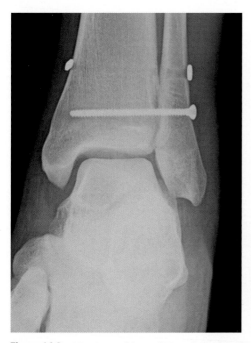

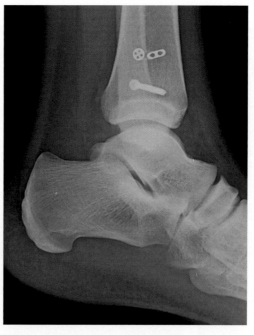

Figure 14.8 Mortise and lateral X-ray following fixation of high fibular fracture (Maissoneuve fracture) with stainless steel 3.5-mm cortical screw and flexible suture button device (Tightrope; Athrex, Maples, Florida).

require removal (Fig. 14.8). Controversy also exists over the necessity and timing for removal of syndesmotic screws; I prefer to leave syndesmotic screws in for 3 to 4 months following operative treatment of a fracture, but patients are allowed to begin weight bearing 6 weeks after operative fixation. Some surgeons routinely leave syndesmotic screws in place.

Results

In general, the results following an anatomic reduction of a displaced ankle fracture are good. Posttraumatic arthritis can develop despite an anatomic reduction, most likely as a result of chondral injury sustained at the time of initial injury. One arthroscopic study found 79% of patients to have some degree of chondral injuries, especially in patients with Weber C–PER fractures. Some degree of stiffness is to be anticipated, with most patients resuming full activities following healing of these fractures. Some studies have noted some functional deficits 1 or even 2 years after an uncomplicated ankle fracture.

PILON FRACTURES

PATHOGENESIS

Tibial pilon fractures involve the weight-bearing surface of the distal tibia or adjacent tibial metaphyses. These fractures are the most serious injuries involving the ankle joint because they disrupt the weight-bearing surface of the joint. The usual mechanism of injury is an axial load, either because of a fall from a height or a motor vehicle accident with the foot hitting the floorboard. Some are because of lower-energy injuries without significant impaction when a significant rotational component splits the articular surface. The complexity of their articular injury and the limited nature of the soft tissue of the distal tibia contribute to a high rate of wound complications following surgical treatment.

DIAGNOSIS

Physical Examination and History

- Most patients who have sustained a tibial pilon fracture present with a history of high-energy trauma to the lower extremity.
- There is a relatively high incidence of associated musculoskeletal and other system trauma owing to the high-energy nature of this injury.
- Occasionally, patients report a severe rotational injury, such as may occur while skiing, that can lead to a split rather than an axial load of the plafond with a better prognosis.
- In addition to delineating the mechanism of injury, the history should evaluate associated medical conditions that may increase the risk of wound-healing problems, such as diabetes or peripheral vascular disease.

- The use of tobacco, which leads to increased wound-healing problems and poorer bone healing, should also be evaluated.

Clinical Features

- Open injuries should be documented and urgently managed with surgical irrigation and debridement.
- Otherwise, the magnitude of soft-tissue swelling and the presence of fracture blisters should be noted. Fracture blisters are of two types:
  - Clear fluid-filled blisters—cleavage injury at the dermal–epidermal junction with areas of retained epithelial cells leading to faster reepithelialization
  - Blood-filled blisters—more significant injury without areas of retained epithelial cells with higher rate of wound complications when surgery is performed through these areas
- In general, blisters should be allowed to reepithelialize before an incision is made through these areas.

Radiologic Features

- Standard AP and lateral radiographs of the ankle are mandatory in all of these patients to assess the degree of damage to the joint surface, fibula, and adjacent metaphyseal–diaphyseal bone.
- Occasionally, oblique radiographs can be helpful to further delineate the fracture anatomy.
- CT scanning is helpful for preoperative and intraoperative planning and treatment and to provide a more accurate prognosis regarding eventual surgical outcome by determining the degree of comminution of the articular surface.

Classification

Two classifications are commonly used to describe tibial pilon fractures—the Rüedi–Allgöwer classification (Table 14.3 and Fig. 14.9) and the AO–OTA classification (Table 14.4 and Fig. 14.10).

TREATMENT

Most tibial pilon fractures are displaced and thus necessitate operative reduction to restore the weight-bearing surface of the tibial plafond. On the rare occasion of a

TABLE 14.3 RÜEDI–ALLGÖWER CLASSIFICATION OF TIBIAL PILON FRACTURES

Type	Description
I	Cleavage fracture, distal tibia, with nondisplaced articular surface
II	Mild-to-moderate displacement of the articular surface with large articular fragments with minimal to no comminution
III	Comminution of articular surface and adjacent metaphysis with significant impaction

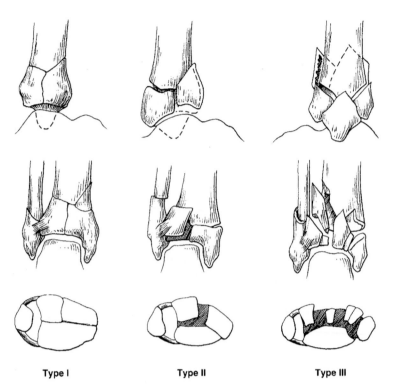

Type I   Type II   Type III

Figure 14.9 Schematic representation of Rüedi–Allgöwer classification system of tibial pilon fractures. (Adapted from Müeller ME, Allgower M, Schneider R, et al., eds. Manual of internal fixation: techniques recommended by the OA–ASIF group, 3rd ed. New York: Springer–Verlag, 1991:279.)

type I Rüedi–Allgöwer fracture with no displacement, it can be treated with a short leg nonwalking cast for approximately 6 weeks before being advanced to weight-bearing protection.

Because of the high rate of wound complications after operative treatment of these complex fractures with an impaired soft-tissue envelope and frequent presence of blisters, definitive surgical reconstruction of the tibial articular surface is usually delayed until soft-tissue swelling has improved. More recent reports have yielded lower wound complication rates by using a transportable external fixator for provisional fixation. This technique involves placing a provisional external fixator along the medial aspect of the ankle to pull the soft tissues out to length, with most surgeons treating the fibula with ORIF at the time of placement of the medial external fixator because the lateral soft tissues are generally not as compromised as the distal pretibial soft-tissue envelope.

Definitive fixation of the plafond is delayed until adequate edema resolution has occurred, which can range from 5 to 21 days in most cases.

TABLE 14.4 AO–OTA CLASSIFICATION OF TIBIAL PILON FRACTURES

Type	Description
A	Extra-articular
B	Partial articular
C	Complete articular

Surgical Treatment

Definitive surgical fixation generally includes open reduction and plate fixation, emphasizing biologic principles of minimal soft-tissue stripping of the soft tissues and bony fragments.

Open Reduction with Plates

This method of treatment has more or less supplanted use of an external fixator associated with problems of pin track infections, less direct control of the bony fragments, and poorer patient acceptance. Recent studies emphasizing biologic principles using indirect reduction techniques that use soft-tissue attachments to facilitate the reduction with distraction across the surgical site intraoperatively, use meticulous soft-tissue technique, emphasizing a tension-free closure, and have lead to acceptable wound complication rates.

- Surgical incisions that allow adequate access to address the various fracture patterns are planned. An anterolateral approach has become the most common one used by many surgeons in the recent times (Fig. 14.11).
- When more than one incision is used, as larger a skin bridge as is feasible is made to minimize the risk of skin necrosis.
- Use of specialized low-profile, locking plates specifically designed for the tibial diaphysis, either anterolaterally or medially, have led to more stability, less soft-tissue tension, lower incidence of symptomatic hardware, and, combined with the aforementioned techniques, a lower wound complication rate (Fig. 14.12).
- The joint surfaces are reconstructed from deep to superficial. As the reduction progresses, the deeper articular structures are no longer visible after the more superficial structures are reduced.

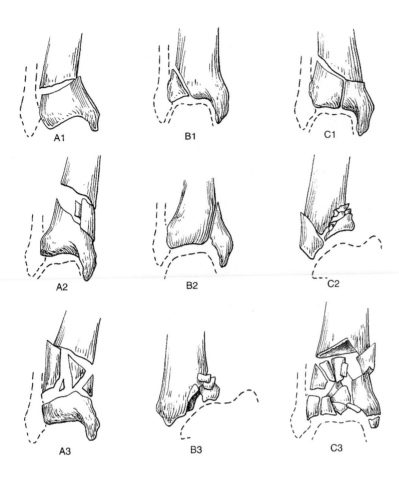

Figure 14.10 Schematic representation of AO–OTA classification of tibial pilon fractures. (Adapted from Orthopaedic Trauma Association Committee for Coding and Classification. Fracture and dislocation compendium. J Orthop Trauma 1996;10(suppl 1):S57.)

- Preoperative CT scans help to localize the incisions directly over a fracture plane to minimize soft-tissue stripping necessary to mobilize the fragment (Fig. 14.13).
- With a significant diaphyseal extension, subcutaneous plating methods wherein a small incision is made distally and a plate is slid along the subcutaneous border of the tibia with percutaneous screws placed into the plate proximally helps to minimize soft-tissue trauma (Fig. 14.14).
- This technique is facilitated by having a high-quality fluoroscopy unit with laser-targeting of the proximal holes to help localize the stab incision sites for proximal screws.

Complications

Wound Complications
- Potentially catastrophic wound complications with subsequent infection and osteomyelitis can develop after treatment of pilon fractures when operating through the compromised soft-tissue envelope.
- The most important concept with regard to wound complications is to avoid them by delaying surgery with a temporary external fixator until the soft-tissue envelope is healthier (blisters are healed and soft-tissue edema is improved), performing a tension-free closure at the time of surgery, and using meticulous soft-tissue technique during the procedure.
- Superficial skin necrosis is treated with local wound care.
- Full-thickness skin loss with exposure of underlying bone and hardware mandates aggressive treatment, most likely with free flap coverage.

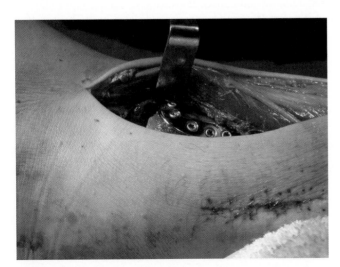

Figure 14.11 Photograph demonstrating anterolateral exposure with anterior locking plate. The superficial peroneal nerve can be seen coursing obliquely across the surgical wound proximally.

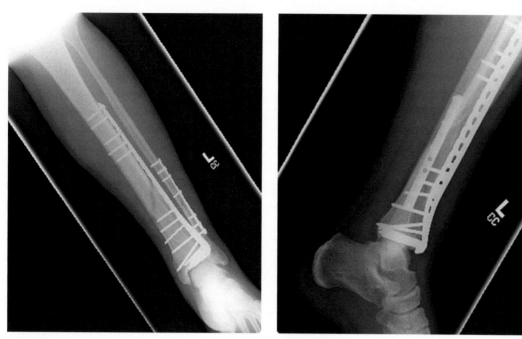

Figure 14.12   AP and lateral radiographs following anterolateral plating of intra-articular type IIC pilon fracture with lateral fibular plating.

Osteomyelitis

■ Osteomyelitis generally develops only in patients with significant wound complications.

■ The best treatment is avoidance by prompt treatment of deep wound dehiscences with exposed bone and hardware.

■ Chronic osteomyelitis must be managed with aggressive debridement and bone grafting, which usually necessitates an ankle fusion in cases that are salvageable.

■ Below-knee amputation is often the best salvage option in patients with chronic osteomyelitis.

Arthrosis and Stiffness

■ Stiffness after tibial pilon fracture is because of a varying amount of posttraumatic fibrosis and arthrosis.

■ Although anatomic reduction and stable fixation allows for early range of motion (ROM) to help minimize stiffness, this is still a relatively common complication. It is a particularly difficult problem to treat, short of fusing the ankle joint.

Nonunion, Delayed Union, and Malunion

■ Nonunion of the metaphyseal–diaphyseal junction is not uncommon in patients with these complex, high-energy injuries.

■ If healing is not evident by 12 weeks, bone grafting of the fracture site should be considered (Fig. 14.15).

■ Malunions are relatively common and are best avoided by creating a stable fracture construct at the time of initial treatment.

Posttraumatic Arthritis

■ Many studies have documented nearly all cases to have some degree of radiographic evidence of varying degrees of posttraumatic arthritis after pilon fractures. Some have shown a correlation between fracture type, incidence of posttraumatic arthritis, and poor results.

■ The quality of the fracture reduction in some studies has correlated with clinical results.

Results and Outcome

In general, results after tibial pilon fractures correlate most closely with the initial displacement, that is, amount of initial trauma. Anatomic reduction without a wound complication postoperatively leads to the greatest likelihood of a good result, but an anatomic reduction does not guarantee a good result. In one prospective randomized study, all patients who had a type II or III Ruedi fracture had some degree of radiographic joint space narrowing at a minimum follow-up of 2 years. In another recent study, at 5 and 12 years after surgery, 27 of 31 patients were unable to run and 14 had changed jobs, but few had secondary reconstructive procedures. On average, these patients improved for 2.4 years after injury.

FRACTURES OF NECK AND BODY OF THE TALUS

PATHOGENESIS

Fractures of the neck and body of the talus account for approximately 50% of significant injuries of the talus.

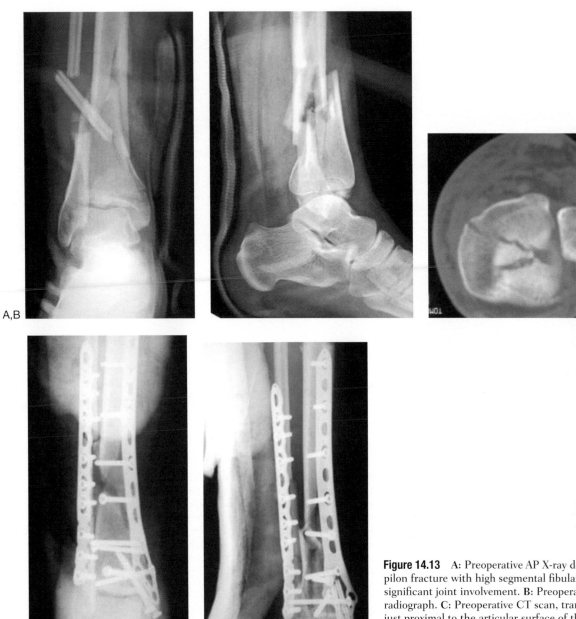

A,B

C

D,E

Figure 14.13 A: Preoperative AP X-ray demonstrating pilon fracture with high segmental fibular fracture with significant joint involvement. **B:** Preoperative lateral radiograph. **C:** Preoperative CT scan, transverse CT cut just proximal to the articular surface of the plafond. **D:** Postoperative AP X-ray demonstrating fixation of tibia and fibula with a low-profile plate. **E:** Postoperative lateral X-ray of the same patient.

Generally, they are associated with high-energy trauma such as motor vehicle accidents or fall from a height. The theoretical mechanism is hyperdorsiflexion of the neck of the talus with impaction of the neck or body against the anterior lip of the tibia, although it is difficult to recreate this fracture in the laboratory with this mechanism.

The vascular anatomy of the talus is pertinent because the limited blood supply to the body can predispose patients to avascular necrosis (AVN) following fracture. With no tendinous attachments and approximately two-thirds of its surface covered with articular cartilage, it has a limited area for blood supply to enter. The arterial blood supply derives from the following:

- Artery of the tarsal canal—a branch of the posterior tibial artery, supplies medial half to two-thirds of the body
- Artery of the sinus tarsi—formed from a branch of the anterior tibial and peroneal arteries, forming an anastomotic sling with the artery of the tarsal canal under the talar neck
- Deltoid arterial branches—branch of the arterial tarsal canal that enters medially with the deep deltoid ligament and may be the only remaining blood supply in displaced fractures of the neck or body of the talus

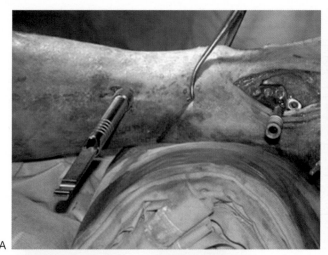

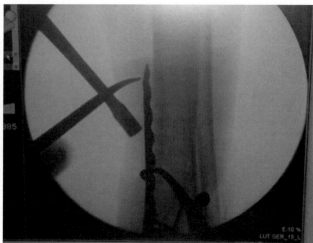

A

B

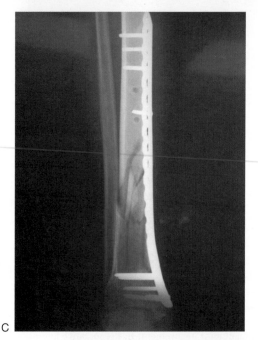

C

Figure 14.14 A: Photograph demonstrating percutaneous incision, approximately 7 cm in length before insertion of this medially based pilon plate. Note percutaneous tenaculum holding plate to bone in center of picture and depth gauge in wound where a percutaneous screw was placed. B: AP fluoroscopic view intraoperatively confirming plate is on bone while localizing screw hole at proximal tip with hemostat. C: AP radiograph of the same patient after placement of percutaneous pilon plate. Note large segment of bone without fixation that was not exposed intraoperatively, which led to rapid fracture consolidation postoperatively owing to lack of periosteal stripping.

DIAGNOSIS

Physical Examination and History

- Patients report a high-energy trauma.
- Many patients have associated musculoskeletal trauma resulting from the high-energy nature of this injury with medial malleolar fractures reported in 20% to 50% of these patients.

Clinical Features

- On examination, fracture displacement and possible dislocation of the talus can be masked by rapid onset of swelling.
- The body of the talus can be palpable subcutaneously in the posteromedial ankle in severe cases.
- Neurovascular structures are usually spared from serious injury.
- There is a relatively high incidence of open injuries in these patients.

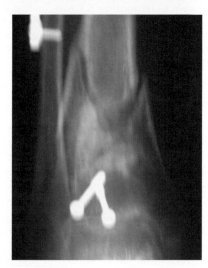

Figure 14.15 Postoperative X-ray 4 months after surgery demonstrating nonunion of metaphyseal–diaphyseal portion of a plafond fracture.

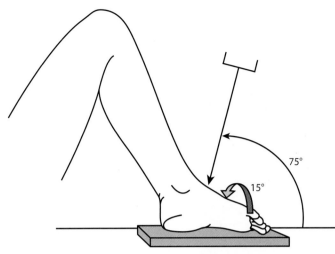

Figure 14.16 Diagram of proper orientation and position of foot for obtaining Canale view that demonstrates varus–valgus alignment of the talar neck. Note the ankle is in maximal plantarflexion, foot pronated is 15°, and X-ray beam is angled cephalad 75° relative to cassette.

Radiologic Features

- The fracture is usually readily apparent from AP and lateral radiographs of the talus.
- Varus or valgus displacement of the talar neck is best seen on a modified Canale view (Fig. 14.16).

Classification

Talar neck fractures are classified with the Hawkins classification (Table 14.5 and Fig. 14.17).

TREATMENT

- In the Hawkins I fracture, the ankle can be placed in neutral position with no evidence of displacement.
  - On these rare occasions, patients can be kept in a cast for approximately 8 weeks followed by an additional

TABLE 14.5 HAWKINS CLASSIFICATION SYSTEM FOR TALAR NECK FRACTURES

Type	Description
Hawkins I	Nondisplaced, stable fracture 0%–10% rate of AVN
Hawkins II	Displaced fracture with subtalar joint incongruity or dislocation 20%–50% rate of AVN
Hawkins III	Incongruity of subtalar and ankle joints, usually dislocation of body of talus posteromedially 80%–100% rate of AVN
Hawkins IV	Rare case with Hawkins III plus talonavicular joint displacement Risk of AVN of head fragment

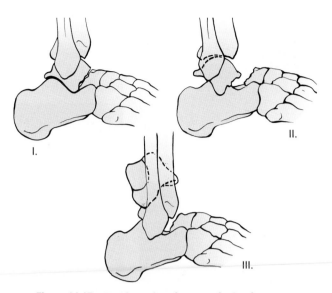

Figure 14.17 Hawkins classification of talus fractures.

month of protection with a controlled active motion walker. An apparent nondisplaced fracture that displaces with the ankle placed in neutral position is actually a Hawkins II fracture.

- A Hawkins II fracture (Fig. 14.18) should be promptly treated with closed reduction.
  - Maximum plantarflexion and traction of the foot will usually realign the head with body fragment.
  - Varus or valgus stress realigns the neck in the transverse plane.
  - A near-anatomic reduction allows a delay in surgical treatment.
- Hawkins III fractures with a dislocated body of the talus should be taken directly to surgery because the likelihood of successful closed reduction is negligible (Fig. 14.19).
  - Operative treatment of these fractures should use a combined anteromedial–anterolateral approach.
  - Anteromedial incision—anterior aspect of the medial malleolus, dorsal aspect of the navicular tuberosity, which exposes the medial neck.

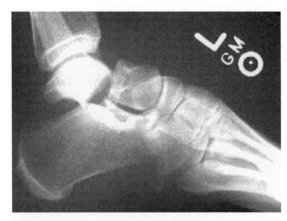

Figure 14.18 Lateral X-ray of displaced Hawkins II fracture before reduction. Note dislocated posterior facet of the subtalar joint with congruent ankle joint.

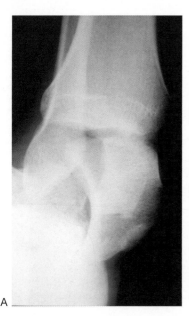

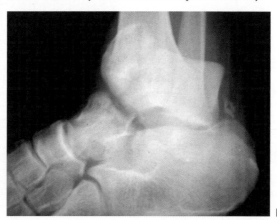

Figure 14.19 A: AP (B) and lateral X-rays of Hawkins III fracture with body of talus dislocated posteromedially.

A ___

B

- [ ] Anterolateral incision—from anterior tip of the fibula to base of the fourth metatarsal, exposing the lateral neck of the talus and allowing access to the subtalar joint.
- [ ] Fixation is generally with 3.5-mm fully threaded cortical screws for neutralization in contrast to lag fixation to prevent displacement into varus if medial comminution is present (Fig. 14.20).
- [ ] Titanium screws allow for postoperative MRI (Fig. 14.21).
- [ ] Although screws inserted from posterior lead to greater biomechanical stability, they necessitate a third incision (which is difficult with the patient in the supine position) as the two anterior incisions are necessary for reduction; in my opinion, this is not necessary.
- [ ] Hawkins III fractures require a longer medial incision and generally require medial malleolar osteotomy to facilitate reduction if the malleolus has not been fractured.
- [ ] A traction pin should be placed in the inferior aspect of the calcaneus to facilitate reduction of the body of the talus into the mortise.

- [ ] With talar body fractures, medial malleolar osteotomies are often necessary to facilitate exposure and reduction of the body of the talus, because the malleoli preclude adequate visualization of the fracture (Fig. 14.22).

Complications

- Skin necrosis and osteomyelitis can occur, especially after Hawkins III fractures if there is a significant delay, with death of the skin overlying the body fragment.
- Nonunion is unusual although malunion is common, especially with medial talar neck comminution. The

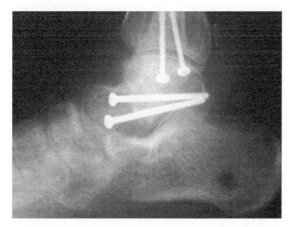

Figure 14.20 Postoperative lateral X-ray following ORIF with talar neck fracture with cortical screws.

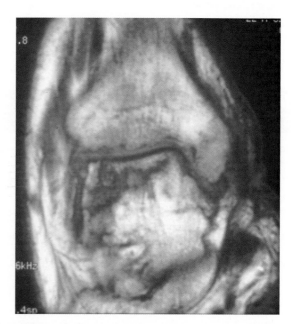

Figure 14.21 Postoperative coronal MRI scan demonstrating subchondral collapse and cystic changes consistent with AVN of the body of the talus. Note titanium screw in medial malleolus minimally scatters image.

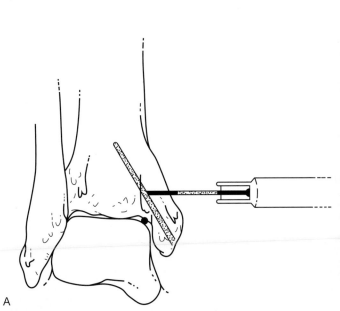

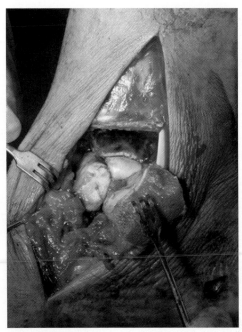

A   B

Figure 14.22 **A:** Schematic diagram demonstrating step cut osteotomy. The saw is cutting transversely into tibia approximately 1 cm above plafond stopping at the level of the axilla. Osteotome is then used to complete the osteotomy from anterior to posterior. Care must be taken to release the anterior joint capsule and the superficial and deep posterior tibial tendon sheath while protecting the deltoid ligament to allow reflection of fragment distally. **B:** Intraoperative photograph demonstrating step cut osteotomy being reflected inferiorly with sharp Senn retractor. Reduced talar dome fracture evident while in proximal aspect of the wound the posterior tibial tendon is visualized.

best treatment is prevention with anatomic reduction and rigid internal fixation.

- Occasionally, in comminuted cases, a small fragment plate along the neck of the talus may be necessary for fixation (Fig. 14.23).

- Varus malunions are difficult to treat and most commonly necessitate a talonavicular fusion or triple arthrodesis with lengthening of the medial column to correct the varus–supination deformity. A few case reports on talar neck osteotomies have been reported but have a risk of talar body AVN.

- Subtalar joint arthritis and arthrofibrosis are the most common complications following talar neck fractures, occurring in more than 60% of patients in some series. Ankle arthrosis and stiffness are less common.

- AVN is the most feared complication of talar neck and body fractures.
  - □ Radiographic evaluation includes looking for a Hawkins sign, which is a subchondral radiolucency evident on the AP view of the ankle 6 to 8 weeks after injury. It indicates active subchondral bony atrophy, reflecting an intact blood supply (Fig. 14.24). Absence of the sign does not confirm AVN.
  - □ MRI scanning performed 6 to 12 weeks following talar neck fractures can document the presence of AVN if titanium implants have been used, which cause little distortion to the MRI scan. One MRI study demonstrated that patients with more than

50% involvement of their body with AVN led to collapse (Fig. 14.21).
  - □ AVN of the talus is difficult to treat because of the uncertain long-term prognosis and the prolonged period of revascularization. Although some studies advocate prolonged non–weight bearing, others have demonstrated no benefit. My personal preference is to allow patients to bear weight after facture healing even in the presence of AVN after counseling the patients of the risk of collapse.

OTHER FRACTURES OF THE TALUS

Fractures of the Lateral Process

- These fractures account for approximately one-fourth of all fractures of the body of the talus and are often overlooked.

- They can be confused with an inversion sprain of the ankle because they frequently have an inversion mechanism.

- Mechanism is either an avulsion fracture following an inversion injury or impaction in an eversion injury.

- It is known to occur frequently in snowboarders and has been termed "snowboarder's ankle."

- Scrutiny of plain radiographs of the ankle generally demonstrates the presence of this fracture on an AP

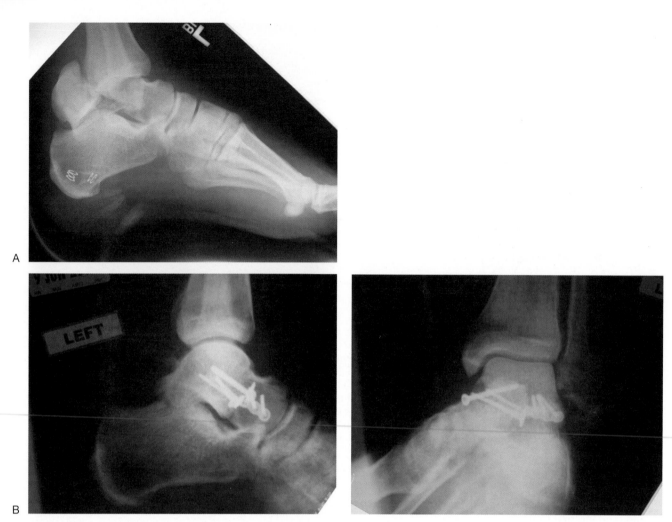

A

B

Figure 14.23 **A:** Lateral radiograph demonstrating Hawkins III fracture of talar neck. Comminution difficult to visualize on this radiograph. **B:** Postoperative AP and lateral ankle radiographs demonstrating medial screw and lateral sinus tarsi mini fragment plate used to fixate this fracture.

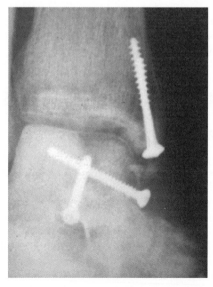

Figure 14.24 AP X-ray demonstrating positive Hawkins sign along the medial aspect of the talar dome, reflecting intact blood supply with sclerotic lateral half of the talar body.

view. CT scans help demonstrate the size and presence of comminution (Fig. 14.25).

- Nondisplaced fractures are treated with immobilization for approximately 3 weeks with displaced fractures usually requiring operative treatment.
- Comminuted fragments are excised. Occasionally, large fragments can be treated with ORIF.

Fractures of the Head

- These are rare injuries and are present in only approximately 5% of fractures of the talus.
- Often, it is a compression fracture caused by impaction against the navicular or longitudinal oblique fracture owing to shearing.
- Most often these result from talonavicular subluxation or dislocation injuries.
- Displaced fractures should be treated with ORIF, which usually necessitates use of headless screws or absorbable pins or screws through the articular cartilage.

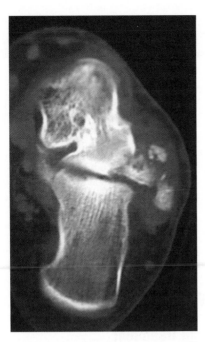

Figure 14.25   CT scan demonstrating comminuted lateral talar process fracture.

Posterior Process Fractures

- Fracture of the posterior process of the talus with impaction can occur from a hyperflexion injury or avulsion-type injury with hyperdorsiflexion. These fractures can be difficult to differentiate radiographically from an os trigonum.
- They are generally small and can be treated with a period of immobilization.
- They are sometimes persistently symptomatic and can necessitate excision. Rarely, they are large and can be treated with ORIF.

CALCANEUS FRACTURES

PATHOGENESIS

Etiology

The calcaneus is the most frequently fractured tarsal bone (approximately 60% of all tarsal fractures). Seventy-five percent are intra-articular. Most of these fractures are high-energy injuries with associated pathology:

- Spine fracture—10%
- Other extremity fractures—25%
- Bilateral—10%
- Open fractures—approximately 5%

Most calcaneus fractures occur from a fall from a height in men aged 35 to 45 years and are frequently work-related. Because of the complex fracture anatomy and compromised

---

- Arthritis or arthrosis of the subtalar ± calcaneocuboid joint
- Peroneal tendon impingement ± calcaneofibular impingement
- Widened heel with subsequent shoe-fitting problems
- Malleoli closer to ground with heel counter irritation by shoe
- Decreased ankle dorsiflexion caused by the relative dorsiflexed position of the talus, leading to an anterior tibiotalar abutment and subsequent arthritic changes
- Elevated Achilles tendon insertion, leading to weakened gastrocnemius–soleus complex
- Limb-length discrepancy
- Shortened calcaneus with decreased lever arm to gastrocnemius–soleus complex, thus weakening it

soft-tissue envelope, ORIF remains a challenging and complicated treatment option. Multiple problems are associated with an unreduced intra-articular calcaneus fracture (Box 14.1).

DIAGNOSIS

Physical Examination and History

- Most patients who present with a calcaneus fracture report a fall from a height or other high-energy injuries such as a motor vehicle accident.
- Patients are unable to walk and frequently have associated injuries as outlined earlier.
- Other important historical factors include associated medical conditions, especially diabetes or peripheral vascular disease because both can lead to increased wound-healing problems.
- Tobacco use is particularly important because smoking leads to an increased rate of wound complications.

Clinical Features

- Physical examination is important to determine the integrity of the soft tissue because some are open fractures.
    - Severe swelling should be documented.
    - One objective test used to assess the amount of soft-tissue swelling is the wrinkle test. The wrinkle test is performed with the ankle in dorsiflexion and eversion. If there is no wrinkling on the anterolateral aspect of the ankle, excessive swelling likely precludes safe open reduction at that time.

Radiologic Features

- The initial radiographic evaluation includes AP, lateral, and axial Harris views of the hindfoot. These give a good initial idea of the amount of fracture displacement with the lateral projection being the most sensitive radiographic measurement of depression of the joint surface.

- Bohler's angle can be measured from the lateral view and usually ranges from 30° to 35°.
- The Harris axial view allows visualization of the amount of varus malalignment of the posterior tuberosity fragment. Broden's views, which are obtained by internally rotating the foot with the ankle in neutral position and angling the X-ray beam from 10° to 40° from vertical, focuses on the posterior facet but is generally used only intraoperatively to assess reduction.
- CT scanning has vastly improved the ability to visualize the fracture anatomy.
  - ☐ The coronal cuts allow visualization of the posterior facet articular surface, and the transverse cuts allow assessment of the amount of shortening and involvement of the calcaneocuboid joint. Sagittal views can show the amount of facet rotation and depression often better than the coronal views (Fig. 14.26).

Classification

Calcaneal fractures can be classified using either radiographs (Table 14.6 and Fig. 14.27) or CT in the Sanders system (Table 14.7 and Fig. 14.28). The latter classification system has prognostic importance because higher grades of fractures have a poorer prognosis and can guide

TABLE 14.6 RADIOGRAPHIC CLASSIFICATION OF CALCANEAL FRACTURES

Type	Description
Joint depression	Secondary fracture line beneath the displaced articular fragment exits along the superior aspect of the posterior tuberosity
Tongue type	Secondary fracture line exits the posterior aspect of the tuberosity, leaving a large piece of the posterior tuberosity attached to the displaced posterior facet fragment (Fig. 14.27)

operative treatment as many surgeons will perform primary subtalar fusion for type IV fractures.

TREATMENT

Nonsurgical Treatment

Although nonreduced fractures cause multiple problems (Box 14.1), many fractures are still treated nonsurgically. Nonoperative treatment includes a compressive Jones dressing initially with non–weight bearing for approximately 6 weeks

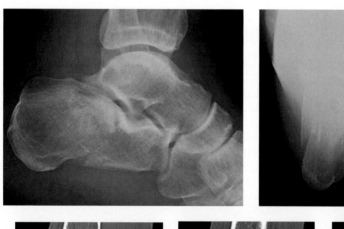
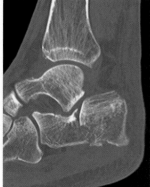
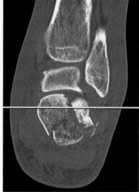
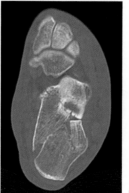

Figure 14.26   Lateral (**A**), axial–Harris X-ray (**B**), sagittal CT (**C**), coronal CT (**D**), and transverse CT (**E**) of a displaced intra-articular calcaneus fracture. Fracture evident on plain lateral X-ray but depression of facet more evident on sagittal CT. Coronal CT shows relatively small but displaced posterior facet fragment.

Lateral

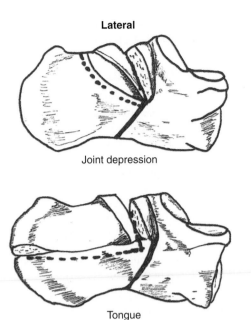

Joint depression

Tongue

Figure 14.27 Schematic diagram of joint depression and tongue-type fractures (see text).

TABLE 14.7 SANDERS' CT CLASSIFICATION OF CALCANEAL FRACTURES

Type	Description
I	Nondisplaced
II	Two major articular fragments in the coronal scan through the sustentaculum tali
III	Three major articular fragments
IV	Highly comminuted with four or more articular fragments

with a gradual progression to weight bearing. An absolute indication for a nonsurgical treatment is a nondisplaced fracture. Relative contraindications include a heavy smoker or having advanced physiologic age, diabetes, massively comminuted fractures, bilateral injuries, or work-related injuries. A large prospective, randomized study demonstrated that bilateral injuries, especially in patients with worker's compensation claims, fared no better with surgery.

Surgical Treatment

- Sanders types II and III fractures can be amenable to surgical reduction.
- Many surgeons recommend an extensile L-shaped lateral approach, elevating the entire soft tissue flap off the lateral side of the calcaneus, holding it with retraction pins with a "no-touch" technique during surgery.

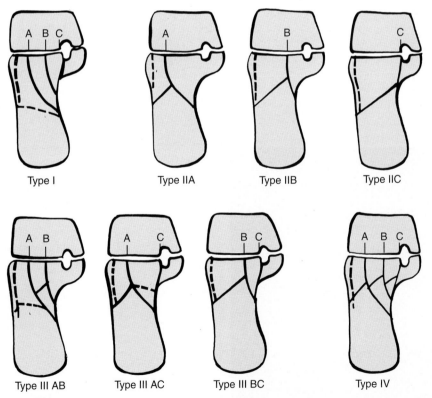

Type I   Type IIA   Type IIB   Type IIC

Type III AB   Type III AC   Type III BC   Type IV

Figure 14.28 Schematic diagram of Sanders classification. (Adapted from Sanders R, Fortin P, Pasquale T, et al. Operative treatment in 120 displaced intra-articular calcaneal fractures: results using a prognostic CT scan classification. Clin Orthop 1993;290:87–95.)

- The fracture is then reduced, generally with the following:
  - ☐ Anterior process reduction
  - ☐ Posterior tuberosity reduction
  - ☐ Posterior facet reduction.
- Appropriate low-profile, frequently locking, plates and screws are placed to maintain the reduction (Fig. 14.29).
- Recently, more surgeons have begun using either a limited sinus tarsi approach or performing the whole procedure percutaneously to minimize postoperative morbidity, specifically pain, swelling and stiffness, and to minimize the risk of wound complications (Fig. 14.30).
- A two-layer closure is used.
- ROM is started after the wound has sealed to minimize postoperative stiffness.

One study demonstrated in the Sanders type IIC fracture—because the posterior facet is in one piece sheared off of the sustentaculum tali—a closed reduction with a large percutaneous pin and subsequent screw fixation can avoid the morbidity of an extensile lateral approach. Some patients with marked comminution of the surface or denuded subchondral bone can be treated with a primary subtalar fusion. Advocates of this treatment report an overall shorter period of disability.

Results and Complications

The literature is contradictory regarding results of surgical versus nonsurgical treatment of calcaneus fractures. Some studies report superior results with nonsurgical treatment, whereas others have demonstrated equivalent or better results with surgery. In a recent large prospective, randomized study, overall equivalent results of surgical and non-surgical treatment were demonstrated. However, when the results were stratified, there was a much higher incidence of secondary fusion for patients treated nonsurgically, and certain patient populations (e.g., females and those with unilateral fractures, non–work-related injuries, reduction with less than a 2-mm stepoff, comminuted fractures, or a light workload) fared better with surgery.

- Wound dehiscence remains the most feared complication in that it frequently leads to osteomyelitis because the bone and hardware are generally exposed with a significant wound complication.

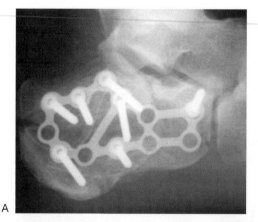

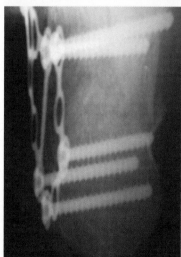

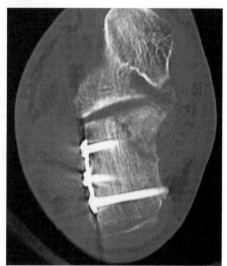

Figure 14.29 Postoperative lateral (A) and axial (B) Harris radiographs and CT scan (C) demonstrating congruent reduction of Sanders type IIB fracture.

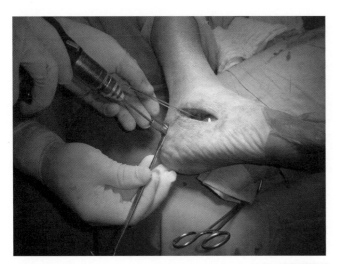

Figure 14.30 Intraoperative photograph demonstrating limited sinus tarsi approach. Note separate small incision over posterior tuberosity of calcaneus to percutaneously anchor the posterior aspect of plate.

- ☐ The best method of treatment is prevention by avoiding surgery until adequate soft-tissue edema resolution has occurred.
- ☐ Smokers and diabetic patients also have a greater risk of wound complications, and it is argued these are relative contraindications to surgical intervention.
- Subtalar arthrosis and arthritis are frequently present to some degree, with most patients losing approximately one-third to one-half of their subtalar motion despite aggressive postoperative rehabilitation.
  - ☐ This stiffness is caused by a combination of nonanatomic joint reduction, or more commonly, intra-articular adhesions or chondral damage that occurred at the time of initial injury.

OTHER CALCANEAL FRACTURES AND SOFT-TISSUE CONDITIONS

Calcaneal Avulsion Fractures

- Although calcaneal fractures usually occur from an axial load during a fall, occasionally they can occur following an avulsion injury from a forceful contraction of the gastrocnemius–soleus complex, avulsing the superior aspect of the calcaneal posterior tuberosity.
- They can involve the posterior aspect of the posterior facet, but they are usually extra-articular.
- Such fractures generally are a surgical emergency because the overlying skin becomes stretched.
- With any significant displacement, these should be treated with operative reduction in a prompt fashion to avoid skin necrosis (Fig. 14.31).
- The reduction can usually be achieved with an indirect reduction maneuver.
- If no skin necrosis occurs, these fractures have a better prognosis than intra-articular fractures because there is a lower rate of significant articular damage.

Anterior Process Fractures of the Calcaneus

- An anterior process fracture of the calcaneus occurs through avulsion with a plantarflexion–inversion injury of the hindfoot.
- A variable-sized piece of bone of the anterior process of the calcaneus attached to the bifurcate ligament is avulsed.
- It is generally visible on plain lateral or oblique radiographs of the hindfoot.
- These fractures can be treated the same as an ankle sprain with rest, ice, compression, and elevation, and if a symptomatic nonunion develops, a small fragment can be excised.
- Less frequently, the fragment is large, more than 1 cm in diameter, and involves a significant portion of the calcaneocuboid joint. These large fragments should be fixed with ORIF if displaced.

Compartment Syndrome

- One soft-tissue condition mandating urgent surgical treatment of a calcaneus fracture is compartment syndrome.
- The foot has five main compartmental spaces susceptible to compartment syndrome in high-energy injuries. The calcaneal compartment is separate.
- The patient complains of severe, increasing pain out of proportion to the injury.
  - ☐ Patients have pain with passive dorsiflexion of the toes, which stretches the ischemic plantar musculature in the arch.
- Compartment pressure should be measured in patients in whom compartment syndrome is suspected or patients with severe swelling or altered mental status.
- The involved compartment should be released and surgical wounds left open when treating this potentially devastating complication.

SUBTALAR DISLOCATION

PATHOGENESIS

Subtalar dislocations generally occur following a high-energy injury. Medial subtalar dislocation occurs with plantarflexion of the foot and forced inversion of the forefoot, which produces dislocation of both the talonavicular and subtalar joints. Medial dislocation can result in the head of the talus buttonholing through the extensor digitorum brevis and the anterior capsule, which can occasionally prevent closed reduction. Lateral dislocation occurs with plantarflexion of the foot accompanied by forceful eversion of the forefoot. Lateral dislocation can result in the head of the talus being forced through the talonavicular capsule with the posterior tibial tendon

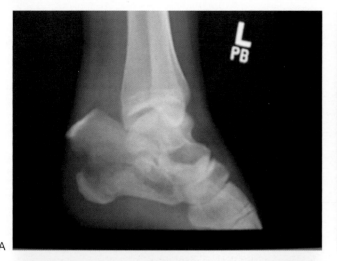

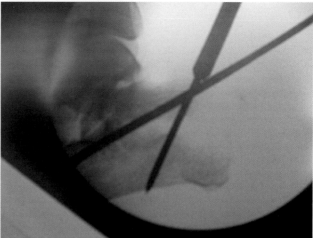

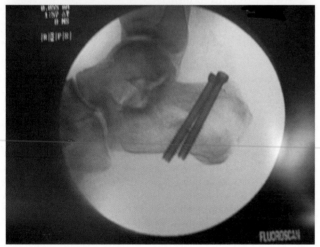

Figure 14.31 **A:** Lateral preoperative radiograph demonstrating avulsion fracture of the calcaneus with bone tenting the skin posteriorly. **B:** Intraoperative fluoroscopic lateral view demonstrating a large smooth pin inserted from posterior to anterior that was used to percutaneously reduce the fracture. Guide pin with depth gauge in place also seen before inserting dorsal to plantar screw through posterior tuberosity. **C:** Postoperative radiograph demonstrating cannulated screws maintaining reduction of fracture. Note the congruent reduction of the posterior facet of the subtalar joint.

lying dorsal to the neck of the talus, which can often preclude successful closed reduction.

DIAGNOSIS

Physical Examination and History

- The history is consistent with the mechanism of injury as outlined earlier.
- The clinical appearance of the foot demonstrates the direction of dislocation.
  - ☐ In a medial dislocation, the foot is plantarflexed, adducted, and supinated.
  - ☐ The overlying skin can be stretched over the head of the talus.
  - ☐ In a lateral dislocation, the foot appears pronated and abducted, and the talar head can be palpable along the medial hindfoot.

Radiologic Features
- AP, lateral, and oblique radiographs of the hindfoot are a minimum for evaluation. The direction of dislocation can generally be determined easily from these three radiographs (Fig. 14.32).

- Occasionally, a double-density sign of the talonavicular joint is the most obvious radiographic finding of a subluxation of dislocation.
- Although not necessary for making the diagnosis, some surgeons advocate a postreduction CT scan to evaluate for intra-articular subtalar joint debris or talar head impaction injury.

Classification

Classification is either medial, if the foot has displaced medially, or lateral, if the foot is displaced laterally.

TREATMENT

- An immediate closed reduction should be performed on priority in a subtalar dislocation to avoid skin breakdown and neurovascular compromise.
- Under general anesthetic or significant sedation, traction and relocation should be attempted.
- Direct pressure over the head of the talus with either of these reduction maneuvers can facilitate the reduction.
- Most medial subtalar dislocations can be reduced closed because the talar head can be reduced through the hole

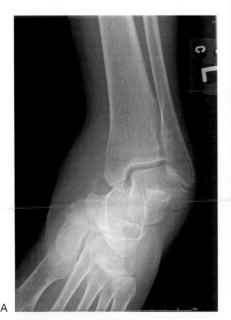
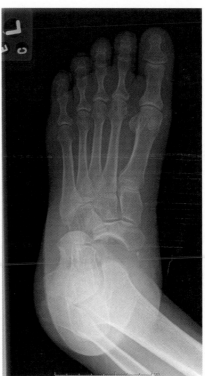
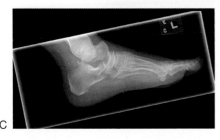

Figure 14.32 **A:** AP ankle radiograph and AP foot demonstrating medial subtalar dislocation. **B:** With obvious medial talonavicular dislocation on AP foot view **C:** lateral view showing the subtalar incongruity clearly.

in the extensor digitorum brevis or talonavicular joint capsule.

■ Lateral subtalar dislocation can be irreducible as a result of the posterior tibial tendon wrapping over the dorsal aspect of the neck of the talus.

■ Failed closed reduction should be treated with open reduction as soon as possible to prevent skin necrosis and neurovascular skin complications.

■ Postreduction radiographs are obtained to confirm an anatomic reduction.

■ CT scans are advocated by some to rule out the presence of intra-articular debris and the presence of a talar head fracture.

■ Fractures should be immobilized for approximately 3 to 4 weeks after reduction, and then gentle mobilization and weight bearing are begun.

■ ROM of the toes can begin immediately after reduction to prevent adhesions to the extensor tendons.

Complications

Although many of these dislocations can be easily reduced and yield good functional results, delay in diagnosis can lead to an increased rate of subtalar arthrosis and subse-

quent stiffness. Impaction fractures of the head of the talus can also lead to increased stiffness and pain following these injuries. AVN is uncommon following subtalar dislocations.

FRACTURES OF THE NAVICULAR

PATHOGENESIS

Fractures of the navicular are relatively uncommon injuries. They can be classified as follows:

■ Avulsion–dorsal lip fracture—the most common fracture but tends to be of little significance because it is more a reflection of ligamentous injury and is managed symptomatically as a sprain.

■ Fracture of the navicular tuberosity—occurs following acute eversion injury of the foot with contraction of the tibialis posterior muscle, usually minimally displaced

owing to complex tibialis posterior insertion. Can be associated with occult midtarsal subluxation, cuboid fracture, or anterior process calcaneus fracture; can be managed symptomatically if nondisplaced with approximately 4 to 6 weeks of walking cast or boot. Rare cases of displacement are treated with ORIF.
- Fractures of the body of the navicular—most severe injury (refer to following section).
- Navicular stress fracture (refer to following section).

The mechanism of injury of a fracture of the body can be direct or indirect. Direct force such as a crush injury frequently results in comminuted fractures. Indirect forces include a fall with the foot in plantarflexion causing axial compression. Indirect mechanism is frequently associated with significant displacement as a result of extensive ligamentous disruption.

The mechanism of a stress fracture, similar to elsewhere in the body, is repetitive stress. Most commonly it is associated with running activities. Such fractures are uncommon and are frequently misdiagnosed with average time to diagnosis being 4 months in some series. A predisposition exists in the midportion of the body in that it is a watershed area of blood supply. Arterial supply comes dorsally from branches of the dorsalis pedis, medially at the tuberosity with the posterior tendon insertion, and plantarly from the medial plantar artery, leaving an avascular central third.

DIAGNOSIS

Physical Examination and History

- Patients with an acute fracture of the body of the navicular present with pain along the medial aspect of the arch with the mechanism of injury consistent with that described.
- Patients with a stress fracture usually present with an insidious onset of medial midfoot pain during running activities.

Clinical Features

- On examination, patients with acute body fractures usually have marked tenderness, swelling, and pain with any attempt at ROM of the hindfoot.
- In displaced fractures, an adduction–supination deformity of the foot can be present.
- Patients with a navicular stress fracture can have mild, diffuse tenderness or no localized tenderness and frequently have no swelling.

Radiologic Features

- Patients with suspected navicular fractures should be evaluated with AP, oblique, and lateral radiographs of the hindfoot.
- In cases of acute fracture, fracture planes are usually relatively obvious.
- For preoperative planning, CT scans with coronal and transverse cuts can better delineate the fracture anatomy and sites of comminution.
- In cases of navicular stress fractures, plain radiographs sometimes demonstrate incomplete fracture lines or they can be normal.

- If a navicular stress fracture is suspected, CT scans are helpful in confirming the diagnosis.
- A bone scan shows increased activity at the site of the stress fracture.
- An MRI scan can also demonstrate the presence of a navicular stress fracture but does not define the fracture anatomy as well as a CT scan.

Classification

One classification system is used commonly for fractures of the body of the navicular (Table 14.8 and Fig. 14.33).

TREATMENT

Body Fractures

- Nondisplaced navicular body fractures can be treated with a short leg nonwalking cast with the ankle in neutral position. Typically, the patient is non–weight bearing for approximately 4 to 6 weeks, followed by 4 to 6 weeks of protected weight bearing in a walking boot.
- Displaced fractures mandate ORIF to achieve anatomic reduction of the essential, mobile talonavicular joint.
- With a significant amount of comminution present, especially in type III fractures, one study defined adequate reduction as having reduced 60% or more of the articular surface owing to the difficulty of fracture repair.
- For surgical repair, the patient is placed supine and an anteromedial approach between the anterior and posterior tibial tendons is used.
- In most cases, a secondary lateral incision helps better expose the proximal articular surface of the navicular because it is difficult to visualize.
- Direct and indirect methods of reduction are used to reduce a fracture.
- In cases of minimal to no comminution, the plantar lateral and dorsal medial fragments can be reduced and secured with lag screws.
- Because the naviculocuneiform joints are essentially immobile, if any significant degree of comminution exists, large navicular fragments can be fixed to their respective

TABLE 14.8 CLASSIFICATION OF FRACTURES OF THE NAVICULAR

Type	Description
1	Fractures occur in the coronal plane with no angulation of forefoot
2	Primary fracture line oriented from dorsal lateral to plantar medial, with the major medial fragment and forefoot displaced medially, leading to an adduction deformity Usually no involvement of the naviculocuneiform joint
3	Comminuted fracture in central portion, usually owing to axial load; most difficult to treat and worst prognosis

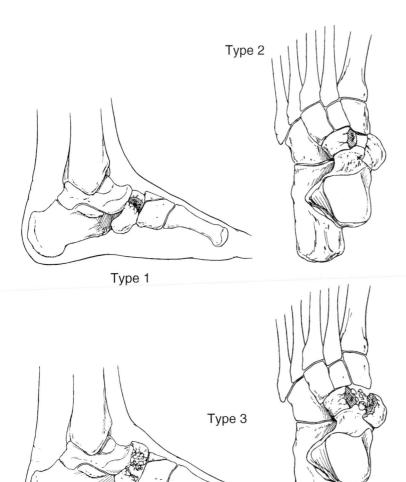

Figure 14.33   Navicular fracture body classifications, types 1 to 3 (see text). (From Thordarson DB. Fractures of the midfoot and forefoot. In: Myerson MS, ed. Foot and ankle disorders, vol 2. Philadelphia: Elsevier, 2000:1282.)

cuneiforms, as it is difficult, or impossible, to place screws across comminuted segments of the navicular (Fig. 14.34).

- Patients are kept in a non–weight-bearing short leg cast until early evidence of radiographic consolidation, which is generally a minimum of 6 weeks of non–weight-bearing followed by an additional 4 to 6 weeks of short leg cast or boot immobilization.

Results

Results depend on the ability to achieve an anatomic reduction. In one study, in all type I fractures and two-thirds of type II injuries, it was possible to achieve an anatomic reduction. In only one-half of type III injuries was a satisfactory reduction obtained. At an average follow-up of almost 4 years, they reported good results in two-thirds of their patients, fair results in 19%, and poor results in 14%, reflecting the gravity of this injury. The most common complication noted was posttraumatic arthritis of the talonavicular joint. However, in one series, AVN of the central third developed in one-third of patients treated with open reduction of a displaced navicular, and AVN of the entire navicular developed in two patients, with one resulting in collapse.

Navicular Stress Fractures

- Almost all of these fractures are nondisplaced (Fig. 14.35).
- Nonoperative treatment includes 6 to 8 weeks of short leg nonwalking cast immobilization. If a nonunion develops, or, rarely, if displacement occurs, lag screw fixation with or without bone grafting in the nonunion plane is advisable.
- Operative treatment of navicular stress fractures in high-performance athletes to minimize their period of disability has been advocated by some but a recent meta-analysis showed best results with short leg cast, non–weight-bearing immobilization.
- In cases with significant sclerosis of the stress fracture site, a limited incision directly overlying the fracture plane dorsally can be made to introduce a small curette into the stress fracture plane, performing either local bone grafting if it is a large enough gap or fenestrating it with a drill bit to encourage healing along with dorsal lag screw fixation.
- Navicular stress fractures tend to do well once healing of the fracture is achieved.

Figure 14.34   AP preoperative X-ray (**A**), transverse CT scan (**B**), and postoperative X-ray (**C**) of comminuted navicular fracture with fixation of large navicular fragments to cuneiforms.

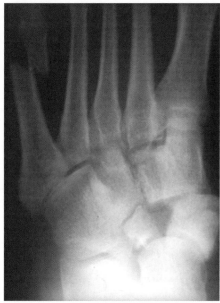
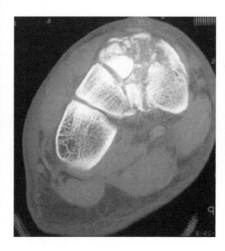
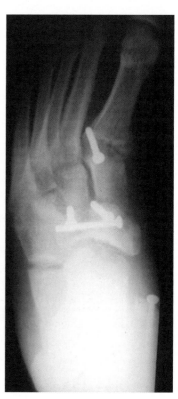

A,B   C

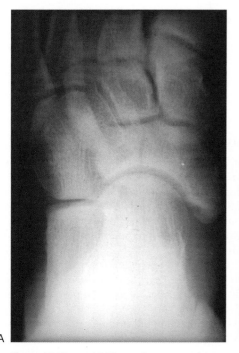
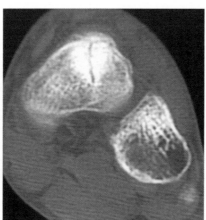

A   B

Figure 14.35   **A:** AP X-ray of patient with a navicular stress fracture with insidious onset of medial midfoot pain. **B:** Coronal CT scan demonstrating incomplete fracture plane with dorsal callus formation.

TARSOMETATARSAL (LISFRANC) INJURIES

PATHOGENESIS

Lisfranc injuries are relatively uncommon, accounting for only about 0.2% of all fractures. Although classically associated with high-energy injuries such as motor vehicle accidents or a fall from a height, some can occur with relatively low-energy twisting injuries.

Two different forces can cause this injury:

▪ Direct—crushing injury such as a foot that is run over by a vehicle. It is frequently associated with soft-tissue injury and can involve compartment syndrome, especially if the intercommunicating arterial branch between the dorsalis pedis and the plantar arterial arch is disrupted between the bases of the first two metatarsals.
▪ Indirect mechanism—axial loading of plantarflexed foot or severe abduction leading to dorsal ligamentous disruption. Examples of this more common injury include the foot hitting the floorboard of a car, falling on the heel of a planted foot, and falling off of a horse with the foot in a stirrup.

The anatomy of the tarsometatarsal joint has functional, and, therefore, treatment implications.

▪ The second metatarsal base is wedge-shaped, wider dorsally, and sits between the bases of the first and third metatarsals, leading to a high degree of stability and minimal motion (Fig. 14.36).
▪ Dense ligamentous attachments secure the metatarsal bases to their respective tarsal bones.
▪ The medial three metatarsal bases articulate with their respective cuneiform, and the fourth and fifth metatarsals articulate with the cuboid.
▪ The stronger ligaments are present across the plantar aspect of the tarsometatarsal joint.
▪ The second through fifth metatarsal bases are attached to one another with the dense intermetatarsal attachments.
▪ No intermetatarsal ligament exists between the first and second metatarsals. Instead, the Lisfranc ligament runs obliquely from the second metatarsal base to the medial cuneiform.

The foot has been described as having three columns:

▪ Medial—includes first ray and its metatarsocuneiform joint.
▪ Middle column—includes second and third rays with second and third metatarsocuneiform joints.
▪ Lateral—includes fourth and fifth rays and cuboid.

The medial three rays have minimal movement, whereas the fourth and fifth tarsometatarsal joints have much greater movement; thus a two-column model of the foot is probably more helpful clinically. Any operative fixation needs to preserve the greater motion of the fourth and fifth tarsometatarsal joints. The ligamentous and osseous anatomy explains

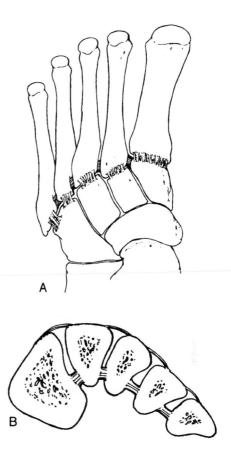

Figure 14.36 Schematic representation of bone and ligamentous architecture of the tarsometatarsal joint. **A:** Dorsal view demonstrates strong ligamentous support between metatarsal bases and adjacent tarsal bones. **B:** Coronal cut demonstrates the keystone configuration of second metatarsal in the transverse arch. (From Thordarson DB. Fractures of the midfoot and forefoot. In: Myerson MS, ed. Foot and ankle disorders, vol 2. Philadelphia: Elsevier, 2000:1266.)

multiple variations of these midfoot injuries. Separations between the first and second metatarsals can be explained by the lack of an intermetatarsal ligament in this area.

DIAGNOSIS

▪ A high index of suspicion is necessary for any patient complaining of midfoot pain.
▪ The mechanism should correlate with the previously described modes of injury.
▪ Polytraumatized patients should have their feet carefully evaluated because 20% of these injuries are missed on initial evaluation in polytrauma patients.

Physical Examination and History

Clinical Features

▪ On examination, these patients have a variable degree of swelling and deformity, depending on the magnitude of injury.
▪ All patients have tenderness along the midfoot in the zone of injury.

■ Attempted ROM through these joints elicits pain.
■ Occasionally, patients have ecchymosis in the midarch region, which can be diagnostic for this injury.

Radiologic Features

■ Radiographic evaluation of midfoot injuries includes a standard AP, 30° oblique, and lateral radiographs of the foot.
■ Care must be taken to orient the X-ray beam perpendicular to the dorsum of the foot, not relative to the floor, because this causes obliquity of the tarsometatarsal joints, thus distorting the normal radiographic relationships.
■ Because of the varying patterns of injury, each of the metatarsals must be evaluated with respect to its corresponding midfoot bone (Fig. 14.37).
  □ AP view: The medial border of the second metatarsal forms a continuous line with the medial border of the middle cuneiform, and the intermetatarsal space between the first and second metatarsals is equal to the space between the middle and medial cuneiforms.
  □ 30° oblique view: The medial border of the fourth metatarsal forms a continuous line with the medial border of the cuboid, and the lateral border of the third metatarsal forms a straight line with the lateral border of the lateral cuneiform. The intermetatarsal space between the second and third metatarsals is also found to be equal and aligned to the intertarsal space between the middle and lateral cuneiforms.
  □ Lateral view: No evidence of dorsal, or less commonly plantar, displacement of the metatarsals relative to the tarsal bones should be evident.

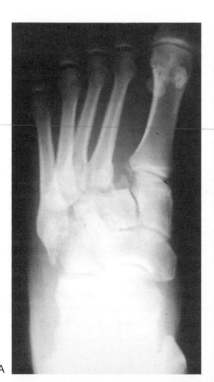
A

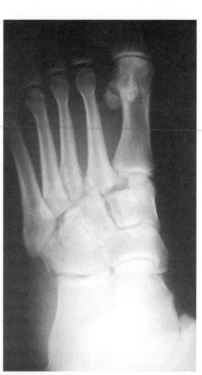
B

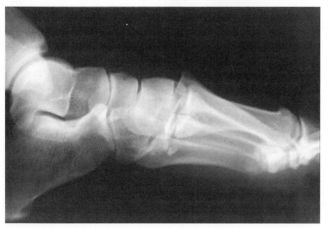
C

Figure 14.37   AP (**A**), oblique (**B**), and lateral (**C**) X-rays of a patient with Lisfranc injury.

- In addition, the intermetatarsal 1-2 space should be evaluated for the presence of a small bony avulsion fragment (fleck sign), which represents an avulsion fracture by the Lisfranc ligament, which is pathognomonic of this injury.
- In uncertain cases, comparison radiographs of the opposite foot can be obtained.
- Stress radiographs can provide additional help in making this diagnosis.
  - ☐ Plantarflexion stress views demonstrate dorsal ligamentous instability with dorsal gapping.
  - ☐ Abduction–pronation and adduction–supination views demonstrate lateral and medial translations, respectively, in unstable cases.
- In subacute settings, standing lateral radiographs can be compared with assess for instability.
- CT scans of the midfoot can define comminution but generally are not necessary to make the diagnosis or for planning treatment.

Classification

Various classification systems have been proposed. The most important determination is to discern whether the fracture is nondisplaced or displaced because displaced fractures require surgical reduction. The most comprehensive classification includes three types with additional subclassifications (Table 14.9 and Fig. 14.38).

TABLE 14.9 CLASSIFICATION OF TARSOMETATARSAL INJURIES

Type	Description
A	Total incongruity in any plane or direction
B1	Partial incongruity in which only the first ray is involved
B2	Partial incongruity with displacement of one or more of the lesser metatarsals
C1	Divergent dislocation with first metatarsal medial and lesser metatarsals partially incongruent
C2	Divergent dislocation with divergent pattern with total incongruity of the lesser metatarsals

TREATMENT

Surgical Indications and Contraindications

Because of the potential long-term morbidity, most displaced fractures are treated surgically. I do not think there is a role for nonoperative treatment in any patient who is medically stable with any visible degree of instability or displacement of the Lisfranc joint.

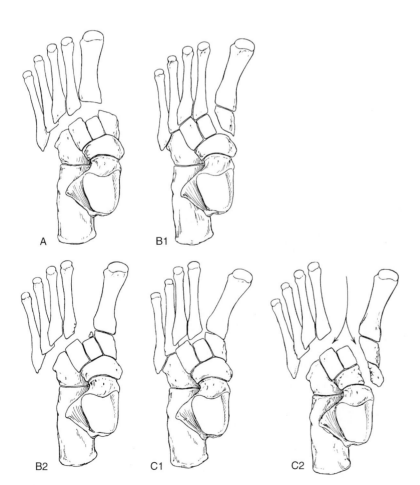

Figure 14.38 Tarsometatarsal fracture classification system (see text). (From Thordarson DB. Fractures of the midfoot and forefoot. In: Myerson MS, ed. Foot and ankle disorders, vol 2. Philadelphia: Elsevier, 2000:1271.)

■ Surgical fixation follows the usual principles of operative fracture treatment, including obtaining an anatomic reduction with rigid internal fixation.

■ Although percutaneous pinning techniques have been described, it is difficult to guarantee an anatomic reduction percutaneously and most surgeons prefer an open approach.

■ Fixation can be achieved with K-wires or screws.

  □ The advantages of K-wire fixation include ease of insertion and removal. The disadvantages are pin migration, risk of infection, and loss of reduction, especially because K-wires are usually removed 6 to 8 weeks after surgery when the soft tissue is not completely healed.

  □ Screw fixation provides improved fixation but is more technically difficult to insert, and most surgeons still routinely remove screws after soft-tissue healing. Some surgeons now recommend plate fixation to minimize iatrogenic chondral injury owing to the screws traversing the articular surface.

Operative Technique

■ Surgery is postponed until adequate soft-tissue edema resolution has occurred.

■ The tarsometatarsal joints are approached through two longitudinal incisions:

  □ One incision over the first intermetatarsal space allows access to the first, second, and third tarsometatarsal joints; it is the only incision necessary for partial incongruity patterns.

  □ Second incision is centered over the base of the fourth metatarsal allowing for reduction and fixation of the third, fourth, and fifth metatarsals.

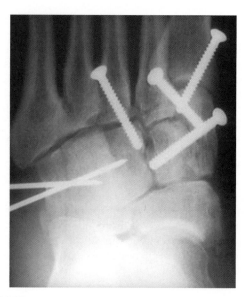

Figure 14.39 Postoperative X-ray of patient following screw fixation of Lisfranc (tarsometatarsal) fracture dislocation with K-wires across cuboid fracture.

■ With the medial incision, the neurovascular bundle is retracted laterally.

■ All joints should be inspected for osteocartilaginous debris because plantar comminution is relatively common.

■ Either the first or second metatarsal can be reduced first.

■ Each joint should be secured with at least two K-wires at 90° to one another or preferably with at least one fully threaded cortical screw or a dorsal plate (Figs. 14.39 and 14.40).

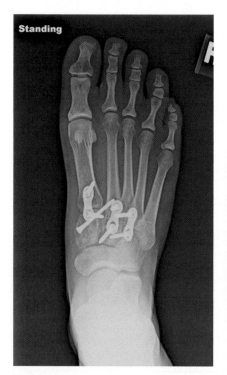

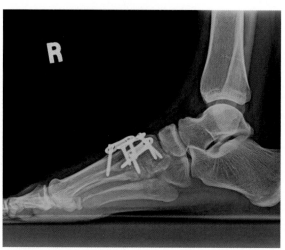

Figure 14.40 Postoperative AP and lateral radiographs demonstrating dorsal plate fixation instead of screw fixation for Lisfranc injury. Some surgeons feel that the lack of screws penetrating the central portion of the articular surface of these joints can potentially lead to less posttraumatic arthritis.

- Because a greater amount of motion is present in the fourth and fifth metatarsocuboid joints, most surgeons use only K-wires across these joints so that they can be removed approximately 6 to 8 weeks after surgery to minimize stiffness of these important joints.
- In some cases, significant shortening of the lateral column occurs with impaction of the cuboid (i.e., nutcracker injury). In these cases, the cuboid needs to be reduced either indirectly with an external fixator or directly with bone grafting and fixation of the cuboid.
- If adequate stability cannot be obtained with bone grafting and internal fixation of the cuboid fracture, a laterally based external fixator or subcutaneous plate between the fifth metatarsal and the calcaneus needs to be kept in place until adequate bone healing occurs.
- Patients are maintained non–weight bearing in a short leg cast for 6 to 8 weeks, at which time any K-wires can be removed.
- A short leg walking cast with a well-molded arch is then applied for an additional 4 to 6 weeks.
- A custom orthotic can be used for another 6 months following injury to help protect the midfoot.

Results

Almost all recent studies advocate operative management of these serious displaced injuries. Results of closed reduction and cast immobilization have been disappointing. Some studies have demonstrated superior results using screws compared with K-wires as a result of the better maintenance of reduction. In general, an anatomic reduction results in a superior result compared with a nonanatomic reduction. However, an anatomic reduction does not guarantee a good or excellent result. Posttraumatic arthritis can be related not only to the adequacy of reduction but also to the amount of damage sustained to the articular surface at the time of initial injury. Despite operative treatment with an anatomic reduction, many of these patients develop some persistent pain and often arthritis. Furthermore, a prospective randomized level I study demonstrated more predictable pain relief with primary fusion versus ORIF.

CUNEIFORM AND CUBOID DISLOCATIONS

- Isolated fractures or dislocations of the cuneiform or cuboid are rare.
- Most of these bony injuries are a component of a tarsometatarsal injury in which the force of injury has been dissipated through the tarsometatarsal joint and the naviculocuneiform or intercuneiform joints.
- Treatment principles for these isolated injuries are the same as for tarsometatarsal injuries.

METATARSOPHALANGEAL AND INTERPHALANGEAL JOINT DISLOCATIONS

PATHOGENESIS

Dislocations of the metatarsophalangeal and interphalangeal joints are uncommon. The most common disorder involves the hallux metatarsophalangeal joint. Hallux metatarsophalangeal dislocations are classified as shown in Table 14.10 and Figure 14.41.

TREATMENT

- After closed reduction, most dislocations are stable and can be treated with a walking cast or boot immobilization limiting dorsiflexion of the great toe for the first 2 to 4 weeks.
- If both sesamoids are avulsed from the base of the proximal phalanx and retract, surgical repair is indicated.

METATARSAL FRACTURES

PATHOGENESIS AND MECHANISM

Metatarsal fractures can occur from direct or indirect forces. A fracture of the first through fourth metatarsals usually results from a direct blow to the dorsum of the foot. Indirect forces such as twisting injuries more commonly cause fractures of the fifth metatarsal, especially the tuberosity.

TABLE 14.10 CLASSIFICATION OF HALLUX MP DISLOCATIONS

Type	Description
I	Plantar plate ruptures such that the hallux with the attached sesamoids displaces over the dorsal metatarsal head, locking the head in a plantar position that is irreducible
IIA[a]	Intersesamoidal ligament ruptures with wide separation of the sesamoids and the proximal phalanx sitting dorsal to the metatarsal head
IIB[a]	Transverse fracture of one or both of the sesamoids occur

[a]Types IIA and IIB can generally undergo closed reduction successfully.

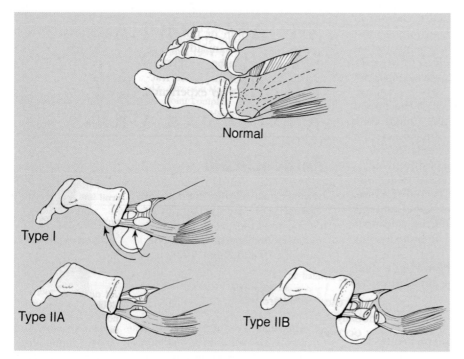

Figure 14.41   Hallux metatarsophalangeal dislocation classification (see text). (From Thordarson DB. Fractures of the midfoot and forefoot. In: Myerson MS, ed. Foot and ankle disorders, vol 2. Philadelphia: Elsevier, 2000:1293; after Jahss MH, ed. Disorders of the foot and ankle: medical and surgical management. Philadelphia: WB Saunders, 1991;1129.)

The bony and ligamentous anatomy of the metatarsals has clinical relevance in that it results in typical displacement patterns. In addition to the dense ligamentous interconnections located at the base of the metatarsals previously described, the metatarsals are interconnected at the level of the metatarsal neck with intermetatarsal ligaments. Therefore, an isolated metatarsal fracture typically does not significantly displace because it is has proximal as well as distal soft-tissue support. In contrast, multiple metatarsal fractures frequently displace significantly as a result of the disruption of the adjacent supporting structures. Because the metatarsals are weight-bearing bones, displacement in the sagittal plane causes alteration in weight bearing across the forefoot. Plantar displacement increases the weight bearing leading frequently to an intractable plantar keratosis and pain. Dorsal displacement can lead to overload of the adjacent metatarsals with possible "transfer metatarsalgia."

DIAGNOSIS

Physical Examination and History

Clinical Features
- The history should be consistent with a mechanism as described earlier for the given injury.
- Physical examination reveals tenderness and a variable degree of swelling localized to the fracture site.

Radiologic Features
- AP, lateral, and oblique radiographs of the involved foot demonstrate the fracture site and displacement, including plantarflexion or dorsiflexion.

- Occasionally, a tangential view of the entire forefoot—an expanded sesamoid view—can help visualize plantar or dorsal displacement.

TREATMENT

Surgical Indications and Contraindications

The goal of treatment of a metatarsal fracture is successful healing and a pain-free foot with normal weight-bearing distribution. Most isolated second through fifth metatarsal fractures can be treated nonoperatively because they do not displace significantly. In general, patients are advanced from either a walking cast or hard-soled shoe to a supportive tennis shoe as pain permits over a 4- to 6-week period.

Fractures of the first metatarsal require more aggressive treatment because they are more likely to displace owing to their lesser ligamentous support and because the first metatarsal supports more weight. Screw and plate fixation can maintain an anatomic reduction of these fractures.

- In patients with multiple metatarsal fractures, significant displacement is common.
- Intramedullary pin fixation allows for appropriate alignment with relative ease of insertion.
- One to three metatarsal fractures can be approached through a single longitudinal incision centered over the area of pathology.
- An appropriately sized intramedullary pin is then drilled retrograde from the fracture site through the plantar skin at the distal forefoot of each of the fractured metatarsals before inserting them across the fracture site (Fig. 14.42).

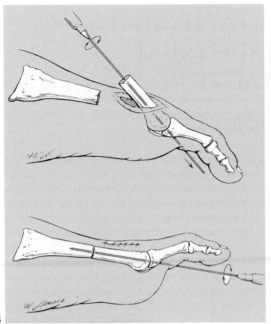

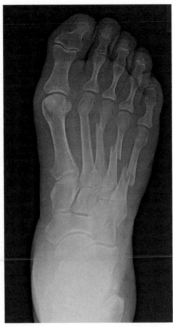

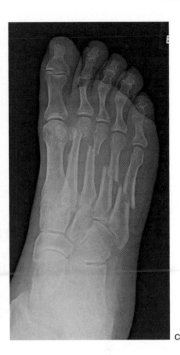

A,B   C

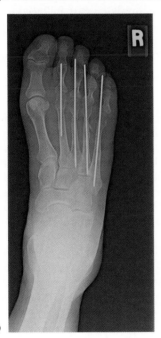

D

Figure 14.42 **A:** Schematic representation of retrograde pinning of K-wire out the metatarsal shaft through the plantar aspect of foot. **B:** Schematic representation demonstrating reduction of the metatarsal fracture with antegrade pinning across the fracture site. **C:** AP and oblique radiographs of forefoot demonstrating displaced fracture of second through fifth metatarsals. **D:** Postoperative AP radiograph demonstrating intramedullary fixation of second through fifth metatarsal fractures.

- After all of the distal metatarsal fragments have a pin placed, the fractures are reduced and the intramedullary pins are inserted across the fracture site.
- In general, a single longitudinal K-wire for a metatarsal provides adequate stability to allow healing without development of altered forefoot weight bearing.
- Patients are kept in a short leg nonwalking cast for approximately 4 to 6 weeks and a walking boot for an additional 4 to 6 weeks.
- K-wires are generally removed 6 to 8 weeks after insertion.
- In general, most metatarsals heal reliably with minimal long-term sequelae.
- The main complication is malunion, resulting in altered weight bearing across the forefoot.

METATARSAL STRESS FRACTURES

- The classic history is an unconditioned military recruit or weekend runner who suddenly increases his activity level.
- The most common lesser metatarsal to sustain a stress fracture is the second metatarsal because it is the longest and stiffest, and is thus exposed to the greatest repetitive stress.
- On examination, the patient has localized tenderness at the fracture site.

- Initial radiographs are usually normal and become positive 2 to 4 weeks after fracture with callus formation.
- A technetium bone scan or MRI can confirm a diagnosis earlier, although generally this is unnecessary because the diagnosis is usually evident.
- Treatment is symptomatic, either with a wood-soled shoe or wrapping of the midfoot and use of an athletic shoe.

AVULSION FRACTURES OF THE BASE OF THE FIFTH METATARSAL

- Avulsion fractures of the fifth metatarsal tuberosity, also known as dancer's fractures, occur frequently (Fig. 14.43).
- The usual mechanism is an inversion injury of the foot.
- The patient develops lateral midfoot pain.
- On examination, patients have tenderness over the fifth metatarsal base.
- Radiographs reveal, in general, a variable-sized piece of the metatarsal tuberosity, which is generally nondisplaced owing to the broad insertion of the peroneus brevis.
- Although one radiographic study suggested that these fractures are because of avulsion by a plantar fascia band, it is more commonly due to avulsion by the peroneus brevis in the author's opinion.
- Treatment of dancer's fractures is generally symptomatic.
- Occasionally, pain is severe enough to require a walking cast or boot for 1 to 2 weeks followed by foot wrapping and a supportive athletic shoe.
- Dancer's fractures almost invariably heal without any sequelae.

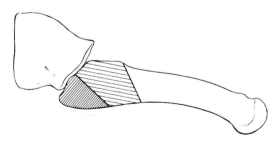

Figure 14.43 Schematic representation of fifth metatarsal base with shaded area demonstrating fractures of the metatarsal tuberosity. Cross-hatched area demonstrates watershed area of blood supply susceptible to stress fracture and nonunion. (From Thordarson DB. Fractures of the midfoot and forefoot. In: Myerson MS, ed. Foot and ankle disorders, vol 2. Philadelphia: Elsevier, 2000:1291.)

METAPHYSEAL–DIAPHYSEAL FRACTURE

PATHOGENESIS

Both acute fractures and stress fractures of the metaphyseal–diaphyseal junction of the fifth metatarsal can occur. Acute fractures generally occur following a significant adduction force across the forefoot. The proximal fifth metatarsal has a unique blood supply with a watershed area at the metaphyseal–diaphyseal junction (Fig. 14.43). A single nutrient artery enters the medial aspect of the metatarsal shaft at approximately the junction of the proximal and the mid third. The blood supply also enters the tuberosity through the peroneus brevis insertion. This watershed area of blood supply predisposes this area to nonunion. With an acute fracture, most surgeons recommend a 6- to 8-week course of short leg nonwalking cast followed by a walking boot for an additional 2 to 4 weeks. If a nonunion develops, it should be treated similar to a stress fracture.

DIAGNOSIS

Stress fractures in this area occur as a result of repetitive trauma and a relatively poor blood supply. Many patients have had some prodrome of dull, activity-related pain before actually sustaining the stress fracture. Plain radiographs generally reveal either sclerosis of the fracture site or a small amount of osteolysis at the fracture. In general, these patients have a slight cavovarus–supinated foot shape, which chronically overloads the lateral border of the foot.

TREATMENT

Because of the high incidence of nonunion following these fractures, controversy exists regarding proper treatment. Conservative treatment requires prolonged use of a short leg nonwalking cast, beginning with a minimum of 6 weeks. Despite prolonged periods of immobilization, nonunion does develop in some patients. High-caliber athletes or other active people are usually treated acutely with intramedullary screw fixation. In addition to more rapid healing and a more predictable period of disability, these patients have a lower rate of refracture. Although intramedullary screw fixation has been described with or without bone grafting, bone graft is generally unnecessary in these patients (Fig. 14.44).

- Surgery begins with an incision approximately 1 to 2 cm in length along the midlateral border of the foot.
- A guide pin for a large cannulated screw can then be inserted along the dorsomedial aspect of the fifth metatarsal base in line with the intramedullary canal.

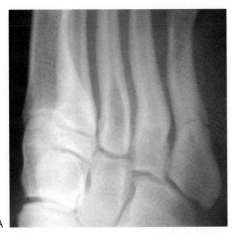
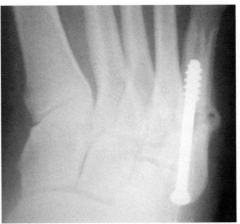

Figure 14.44 **A:** AP X-ray of Division I college basketball player following twisting injury of the foot shows completed stress fracture. **B:** Postoperative X-ray demonstrating intramedullary screw fixation with subsequent fracture healing.

- The size of the thread of the screw can be determined from preoperative radiographs to obtain good canal fill.
- In general, use of an intramedullary screw leads to predictable healing of these fractures.
- Symptomatic hardware should be removed, as needed.
- Most patients should be protected with an orthotic postoperatively to unload the fifth metatarsal or correct a cavovarus foot deformity, if supple.

SESAMOID FRACTURES

PATHOGENESIS

Sesamoid fractures can occur from direct or indirect trauma. Direct trauma with a crushing injury from an object falling on the foot or a fall from a height is more common. Indirect trauma from hyperdorsiflexion of the great toe can cause an avulsion-type fracture.

DIAGNOSIS

Physical Examination and History

- Patients report a direct or indirect trauma as outlined above.

Clinical Features
- On examination, patients have point tenderness over the involved sesamoid with the medial being most commonly injured.
- Dorsiflexion exacerbates the pain.

Radiologic Features
- AP, lateral, and sesamoid (tangential) views are necessary.
- Acute fractures reveal irregular fracture margins compared with the smooth margins of a bipartite sesamoid.

TREATMENT

- Approximately 4 to 6 weeks of immobilization in a short leg walking cast or boot followed by use of a supportive shoe for 4 to 6 more weeks is generally necessary.
- Symptom resolution frequently takes 4 to 6 months.
- Delayed union or nonunion occurs relatively frequently owing to a relatively poor blood supply, especially of the medial sesamoid.
- Further treatment of sesamoid fractures is discussed in Chapter 6.

TOE FRACTURES

PATHOGENESIS

- Fractures of the great toe and lesser toes are usually the result of direct trauma.
- Fractures of the great toe are generally due to an object being dropped on the toe or occasionally kicking a stationary object.
  - □ These fractures are generally nondisplaced and can be treated adequately with a wood-soled shoe until pain resolution allows use of an athletic shoe.
  - □ Occasionally, significant displacement of a large fragment extending in the interphalangeal or metatarsophalangeal joint exists, and ORIF should be performed.
- Lesser toe fractures are common and generally occur as a result of a direct trauma from kicking an immobile object such as a leg of a chair or a table at night while barefooted ("night walker fracture").
- These fractures heal essentially invariably without surgery and simply require taping of the affected toe to the adjacent toe for protection ("buddy taping").
- Fracture tenderness generally subsides over approximately 3 to 4 weeks.

SUGGESTED READINGS

Arntz CT, Veith RG, Hansen ST. Fractures and fracture dislocations of the tarsometatarsal joint. J Bone Joint Surg Am 1988;70:173–181.

Bibbo C, Anderson RB, Davis WH. Injury characteristics and the clinical outcome of subtalar dislocations: a clinical and radiographic analysis of 25 cases. Foot Ankle Int 2003;24:158–163.

Boden SD, Labropoulos PA, McCowin P, et al. Mechanical considerations for the syndesmotic screw—a cadaveric study. J Bone Joint Surg Am 1989;19:1548.

Buckley R, Tough S, McCormack R, et al. Operative compared with nonoperative treatment of displaced intra-articular calcaneal fractures: a prospective, randomized, controlled multicenter trial. J Bone Joint Surg Am 2002;84:1733–1744.

Canale ST, Kelly FB. Fractures of the neck of the talus. J Bone Joint Surg Am 1978;60:143–156.

Goldie I, Peterson L, Lindell D. The arterial supply of the talus. Acta Orthop Scand 1974;45:260.

Hawkins LG. Fractures of the neck of the talus. J Bone Joint Surg Am 1970;52:991–1002.

Jahss MH. Traumatic dislocations of the first metatarsophalangeal joint. Foot Ankle 1980;1:15–21.

Joy G, Patzakis M, Harvey J. Precise evaluation of the reduction of severe ankle fractures. J Bone Joint Surg Am 1974;56:979.

Lauge-Hansen N. Fractures of the ankle. Combined experimental surgical and experimental rank analogic investigation. Arch Surg 1950;60:957.

Lindvall E, Haidukewych G, DiPasquale T, et al. Open reduction and stable fixation of isolated, displaced talar neck and body fractures. J Bone Joint Surg Am 2004;86(10):2229–2234.

Ly TV, Coetzee C. Treatment of primary ligamentous Lisfranc joint injuries: primary arthrodesis compared with open reduction internal fixation. A prospective, randomized study. J Bone Joint Surg Am 2006;88(3):514–520.

Marsh JL, Weigel DP, Dirschl DR. Tibial plafond fractures. How do these ankles function over time? J Bone Joint Surg Am 2003;85:287–295.

Michelson JD. Fractures about the ankle. J Bone Joint Surg Am 1995;77:142.

Myerson MS, Fisher RT, Burgess AR, et al. Fracture dislocations of the tarsometatarsal joints: end results correlated to pathology and treatment. Foot Ankle 1986;6:225–242.

Ruedi TP, Allgower M. Fractures of the lower end of the tibia into the ankle-joint. Injury 1969;1:92–99.

Sanders R, Fortin P, DiPasquale T, et al. Operative treatment in 120 displaced intraarticular calcaneal fractures. Results using a prognostic computed tomography scan classification. Clin Orthop 1993;290:87–95.

Sangeorzan BJ, Benirschke SK, Mosca V, et al. Displaced intra-articular fractures of the tarsal navicular. J Bone Joint Surg Am 1989;71:1504–1510.

Shereff MJ. Complex fractures of the metatarsals. Orthopedics 1990;13:875–882.

Teeny SW, Wiss DA. Open reduction and internal fixation of tibial plafond fractures: variables contributing to poor results and complications. Clin Orthop 1993;292:108–117.

Thordarson DB. Complications after treatment of tibial pilon fractures: prevention and management strategies. J Am Acad Orthop Surg 2000;8:253–265.

Thordarson DB. Talus fractures. Foot Ankle Clin 1999;4:555–570.

Thordarson DB, Krieger LE. Operative vs. nonoperative treatment of intra-articular fractures of the calcaneus: a prospective randomized study. Foot Ankle Int 1996;17:2–9.

Thordarson DB, Motamed S, Hedman T, et al. The effect of fibular malreduction on contact pressures in an ankle fracture malunion model. J Bone Joint Surg Am 1997;79:1809–1815.

Torg JS, Moyer J, Gaughan JP, et al. Management of tarsal navicular stress fractures: conservative versus surgical treatment: a meta-analysis. Am J Sports Med 2010;38(5):1048–1053.

Torg JS, Pavlov J, Cooley LH, et al. Stress fractures of the tarsal navicular. J Bone Joint Surg Am 1982;64:700–712.

Wyrsch B, McFerran MA, McAndrew M, et al. Operative treatment of fractures of the tibial plafond: a randomized, prospective study. J Bone Joint Surg Am 1996;78:1646–1657.

Yablon IG, Heller FG, Shouse L. The key role of the lateral malleolus in displaced fractures of ankle. J Bone Joint Surg Am 1977;59:169.

INDEX

Note: Page numbers followed by *f* indicate figures, those followed by *t* indicate tables, and those followed by *b* indicate boxes.